# Pediatric Fundamentals of Critical Care Support

## Second Edition

> Maintenance Fluid Calculation (peds): **1.5 X**
> 4 mL/kg → 1st 10 kg
> 2 mL/kg → 2nd 10 kg
> 1 mL/kg → remaining kg

Copyright © 2013 Society of Critical Care Medicine, exclusive of any U.S. Government material.

All rights reserved.

**No part of this book may be reproduced in any manner or media, including but not limited to print or electronic format, without prior written permission of the copyright holder.**

*The views expressed herein are those of the authors and do not necessarily reflect the views of the Society of Critical Care Medicine.*

Use of trade names or names of commercial sources is for information only and does not imply endorsement by the Society of Critical Care Medicine.

This publication is intended to provide accurate information regarding the subject matter addressed herein. However, it is published with the understanding that the Society of Critical Care Medicine is not engaged in the rendering of medical, legal, financial, accounting, or other professional service and THE SOCIETY OF CRITICAL CARE MEDICINE HEREBY DISCLAIMS ANY AND ALL LIABILITY TO ALL THIRD PARTIES ARISING OUT OF OR RELATED TO THE CONTENT OF THIS PUBLICATION. The information in this publication is subject to change at any time without notice and should not be relied upon as a substitute for professional advice from an experienced, competent practitioner in the relevant field. NEITHER THE SOCIETY OF CRITICAL CARE MEDICINE, NOR THE AUTHORS OF THE PUBLICATION, MAKE ANY GUARANTEES OR WARRANTIES CONCERNING THE INFORMATION CONTAINED HEREIN AND NO PERSON OR ENTITY IS ENTITLED TO RELY ON ANY STATEMENTS OR INFORMATION CONTAINED HEREIN. If expert assistance is required, please seek the services of an experienced, competent professional in the relevant field. Accurate indications, adverse reactions, and dosage schedules for drugs may be provided in this text, but it is possible that they may change. Readers must review current package indications and usage guidelines provided by the manufacturers of the agents mentioned.

Managing Editor: Katie Brobst

Printed in the United States of America
First Printing, June 2013

**Society of Critical Care Medicine**
Headquarters
500 Midway Drive
Mount Prospect, IL 60056 USA
Phone +1 847 827-6869
Fax +1 847 827-6886
www.sccm.org

International Standard Book Number: 978-0-936145-90-7

**Pediatric Fundamental Critical Care Support**
**Second Edition**

*Editor*

**Maureen A. Madden, MSN, CPNP-AC, CCRN, FCCM**
Assistant Professor of Pediatrics
UMDNJ-Robert Wood Johnson Medical School
Pediatric Critical Care Nurse Practitioner
RWJUH- Bristol Myers Squibb Children's Hospital
New Brunswick, New Jersey, USA
*No disclosures*

*PFCCS Second Edition Planning Committee and Authors*

**Colonel Daniel B. Bruzzini, MD, FAAP, FCCM**
United States Air Force
Wright-Patterson Air Force Base
Ohio, USA
*No disclosures*

**Edward E. Conway, Jr, MD, MS, FAAP, FCCM**
Professor and Chairman Chief, Pediatric Critical
Care Medicine
Pediatrician-in-Chief
Milton and Bernice Stern Department
of Pediatrics
Beth Israel Medical Center
New York, New York, USA
*No disclosures*

**Michael O. Gayle, BS, MB, FCCM**
Associate Professor, Pediatrics
University of Florida College of Medicine
Chief, Division of Hospital Pediatrics
Chief, Division of Pediatric Critical Care Medicine
Medical Director, Wolfson Children's Hospital
Outreach Program
Jacksonville, Florida, USA
*No disclosures*

**Rodrigo Mejia, MD, FCCM**
Director, Pediatric Critical Care Service
Professor of Pediatrics
Children's Cancer Hospital at
The University of Texas MD Anderson Cancer Center
Houston, Texas, USA
*No disclosures*

**Mohan R. Mysore, MD, FAAP, FCCM**
Director/Clinical Service Chief
Pediatric Critical Care Medicine
Professor of Pediatrics, UNMC College of Medicine
Children's Hospital & Medical Center
Omaha, Nebraska, USA
*No disclosures*

**Ellen J. Pringle, RRT-NPS, RPFT, CNE**
Education Coordinator, Simulation Center
University of Texas MD Anderson Cancer Center
Office of Performance Improvement
Houston, Texas, USA
*No disclosures*

**Karl L. Serrao, MD, FAAP, FCCM**
Professor of Anesthesiology and Pediatrics
University of Texas Medical Branch at Galveston
Pediatric Critical Care Medicine
Driscoll Children's Hospital
Corpus Christi, Texas, USA
*No disclosures*

# Pediatric Fundamental Critical Care Support
## Second Edition

*Authors*

**Joseph R. Angelo, MD**
Assistant Professor
Department of Pediatrics
Division of Pediatric Nephrology
University of Texas Health Center at Houston
University of Texas MD Anderson Cancer Center
Houston, Texas, USA
*No disclosures*

**Beth A. Ballinger, MD**
Assistant Professor
Medical Director, General Surgical and Trauma
Intensive Care Unit
Trauma, Critical Care and General Surgery
Mayo Clinic
Rochester, Minnesota, USA
*No disclosures*

**Gregory H. Botz, MD, FCCM**
Distinguished Teaching Professor
Professor of Anesthesiology and Critical Care
Medicine
University of Texas MD Anderson Cancer Center
Houston, Texas, USA
*No disclosures*

**Dana A. Braner, MD, FCCM**
Chief, Division of Critical Care
Alice K. Fax Professor of Pediatric Critical Care
Vice Chair Inpatient
Doernbecher Children's Hospital
Portland, Oregon, USA
*No disclosures*

**Joseph A. Carcillo, MD**
Professor of Critical Care Medicine and Pediatrics
University of Pittsburgh School of Medicine
UPMC-Children's Hospital of Pittsburgh
Pittsburgh, Pennsylvania, USA
*No disclosures*

**Linda C. Carl, EdD, MSN, RN**
Professor, Graduate Nursing School
Kaplan University
Chicago, Illinois, USA
*No disclosures*

**Arthur Cooper, MD, MS, FACS, FAAP, FAHA, FCCM**
Professor of Surgery
Columbia University College of Physicians
and Surgeons
Director of Trauma and Pediatric
Surgical Services
Harlem Hospital Center
New York, New York, USA
*No disclosures*

**Jose Cortes, MD**
Assistant Professor
Division of Pediatrics
The University of Texas MD Anderson
Cancer Center
Houston, Texas, USA

**Guillermo De Angulo, MD, FAAP**
Clinical Associate Professor of Pediatrics
Herbert Wertheim College of Medicine
Florida International University
Miami Children's Hospital
Miami, Florida, USA
*No disclosures*

**Werther Brunow de Carvalho, MD, PhD**
Full Professor of Intensive Care/Neonatology
at the Children's Institute
University of São Paulo Faculty of Medicine
Clinics Hospital
São Paulo, Brazil
*No disclosures*

**Aaron J. Donoghue, MD, MSCE**
Assistant Professor of Pediatrics and
Critical Care Medicine
Perelman School of Medicine at the
University of Pennsylvania
Philadelphia, Pennsylvania, USA
*No disclosures*

**Elizabeth A. Farrington, PharmD, FCCM, BCPS**
Pediatric Pharmacist III
New Hanover Regional Medical Center
Wilmington, North Carolina, USA
*No disclosures*

**Kate Felmet, MD**
Assistant Professor of Critical Care Medicine
and Pediatrics
Children's Hospital of Pittsburgh
Pittsburgh, Pennsylvania, USA
*No disclosures*

**Jose Roberto Fioretto, MD, PhD**
Associate Professor of Pediatrics
Pediatric Critical Care Medicine
Botucatu Medical School
São Paulo State University
São Paulo, Brazil
*No disclosures*

**Jeremy S. Garrett, MD**
Associate Professor of Pediatrics
Pediatric Critical Care Medicine
Saint Louis University School of Medicine
Cardinal Glennon Children's Medical Center
St. Louis, Missouri, USA
*No disclosures*

**Ana Lía Graciano, MD, FAAP**
Associate Clinical Professor
Academic Division Chief, Pediatric Critical Care
University of California San Francisco-Fresno
Children's Hospital of Central California
Fresno, California, USA
*No disclosures*

**Chhavi Katyal, MD**
Pediatric Critical Care Medicine
Children's Hospital at Montefiore
Assistant Professor of Pediatrics
Albert Einstein College of Medicine
Bronx, New York, USA
*No disclosures*

**Keith C. Kocis, MD, MS, FAAP, FACC, FCCM**
Professor of Anesthesia, Pediatrics and
Biomedical Engineering (Adjunct)
Division of Pediatric Cardiology
PCCM Fellowship Director
The University of North Carolina at Chapel Hill
Chapel Hill, North Carolina, USA
*No disclosures*

**Robert E. Lynch, MD, PhD, FCCM**
Director, Pediatric Critical Care
Mercy Children's Hospital
Creve Coeur, Missouri, USA
*No disclosures*

**Vinay M. Nadkarni, MD, FCCM**
Medical Director, Center for Simulation,
Advanced Education and Innovation
The Children's Hospital of Philadelphia
Philadelphia, Pennsylvania, USA
*No disclosures*

**Regina S. Okhuysen-Cawley, MD**
University of Texas MD Anderson Cancer Center
Houston, Texas, USA
*No disclosures*

**Pascal Owusu-Agyemang, MD**
Assistant Professor
University of Texas MD Anderson Cancer Center
Houston, Texas, USA
*No disclosures*

**Michele C. Papo, MD, MPH, FCCM**
Medical Director, Pediatric ICU
Medical City Children's Hospital
Dallas, Texas, USA
*No disclosures*

**Sujatha Rajan, MD**
Assistant Professor, Pediatric Infectious Diseases
Cohen Children's Medical Center of New York
Hofstra/North Shore-LIJ School of Medicine
New Hyde Park, New York, USA
*No disclosures*

**Elizabeth Rebello, MD**
Assistant Professor
Department of Anesthesiology and Perioperative Medicine
Division of Anesthesiology and Critical Care
University of Texas MD Anderson Cancer Center
Houston, Texas, USA
*No disclosures*

**Ramon J. Rivera, MD**
Associate Professor of Anesthesiology
University of Texas Medical Branch at Galveston
Pediatric Intensivist
Anesthesiology Associates
Driscoll Children's Hospital
Corpus Christi, Texas, USA
*No disclosures*

**Lorry G. Rubin, MD**
Chief, Pediatric Infectious Diseases
Cohen Children's Medical Center of New York
Hofstra/North Shore-LIJ School of Medicine
New Hyde Park, New York, USA
*No disclosures*

**James Schneider, MD**
Pediatric Critical Care Medicine
Cohen Children's Medical Center of New York
Hofstra/North Shore-LIJ School of Medicine
New Hyde Park, New York, USA
*No disclosures*

**Kevin Schooler, MD, PhD**
Assistant Professor of Anesthesiology and Pediatrics
University of Texas Medical Branch
Galveston, Texas, USA
Pediatric Critical Care Driscoll Children's Hospital
Corpus Christi, Texas, USA
*No disclosures*

**Shinpei Shibata, MD**
Assistant Professor
Division of Pediatric Critical Care
Oregon Health & Science University
Portland, Oregon, USA
*No disclosures*

**Jayesh Thakker, MD**
Associate Professor, Department of Pediatrics
University of Nebraska Medical Center
Medical Director, PICU
The Nebraska Medical Center
Pediatric Critical Care Medicine
Children's Specialty Physicians
Children's Hospital & Medical Center
Omaha, Nebraska, USA
*No disclosures*

**Alexis A. Topjian, MD**
Assistant Professor of Anesthesiology
and Critical Care
Attending Physician
The Children's Hospital of Philadelphia
Philadelphia, Pennsylvania, USA
*Grants: National Institutes of Health U01 for Therapeutic Hypothermia After Pediatric Cardiac Arrest Trial National Institute of Neurological Disorders and Stroke K23 Scientist Development Program (Subawards)*

**Henry Michael Ushay, MD, PhD, FCCM**
Medical Director, Pediatric Critical Care Unit
Children's Hospital at Montefiore
Bronx, New York, USA
*No disclosures*

# Acknowledgments

*The following individuals contributed to the development of* Pediatric Fundamental Critical Care Support, Second Edition, *by reviewing the material and offering valuable insight.*

**M. Ruth Abelt, MS, CPNP-AC**
Director of Advanced Level Practitioners
Baylor College of Medicine
Texas Children's Hospital
Houston, Texas, USA
*No disclosures*

**Adeyinka Adebayo, MD, FAAP**
Division of Pediatric Critical Care
The Brooklyn Hospital Center
Brooklyn, New York, USA
Assistant Professor of Clinical Pediatrics
Weill Medical College of Cornell University
New York, New York, USA
*No disclosures*

**Ayman Al Eyadhy, MD**
Head, Pediatric Intensive Care Unit
Assistant Professor & Consultant Department of Pediatrics
College of Medicine, King Saud University
Riyadh, Saudi Arabia
*No disclosures*

**Grace M. Arteaga, MD, FAAP**
Pediatric Critical Care Medicine
Pediatric Transport Medical Director
Mayo Clinic
Rochester, Minnesota, USA
*No disclosures*

**Sangita Basnet, MD, FAAP**
Assistant Professor of Clinical Pediatrics
Chief, Division of Pediatric Critical Care Medicine
Southern Illinois University School of Medicine
Medical Director, Pediatric Critical Care Unit
St. John's Children's Hospital
Springfield, Illinois, USA
*No disclosures*

**Rahul Bhatia, MD**
Assistant Professor
Pediatrics, Pediatric Critical Care
Associate Residency Program Director, Pediatrics
Loyola University Medical Center
Maywood, Illinois, USA
*No disclosures*

**Bronwyn Bishop**
Senior Registered Nurse, NICU
Royal Darwin Hospital
Tiwi, Northern Territory, Australia
*No disclosures*

**Naomi B. Bishop, MD**
Assistant Professor
Division of Critical Care Medicine
Department of Pediatrics
Weill Cornell Medical College
New York, New York, USA
*No disclosures*

**Yonca Bulut, MD**
Professor of Pediatrics
Division of Pediatric Critical Care
Department of Pediatrics
Mattel Children's Hospital, UCLA
Los Angeles, California, USA
*No disclosures*

**Andrew Clift, MD, MBBS (Hon), BMedSci (Hon), MPH, FACTM, AFFTM, FACRRM, DRANZCOG, DCH, JCCA, PostGradDip US (echocardiography), CCPU**
President & Founder
The Children's Sanctuary
Siem Reap, Kingdom of Cambodia
*No disclosures*

**Michael Karadsheh, MD, FAAP**
Assistant Professor of Pediatrics
Division of Pediatric Critical Care
University of Arizona
Tucson, Arizona, USA
*No disclosures*

**Martha C. Kutko, MD, FAAP, FCCM**
Attending Physician, Pediatric Critical Care Medicine
Hackensack University Medical Center
Hackensack, New Jersey, USA
Associate Professor, Department of Pediatrics
UMDNJ-New Jersey Medical School
Newark, New Jersey, USA
*No disclosures*

**Jong Lee, MD, FACS, FCCM**
Associate Professor of Surgery
Annie Laurie Howard Chair in Burn Surgery
Associate Director of Burn Services
Program Director, Surgical Critical Care Fellowship
University of Texas Medical Branch
Galveston, Texas, USA
*No disclosures*

**David Markenson, MD, MBA, FAAP, FACEP**
Medical Director, Disaster Medicine and Regional Emergency Services
Westchester Medical Center
Valhalla, New York
Professor of Pediatrics, Maria Fareri Children's Hospital
New York Medical College
Director, Center for Disaster Medicine
Professor of Clinical Public Health
School of Health Sciences and Practice and Institute of Public Health
New York Medical College
Valhalla, New York, USA
*No disclosures*

**Riza V. Mauricio, PhD, RN, CPNP-AC, CCRN**
Pediatric ICU Nurse Practitioner
The Children's Hospital of the University of Texas
MD Anderson Cancer Center
Houston, Texas, USA
*No disclosures*

**Michael P. Miller, MD, FAAP, FCCP**
Director Pediatric Critical Care
New Hampshire's Hospital for Children
Manchester, New Hampshire, USA
*No disclosures*

**Suzi Nou, MBBS, BMedSci, FANZCA**
Specialist Anaesthetist
Royal Darwin Hospital
Tiwi, Northern Territory, Australia
*No disclosures*

**Toni M. Petrillo-Albarano, MD, FAAP, FCCM**
Associate Professor of Pediatrics
Emory University School of Medicine
Director, PICU
Director, Pediatric Critical Care Medicine Fellowship
Co-medical Director, Children's Transport
Children's Healthcare of Atlanta at Egleston
Atlanta, Georgia, USA
*No disclosures*

**Louisdon Pierre, MD, MBA, FAAP, FCCM**
Director, Pediatric Critical Care
The Brooklyn Hospital Center
Brooklyn, New York, USA
Assistant Professor of Clinical Pediatrics
Weill Medical College of Cornell University
New York, New York, USA
*No disclosures*

**Brad Poss, MD, MMM**
Professor of Pediatrics
Division of Pediatric Critical Care
University of Utah School of Medicine
Salt Lake City, Utah, USA
*No disclosures*

**Hariprem Rajasekhar, MD**
Pediatric Critical Care
Robert Wood Johnson University Hospital
New Brunswick, New Jersey, USA
*No disclosures*

**Alexandre T. Rotta, MD, FAAP, FCCM**
Chief, Division of Pediatric Critical Care
Rainbow Babies & Children's Hospital
Professor of Pediatrics
Case Western Reserve University
School of Medicine
Cleveland, Ohio, USA
*No disclosures*

**Brian Spain, MBBS, MRCA, FANZCA**
Director, Department of Anaesthesia
Royal Darwin Hospital
Tiwi, Northern Territory, Australia
*No disclosures*

**Fernando Stein, MD, FCCM**
Associate Professor
Baylor College of Medicine
Texas Children's Hospital
Houston, Texas, USA
*No disclosures*

**Todd Sweberg, MD**
Attending Physician
Pediatric Critical Care Medicine
Cohen Children's Medical Center of New York
Hofstra/North Shore-LIJ School of Medicine
New Hyde Park, New York, USA
*No disclosures*

**M. Hossein Tcharmtchi, MD**
Associate Professor
Director, Fellowship Training Program
Pediatric Critical Care Medicine
Department of Pediatrics
Baylor College of Medicine
Texas Children's Hospital
Houston, Texas, USA
*No disclosures*

**Christopher M. Watson, MD, MPH**
Department of Anesthesiology and
Critical Care Medicine
Johns Hopkins University School of Medicine
Baltimore, Maryland, USA
*No disclosures*

# Pediatric Fundamental Critical Care Support
## Second Edition

### *Contents*

| Chapter | Title | Page |
|---|---|---|
| 1 | Assessment of the Critically Ill Child | 1-1 |
| 2 | Airway Management | 2-1 |
| 3 | Pediatric Cardiac Arrest | 3-1 |
| 4 | Diagnosis and Management of the Child With Acute Upper and Lower Airway Disease | 4-1 |
| 5 | Mechanical Ventilation | 5-1 |
| 6 | Diagnosis and Management of Shock | 6-1 |
| 7 | Acute Infections | 7-1 |
| 8 | Fluids, Electrolytes, and Neuroendocrine Metabolic Derangements | 8-1 |
| 9 | Traumatic Injuries in Children | 9-1 |
| 10 | Pediatric Burn Injury | 10-1 |
| 11 | Nonaccidental Injuries: Diagnosis and Management | 11-1 |
| 12 | Pediatric Emergency Preparedness | 12-1 |
| 13 | Management of the Poisoned Child and Adolescent | 13-1 |
| 14 | Transport of the Critically Ill Child | 14-1 |
| 15 | Neurologic Emergencies | 15-1 |
| 16 | Management of the Child With Congenital Heart Disease | 16-1 |
| 17 | Oncologic and Hematologic Emergencies and Complications | 17-1 |
| 18 | Acute Kidney Injury | 18-1 |
| 19 | Postoperative Management | 19-1 |
| 20 | Sedation, Analgesia, and Neuromuscular Blockade | 20-1 |
| 21 | Invasive Medical Devices | 21-1 |

| Appendix | Title | Page |
|---|---|---|
| 1 | Pediatric Normal Values | Appendix 1-1 |
| 2 | Intraosseous Needle Insertion | Appendix 2-1 |
| 3 | Acid-Base Balance and Arterial Blood Gas Analysis | Appendix 3-1 |
| 4 | Oxygen Delivery Devices | Appendix 4-1 |
| 5 | Airway Adjuncts | Appendix 5-1 |
| 6 | Endotracheal Intubation | Appendix 6-1 |
| 7 | Common Medications | Appendix 7-1 |
| 8 | Difficult Airway Algorithm | Appendix 8-1 |
| 9 | Advanced Life Support Algorithms | Appendix 9-1 |
| 10 | Defibrillation/Cardioversion | Appendix 10-1 |
| 11 | Temporary Transcutaneous Cardiac Pacing | Appendix 11-1 |
| 12 | Thoracostomy | Appendix 12-1 |
| 13 | Central Venous Access | Appendix 13-1 |
| 14 | Handoff Mnemonics for Transport and Trauma | Appendix 14-1 |
| 15 | Pediatric Transport Form | Appendix 15-1 |
| 16 | Arterial Catheter Insertion | Appendix 16-1 |

**Index**

# Chapter 1

# ASSESSMENT OF THE CRITICALLY ILL CHILD

## ✓ Objectives

- Review anatomic and physiologic differences between pediatric and adult patients.
- Apply the DIRECT methodology — detection, intervention, reassessment, effective communication, and teamwork.
- Recognize respiratory failure and describe the clinical features of the different types of shock.
- Discuss the role of ancillary tests in the cardiopulmonary evaluation of a child.
- Explain how to perform a rapid evaluation of a child's physiological status.
- Apply the Pediatric Early Warning Score (PEWS) system to detect clinical deterioration early.
- Discuss the early recognition and treatment of sepsis.

## Case Study

A 3-month-old infant girl with a history of prematurity is brought to the emergency department by her father and mother following a 1-week history of nasal congestion, cough, wheezing, post-tussive emesis, poor fluid intake, tachypnea, and fever. On arrival, the infant's vital signs are: heart rate, 182 beats/min; respiratory rate, 72 breaths/min; pulse oximetry, 87% in room air; and temperature, 101.7°F (38.7°C). She is irritable, grunting, and tachypneic with subcostal and intercostal retractions. Capillary refill is delayed at 3 seconds. She is given an albuterol (salbutamol) nebulizer treatment followed by 45% oxygen via an air-entrainment Venturi mask by the emergency department staff. You have been asked to assist in her management.

**Detection**

- What is this child's physiologic status based on the Pediatric Early Warning Score (PEWS) (**Table 1-1**)?
- What are the most likely and worst possible diagnoses?

**Intervention**

- What are the most immediate treatment strategies?

### Reassessment
- Is the current treatment strategy effective?
- Does she need more albuterol (salbutamol) nebulization and/or other therapeutic interventions?

### Effective Communication
- When the patient's clinical status changes, who needs to know and how will the information be disseminated?
- Where is the best place to manage the care of this patient?

### Teamwork
- How are you going to implement the treatment strategy?
- Who is to do what and when?

**Table 1-1. Pediatric Early Warning Score (PEWS)[a]**

| | 0 | 1 | 2 | 3 | Score |
|---|---|---|---|---|---|
| Behavior | Playing/appropriate | Sleeping | Irritable | Lethargic/confused OR reduced response to pain | |
| Cardiovascular | Pink OR capillary refill 1-2 s | Pale or dusky OR capillary refill 3 s | Gray or cyanotic OR capillary refill 4 s OR tachycardia of 20 beats/min above normal rate | Gray or cyanotic AND mottled OR capillary refill >5 s OR tachycardia of 30 beats/min above normal rate OR bradycardia | |
| Respiratory | Within normal parameters, no retractions | >10 above normal parameters OR using accessory muscles OR >30% $F_{IO_2}$ or >3 L/min | >20 above normal parameters OR retractions OR >40% $F_{IO_2}$ or >6 L/min | ≥5 below normal parameters with retractions or grunting OR >50% $F_{IO_2}$ or >8 L/min | |
| **Total Score** | | | | | |

[a]Score by starting with the most severe parameters. Score 2 extra for every 15-minute nebulization (including continuous) or persistent postoperative vomiting. Use L/min to score regular nasal cannula. Use $F_{IO_2}$ to score high-flow nasal cannula.

| | Age | Heart Rate at Rest (beats/min) | Respiratory Rate at Rest (breaths/min) |
|---|---|---|---|
| Newborn | Birth - 1 mo | 100-180 | 40-60 |
| Infant | 1 - 12 mo | 100-180 | 35-40 |
| Toddler | 13 mo - 3 y | 70-110 | 25-30 |
| Preschool | 4 - 6 y | 70-110 | 21-23 |
| School age | 7 - 12 y | 70-110 | 19-21 |
| Adolescent | 13 - 19 y | 55-90 | 16-18 |

Reproduced with permission. © 2010 American Academy of Pediatrics. Akre M, Finkelstein M, Erickson M, Liu M, Vanderbilt L, Billman G. Sensitivity of the pediatric early warning score to identify patient deterioration. *Pediatrics*. 2010;125:e763-e769.

# I. INTRODUCTION

This chapter will discuss the maturational, anatomical, and physiological differences of children and their responses to shock, trauma, and illness as contrasted to those of an adult. This chapter also introduces the key PFCCS course learning and management concept, **DIRECT**: detection, intervention, reassessment, effective communication, and teamwork (**Figure 1-1**).

**Figure 1-1.** DIRECT Methodology

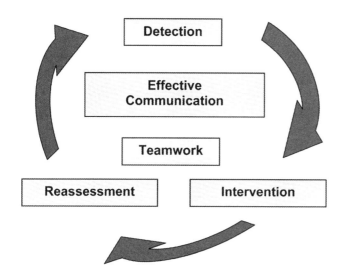

**Detection:** Using the history, physical exam, and PEWS system alerts the critical care team to the physiological status of the child. These items then guide appropriate laboratory and radiographic evaluations to establish a working/presumptive diagnosis, differential diagnoses, and worst possible diagnoses.

**Intervention:** This is the process of treating and correcting the disease or injury while keeping in mind the critical care maxim to minimize morbidity and prevent mortality.

**Reassessment:** This ensures the treatment is appropriate for the severity of the disease and/or injury.

**Effective Communication:** The greatest source of injury and death in healthcare is due to communication errors. The more complicated the patient, the more important it is for everyone to communicate their perspective to the team so multiple and often time-sensitive tasks can be done expertly and promptly.

**Teamwork:** The patient does best when all disciplines on the healthcare team bring their specialized training to work together synergistically to care for the needs of the critically ill or injured pediatric patient.

In the case presented, the patient's PEWS is 5 (behavior irritable = 2 points, cardiovascular capillary refill 3 seconds = 1 point, and respiratory 45% oxygen and respiratory rate >20 above normal = 2 points). A critical PEWS is defined as >4, a score that facilitates the early identification of physiologic deterioration. The team must recognize this, intervene by providing respiratory support, and continually reassess the patient's response to intravenous (IV) fluids and albuterol (salbutamol) nebulization therapy. It takes a team of individuals communicating and working together to obtain the best clinical outcomes.

# II. THE GENERAL EXAMINATION

The general examination is probably the most important part of the physical exam. It begins the moment one sees a pediatric patient and is summed up nicely in the answer to this simple but essential question: "Does this child look sick?" PEWS expedites the evaluation process by focusing on the behavioral, cardiovascular, and respiratory status of the pediatric patient. Because young children are unable to verbalize specific complaints, evaluation by the healthcare provider depends upon general and specific features of the examination in addition to information obtained from a parent or guardian. Although many of the early signs of distress are subtle, their recognition can increase the likelihood that timely interventions will be successful and more serious disease progression will be prevented. If healthcare providers initially miss the more elusive signs of illness, they may later assume a child's condition has suddenly deteriorated when, in fact, a seemingly abrupt change reflects an advanced point along a continuum of physiologic compromise. Important aspects to be considered in the general examination of a pediatric patient are listed in **Table 1-2.**

> *A child's general appearance will immediately help the observer discern the presence of serious illness.*

During the clinical exam, children should be allowed to remain in the position they spontaneously assume for comfort. For children younger than 1 year, this is often in the arms of their parent or primary caregiver. Illness may be marked by a child's inability to find a position of comfort. Pediatric patients should not be forced to assume a different position than the one they decide upon because doing so could potentially compromise a tenuous airway as in epiglottitis, severe laryngotracheobronchitis (croup), or foreign body obstruction.

> *A child's level of reactivity and responsiveness is usually a reflection of the level of cerebral perfusion.*

### Table 1-2  General Examination

**Skin**
- Loss of normal pink coloration of mucosa and nail beds
- Mottling
- Skin warmth or coolness
- Prolonged capillary refill, determined with extremity above the level of the patient's heart to prevent mistaken assessment of venous refill

**Signs of Dehydration**
- Sunken fontanelle in infants
- Absent tears
- Sunken eyes
- Skin tenting
- Dry mucous membranes

**Color**
- Cyanosis
- Acrocyanosis (may be present if room temperature is cool)
- Central cyanosis
- Jaundice
- Pallor

**Breathing**
- Bradypnea/tachypnea
- Stridor
- Audible wheezing
- Nasal flaring/grunting
- Intercostal retractions

**Level of Alertness**
- Awake and alert
- Responds to verbal commands
- Responds only to painful stimulation
- Unresponsive

An ill child may initially have increased irritability, followed by decreasing responsiveness, increasing flaccidity, and lethargy. This is observed in conditions such as hypoxia, hypercarbia, uncompensated shock, traumatic brain injury, and hypoglycemia. Depressed mental status requires rapid evaluation of the respiratory and cardiovascular status. In children, respiratory failure most often precedes cardiovascular failure in the absence of an underlying congenital heart defect or trauma. Signs of physical injury can be very subtle to nonexistent, especially in cases of "shaken baby syndrome" (i.e., nonaccidental trauma). In most infants, alertness can be evaluated by observing their ability to fixate on objects, particularly a parent's face. The infant should turn toward sound and should follow an object horizontally and, starting at 1 month of age, should follow an object vertically as well. Older children, 8 months to 2 years, should exhibit anxiety toward strangers and show clear recognition of their parents or caregivers.

# III. RESPIRATORY SYSTEM AND AIRWAY

Respiratory failure is particularly common in infants due to variable maturation in 3 areas:

- Central nervous system receptor and effector mechanisms for the respiratory drive
- Chest wall stability and respiratory muscular strength
- Conducting airways and the alveolar-capillary complex

The respiratory response to hypoxemia in neonates may be biphasic — hyperpnea initially, followed by hypopnea and hypoventilation. This response occurs despite apparently normal central and peripheral chemoreceptors to oxygen and carbon dioxide. The hyperpnea-followed-by-hypopnea response is potentially preventable by early detection and intervention when airway and breathing compromise begin.

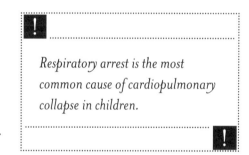

*Respiratory arrest is the most common cause of cardiopulmonary collapse in children.*

## A. Anatomic and Physiologic Considerations

The thorax is more cartilaginous in infants and young children and, therefore, is more compliant than in an adult. Infants with respiratory distress are less successful in augmenting tidal volume with increasing respiratory effort because the compliant chest wall retracts inward under the increased negative intrathoracic pressure. This results in reduced tidal volume ventilation and indirectly increases the work of breathing and soft tissue retractions. In addition, because an infant's ribs are aligned on a more horizontal plane, the inspiratory displacement of the thorax on the anteroposterior plane is decreased, further reducing the efficiency of the bellows effect of the thorax.

The horizontal muscular insertion points of the pediatric diaphragm on the thorax resemble those of an adult with obstructive lung disease and its associated flattened diaphragm. Therefore, the lower thorax may be drawn inward during inspiration, causing reduced inspiratory volume. Immature intercostal muscles cannot assist active ventilation for several years after birth; thus, more dependency is placed upon diaphragmatic function and excursion. Compromise of diaphragmatic excursion by gastric distention, abdominal distention, surgery, and other factors may quickly evolve into impaired respiratory function.

Pediatric lungs are not fully mature until 6 to 8 years of age. Alveolar size and number increase substantially during childhood; lung compliance also increases. Tidal volume as a fraction of total lung capacity remains fairly constant through childhood at 6 to 8 mL/kg of ideal body weight. High intrinsic or externally supplied flow rates are required to deliver this tidal volume because children have a short inspiratory duration. Smaller anatomic conducting airways may produce high resistance if further narrowed by inflammation, edema, mucus, bronchospasm, bronchiolitis, and other conditions. Poiseuille's law states the resistance in an airway is inversely related to its radius to the 4th power, so reducing the airway radius by 50% would increase the resistance sixteen times — $1/(1/2)^4$ (**Chapter 2, Figure 2-1**). Such high peripheral airway resistance may also alter exhalation and induce dynamic closure of the airways and auto–positive end-expiratory pressure. Closing capacity in infants and small children is within their functional residual capacity, thereby making them more susceptible to airway closure during tidal volume breathing. These factors combine to produce less respiratory reserve in the pediatric patient. Consequently, children may decompensate rapidly, leading to cardiopulmonary arrest if there is no intervention.

The majority of deaths in children (especially those younger than 1 year) involve respiratory disorders resulting from infection, poisonings, trauma, submersion, suffocation, or sudden infant death syndrome.

## B. Physical Examination

Nasal flaring (increases the nares radii to reduce resistance to the 4th power), tachypnea, grunting (exhalation against a partially closed glottis to prevent collapse of alveoli), and retractions are signs of increased work of breathing as the patient attempts to maintain adequate minute ventilation and oxygenation in response to pulmonary or airway compromise. Given the compliant nature of a child's chest wall, retractions can be profound, with evidence of subcostal, intercostal, and suprasternal retractions. Tachypnea is an important sign of illness in infants and young children, and bradypnea is an ominous precursor of impending respiratory arrest.

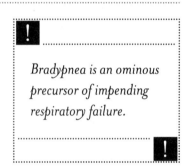

*Bradypnea is an ominous precursor of impending respiratory failure.*

Such extreme variations in respiratory rate have many etiologies (**Table 1-3**). The normal respiratory rate of an infant or child is age dependent (**Appendix 1**). Always be wary of "normal" respiratory rates in a lethargic or poorly responsive pediatric patient. The pediatric brain is more metabolically active than the adult brain. Mental status is a sensitive indicator of inadequate oxygenation, ventilation, and perfusion. As previously mentioned, a patient's position of comfort is usually one allowing adequate gas exchange. For example, a child with upper airway obstruction (e.g., epiglottitis) will usually attempt to sit forward or assume a tripod position. According to Poiseuille's law, lower airflow velocity and less viscous inspired air promote laminar airflow, not turbulent airflow, thereby decreasing airflow resistance and subsequent work of breathing. If a child becomes agitated when separated from the parent to facilitate clinical examination, the increase in velocity of airflow (i.e., crying) can lead to turbulent airflow, thereby increasing

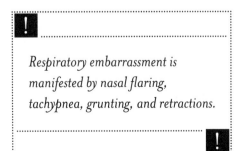

*Respiratory embarrassment is manifested by nasal flaring, tachypnea, grunting, and retractions.*

airway resistance and possibly converting a partially obstructed airway (e.g., epiglottitis or foreign body obstruction) into a completely obstructed airway.

The shape and movement of the chest during respiration will alert the observer to underlying respiratory problems. A rib-cage deformity, such as pectus excavatum, pectus carinatum, or scoliosis, may suggest the presence of restrictive lung disease, pulmonary hypoplasia, and/or abnormal respiratory mechanics. Asymmetry of chest rise can be noted visually and by laying one's palms on each side of the patient's chest and noting differential hand rise. Asymmetry is indicative of unequal air entry and serious underlying pathology (**Table 1-4**). Auscultation of breath sounds will reveal the adequacy and symmetry of air entry and allow detection of any other sounds, such as wheezes, crackles, and rubs. Auscultation may be difficult or easy, depending on the child's level of cooperation and environmental surroundings. Because children have thinner chest walls than adults, breath sounds are easily audible but less easily localized, and other transmitted sounds often interfere with accurate auscultation. When checking for symmetric breath sounds after intubation, it is best to auscultate in the anterior axillary line as opposed to the midclavicular line to minimize contralateral breath sound transmission and false identification of equal breath sounds bilaterally. Nevertheless, when a child is agitated and crying, adequate auscultation may not be possible.

### Table 1-3 Causes of Variations in Respiratory Rate

| Tachypnea | Bradypnea |
| --- | --- |
| • Fever | • Hypothermia |
| • Pain and anxiety | • Central nervous system injury |
| • Hypovolemia | • Drug-induced depression |
| • Respiratory disease | • Neuromuscular disease |
| • Metabolic acidosis | • Severe shock |
| • Heart failure | • Metabolic disorders |
| • Adverse drug effect | |
| • Hyperviscosity syndromes | |

### Table 1-4 Causes of Asymmetrical Chest Movement

- Unilateral pneumothorax
- Unilateral pleural effusion
- Foreign body aspiration with hyperinflation
- Mucous plugging of main-stem bronchus
- Lobar atelectasis

In general, cyanosis of the skin and nail beds, if present, is indicative of hypoxemia, but may be a late finding in the hypoxemic child. Cyanosis is dependent upon the patient's total hemoglobin concentration because >5 g/dL must be desaturated for cyanosis to be clinically observed. Because children have lower hemoglobin concentration than adults or in the setting of actual blood loss due to trauma, the blood oxygen content must fall to very low levels before cyanosis is clinically evident. Oxygenation is dependent upon the mean airway pressure and the percentage of inspired oxygen.

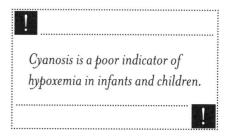

*Cyanosis is a poor indicator of hypoxemia in infants and children.*

The advent of pulse oximetry has enabled the noninvasive measurement of hemoglobin oxygen saturation. Pulse oximetry does not accurately assess ventilation status, but end-tidal $CO_2$ capnography does. See **Table 1-5** for the advantages of capnography.

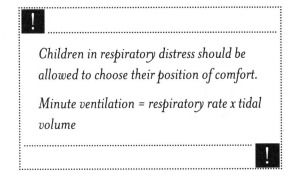

*Children in respiratory distress should be allowed to choose their position of comfort.*

*Minute ventilation = respiratory rate x tidal volume*

Alveolar ventilation is primarily responsible for removal of $CO_2$ and is represented by minute ventilation, which is the product of the respiratory rate and tidal volume.

A patient may maintain adequate oxygen saturation in the face of inadequate minute ventilation, especially if supplemental oxygen is provided. Therefore, clinical assessment, including attention to mental status, chest movement, respiratory rate, work of breathing, and capnography, is crucial to determine the adequacy of $CO_2$ minute ventilation. Another essential respiratory monitoring adjunct to the clinical examination is arterial blood gas sampling, as well as transcutaneous $CO_2$ monitoring if available.

### Table 1-5  Advantages of Capnography

- Noninvasive monitoring of ventilation
- Measure of respiratory rate and regularity of breathing
- Confirms and continuously monitors endotracheal tube placement in the trachea
- Alarms first when endotracheal tube becomes dislodged or obstructed
- Alveolar $CO_2$ correlates with arterial $CO_2$
- Detection of lower-airway obstruction with waveform

## C. Airway Evaluation

###  Case Study

A 15-month-old boy was brought into the emergency department with sudden-onset tachypnea (respiratory rate of 45 breaths/min), chest wall retractions, and irritability after a choking episode. The patient was noted to be wheezing on auscultation. He is not cyanotic and his capillary refill is 1 to 2 seconds. A chest radiograph reveals hyperinflation of the right lung in the anteroposterior and right lateral decubitus position. The patient is taken to the operating room for bronchoscopy for possible foreign body removal.

**Detection**

- Why is this patient wheezing?
- What is his PEWS?
- What noninvasive monitoring might be useful in evaluating this patient?

**Intervention**

– What might happen if this child was not allowed to choose his own position of comfort?

– Should he stay with his parent en route to the operating room to keep him calm?

**Reassessment**

– Is bronchoscopy the best initial course of action?

**Effective Communication**

– It is important for all team members to keep the child calm and to allow him to assume his own position of comfort.

**Teamwork**

– The ability to secure the airway should it become completely obstructed.

– Stabilize the child's condition until the foreign body can be removed by bronchoscopy.

In the case presented, the patient's PEWS is: behavior irritable = 2, cardiovascular pink = 0, respiratory retractions = 2, total = 4. This is a case of aspirated foreign body resulting in airway obstruction and respiratory compromise. Sometimes these same signs and symptoms have been misinterpreted as indicators of reactive airway disease.

The first consideration is to allow the pediatric patient to find a position of comfort. A child with impending airway obstruction (e.g., chemical burn ingestion) often prefers to sit forward leaning on the outstretched arms (i.e., tripod position). If the child is unconscious or obtunded, head position is paramount. In the setting of trauma, stabilization of the cervical spine with immobilization – to avoid incidental movement, hyperextension, or flexion – is essential to decrease the risk of iatrogenic spinal cord injury. The child younger than 2 years has a relatively large occiput which causes the neck to flex forward, potentially obstructing the airway and/or further exacerbating a cervical spine injury, when the child is placed on a firm mattress or rigid backboard. The sniffing position is preferred and can be accomplished by tilting the head back slightly and/or placing a rolled towel beneath the shoulders in those younger than 2 years. Placing a folded towel or sheet under the child's occiput can accomplish the sniffing position in patients older than 2 years. Infants, particularly those younger than 2 months, are obligate nasal breathers. Simple suctioning is often an important intervention to relieve an airway obstruction, especially in an infant with respiratory syncytial virus infection. In the case of congenital choanal atresia, the neonate has difficulty eating and is cyanotic at rest but pink when crying. An oral airway and/or prone positioning are oftentimes all that is needed to maintain an open airway at rest until the anomaly can be surgically corrected. In the setting of trauma, a length-based weight, equipment, and emergency medications tape (e.g., Broselow tape) are invaluable in quickly ascertaining the appropriately sized equipment and medication doses needed to assist intubation. Exercise caution regarding the quality and clinical accuracy of smartphone pediatric medication dosing applications and treatment protocols.

The first intervention for respiratory compromise (cyanosis, tachypnea, nasal flaring, and chest wall retractions) is to administer oxygen. This can be done using any number of devices: non-rebreathing mask, face mask, air-entrainment Venturi face mask, nasal cannula, oxygen hood, or face tent (**Chapter 2**). Pulse oximetry and arterial blood gas measurements can be used to assess for an adequate or excessive amount of oxygen supplementation. Capillary blood gas measurements approximate arterial blood gas pH and arterial $CO_2$ levels well, but do not provide an accurate arterial oxygen concentration. Hypoxia and hyperoxia are deleterious and should be avoided.

A child has two to three times the oxygen consumption rate and resting energy expenditure of an adult. When a child presents in respiratory distress, one should first administer 100% oxygen using a non-rebreathing face mask and then titrate the percentage of oxygen delivered. The usual arterial oxygenation goal is 80 to 100 mm Hg on arterial blood gas analysis, which corresponds approximately to a pulse oximetry of 94% to 98%. Using the most appropriate and best tolerated oxygen delivery device, supplemental oxygen ought to be heated and humidified to avoid drying the mucosa of the oro- and nasopharynx. Airway obstruction, aspiration, and apnea are serious hazards to respiratory function.

> *Nasal flaring is a sensitive indicator of respiratory distress in infants. Simply suctioning the nasal passages can be an important intervention in establishing airway patency.*

The anatomy of the pediatric airway, especially in infants and young children, predisposes these patients to airway obstruction when they are positioned incorrectly. In addition to a large occiput, children younger than 2 years have a relatively large tongue, a larger and more floppy epiglottis, and an anteriorly placed larynx. These factors, combined with decreased hypopharyngeal tone, lead to the loss of airway patency in obtunded patients because they are unable to keep these soft tissue structures apart. (See **Chapter 2**, which details the factors affecting pediatric endotracheal intubation.)

In young children, common causes of airway obstruction are viral croup, bacterial tracheitis, foreign body, and, less commonly, epiglottitis in countries with successful *Haemophilus influenzae* type B immunization programs. Clinical examination may help identify the site of obstruction. Airway obstruction above the thoracic inlet tends to cause stridor (inspiratory noise), as in viral croup or post-extubation laryngeal edema. These stridulous patients may respond to nebulized racemic epinephrine (adrenaline) (0.05 mg/kg, maximum 0.5 mg in 3 mL normal saline) and IV steroids (dexamethasone, 0.5 mg/kg; maximum dose, 10 mg every 6 h).

Asthma is not the sole reason for wheezing and intrathoracic lower-airway obstruction. Infants with respiratory syncytial virus bronchiolitis may present similarly and sometimes respond to bronchodilators. Those children wheezing from asthma should receive supplemental oxygen, inhaled beta-agonist, corticosteroid (methylprednisolone, 1-2 mg/kg, maximum 60 mg per dose), and possibly ipratropium bromide, a nebulized anticholinergic. Children with both upper and lower airway obstruction and low oxygen requirements (e.g., asthma, bronchiolitis) may benefit from improved laminar flow through the narrowed passages by breathing heliox, a mixture of oxygen and helium (typically 30% oxygen, 70% helium). The less viscous or less dense the inhaled mixture, the less likely it is to have obstructive turbulent flow at higher velocities through disease-narrowed airway passages.

If there is no response to these therapies, then the diagnoses of foreign body or vascular ring obstruction, in which the aorta and/or its branches encircle the trachea, must be entertained. Vascular rings usually present between 2 and 5 years of age. Foreign bodies do not allow the affected lung to deflate on exhalation due to the ball-valve action, whereby air can get in past the obstruction but can't get out. Both foreign body aspiration and vascular rings need a high index of suspicion in the pediatric age group to make the correct diagnosis.

## D. Respiratory Failure

Children in respiratory distress progressing to respiratory failure will exhibit increased work of breathing until they experience muscle fatigue or are no longer able to compensate. Causes of respiratory failure in children can usually be grouped by age. In premature neonates, respiratory failure results from apnea of prematurity or neonatal respiratory distress syndrome, in which atelectasis and impaired gas exchange occur as a result of surfactant deficiency and ineffective chest bellows. In term neonates, bacterial pneumonia, sepsis, meconium aspiration, and congenital airway abnormalities are most common. In infants and toddlers, lower-respiratory disease from pneumonia, bronchiolitis, asthma, foreign-body aspiration, and upper-airway obstruction related to infection are common. The causes of respiratory failure in older children are similar to those found in adults. Treatment of respiratory failure begins with early recognition and securing the airway. It is critically important to have all the equipment necessary and function checked for a safe and successful intubation (**Chapter 2**).

Noninvasive monitoring has become indispensable in the evaluation of patients in respiratory distress. With pulse oximetry and end-tidal $CO_2$ capnography, oxygenation and ventilation can be objectively monitored. Ancillary investigative tests, such as chest radiograph, arterial blood gas examination, and other studies summarized in **Table 1-6**, are useful in confirming respiratory failure, elucidating its etiology, and monitoring response to therapy. These tools are not substitutes for clinical examination. The clinical assessment and judgment of the healthcare provider are the most valuable tools for recognizing a patient in impending respiratory failure.

## E. Mechanical Ventilation

When supporting oxygenation and ventilation with positive pressure bag-valve-mask or a mechanical ventilator, volutrauma – damage to a lung caused by lung overdistention – must be avoided. It is very easy to hypo- or hyperventilate a patient. Close attention to chest rise can ensure adequate, not excessive, chest expansion during bag-valve-mask/endotracheal tube ventilatory support. When selecting the tidal volume for mechanical ventilation, the ideal body weight should be used, especially if the patient is obese. Furthermore, it is important to avoid volutrauma by first selecting a lower volume and advancing to higher volumes as dictated by chest rise, auscultation of breath sounds from superior to inferior lobes, and clinical improvement. The typical tidal volume for a pediatric patient will range from 6 to 8 mL/kg. Conventional mechanical ventilation is usually divided into pressure and volume ventilation. Traditionally, pressure ventilation was used in small children and neonates because the mechanical ventilators at the time could not deliver small tidal volumes accurately. With miniaturization and advances in technology, ventilators are capable of delivering tidal volumes as low as 3 mL for use in extremely premature infants (**Table 1-7**). Furthermore, the line between pressure and volume ventilation has been blurred in new modes of mechanical ventilation (e.g., pressure-regulated volume control) to take advantage of their differences in the hopes of minimizing ventilator-induced lung injury (**Chapter 5**).

In pediatric patients, the respiratory system receives most of the critical care attention because most cardiovascular failure is preceded by respiratory failure. It is vitally important to detect, intervene, and reassess the pediatric airway continuously and to communicate effectively as a team to minimize pediatric morbidity and to prevent mortality.

### Table 1-6. Ancillary Studies to Evaluate Respiratory Status

| Study | Evaluation |
|---|---|
| Arterial blood gas (in room air) | Hypoxemia = low $Pa_{O_2}$ (<60 mm Hg [<8.0 kPa]) |
| | Hypercarbia = high $Pa_{CO_2}$ (>45 mm Hg [>6.0 kPa]) |
| | Acidosis = pH <7.35 |
| | Alkalosis = pH >7.45 |
| | Adequate $Pa_{O_2}$ does not mean adequate oxygenation if the Hgb is low |
| | pH >7.35 and $Pa_{CO_2}$ 35-45 mm Hg in a child with severe increased work of breathing is sign of impending respiratory failure |
| Pulse oximetry ($Sp_{O_2}$) | Noninvasive measure of oxyhemoglobin |
| | Goal: 94%-98% when supplemental oxygen is used |
| | Monitor oxygenation in response to treatment; avoid hypoxia and hyperoxia |
| Hemoglobin | $Ca_{O_2}$ = (Hgb x 1.34 x $Sa_{O_2}$) + dissolved oxygen (0.0031 x $Pa_{O_2}$) |
| | $D_{O_2}$ = $Ca_{O_2}$ x cardiac output |
| Capnography | Measure exhaled $CO_2$ from nasal cannula, ETT, or tracheostomy tube |
| | Noninvasively monitors adequacy of ventilation alveolar $CO_2$ correlates with arterial $CO_2$ |
| | Confirms and monitors tracheal placement of ETT |
| | Detect lower-airway obstruction with waveform appearance |
| | Determines physiological dead space |
| Peak expiratory flow rate | Generates maximum flow during forced exhalation |
| | Decreases with lower-airway obstruction (asthma) |
| | Monitors bronchodilator therapy |
| | Requires cooperation to perform, and therefore may be useful only in older children |
| Chest radiograph | Airway obstruction |
| | Pneumothorax and/or pleural effusion |
| | Parenchymal lung disease |
| | Atelectasis |
| | Volutrauma |

Hgb, hemoglobin; ETT, endotracheal tube; $Ca_{O_2}$, concentration determinant of arterial oxygen content; $Sa_{O_2}$, arterial oxygen percent saturation; $D_{O_2}$, oxygen delivery

### Table 1-7. Initial Mechanical Ventilator Settings for Infants Weighing <5 kg

| Initial Mode | Choose between Volume-Controlled and Pressure-Limited |
|---|---|
| Tidal volume | 4-6 mL/kg; set directly based on ideal body weight in volume controlled and indirectly by selecting a peak inspiratory pressure limit, usually 20-24 cm $H_2O$ pressure |
| Time limit | Inspiratory time: neonates, 0.25-0.4 s; infants, 0.5-0.6 s. Less compliant lungs can tolerate longer inspiratory time as the exhalation time constant in stiff lungs is short. |
| Respiratory rate | 30-40 breaths/min as a back-up rate in case of apnea |
| Positive end-expiratory pressure | 5-7 cm $H_2O$ to prevent atelectasis at the end of exhalation |

# IV. CARDIOVASCULAR SYSTEM

## A. Anatomic and Physiologic Considerations

The circulating blood volume per kilogram is higher in children than in adults, but the absolute volume is lower in children due to their small body size. Consequently, children are less able to tolerate small amounts of blood loss compared to adults. Blood replacement is dependent upon the patient's clinical status, vital signs, ongoing blood loss, risks of transfusing packed red blood cells, and current hematocrit relative to expected hematocrit (**Table 1-8**).

### Table 1-8. Pediatric Hemoglobin/Hematocrit Values by Age and Gender

**Hematocrit**
Calculated from mean corpuscular volume and red blood cell count
(electronic displacement or laser)

| Age | Reference Values (conventional) % of packed red cells (red cells/whole blood cells × 100) | Reference Values (SI) Volume fraction (red cells/whole blood) |
|---|---|---|
| 0-30 d | 44-70% | 0.44-0.70 |
| 1-23 mo | 32-42% | 0.32-0.42 |
| 2-9 y | 33-43% | 0.33-0.43 |
| 10-17 y (male) | 36-47% | 0.36-0.47 |
| 10-17 y (female) | 35-45% | 0.35-0.45 |
| >18-99 y (male) | 42-52% | 0.42-0.52 |
| >18-99 y (female) | 37-47% | 0.37-0.47 |

**Hemoglobin**

| Age | g/dL | mmol/L |
|---|---|---|
| 0-30 d | 15.0-24.0 | 2.32-3.72 |
| 1-23 mo | 10.5-14.0 | 1.63-2.17 |
| 2-9 y | 11.5-14.5 | 1.78-2.25 |
| 10-17 y (male) | 12.5-16.1 | 1.93-2.50 |
| 10-17 y (female) | 12.0-15.0 | 1.86-2.32 |
| >18-99 y (male) | 13.5-18.0 | 2.09-2.79 |
| >18-99 y (female) | 12.5-16.0 | 1.93-2.48 |

Adapted with permission. © 2011 Elsevier. Table 708-6. In: Kliegman RM, Stanton BF, Geme III JW, et al, eds. *Nelson Textbook of Pediatrics*. 19th ed. Philadelphia, PA: Saunders; 2011.

Cardiac output is dependent upon heart rate and stroke volume, as shown in the formula: cardiac output = heart rate x stroke volume. Stroke volume is dependent upon preload, contractility, and afterload. The ability of the heart to change its force of contraction in response to changes in preload (venous return) is described by the Frank-Starling curve (**Figure 1-2**).

**Figure 1-2.** Frank-Starling Curve: Relationship of Myocardial Force of Contraction and Filling Pressure

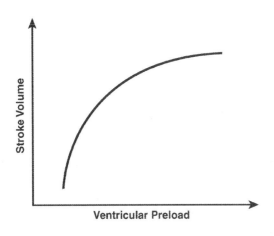

Vagal tone is increased in children but especially in infants younger than 1 year. When a laryngoscope touches the posterior pharynx or if an endotracheal tube suction catheter contacts the pediatric carina, these stimulate the vagus nerve, which innervates the heart's atrial-ventricular (A-V) conduction node. This increased vagal nerve parasympathetic discharge can precipitate a rapid decline in heart rate, resulting in a dramatic decrease in cardiac output, which may precipitate cardiac arrest. Appropriate use of atropine before intubation and care in not passing the endotracheal tube suction catheter past the end of the endotracheal tube will minimize this risk.

The myocardium of an infant younger than 8 weeks has limited ability to stretch, thereby limiting his/her ability to increase cardiac output in response to increased preload from blood or fluid boluses. The fetal right heart is dominant *in utero* and is responsible for approximately 60% of the systemic cardiac output through the ductus arteriosus. After birth, the lungs expand and the ductus arteriosus gradually closes, typically over 2 days. Right-sided resistance gradually falls to adult levels by 8 weeks of age. Newborn myocardial anatomy changes so that the initially larger right ventricle decreases in mass and the left ventricle increases in size and mass. Illness, hypoxemia, hypothermia, acidosis, or congenital heart defects may interrupt this physiological transition by maintaining elevated pulmonary blood pressure and a patent ductus arteriosus.

In neonates, exercise caution regarding central venous pressure monitoring interpretation because it does not necessarily reflect circulatory blood volume or left ventricular efficiency. Left and right heart function may be disparate, and each side may fail independently. Therefore, pulmonary artery catheters may occasionally be required to monitor left and right heart filling pressures. The neonatal myocardium exhibits a limited response to catecholamines due to immaturity of sympathetic nervous system innervation, as well as a reduced number of $\beta_1$-receptors, both of which increase over the first several weeks of life. The physiologic effects of exogenous catecholamine administration, therefore, may be quite variable; careful titration to the individual infant's response is essential.

Any augmentation of pediatric cardiac output is dependent upon the patient's heart rate and diastolic filling time. The absolute amount of cardiac output is small (~600 mL/min); however, the cardiac output per kilogram of weight in the newborn (>200 mL/kg/min) is higher than that of adults, with the cardiac index at birth (4 L/min/m$^2$) gradually falling to adult normative values (2.5 to 3 L/min/m$^2$) in adolescence. This occurs because oxygen consumption is dependent on cardiac output, and oxygen consumption per kilogram of body weight is greater in infants than in adults. Familiarity with the normative ranges of heart rates is important because those ranges vary with age (**Appendix 1**). Rarely do arrhythmias produce significant changes in cardiac output with the exception of sustained supraventricular tachycardia. Severe tachycardia will decrease diastolic filling time, resulting in a rapid fall in stroke volume. Ventricular arrhythmias are uncommon, but may signify congenital heart disease, myocarditis, cardiomyopathy, or electrolyte imbalance when present. Bradycardia will result in decreased cardiac output and therefore decreased oxygen delivery, and is most often an ominous sign of significant hypoxemia or acidosis.

## B. Physical Examination

The physical examination of the cardiovascular system should focus on assessing tissue perfusion as it relates to circulation and end-organ function. This includes evaluation of mental status, skin color, temperature, capillary refill, pulse character, heart rate, rhythm, and blood pressure.

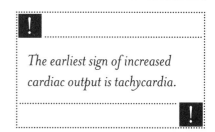

*The earliest sign of increased cardiac output is tachycardia.*

Cardiac output in children, especially infants, is dependent on the patient's heart rate. Blood pressure varies with age, height, and gender. Hypotension can be defined as a systolic blood pressure or mean arterial blood pressure <5th percentile. In children aged 1 to 10 years who are at the 50th percentile for height, the predicted 5th percentile systolic blood pressure and mean arterial blood pressure can be quickly determined using the following formulas:

Systolic blood pressure (mm Hg) 70 + (age in years × 2)

Mean arterial pressure (mm Hg) <40 + (age in years × 1.5)

The end-organ systems of special relevance are the brain and the kidneys because the body's homeostatic mechanisms give priority to preservation of perfusion to these tissues. Brain and kidney function are assessed by evaluating the patient's mental status and urine output. Deterioration of end-organ function is a precursor to circulatory arrest. In addition to the clinical exam, several ancillary studies (**Table 1-9**) should be used to fully evaluate and monitor the critically ill child.

## C. Shock

Shock may be defined as a state of cardiopulmonary dysfunction that fails to provide sufficient oxygen and nutrients to meet the metabolic needs of vital organs and peripheral tissues. For example, when a patient with hemorrhage continues to lose blood, the body compensates by trying to maintain adequate perfusion pressure to essential organs. The heart rate increases in an attempt to maintain adequate cardiac output as venous return diminishes along with a compensatory increase in systemic vascular resistance. This results in preservation of a normal blood pressure during the early phase (compensated phase) of shock, with hypotension occurring when the circulatory compensatory mechanisms are overwhelmed by uncorrected, ongoing blood loss. When hypotension is present, the patient is in late-stage (decompensated) shock, which is accompanied by weak, thready pulses, markedly prolonged capillary refill time, mottled extremities, and obtunded sensorium. Timely recognition of the shock state and aggressive intervention are essential to obtaining an optimal outcome. As soon as the diagnosis of shock is considered, early cardiopulmonary monitoring, vascular access, and treatment must be implemented.

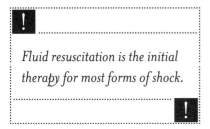

*Fluid resuscitation is the initial therapy for most forms of shock.*

### Table 1-9  Ancillary Studies to Evaluate Cardiovascular System

| Study | Evaluation |
| --- | --- |
| Blood gas | May use both arterial and venous blood gases if necessary<br>Detects acid-base imbalances |
| Serum lactate | Forms as result of tissue hypoxia and anaerobic metabolism<br>Reflects poor tissue perfusion<br>Serves as a prognostic indicator to assess response to therapy |
| Total serum $CO_2$ | Measures all forms of $CO_2$ (primarily bicarbonate)<br>Measures severity of metabolic acidosis |
| Hemoglobin concentration | Gauges arterial oxygen content and therefore oxygen delivery<br>Monitors ongoing blood loss in hemorrhagic shock |
| Urinary catheter | Continuously monitors urine output<br>Children: 1-2 mL/kg/h<br>Adolescents: 0.5-1 mL/kg/h |
| Continuous arterial pressure monitoring | Provides ongoing evaluation of blood pressure<br>Supplies information on systemic vascular resistance and cardiac output through waveform analysis<br>Monitors fluid resuscitation and inotropic/vasopressor therapy<br>Facilitates arterial blood gas sampling |
| Central venous pressure monitoring | Assesses preload and guides fluid therapy<br>Increases in obstructive forms of shock<br>Measures central venous oxygen saturation<br>Evaluates cardiac output and oxygen delivery |
| Chest radiograph | Assesses for congestive heart failure<br>Cardiomegaly<br>Pulmonary edema<br>Pleural effusion |
| Echocardiography | Shows contractility<br>Measures estimated ventricular pressures<br>Displays chamber size and wall thickness<br>Demonstrates congenital anomalies<br>Shows pericardial effusion |

Rapid restitution of circulating intravascular volume is critical if end-organ damage is to be avoided. Hepatomegaly can be a sign of fluid overload in the pediatric patient; however, it must be viewed with caution. Disease processes common to children (e.g., asthma, respiratory syncytial virus, bronchiolitis, and pneumonitis) can cause lung hyperinflation, resulting in downward displacement of the liver. Other signs of volume overload should also be considered in the evaluation of these patients. If a child with an enlarged liver fails to respond to the initial fluid administration, radiological examination of the chest may help to evaluate heart size.

Crackles may occur late in children who are developing congestive failure, and a gallop may be difficult to discern in infants owing to their rapid heart rate. (See **Chapter 6** for a more extensive discussion.)

## 1. Hypovolemic Shock

 **Case Study**

A previously healthy 4-month-old girl presents to the emergency department with a 4-day history of vomiting, loose watery stools, and low-grade fever. She became lethargic 24 hours earlier and has refused to drink water or tea offered by her parents. On physical exam, her heart rate is 200 beats/min, capillary refill is prolonged at 4 seconds, and she has a respiratory rate of 35 breaths/min.

**Detection**
- What is the etiology of shock in this scenario?
- What is her PEWS?

**Intervention**
- Would isotonic (e.g., normal saline) or hypotonic (e.g., 5% dextrose in water) IV fluid be best?
- Would a trial of oral rehydration therapy be appropriate in this context?

**Reassessment**
- If large volumes of warmed fluid are needed rapidly, would a rapid infuser be the best way to administer them?

**Effective Communication**
- What type of access is needed? Peripheral and/or central? Intravenous? Intraosseous? Facilitated subcutaneous using recombinant human hyaluronidase?

**Teamwork**
- How long and how many times should team members try for IV access before attempting intraosseous access? (See **Appendix 2**.)

This patient's PEWS is: behavior lethargic = 3, cardiovascular capillary refill of 4 seconds = 2, respiratory rate within normal limits = 0, total = 5. The most common cause of shock in the pediatric patient is acute hypovolemia resulting from increased fluid and electrolyte losses (gastrointestinal disorders) or blood loss resulting from severe trauma. Globally, approximately 2 billion gastroenteritis cases occur each year. Acute gastroenteritis is the second leading cause of death in children younger than 5 years, with over 2 million deaths worldwide.

A detailed medical history should be obtained from the child's parent or caregiver and referring institution. A history of increased fluid losses (vomiting and diarrhea), lethargy, and decreased urine output is found in infants with hypovolemic shock. Blood pressure is maintained longer in hypovolemic children than in adults; thus, blood pressure is not a clear indicator of volume and perfusion status. Tachycardia, mental status, capillary refill, decreased urine output, and temperature of extremities are much more reliable indicators of hypovolemia because they may become abnormal much earlier than hypotension in a child. The primary treatment is appropriate intravascular fluid volume resuscitation with isotonic solutions (**Chapters 6** and **8**). In resource-limited environments, oral rehydration therapy using oral rehydration salts, as recommended by the World Health Organization, has been shown to be effective, especially in cases of diarrhea caused by *Vibrio cholerae*.

## Case Study

A 5-year-old boy who was riding a bicycle without a helmet was hit by an automobile. A bystander picked him up and drove him to the emergency department. The boy's eyes are closed; he is moaning and won't respond to verbal commands or painful stimuli (e.g., nail bed pressure). His torso is markedly bruised and has a profusely bleeding open femur fracture. His heart rate is 200 beats/min, blood pressure is 70/30 mm Hg, capillary refill is 4 seconds, and pulse oximetry is 88% on room air.

**Detection**
- What is your first priority?
- What is the child's mental status?

**Intervention**
- What equipment do you need? How do you determine the appropriate size?
- What fluids should be administered and how?
- Would applying a tourniquet be appropriate management of his ongoing blood loss? Is he a candidate for damage control resuscitation?

**Reassessment**
- What is his response to the fluid administration? Is there any response?
- What is his mental status now?

**Effective Communication**
- Identification of problems and the success of a particular intervention have to be communicated amongst team members.
- Monitoring systems have to be attached and interpreted.

**Teamwork**
- What medical/surgical specialties need to be involved in the care of this patient?

This child is in obvious hypovolemic shock as a result of trauma. Many steps must be done in parallel as part of the primary survey (**Table 1-10**). Ideally, the traumatically injured child is evaluated and treated at the closest appropriate facility. This decision begins at the scene of injury and is reevaluated continuously along the levels of care. Laboratory investigations and radiological imaging studies must not delay the evaluation, treatment, or transport of the critically injured child to the center for appropriate definitive care (**Chapter 9**).

## Table 1-10  Primary Survey, Adjuncts, and Secondary Survey Mnemonics

**Primary Survey: SCABDE**
S – Safety: standard precautions, scene safety, patient and parent safety
C – Circulation: stop obvious bleeding (tourniquet) and start volume resuscitation
A – Airway: secure the airway with cervical spine stabilization
B – Breathing: oxygenate and ventilate; apply pulse oximetry and capnography
D – Disability: pupillary response, Glasgow Coma Scale, and point-of-care glucose test
E – Exposure: remove clothes, log roll, look behind cervical collar, keep warm (blankets, warm fluids, radiant warmer, warming blanket)

**Adjuncts to the Primary Survey: FFG**
F – Foley: after rectal exam to check for high-riding prostate in males, suggestive of urethral injury
F – Focused Assessment Sonography in Trauma (F.A.S.T.) exam
G – Gastric tube: place orally if unconscious and until face and basilar skull fractures are ruled out

**Secondary Survey: HEELPP MEE!**
H – History – AMPLE: allergies, medications, past medical history, last meal, and event details
E – Electrocardiographic monitoring: ensure chest leads are placed as soon as possible
E – End-tidal $CO_2$ monitoring
L – Laboratory tests: minimum prothrombin time/partial prothrombin time, blood typing and cross matching, arterial blood gas
P – Pulse oximetry
P – Photography: plain film radiographs minimum (anterior-posterior chest and pelvis) and computed tomography of head and neck as indicated
M – Medications: tetanus vaccine and/or immunoglobulin depending on vaccination status; antibiotics and other medications as needed
E – Evaluate: examine entire patient
E – Evacuate: consider transport if patient needs exceed your or the institution's capabilities

Reproduced with permission. © 2009 Kristen B. Bruzzini, PhD, and Col. Daniel B. Bruzzini, MD.

## 2. Cardiogenic Shock

### Case Study

A 9-year-old, usually active boy, who had a mild case of gastroenteritis 10 days ago, presents with a sudden decrease in activity, fever, difficulty breathing, chest pain, and swollen feet. On physical exam, he is ill-appearing, gray in color, listless, tachypneic at 35 breaths/min, and has an enlarged liver and new-onset heart murmur.

### Detection
- What is his PEWS?
- What studies should you perform to confirm your diagnosis?

### Intervention
- What medications and/or procedures are required?

### Reassessment
- How will you measure this child's response?

### Effective Communication
- What should the team be accomplishing first?

### Teamwork
- What other specialists should be involved?

This patient's PEWS is: behavior listless = 3, cardiovascular gray color = 3, tachypnea >10 above normal = 1, total = 7. Congestive heart failure in children is most often due to underlying congenital heart anomalies and often precedes cardiogenic shock. This can often be the result of acute or chronic changes in the heart's preload, afterload, contractility, rate, and/or rhythm. In the case of congenital heart disease, signs and symptoms vary depending on the type of lesion (**Chapter 16**). Myocarditis should be considered in all children with new-onset congestive heart failure. The usual symptoms of heart failure are fatigue, dyspnea on exertion, poor feeding in infants, acute onset edema, and fever. In this patient, there is also an antecedent history of a viral illness (upper respiratory infection or acute gastroenteritis) within 2 weeks of presentation. Early transfer to a pediatric intensive care unit for further monitoring, inotropic support, and a complete evaluation by a pediatric cardiologist is recommended. Other common etiologies of cardiogenic shock include hypoxic-ischemic episodes after acute life-threatening events, near drowning, or strangulation.

### 3. Distributive Shock

## Case Study

A 7-year-old girl with a peanut allergy is at a birthday party. She eats a chocolate chip cookie with nuts in it. Ten minutes later, she is not feeling well and complains of difficulty breathing. First responders (emergency medical services) are called. Just before they arrive, she becomes unresponsive with labored breathing and audible wheezing. She appears flushed and has an urticarial rash; her eyes are swollen shut from facial edema. She is warm, tachycardic with a heart rate of 160 beats/min, and has bounding pulses. Her blood pressure is 80/20 mm Hg.

### Detection
- What is her PEWS?
- What is the etiology of shock in this scenario?

### Intervention
- What would be your immediate response?
- What medications does she need?

### Reassessment
- Does her airway need to be secured?
- Is her breathing improving?

**Effective Communication**
- Who needs to know of her anaphylactic reaction? Family? School?
- How would you help the family prevent it in the future? Medical alert bracelet?

**Teamwork**
- Many steps are needed to be done simultaneously and quickly to evaluate and treat her circulatory, airway, and respiratory compromise.

This girl's PEWS is: behavior unconscious = 3, cardiovascular heart rate >30 above normal = 3, respiratory labored breathing = 2, total = 8. Distributive shock occurs as a result of an abnormality of vasomotor tone. This has the effect of redistributing blood volume and flow to the periphery, causing relative hypovolemia. In essence, the intravascular space has increased size without a corresponding increase in intravascular volume. Patients appear flushed and have warm extremities with bounding pulses. They are typically tachycardic with a wide pulse pressure and brisk capillary refill. In anaphylaxis, histamine is released from the mast cells and basophils in the lung and gastrointestinal tract. The signs of anaphylaxis include wheezing, respiratory distress, urticaria, vomiting, swelling of the face and tongue, and hypotension. Neurogenic shock is accompanied by a loss of sympathetic tone, which results in decreased peripheral vasomotor tone, vasodilatation, and a lack of compensatory rise in heart rate in response to shock. Neurogenic shock is resistant to fluid resuscitation but is responsive to appropriate α-adrenergic agents (e.g., phenylephrine, 0.1-0.5 μg/kg/min).

Anaphylaxis is an acute, potentially life-threatening syndrome, with multisystem manifestations resulting from the rapid release of inflammatory mediators. Foods – most commonly, milk, eggs, wheat, and soy – can be a significant trigger for immunoglobulin E-mediated anaphylaxis in children. Peanuts and fish are among the most potent triggers, but other common stimuli include preservatives in food and drugs, medications (antibiotics), insect venom (bee sting), and bioactive substances (blood products).

## Case Study

A 4-year-old boy is brought into the pediatric intensive care unit from a referring hospital where he presented 2 days ago with fever, tachypnea, and an oxygen requirement caused by influenza A pneumonia. He initially improved until the day of transfer when he was found to be poorly responsive, hypothermic, hypotensive, and tachycardic. A chest radiograph revealed a large left pleural effusion. Blood culture revealed Gram-positive cocci in clusters consistent with *Staphylococcus aureus.*

**Detection**
- What type of shock does this patient have?

**Intervention**
- What monitoring, IV access, and medications does this patient need?

**Reassessment**
- After starting vasoactive medications, how does one measure effectiveness?

**Effective Communication**

- How should the life-threatening nature of this illness be communicated to all his caregivers?

**Teamwork**

- Fluid resuscitation, central access for vasoactive medications, and possible chest pleurocentesis must be accomplished quickly by healthcare providers working together to obtain the best possible clinical outcome for this child and family.

As in adults, the most common cause of distributive shock in pediatric patients is sepsis. Septic shock is characterized by changes in mental status, fever or hypothermia, and perfusion abnormalities such as vasodilation (warm shock) early in septic shock followed by vasoconstriction (cold shock).

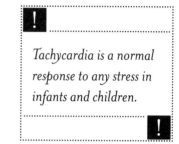

*Tachycardia is a normal response to any stress in infants and children.*

The clinical presentation of "warm shock" is vasodilation, tachycardia, bounding pulses, brisk capillary refill, and widened pulse pressure. These patients have low systemic vascular resistance and high cardiac output. "Cold shock" reflects a low cardiac output state with poor peripheral perfusion and high systemic vascular resistance. These individuals will present with tachycardia, prolonged capillary refill, mottled skin, and weak pulses. The therapeutic goal in septic shock is to restore and maintain optimal organ perfusion and oxygenation as evidenced by normal mentation and adequate urine output (≥1 mL/kg/h). Children in shock are usually severely hypovolemic and will respond to aggressive fluid resuscitation (**Chapter 6**). Isotonic fluid boluses in 20 mL/kg increments are usually helpful. Crystalloids (e.g., normal saline or Ringer lactate solution) or colloids (5% albumin or dextran) may be used. Typical fluid requirements range from 40 to 200 mL/kg during the initial phase of resuscitation.

After fluid resuscitation, the first choice of vasopressor support in warm shock is norepinephrine (noradrenaline) (0.05 to 0.3 µg/kg/min), then epinephrine (adrenaline) (0.05 to 0.3 µg/kg/min). Dopamine (5 to 10 µg/kg/min) is recommended as the first choice in patients with fluid-refractory cold shock, followed by epinephrine if unresponsive to dopamine. Dobutamine, a $\beta_1$-agonist, may be given to patients with low cardiac output and elevated systemic vascular resistance states (vasoconstricted) after fluid resuscitation. These continuous IV medications are best delivered through a central access line to avoid extravasation injury from a peripherally inserted catheter. Use of corticosteroids (hydrocortisone, 1 to 2 mg/kg/day) is indicated in patients with vasopressor-resistant shock, purpura fulminans, or suspected adrenal insufficiency (chronic corticosteroid use, malignant disease, collagen vascular disorders, etomidate for intubation). The pathophysiology of septic shock is complex and exhibits the features of hypovolemic, distributive, and cardiogenic shock. The therapeutic goal in septic shock is to expeditiously restore and maintain optimal organ perfusion.

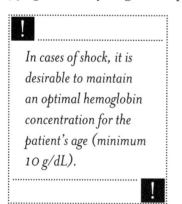

*In cases of shock, it is desirable to maintain an optimal hemoglobin concentration for the patient's age (minimum 10 g/dL).*

## 4. Obstructive Shock

###  Case Study

A full-term 2-week-old male neonate who had been breastfeeding well for the first 10 days presents to his pediatrician with a 4-day history of poor feeding, decreased number of wet diapers, and poor weight gain. On physical exam, he is lethargic with tachypnea, cyanosis, an enlarged liver, no femoral pulses, and a heart murmur. The pediatrician promptly refers him to the hospital for further evaluation.

**Detection**
- What is his PEWS?
- What studies should you perform to confirm your diagnosis?

**Intervention**
- What medications and/or procedures are required?
- What are the side effects of prostaglandin $E_1$ ($PGE_1$; alprostadil) therapy?

**Reassessment**
- How will you measure the child's response?
- How will you prevent adverse complications as a result of $PGE_1$ therapy?

**Effective Communication**
- What should the team be accomplishing first?

**Teamwork**
- What other specialists should be involved?

The patient's PEWS is: behavior lethargic = 3, cardiovascular cyanosis = 2, tachypnea = 1, total = 6. Patients presenting with obstructive shock will exhibit a rapid and often precipitous deterioration in hemodynamic status. Neonates (up to 28 days) with ductal-dependent lesions (e.g., coarctation of the aorta, hypoplastic left heart, aortic stenosis) will typically present in the first few weeks of life in profound shock and have a history of poor feeding, tachypnea, lethargy, cyanosis, thready or absent femoral pulses, and poor or absent urine output (obstructive shock). Prompt initiation of $PGE_1$ (alprostadil; 0.05 to 0.1 µg/kg/min), inotropes, and isotonic fluids are lifesaving. Administration should not be delayed to await a confirmatory echocardiogram. Common side effects of $PGE_1$ are fever, flushing, and apnea. Apnea from $PGE_1$ may occur without warning and at anytime during therapy. When transferring a patient receiving $PGE_1$ to another facility, it is strongly recommended to secure the airway with an endotracheal tube. Once the ductus arteriosus has reopened, the amount of $PGE_1$ can be reduced. Hyperventilation and hyperoxia must be avoided to prevent excessive pulmonary vascular bed dilation leading to preferential pulmonary blood flow away from the systemic side (aorta) across the now patent ductus arteriosus to the pulmonary side (pulmonary artery). This will worsen systemic perfusion and exacerbate systemic shock.

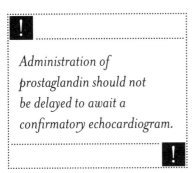

*Administration of prostaglandin should not be delayed to await a confirmatory echocardiogram.*

Patients with nonductal-dependent lesions present outside the neonatal period with a history of tachycardia, gallop rhythm, heart murmur, tachypnea, hepatomegaly, and failure to thrive. These patients will often respond to diuresis with a loop diuretic (furosemide 0.5 to 1 mg/kg) and to inotropic support (milrinone [amrinone] 0.5 to 1 µg/kg/min, or dobutamine 5 to 10 µg/kg/min) and/or afterload reduction with an angiotensin-converting-enzyme inhibitor rather than fluid resuscitation (**Chapter 16**).

# V. NERVOUS SYSTEM

 ## Case Study

A 3-month-old girl with history of colic is brought into the emergency department by her mother after the infant apparently fell from her crib to the floor. On physical examination, she is unresponsive to stimulation. She has multiple bruises to the head, chest, and abdomen. Eye examination reveals retinal hemorrhages. A head computed tomographic scan reveals a subdural blood collection on the left parietal area, and a chest radiograph reveals rib fractures.

**Detection**
- Are the clinical findings consistent with the history provided?
- What are the most life-threatening injuries?

**Intervention**
- What steps must be taken first?

**Reassessment**
- Is the infant responding to therapy?
- Does intracranial pressure need to be monitored directly?

**Effective Communication**
- How should the team interact with the mother, father, and other caregivers?
- What needs to be documented and recorded at the time of presentation and by whom?

**Teamwork**
- What is the role of medical and nursing personnel in cases of suspected nonaccidental trauma?
- When should law enforcement and social services be contacted in suspected cases of nonaccidental trauma?

Any infant or young child with a depressed level of consciousness, seizures, and/or coma should be evaluated for the possibility of nonaccidental trauma (e.g., child abuse, "shaken baby syndrome") even if there are no outward signs of injury. Because of the pliability of their bones, children can sustain internal injury without significant external bruising or rib fractures. Furthermore, infants can lose a significant amount of blood in the cranium, resulting in hypovolemic shock. Unfortunately, the infant in this case is a victim of abuse and has sustained a closed head injury as a result of nonaccidental head trauma.

The Glasgow Coma Scale is frequently used to evaluate a child's neurological status and level of consciousness. This scale is difficult to apply in children, even when it is adapted for age (**Chapter 15**, **Table 15-1**). When assessing the need for further intervention, careful attention should be paid to the pediatric patient's ability to maintain the airway, pupillary reaction, verbal responses, motor system reaction, and the fontanelle status in infants. The fontanelle, which usually closes by 24 months of age, is best examined when the child is calm and sitting up. If the child is supine and/or crying, the anterior fontanelle may feel full and tense, thereby giving a false impression of increased intracranial pressure.

The pupillary response is used to rapidly evaluate brainstem function, but abnormalities in pupillary response, such as miosis and mydriasis, may also be found in many toxidromes. Other pertinent physical signs include muscle tone, muscle strength, facial symmetry, ataxia, and any abnormal movements of extremities and facial musculature. In infants, seizures may be characterized by decreased alertness (the infant does not regard parents or track an object across the visual field), autonomic changes (tachycardia, elevated blood pressure, and dilated pupils), apnea, cyanosis, and subcortical muscle activity (bicycling movements of the legs, swimming movements of the arms, sucking, or tongue thrusting). Tonic-clonic muscle motion may not occur during seizures in infants because neuronal myelination and connections have not fully developed. The treatment of seizures is covered in depth in **Chapter 15**. If the seizure or the medications used to treat the seizure significantly compromise the patient's airway and breathing, an endotracheal tube should be inserted. Neuromuscular blocking agents do not treat seizures and will obscure their physical manifestations. Neuromuscular blocking agents should only be used to facilitate endotracheal intubation. The pediatric intensivist and pediatric neurologist should be involved early in the care of status epilepticus.

Hyponatremia and hypoglycemia should be considered in infants and small children presenting with coma and/or seizures. A point-of-care glucose test is needed as part of the primary survey to rule out hypoglycemia as a cause of altered mental status. Hypocalcemia will cause seizures in infants and is commonly associated with tetany. Treatment of severe symptomatic hypocalcemia with IV calcium chloride or calcium gluconate through a centrally placed catheter is preferred so as to avoid peripheral subcutaneous tissue extravasation and resultant injury. For treatment of electrolyte abnormalities, see **Chapter 8**.

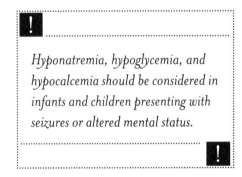

*Hyponatremia, hypoglycemia, and hypocalcemia should be considered in infants and children presenting with seizures or altered mental status.*

# VI. SEPSIS

Because of their incompletely developed immune systems, children and neonates are treated with empiric antibiotic therapy more frequently than are adults. The positive predictive value of blood cultures in the pediatric population is limited and dependent on the number performed, amount of blood obtained, and pathogen involved. The neonatal population is especially vulnerable, and the following factors increase their risk of infection:

- Decreased polymorphonuclear white cell function and storage reservoir
- Poor ability for antibody synthesis
- Reduced delivery of phagocytes to inflammatory sites
- Passive maternal immunity depleted by 6 months after birth

Most maternal antibodies are transported across the placenta in the third trimester of pregnancy, limiting passive maternal immunity in premature neonates. Adult levels of immunoglobulin are not reached until 4 to 7 years of age.

Fever always suggests the possibility of serious bacterial disease. In the febrile infant younger than 2 months, antibiotics are considered an emergency drug and often begun before a source of infection is identified. In these infants, the most common causes of life-threatening bacterial infections in the United States are group B streptococci (*Streptococcus agalactiae*), *Escherichia coli*, *Listeria monocytogenes*, and *Enterococcus*. Before the age of 3 years, the risk of occult bacteremia is increased if the temperature is >104°F (>40°C) or the white blood cell count is <500 cells/mm$^3$ or >15,000 cells/mm$^3$. Absolute neutrophil count <1,000 cells/mm$^3$ and significant neutrophil bandemia of 25% to 30% are also markers of severe bacterial infection in children. A full workup is recommended: blood culture, urine culture, and lumbar puncture for cerebral spinal fluid culture as clinically indicated. In children aged 2 months to 2 years, *Streptococcus pneumoniae*, *Staphylococcus aureus* (methicillin-sensitive or -resistant), *Haemophilus influenzae*, *Neisseria meningitidis*, and *Salmonella* are the organisms most associated with serious infections. Clinical signs of sepsis may involve respiratory distress, temperature instability (including hypothermia), and gastrointestinal distress.

An exanthema or rash is often seen, and its characteristic color and distribution pattern may be specific to a particular infection. Examples of such exanthemas would be petechiae or purpura suggestive of meningococcemia, vesicular lesions indicative of herpes simplex or Coxsackie viral infections, or erythematous rash with evidence of peeling secondary to staphylococcal or streptococcal infections. Definitions for sepsis and organ dysfunction in pediatric patients are discussed at length in **Chapter 7**.

The features unique to the care of infants and children, as discussed in this chapter, severely limit the margin for error in the treatment of critically ill or injured pediatric patients. Therefore, specialty consultation should be requested early. Children tend to deteriorate and recover more quickly than their adult counterparts. It is incumbent on those caring for critically ill children to **DIRECT** their care: **detect** a child with a severe injury or illness; **intervene** in a timely manner; **reassess** each intervention with appropriate monitoring and diagnostic tests; **effectively communicate** with each other so that key information is relayed and lifesaving therapies implemented; and practice **teamwork**, for no one person has all the requisite knowledge, training, and capability to care for a severely ill or injured child.

## Assessment of the Critically Ill Child

- A question that should be asked and answered in every healthcare provider's mind is, "Does this child look sick?" If the answer is yes, the child likely is critically ill.

- The Pediatric Early Warning Score (PEWS) is an evaluation tool utilized as an early indicator of impending clinical deterioration.

- Children should always be examined in the position they spontaneously assume for comfort. Forcing a child into a different position may worsen their respiratory distress and even precipitate respiratory arrest.

- Early signs of respiratory distress in children include tachypnea, grunting, and nasal flaring.

- Ensuring a patent airway is the most important initial step in treating a child with respiratory compromise. Chest movement does not ensure a patent airway.

- A child's perfusion status is best assessed initially by mental status, capillary refill, urine output, and temperature of extremities. Hypotension is a late finding in pediatric shock. Timely recognition of the shock state and aggressive intervention are essential to obtaining an optimal outcome.

- Infants and young children presenting with seizures should be evaluated for electrolyte imbalances and hypoglycemia.

- Young infants face an increased risk of infection due to their immature immune systems. Empiric antibiotics are considered emergency drugs for febrile infants younger than 2 months.

## Suggested Readings

1. Agency for HealthCare Research and Quality. TeamSTEPPS. http://teamstepps.ahrq.gov. Accessed May 13, 2013.

2. Akre M, Finkelstein M, Erickson M, Liu M, Vanderbilt L, Billman G. Sensitivity of the pediatric early warning score to identify patient deterioration. *Pediatrics*. 2010;125:e763-e769.

3. Allen CH, Etzwiler LS, Miller MK, et al. Recombinant human hyaluronidase-enabled subcutaneous pediatric rehydration. *Pediatrics*. 2009;124:e858-e867.

4. Borgman M, Spinella PC, Perkins JG, et al. The ratio of blood products transfused affects mortality in patients receiving massive transfusions at a combat support hospital. *J Trauma*. 2007;63: 805-813.

5. Frauenfelder C, Raith E, Griggs W. Damage control resuscitation of the exsanguinating trauma patient: pathophysiology and basic principles. *J Mil Veterans Health*. 2011;19.

6. Fuenfer M, Creamer K, Lenhart MK, eds. *Pediatric Surgery and Medicine for Hostile Environments.* Washington, DC: Office of the Surgeon General; 2010.

7. Haque IU, Zaritsky AL. Analysis of the evidence for the lower limit of systolic and mean arterial pressure in children. *Pediatr Crit Care Med.* 2007;8:138-144.

8. Hsu JM, Pham TN. Damage control in the injured patient. *Int J Crit Illn Inj Sci.* 2011;1:66-72

9. Jansen J, Thomas R, Loudon MA, Brooks A. Damage control resuscitation for patients with major trauma. *BMJ.* 2009;338:b1778.

10. Steele SR, Peoples GE. Damage control in the war wounded. *Adv Wound Care (New Rochelle).* 2012;1:31-37.

11. United States Army Institute of Surgical Research (USAISR). Damage Control Resuscitation: Joint Trauma System. http://www.usaisr.amedd.army.mil/clinical_practice_guidelines.html. Updated February 1, 2013. Accessed May 13, 2013.

12. World Health Organization Global Task Force on Cholera Control. First steps in managing an acute outbreak of diarrhoea. http://www.who.int/cholera/publications/firststeps/en/index.html. Accessed May 13, 2013.

# Chapter 2

# Airway Management

## ✓ Objectives

- Recognize the signs and symptoms of an unstable airway.
- Detect the signs and symptoms of respiratory failure.
- Identify anatomic and physiologic variables involved in the management of the pediatric airway.
- Describe how to open and maintain an airway manually and with the help of airway adjuncts.
- Explain how to support a patient with bag-mask ventilation.
- Relate the preparation and sequence of intubating pediatric patients.
- Determine the potential for difficult intubation and discuss alternative methods of establishing a stable airway.

## 📁 Case Study

A 3-year-old boy with a 2-day history of a barking cough has worsening retractions and desaturations over the last hour.

**Detection**
- What is this child's physiologic status?
- What signs and symptoms are indicative of respiratory distress?
- What are the most likely diagnosis and the worst possible diagnoses?

**Intervention**
- What are the most immediate treatment strategies?
- What initial treatment options may be attempted to maintain the airway?
- If you decide to intubate the patient, what steps must be taken to ensure that the intubation is as safe as possible?
- What size and type of laryngoscope blade would you select?
- What size of endotracheal tube would you select, and what would be the appropriate depth of tube placement?

**Reassessment**
- Is the current treatment strategy effective?
- Does the patient need other therapeutic interventions?

**Effective Communication**
- When the patient's clinical status changes, who needs the information and how will it be disseminated?
- Where is the best place to manage the care of this patient?

**Teamwork**
- How are you going to implement the treatment strategy?
- Who is to do what and when?

# I. INTRODUCTION

Respiratory distress, a frequent occurrence in children, can develop from problems at all levels of the respiratory tract. The majority of cardiopulmonary arrests in children are heralded by respiratory failure. Recognition and interruption of the progression from respiratory compromise to respiratory failure is fundamental to pediatric airway management. The ability to recognize airway compromise and to establish and maintain a patent airway, despite age-related anatomic differences, is essential.

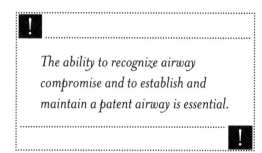
*The ability to recognize airway compromise and to establish and maintain a patent airway is essential.*

# II. ANATOMIC AND PHYSIOLOGIC CONSIDERATIONS

The airway of a child changes dramatically from birth to adulthood. To assess and manage airway emergencies, it is necessary to understand certain anatomic and developmental aspects of a child's airway.

- In children, the nose provides nearly half of the total airway resistance. The infant's nose is short, soft, and small with nearly circular nares. Infants younger than 2 months are obligate nasal breathers. Although the nares double in size from birth to 6 months, they can be easily occluded by edema, secretions, or external pressure. Clearing the nasal passages by suctioning can significantly improve an infant's respirations.

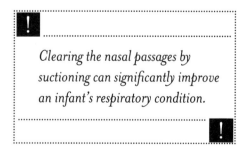
*Clearing the nasal passages by suctioning can significantly improve an infant's respiratory condition.*

- A child's tongue is large in relation to the oral cavity. This relative disproportion is increased in developmental disorders such as Pierre Robin sequence and severe micrognathia. A large tongue in a relatively small oral cavity increases the difficulty of visualizing the larynx during laryngoscopy. Backward displacement of the tongue into the posterior pharynx as a result of decreased muscle tone in sleep, depressed level of consciousness from head injury, sedation, or other nervous system dysfunction can result in upper airway obstruction.

- The level of the larynx in the neck changes from C2 in neonates to C3 to C4 in children and ends up at C5 to C6 in adults. In infants, the epiglottis is at the level of the first cervical vertebrae and overlaps the soft palate. The high position of the larynx, combined with a large tongue and a small mandible, contributes to an infant's susceptibility to airway obstruction.

    The high position of the larynx makes the angle between the base of the tongue and the glottic opening more acute, which increases the difficulty of visualizing the vocal cords during laryngoscopy. Therefore, a straight laryngoscope blade, such as a Miller blade, may be superior for creating a straight plane from the mouth to the glottis.

- An infant's epiglottis is long, soft, and omega ($\Omega$)-shaped, whereas an adult's epiglottis is shorter, more rigid, and flatter. A longer and softer epiglottis is more difficult to control during laryngoscopy. Using a straight laryngoscope blade, which directly lifts the epiglottis and exposes the vocal cords, can overcome this difficulty.

- A pediatric larynx is funnel-shaped, with the subglottic portion angled posteriorly to the supraglottic portion. Consequently the narrowest portion of the larynx is in the subglottic space. As a result, inflating the cuff of an endotracheal tube could lead to subglottic edema. The adult larynx is barrel-shaped, with the narrowest portion at the level of the vocal cords, and less prone to this complication.

    > *A pediatric larynx is funnel-shaped; the narrowest portion is the cricoid cartilage. An adult larynx is barrel-shaped; the narrowest portion is the vocal cords.*

- The internal diameter of a pediatric trachea is approximately one-third that of an adult, resulting in higher airflow resistance. Resistance to airflow is a function of $1/r^4$, where r is the airway radius. A small decrease in airway diameter (2 × radius) due to edema or secretions causes a far greater increase in resistance in a child than in an adult (**Figure 2-1**).

**Figure 2-1.** Airway Resistance Proportionate to Airway Radius

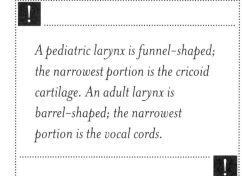

- The length of a newborn's trachea is approximately 5 cm, and that of an 18-month-old infant is approximately 7 cm. Given this short length, both right main-stem bronchus intubation and accidental extubation are common.

- The chest wall of infants is easily compressible due to the higher elasticity of its cartilaginous structures.

    - The use of abdominal muscles leads to a characteristic see-saw, or abdominal, breathing pattern.
    - Intercostal, subcostal, and suprasternal retractions become prominent as airway obstruction or lung disease increases the work of breathing.
    - Respiratory muscle fatigue may lead to decreased respiratory effort as respiratory failure progresses.

# III. ASSESSING RESPIRATORY STATUS

In children, as in adults, assessment of airway patency and spontaneous respiratory effort is a crucial first step. The clinician must recognize signs of distress as well as look, listen, and feel for diminished or absent air movement.

## A. Observe the General Appearance of the Child

Give careful attention to:

- Muscle tone and spontaneous and reactive movement
- Alertness/interaction with the environment or caregiver
- Inconsolable crying or agitation
- Ability to speak or cry (phonation and crying require air movement)
- Injury to the airway or other conditions (e.g., cervical spine fracture or facial burns) that will affect assessment and manipulation of the airway
- Signs of congenital malformations of the face, mouth, or tongue that might contribute to respiratory problems
- Signs of airway obstruction due to decreased level of consciousness

Ventilation may be adequate with minimal thoracic excursion, but respiratory muscle activity and even vigorous chest movement do not ensure that tidal volume is adequate.

# Airway Management 2

## B. Assess the Child's Respiratory Rate

Keep in mind these facts:

- The normal respiratory rate varies with age (**Table 2-1** and **Appendix 1**).

- The respiratory rate is best assessed by observation. Expose the child's chest and watch the rise and fall of the chest and abdomen.

- A respiratory rate >60 breaths/min is abnormal in a child of any age.

- An abnormally slow rate may herald respiratory failure.

> *A respiratory rate >60 breaths/min is abnormal in a child of any age.*

## C. Consider the Work of Breathing

- Intercostal, subcostal, and suprasternal retractions increase with progressive respiratory distress. Decreasing respiratory rate and diminished retractions in a child with a history of distress may signal severe fatigue.

- Increased inspiratory effort often amplifies airway resistance, causing collapse of the compliant upper airway and producing stridor.

### Table 2-1  Age-Normal Respiratory Rates

| Age | Respiratory Rate (breaths/min) |
|---|---|
| Newborn | 30-60 |
| Infant (1-12 months) | 30-60 |
| Toddler (1-2 years) | 24-40 |
| Preschooler (3-5 years) | 22-34 |
| School age (6-12 years) | 18-30 |
| Adolescent (13-17 years) | 12-16 |

- Nasal flaring is an effort to increase airway diameter and is often seen with hypoxemia.

- Grunting is an expiratory noise produced by an effort to prevent airway collapse by generating positive end-expiratory pressure.

> *Auscultate over the mouth, nose, and neck as well as the central and peripheral chest. Listen for quality, pitch, right-to-left symmetry, and magnitude of breath sounds.*

- Obstruction or narrowing of the extrathoracic airway (nose, posterior pharynx, larynx, and subglottic space) causes high-pitched inspiratory noise (stridor) and retractions.

- Obstruction or narrowing of the intrathoracic airways results in signs and symptoms that occur predominantly during expiration. Wheezing (high-pitched expiratory sounds) is caused by expiratory obstruction.

- Incomplete obstruction (during which a limited amount of air can be inspired and expired from the lungs) due to pharyngeal soft-tissue collapse, a mass, or a foreign body in the airway may be associated with snoring, stridor, gurgling, or noisy breathing.

- Complete airway obstruction (during which no air can be inspired or expired) is likely when respiratory effort is visible but breath sounds are absent.

- Crackles are end-inspiratory noises usually heard with parenchymal lung diseases, such as pneumonia and bronchiolitis, and are loudest in the peripheral lung fields.

- Asymmetry of breath sounds is an important clue. Breath sounds may be diminished or absent on one side in the presence of pneumothorax or pleural effusion or when a tracheal tube is placed in the opposite main bronchus.

## D. Evaluate Mental Status

- Agitation and irritability may indicate hypoxemia. Lethargy in the presence of acceptable oxygen saturation may reflect an elevated carbon dioxide tension.

- The presence and strength of protective airway reflexes (i.e., cough and gag) must be assessed cautiously. Overly aggressive stimulation of the posterior pharynx while assessing those reflexes may precipitate emesis and aspiration of gastric contents. Moreover, stimulation of the posterior pharynx may convert partial upper airway obstruction (due to illnesses such as epiglottitis) to complete airway obstruction.

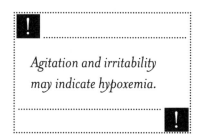

*Agitation and irritability may indicate hypoxemia.*

If respiratory efforts are absent and an immediate remedy is not available, proceed to manual support and assisted ventilation while preparing to establish an artificial airway.

# IV. MONITORING RESPIRATORY FUNCTION

## A. Longitudinal Physical Assessment

Once a patient is found to be in respiratory distress, close monitoring of respiratory function is essential. Auscultation and observation are important components of this monitoring. Alarms indicating inadequate ventilation and oxygenation should be set. Constant vigilance is required once a patient is intubated and placed on a mechanical ventilator.

## B. Arterial Blood Gas

Arterial blood gas measurement may be helpful when either the etiology or the degree of respiratory insufficiency is unknown. Careful consideration should be given to the fact that arterial puncture is a painful procedure; the resultant agitation might worsen the respiratory distress of some children.

A systematic approach to arterial blood gas interpretation consists of:

- Determining the degree of alveolar ventilation based on the $Pa_{CO_2}$
- Assessing whether the patient's pH can be explained solely on the basis of $Pa_{CO_2}$ or if a metabolic component exists
- Determining whether the ventilatory or metabolic event was primary or compensatory
- Assessing the effectiveness of correction of any hypoxemic state

Arterial blood gas disorders are classified into 4 main categories: hypoventilation, alveolar hyperventilation, metabolic acidosis, and metabolic alkalosis.

### 1. Hypoventilation

Hypoventilation (respiratory acidosis) results in an elevation of $P_{CO_2}$, which causes the $HCO_3^-$:$P_{CO_2}$ ratio to decrease and results in a decrease in pH. Carbon dioxide retention can be caused by hypoventilation or a ventilation-perfusion inequality. Increasing ventilation in most cases will correct respiratory acidosis. If the patient is unstable, manual bag-mask ventilation is indicated until the underlying problem can be addressed.

If respiratory acidosis persists (as seen in chronic ventilatory failure), the kidneys respond by conserving $HCO_3^-$. Renal compensation is typically not complete, and so the pH approaches but does not fully return to 7.4.

### 2. Alveolar Hyperventilation

Alveolar hyperventilation (respiratory alkalosis) results in decreased $P_{CO_2}$, which in turn elevates the pH. Bicarbonate and base excess remain in the normal range because the kidneys have not had time to establish adequate compensation. Pain and anxiety may cause acute hyperventilation and alkalosis in children. Hypoxemia may lead to increased minute ventilation and respiratory alkalosis.

### 3. Metabolic Acidosis

A primary decrease in $HCO_3^-$ in turn leads to a decreased pH. Bicarbonate can be lowered by an accumulation of acids in the blood, as in uncontrolled diabetes mellitus, and production of lactic acid in the setting of tissue hypoxia. Respiratory compensation occurs by an increase in ventilation that lowers the $P_{CO_2}$ and in turn raises pH. Respiratory insufficiency in the presence of metabolic acidosis is concerning due to the degree of acidosis that results when a patient is unable to increase ventilation.

### 4. Metabolic Alkalosis

An increase in $HCO_3^-$ raises the $HCO_3^-$:$P_{CO_2}$ ratio and thus the pH. Compensation occurs by hypoventilation and $CO_2$ retention. Metabolic alkalosis is seen in the child with pyloric stenosis who loses large amounts of stomach acid due to vomiting. The child's ability to compensate for metabolic alkalosis by hypoventilation is limited by hypoxia.

For additional information, please see **Appendix 3**.

## C. Pulse Oximetry

Pulse oximetry provides continuous, noninvasive measurement of arterial oxyhemoglobin saturation ($Sao_2$). **Figure 2-2** shows the oxyhemoglobin saturation curve, which is a graph of $Sao_2$ versus partial pressure of oxygen ($Pao_2$). Under normal conditions, hemoglobin is 90% saturated with oxygen at a $Pao_2$ of about 60 mm Hg (8 kPa). Raising the $Pao_2$ above 60 mm Hg does not result in an appreciable increase in hemoglobin saturation. However, due to the sigmoidal shape of the oxyhemoglobin saturation curve, once the $Pao_2$ drops below 60 mm Hg, the saturation changes rapidly with small changes in $Pao_2$.

> *Normally, hemoglobin is 90% saturated with oxygen at a $Pao_2$ of about 60 mm Hg (8 kPa). Raising the $Pao_2$ above 60 mm Hg does not result in an appreciable increase in hemoglobin saturation.*

**Figure 2-2.** Oxyhemoglobin Saturation Curve

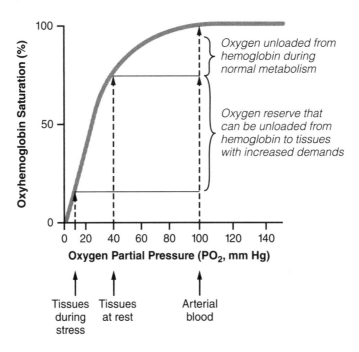

The oxyhemoglobin dissociation curve relates $Po_2$ to oxyhemoglobin saturation. Near-maximal saturation of hemoglobin occurs at a $Po_2$ of 60 mm Hg (8 kPa). $Po_2$ values above this point provide only a modest increase in oxyhemoglobin saturation. Note, however, that a rapid decrease in oxyhemoglobin saturation occurs when the $Po_2$ drops below 60 mm Hg (8 kPa).

The limitations to pulse oximetry in managing critically ill patients include the following:

- Pulse oximetry requires pulsatile blood flow. In the presence of shock and poor perfusion, the accuracy and signal strength become unreliable.

- In carbon monoxide poisoning, most pulse oximeters will read falsely high for oxyhemoglobin saturation because carboxyhemoglobin absorbs light at a similar wavelength as oxyhemoglobin. Blood gas measurement with co-oximetry is the only way to determine the true oxyhemoglobin and carboxyhemoglobin saturations.

- Pulse oximetry is not accurate in methemoglobinemia.

- Oxygen saturation may be underestimated in patients with sickle cell disease and acute vaso-occlusive crisis.

- Intravenous dyes and certain colors of nail polish falsely lower pulse oximetry readings.

- The accuracy of the pulse oximeter should be questioned when a patient's appearance and heart rate do not correlate with the pulse oximeter reading.

- It is always safer to question elevated saturations and accept decreased saturations as accurate until proven otherwise.

## D. Exhaled Carbon Dioxide

End-tidal $CO_2$ monitoring can be used to estimate the arterial $CO_2$ tension. Quantitative continuous capnography can be performed via nasal cannula or with devices that attach to the tracheal tube. Qualitative (colorimetric) devices that change color when exhaled $CO_2$ is present are generally used for confirmation of tracheal tube placement and are discussed later in this chapter.

In the presence of ventilation-perfusion mismatch, airway obstruction, or tracheal tube leak, end-tidal $CO_2$ values may not accurately reflect true arterial $CO_2$ levels.

# V. AIRWAY MANAGEMENT

## A. Oxygen Delivery Systems

Oxygen should be administered immediately in virtually every setting where respiratory difficulty is suspected. Infants and children consume 2 to 3 times more oxygen per kilogram of body weight than adults under basal conditions and even more when they are ill or stressed. Several key points regarding administration of oxygen to children are as follows:

- When administering oxygen to an alert child, the need to increase oxygen delivery must be balanced against the potential for agitation, which increases oxygen consumption.

- If a child is intolerant of one method of oxygen delivery (e.g., nasal cannula), another method should be tried (e.g., face tent). It is often helpful to have a parent hold the child and assist with placement of oxygen delivery devices (**Appendix 4**).

- Children will often assume a position that maximizes airway patency and minimizes respiratory effort. They should be allowed to remain in their position of comfort.

- Oxygen administration will have limited effect in the presence of airway obstruction. In a somnolent or obtunded child, the airway can be obstructed due to neck flexion, relaxation of the jaw, posterior displacement of the tongue against the pharynx, and collapse of the hypopharynx. Before using airway adjuncts, attempt to open the airway using manual methods. The airway should be cleared of secretions to optimize the patient's effort.

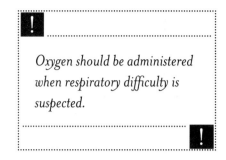

*Oxygen should be administered when respiratory difficulty is suspected.*

- In patients who are making respiratory efforts but are not moving an adequate amount of air, spontaneous respiratory efforts can be assisted with a bag-mask device. These patients can then be transitioned to noninvasive or invasive forms of ventilation. See **Appendix 5** for additional discussion on airway adjuncts.

### 1. Simple Oxygen Mask

The simple oxygen mask is a low-flow device that delivers oxygen with a flow rate of 6 to 10 L/min. The oxygen concentration delivered to the patient can reach a maximum of 60% due to entrainment of room air through the exhalation ports of the mask. An oxygen flow rate of at least 6 L/min should be maintained to sustain an optimal inspired oxygen concentration and prevent rebreathing of exhaled carbon dioxide.

### 2. Partial Rebreathing Mask

A partial rebreathing mask consists of a simple face mask with a reservoir bag. It provides oxygen concentrations of 50% to 60%. During inspiration, the patient draws gas predominantly from the fresh oxygen inflow and the reservoir bag, so entrainment of room air through the exhalation ports is minimized. An oxygen flow rate of 10 to 12 L/min is usually required.

### 3. Non-rebreathing Mask

A non-rebreathing mask consists of a face mask and reservoir bag with a valve incorporated into one or both exhalation ports to prevent entrainment of room air during inspiration. Another valve between the reservoir bag and the mask prevents flow of exhaled gas into the reservoir. An inspired concentration of 95% can be achieved with an oxygen flow rate of 10 to 15 L/min and use of a well-sealed mask.

### 4. Face Tent

A face tent is a high-flow soft plastic bucket that children often tolerate better than a face mask. Even with a high oxygen flow rate, inspired concentrations over 40% cannot be reliably provided. A face tent permits access to the face without interrupting oxygen flow.

### 5. Nasal Cannula

A nasal cannula is a low-flow oxygen delivery system that is useful when low levels of supplemental oxygen are required. The net $F_{IO_2}$ depends on the child's respiratory effort, size, and minute ventilation in comparison with the nasal cannula flow.

# B. Maneuvers to Open and Maintain the Airway

The airway has oral, pharyngeal, and tracheal components. Maximal opening of the airway is obtained by aligning the axes of these components, as shown in **Figure 2-3**. Children younger than 2 years have relatively large heads for their body size, which results in slight neck flexion when they are in the supine position. Children in this age group usually benefit from a small roll placed under the shoulders that allows the head to fall back into proper position. A thin towel or blanket is usually sufficient for this purpose. Care must be taken to avoid overextension of the neck, which will result in obstruction. Smaller rolls of towels on either side of the head will also prevent the head from rolling from side to side. In older children, a small roll under the back of the head helps facilitate proper alignment of the axes.

**Figure 2-3.** Aligning the Oral, Pharyngeal, and Tracheal Axes

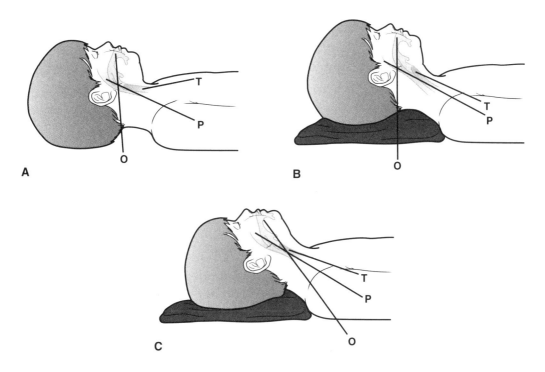

**A**, Maximal opening and visualization of the airway is obtained by aligning the oral (O), pharyngeal (P), and tracheal (T) axes. This is accomplished by placing a patient in the sniffing position. **B**, A folded sheet or towel placed under the occiput aligns the pharyngeal and tracheal axes. **C**, Extension of the neck into the sniffing position then results in approximate alignment of all 3 axes. Proper positioning places the external ear canal anterior to the shoulder. In children younger than 2 years, a folded towel or sheet is placed under the shoulder rather than under the occiput due to the relatively large forehead-to-occiput distance in this age group.

Partial or complete airway obstruction caused by pharyngeal soft tissue collapse or posterior movement of the tongue can usually be relieved by manual maneuvers, including positioning the patient to maximize airway patency and manipulating the jaw and head to open the airway. The first and simplest intervention is the jaw-thrust maneuver illustrated in **Figure 2-4**. The clinician's fingers are placed along the posterior rami of the mandible and the mandible is lifted upward or forward. The jaw-thrust maneuver can be performed safely in a patient with a suspected cervical spine injury because neck alignment is not altered. The jaw-thrust maneuver may be cause discomfort in the awake patient.

**Figure 2-4.** Jaw-Thrust Maneuver

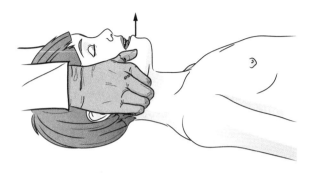

Place fingers on the posterior rami of both mandibles and lift in an anterior direction.

A complementary maneuver for opening an obstructed airway is the head-tilt/chin-lift maneuver. The clinician slightly hyperextends the head to place the patient in the sniffing position. In this position, the ear canal is just above or even with the top of the shoulder when viewed from the side.

> *Airway obstruction caused by pharyngeal soft tissue collapse or posterior movement of the tongue can usually be relieved by a jaw-thrust or chin-lift maneuver.*

Jaw-thrust and chin-lift maneuvers ease obstruction in spontaneously breathing patients but should also be used to provide an unobstructed airway when supporting a patient with bag-mask ventilation.

When a cervical spine injury is suspected, the patient's head should remain in the neutral position at all times, by active stabilization if necessary. Lateral rotation of the head must be avoided. The potential or actual presence of cervical spine injury should not prevent efforts to maintain an unobstructed airway.

## C. Oropharyngeal and Nasopharyngeal Airways

An oropharyngeal (OP) airway consists of a flange, a short bite-block segment, and a curved body, usually made of plastic and shaped to provide an air channel and a suction conduit through the mouth. The curve of the oropharyngeal airway is designed to fit over the back of the tongue to hold it and the soft hypopharyngeal structures away from the posterior wall of the pharynx. The plastic flange should rest against the outer surface of the teeth while the distal end curves around the base of the tongue. If the oropharyngeal airway is too small, it may push the tongue back over the glottic opening; if it is too large, it may stimulate gagging and emesis or push the epiglottis down, further obstructing the airway.

An OP airway can be used to maintain an open airway during bag-mask ventilation, but it is used only in unconscious patients. In conscious or semiconscious patients, it will stimulate gagging, vomiting, and possibly laryngospasm. The technique for inserting an OP airway is described in **Table 2-2** and illustrated in **Figure 2-5**.

# Airway Management

## Table 2-2. Insertion of an Oropharyngeal Airway

- Select the proper size airway. As shown in **Figure 2-5**, the correct size extends from the corner of the mouth to the earlobe.
- If the airway is too short, it won't hold the tongue out of the way.
- If it is too long, it may obstruct breathing.
  - Open the patient's mouth.
  - Insert the airway upside down so the tongue does not obstruct the airway.
  - Advance the airway gently until resistance is encountered.
  - Turn the airway 180° so that it comes to rest with the flange on the patient's teeth.

**Note:** An alternative method, preferable in small infants, is to press the tongue down and forward with a tongue depressor. The oral airway can then be passed, in its final alignment, into position over the tongue.

**Figure 2-5.** Oral Airway Placement

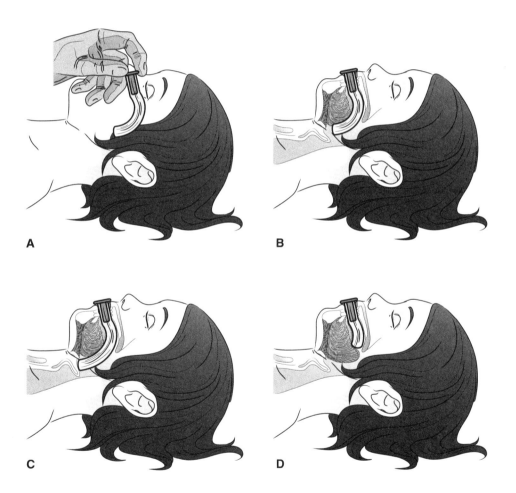

An airway of proper size will relieve obstruction caused by the tongue without damaging laryngeal structures. **A**, The appropriate size can be estimated by holding the airway next to the child's face. The tip of the airway should end just cephalad to the angle of the mandible. **B**, Example of an oropharyngeal airway in correct position and its relationship to airway structures. **C**, If the airway is too big, its tip will hit the epiglottis, pushing it downward and obstructing the glottic opening. **D**, If the airway is too small, it will worsen obstruction by pushing the tongue backwards into the posterior pharynx.

A nasopharyngeal (NP) airway is a soft rubber or plastic tube that provides a conduit for airflow between the nares and the pharynx. It pushes the tongue forward, which relieves airway obstruction. The diameter of an NP airway should be the largest that will easily pass through the nostril, and its length should extend to the nasopharynx, but not be so long that it obstructs gas flow through the mouth or touches the epiglottis.

NP airways are less likely to stimulate vomiting and may be used in patients who are responsive but need assistance in keeping the tongue from obstructing the airway. They are especially helpful in facial and airway deformities such as Pierre-Robin syndrome.

Relative contraindications to NP airways include coagulopathy, basilar skull fracture, and nasal infection or deformity. Unlike OP airways, they may be used in conscious patients. The technique for placing an NP airway is described in **Table 2-3** and illustrated in **Figure 2-6**.

### Table 2-3  Insertion of a Nasopharyngeal Airway

- Choose an airway of the proper size. The length of the airway should be roughly the distance from the tip of the nose to the meatus of the ear.
- Lubricate the airway with surgical lubricant.
- Alleviate vasoconstriction with phenylephrine nose drops (and topical anesthesia with lidocaine if the patient is awake) if possible before any nasal instrumentation. In an acute situation, the lubricating qualities of lidocaine ointment may suffice.
- Insert the tip of the airway perpendicular to the face, not upward toward the cribriform plate. The bevel should point toward the base of the nares or toward the septum. If the airway cannot be inserted into one nostril, try the other.
- Listen by ear or stethoscope for air movement through the airway as it is placed. It is correctly positioned when airflow through the tube is present.
- Secure the airway, then attend to maintaining its patency and position. A nasopharyngeal airway should be treated like an endotracheal tube with regard to suctioning and patency. If airflow cannot be auscultated, the tube is either obstructed or malpositioned.

*Note:* If a commercial nasopharyngeal airway of the proper size is not available, an endotracheal tube of appropriate size can be used instead. Measure the distance from the tip of the patient's nose to the meatus of the ear and use that measurement to determine how much extra length should be cut from the tube prior to insertion.

**Figure 2-6.** Endotracheal Tube Used as a Nasopharyngeal Airway

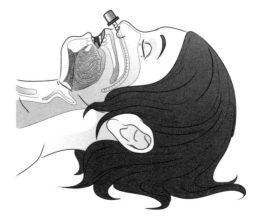

Example of an endotracheal tube used as a nasopharyngeal airway. The insertion technique is described in **Table 2-3**. Note that the 15-mm adapter must be inserted firmly and that the tube must be taped securely to prevent inadvertent advancement.

## D. Bag-Mask Ventilation

Bag-mask ventilation is used to help apneic patients and those with inadequate spontaneous ventilation. Knowing how to provide adequate bag-mask ventilation is the most important airway skill that any healthcare provider can possess.

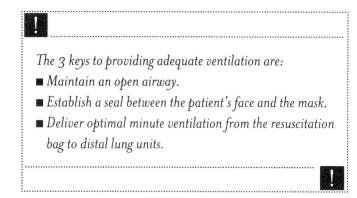

*The 3 keys to providing adequate ventilation are:*
- *Maintain an open airway.*
- *Establish a seal between the patient's face and the mask.*
- *Deliver optimal minute ventilation from the resuscitation bag to distal lung units.*

Positioning the patient appropriately is an essential first step. Maintaining a jaw thrust by positioning the last 3 fingers of one hand under the bony part of the mandible will facilitate ventilation. Keep these fingers off the soft tissue below the mandible to avoid occluding the airway. It may be necessary to move the patient's head and neck gently through a variety of positions to determine the optimum position for airway patency and effective ventilation. A neutral sniffing position without hyperextension is appropriate for infants and toddlers.

The technique for bag-mask ventilation is illustrated in **Figure 2-7**. The hand position is called the *E-C clamp technique*. The thumb and forefinger form a C shape and exert downward pressure on the mask while the remaining fingers of the same hand, forming an E, lift the jaw and pull the face toward the mask. This should create a tight seal. Once the mask is correctly applied, the other hand is used to compress the bag until the chest rises. Ventilation should synchronize with the patient's respiratory effort if the patient is spontaneously breathing; this will prevent gagging. It is better to lift the patient's face into the mask than to push the mask onto the patient's face.

**Figure 2-7.** Bag-Mask Ventilation

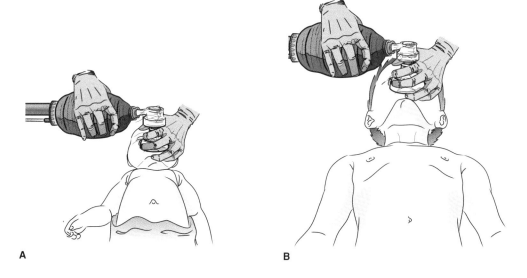

A        B

Note the E-C clamp technique as described in the text. Gentle cricoid pressure (**Figure 2-10**) applied by another rescuer may reduce gastric inflation and decrease the risk of aspiration during bagging. Such pressure should be used only in an unconscious victim. Excessive pressure on the cricoid cartilage should be avoided; only 1 finger is necessary in a young child or infant.

Ventilation provided by 2 rescuers (**Figure 2-8**) can be more effective when there is significant airway obstruction or poor lung compliance. In this technique, 1 rescuer uses both hands to open the airway by placing 3 fingers of each hand on both posterior rami of the patient's mandible and maintains a tight mask-to-face seal while the other rescuer compresses the ventilation bag. Again, the rescuer holding the face mask should concentrate on lifting the jaw and face into the mask in preference to pushing the mask onto the face.

**Figure 2-8.** Two-person Bag-Mask Ventilation

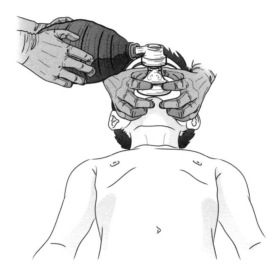

To maintain a tight seal, avoid pushing the mask onto the face but instead use both hands to lift the mandibular rami anteriorly into the mask.

The 2-rescuer technique may be essential in children with difficult airways (e.g., epiglottitis or foreign body aspiration with complete obstruction). If a patient has any respiratory effort at all, rescuer ventilations should be timed with them. Allowing expiration to occur fully prior to providing another breath avoids hyperinflation with consequent hemodynamic and oxygenation problems. Use only the force and tidal volume necessary to make the chest rise. Excessive volumes may compromise cardiac output, distend the stomach, increase the risk of vomiting and aspiration, and add to the risk of barotrauma.

> *To assess the adequacy of bag–mask ventilation:*
> - *Evaluate chest rise and presence of bilateral breath sounds.*
> - *Evaluate clinical response, including improved heart rate and return of good color.*
> - *Monitor oxygen saturation.*

## E. Ventilation Bags

There are 2 types of ventilation bags: self-inflating and flow inflating. Ventilation bags used for resuscitation should be self-inflating and a suitable size for the child. Neonatal bags (250 mL) hold only enough volume to be used with neonates. Pediatric bags (450-500 mL) are adequate for infants and children.

# Airway Management

Many self-inflating bags are equipped with pressure-limited pop-off valves set at 35 to 40 cm $H_2O$. In patients with significant pulmonary disease or anatomic obstruction of the airway, these valves may need to be inactivated to achieve adequate chest rise. Flow-inflating bags require additional expertise.

## F. Troubleshooting

When adequate chest rise does not occur:

- Reposition the head. Make sure the head and neck are not hyperextended and thus causing airway obstruction.
- Ensure that the mask is the appropriate size and applied snugly on the patient's face.
- Make sure that you are lifting the child's jaw to the mask, not pushing the mask onto the child's face.
- Suction the airway if excessive secretions are noted.
- Place an OP airway.
- Disable the pop-off feature of the ventilator bag.
- Use the Sellick maneuver to decrease abdominal distension.
- Assess the need for a nasogastric tube to decompress the stomach and protect against aspiration.
- Check for the presence of a foreign body.

When chest rise is appropriate, but oxygen saturation remains low:

- Check if the bag is connected to an appropriate oxygen source.
- Assess the need for higher pressures and the need to disable the pop-off valve.
- Consider using a positive end-expiratory pressure valve. Patients with lung disease might require additional pressure for improved oxygenation.
- In children with partial airway obstruction, application of 5 to 10 cm $H_2O$ of continuous positive airway pressure may maintain adequate airway patency.

# VI. TRACHEAL INTUBATION

Tracheal intubation is required when less invasive methods of airway management prove inadequate. Many indications signal the need for intubation. The most common is respiratory failure. This is typically due to lower airway or parenchymal disease, such as bronchiolitis or pneumonia, and may result in failure of oxygenation, ventilation, or both. Upper airway obstruction due to foreign bodies, infectious processes, tracheomalacia, tracheal stenosis, or extrinsic compression all may require intubation. Intubation also may be needed to provide cardiovascular and neurologic support. Indications for tracheal intubation are summarized in **Table 2-4**. See **Appendix 6** for discussion of endotracheal intubation.

### Table 2-4 Indications for Tracheal Intubation

- Respiratory failure
- $Pa_{O_2}$ <60 mm Hg (8.0 kPa) with $F_{IO_2}$ >0.6 (excludes cyanotic heart disease)
- $Pa_{CO_2}$ >55 mm Hg (7.3 kPa)
- Excessive work of breathing
- Upper airway obstruction
- Hemodynamic instability (shock)
- Loss or inadequacy of airway protective reflexes
- Neuromuscular weakness
- Severe metabolic acidosis
- Head trauma (intracranial hypertension)
- Need for deep sedation
- Airway protection
- Therapeutic purposes

## A. Tracheal Tubes

Tracheal tubes are sterile polyvinyl chloride tubes with a standard 15-mm adapter for attachment to a bag-mask device or ventilator tubing. They typically have centimeter markings on the side to document the depth of insertion as well as a vocal cord mark at the distal end to help approximate placement while intubating. Tubes are available in cuffed and uncuffed varieties. Historically, uncuffed tubes were recommended for children younger than 8 years because the trachea is narrowest at the cricoid ring in that age group. Uncuffed tubes allow a snug fit but avoid tracheal wall trauma from excessive cuff inflation. Cuffed tubes are constructed with a low-pressure cuff designed to minimize trauma to the tracheal mucosa. These tubes are very helpful in patients with severe lung disease who may require high peak inspiratory pressure or positive end-expiratory pressure. A cuffed tracheal tube should be inflated only to the minimum amount necessary to eliminate any air leak around the tube. In many cases, there will be no air leak, even with the cuff deflated.

Whether a tracheal tube is cuffed or uncuffed, proper fit is essential. When inserted, the tube should fit snugly into the trachea but should pass smoothly, without the need for excessive force. There are several methods of determining proper tube size based upon a patient's age and size. A commonly used formula to calculate uncuffed tube size based on age is:

$$\text{Tube size (mm inner diameter)} = [\text{Age (years)}]/4 + 4$$

Cuffed tubes should be downsized by 0.5 mm when using this formula. The depth of insertion can be estimated by using the formula:

$$\text{Depth of insertion at lip} = \text{Inner diameter of selected tube} \times 3$$

These formulas yield estimates, and adjustments may be needed for specific patients. In all cases, tubes a size above and a size below the estimated one should be available during intubation. Depth of insertion should be assessed by auscultation of breath sounds and with a chest radiograph as soon as possible after intubation.

## B. Laryngoscopes

The laryngoscope displaces the tongue and permits direct visualization of the larynx, vocal cords, and trachea. It consists of a handle (with battery) and a blade that has a light source at its tip. The 2 types of blades, straight (e.g., Miller, Robertshaw) and curved (e.g., Macintosh), are shown in **Figure 2-9**. Each is used in a slightly different manner during intubation. Straight blades are typically used in infants and toddlers and are designed to directly lift the epiglottis out of the way, thus revealing the larynx and vocal cords. Curved blades are typically used in older children and adults, and are placed into the vallecula. Lifting the blade in the anterior direction indirectly lifts the epiglottis and reveals the vocal cords and related structures.

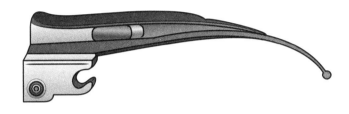
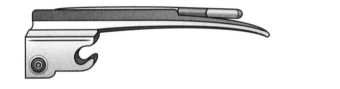

**Figure 2-9.** Laryngoscope Blades

## C. Sedation and Analgesia

Most patients require sedation prior to laryngoscopy and intubation. The goal is to depress the child's level of consciousness sufficiently to produce appropriate conditions for intubation. Those conditions include adequate sedation, analgesia, and amnesia plus blunting of the physiologic responses to airway manipulation, all with a minimum of hemodynamic compromise. Factors that play a role in the selection of sedating agents include, but are not limited to, the agent's rapidity of onset, the patient's hemodynamic status, the need to prevent increases in intraocular or intracranial pressure that may be caused by intubation, and whether the patient is in a fasting state. In many cases, it is ideal to allow for the maintenance of spontaneous ventilatory drive during intubation. A wide variety of medications may be used for sedation, each with its own risks and benefits. In general, medications that act rapidly and are cleared quickly are best. Rapid clearance helps to limit the duration of potential complications. However, the short duration of some agents can result in a patient being intubated (which is painful and frightening) with inadequate sedation and analgesia. Thus, the child's level of consciousness should be continually assessed during and after intubation, giving additional medication as appropriate. Providers should be familiar with the medications used at their institution so as to anticipate side effects that may occur and be prepared to address them. A brief overview of some of the medications commonly used in tracheal intubation is presented in **Table 2-5**. (See **Appendix 7**.)

### Table 2-5  Medications Used to Facilitate Tracheal Intubation

| Agent | Dosing | Onset and Duration | Benefits | Cautions |
|---|---|---|---|---|
| Fentanyl | 1-2 µg/kg IV bolus every 2 min titrated to effect | Onset: Immediate Duration: 30-60 min | • Rapid onset<br>• Short acting<br>• Reversible<br>• Relatively stable hemodynamic profile | • Rigid chest syndrome<br>• Respiratory depression<br>• Lacks amnestic properties |
| Midazolam | 0.05-0.1 mg/kg IV bolus every 5 min titrated to effect | Onset: 1-5 min Duration: 20-30 min | • Rapid onset<br>• Short acting<br>• Provides amnesia<br>• Reversible | • Lacks analgesic properties<br>• Respiratory depression<br>• Hypotension and bradycardia |
| Ketamine | 1 mg/kg IV bolus every 5 min titrated to effect | Onset: 1-2 min Duration: 10-30 min | • Rapid onset<br>• Airway-protective reflexes remain intact<br>• No hypotension or bradycardia | • Increases airway secretions and laryngospasm (blunted with atropine)<br>• Elevates intracranial and ocular pressure<br>• Emergence reactions (blunted with benzodiazepines) |
| Etomidate | 0.3 mg/kg IV bolus initially; 0.1 mg/kg bolus every 5 min thereafter, titrated to effect | Onset: 10-20 s Duration: 4-10 min | • Rapid onset<br>• Short acting<br>• Stable hemodynamic profile | • Potential for adrenal inhibition<br>• May cause myoclonus<br>• Not recommended for children under 10 y |
| Thiopental | 2-3 mg/kg IV bolus, repeat as needed | Onset: 30-60 s Duration: 5-30 min | • Ultra short-acting barbiturate<br>• Decreases intracranial pressure | • Cardiovascular and respiratory depression<br>• Not approved by FDA for children |
| Propofol | 1-3 mg/kg IV bolus initially; 0.5-2 mg/kg bolus every 3-5 min thereafter, titrated to effect | Onset: 30-60 s Duration: 5-10 min | • IV general anesthetic<br>• Rapid onset and recovery | • Cardiovascular and respiratory depression<br>• Contraindicated in patients with egg allergy |

IV, intravenous; FDA, U.S. Food and Drug Administration

## D. Neuromuscular Blockade

Patients with inadequate relaxation despite adequate sedation may require neuromuscular blockade (or paralysis) as an adjunct to intubation. Therefore, it is vitally important to understand the power and risks of pharmacologic paralysis. Once neuromuscular blockers have been administered, all spontaneous respiratory effort ceases. Moreover, in patients with partial airway obstruction, neuromuscular blockade may worsen pharyngeal collapse, potentially resulting in complete airway obstruction. It is thus imperative to be able to maintain patency of the airway with bag-mask ventilation prior to neuromuscular blockade. If adequate chest rise and oxygen saturations cannot be readily maintained with bag-mask ventilation, neuromuscular blockers should not be given until a clinician highly skilled in advanced airway management is present. For the same reason, it is advisable to use, whenever possible, a rapidly acting and quickly cleared neuromuscular blocker. Some frequently used neuromuscular blockers are shown in **Table 2-6**.

### Table 2-6 Neuromuscular Blockade Agents

| Agent | Dosing | Onset and Duration | Benefits | Cautions |
|---|---|---|---|---|
| Succinylcholine (depolarizing neuromuscular blockade) | 1 mg/kg IV | Onset: 30-60 s<br>Duration: 4-6 min | • Rapid onset<br>• Short duration | • Causes muscle fasciculations (blunted with low-dose non-depolarizing neuromuscular blocker)<br>• Potentiates hyperkalemia (contraindicated in head trauma, crush injury, burns, hyperkalemia)<br>• May induce neuroleptic malignant syndrome |
| Vecuronium (non-depolarizing neuromuscular blockade) | 0.1 mg/kg IV | Onset: 1-3 min<br>Duration: 30-40 min | • No fasciculations | • Slower onset<br>• Longer duration of action |
| Rocuronium (non-depolarizing neuromuscular blockade) | 0.6-1.0 mg/kg IV | Onset: 30-60 s<br>Duration: 30-40 min | • No fasciculations | |
| Cisatracurium (non-depolarizing neuromuscular blockade) | 0.1-0.2 mg/kg IV | Onset: 2-3 min<br>Duration: 35-45 min | • Can be used in renal failure<br>• Metabolized through Hoffman elimination | • Potential histamine release |
| Atracurium (non-depolarizing neuromuscular blockade) | 0.3-0.5 mg/kg | Onset: 3-5 min<br>Duration: 20-35 min | • Can be used in renal failure<br>• Metabolized through Hoffman elimination | • Potential histamine release |

IV, intravenous

As with sedatives, it is necessary to be familiar with the pharmacology and side effects of neuromuscular blocking agents prior to using them. Succinylcholine (suxamethonium chloride), in particular, can cause hyperkalemia and malignant hyperthermia. Neuromuscular blockers provide no sedation or analgesia. Long-acting blockers, like vecuronium, often last longer than the short-acting sedative and analgesic medications given prior to intubation. Additional sedation should be provided at regular intervals to ensure that the patient does not awaken during neuromuscular blockade.

## E. Rapid Sequence Intubation

Rapid sequence intubation is employed when there is increased concern about aspiration (e.g., full stomach) and no suspicion of a difficult intubation. The goal is to obtain airway control with a tracheal tube as quickly as possible, thus minimizing aspiration risk. Pre-oxygenation by face mask is provided to increase the available oxygen in the lungs during the procedure. When all necessary intubation equipment and personnel are prepared, rapidly acting sedative, analgesic, and paralytic drugs are given simultaneously. Cricoid pressure is applied at the outset and maintained until the trachea is intubated and adequate confirmatory maneuvers are completed.

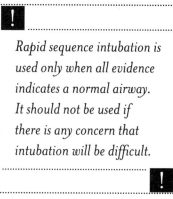

*Rapid sequence intubation is used only when all evidence indicates a normal airway. It should not be used if there is any concern that intubation will be difficult.*

## F. Other Intubation Equipment

Appropriate intubation supplies and equipment (**Table 2-7**) should be assembled at the bedside before beginning an intubation procedure. Cardiopulmonary monitoring and pulse oximetry should be used throughout the procedure. Suction equipment with a large-bore, rigid suction device (such as a Yankauer suction tip) should be used to suction the oropharynx of mucus, blood, and particulate matter. A flexible suction catheter to suction the tracheal tube is helpful as well.

### Table 2-7  Intubation Supplies and Equipment

| Supplies | Comments |
| --- | --- |
| Cardiopulmonary monitor and pulse oximeter | Monitor continuously before, during, and after intubation |
| Suction devices | Test oral (Yankauer) and tracheal tube suction beforehand |
| Stylet | Ensure appropriate size and ease of removal |
| Bag, face mask, and oxygen supply | Test size and function beforehand |
| Oro- or nasopharyngeal airway | |
| Tracheal tubes | Have size above and size below the anticipated size at bedside |
| Syringe, 3 mL, to inflate the endotracheal tube cuff | Ensure cuff is functioning properly |
| Laryngoscope | Ensure light is functioning properly; have various sizes and types of blades at bedside (Miller and Macintosh) |
| End-tidal $CO_2$ detector | Turns yellow when carbon dioxide detected |
| Magill forceps | Use for grasping and advancing tracheal tube during nasotracheal intubation |
| Oxygenating stylet | May be used to insufflate oxygen and as guide for tracheal tube placement |
| Tape or tube-securing device | Adhesive |
| Stethoscope | |
| Medications for intubation, if indicated | |

A stylet should be used to add rigidity to the tracheal tube. To avoid airway trauma, ensure that the stylet does not protrude from the distal end of the tube. Also make sure the stylet can be removed easily once it is in position. Many successfully placed tracheal tubes have become dislodged in the process of removing tight stylets.

An end-tidal $CO_2$ detector should be attached to the tracheal tube after intubation to confirm proper placement. Colorimetric end-tidal $CO_2$ devices change color from purple to yellow to confirm the presence of exhaled $CO_2$ and tracheal placement. The endotracheal tube should be secured with tape or a tracheal tube-securing device with attention to the depth; inadvertent displacement can compromise oxygenation and ventilation.

## G. Intubation

All age-appropriate supplies and equipment should be assembled and checked for proper function before attempting an intubation. Various sizes and shapes of laryngoscope blades should be readily available. Once endotracheal tube size is selected, additional tubes that are one size below and above the calculated endotracheal tube size should be available. Proper positioning is a key element of successful intubation. To visualize the glottis clearly, the oral, pharyngeal, and tracheal axes must be brought into alignment as described earlier and shown in **Figure 2-3**. Alignment of the 3 airway axes can be achieved with slight hyperextension of the head into the sniffing position, with the ear canal just above or even with the top of the shoulder when visualized from the side.

Children younger than 2 years have relatively large heads for their body size, which results in slight neck flexion when they are in the supine position. These children usually benefit from a small roll (thin towel or blanket) placed under the shoulders, which allows the head to fall back into proper position but avoids hyperextension. In older children, a small roll under the occiput helps facilitate proper alignment of the axes. In patients with suspected cervical spine injury, the head should remain in the neutral position at all times and the spine should be stabilized while intubating.

When possible, it is advantageous to pre-oxygenate patients to 100% oxygen saturation with bag-mask ventilation before attempting intubation. Each laryngoscopy and tracheal tube placement attempt should be limited to approximately 30 seconds. An assistant should monitor vital signs continuously. All attempts must be expedient, and failed attempts should be terminated prior to desaturation. After each unsuccessful attempt, the patient should again receive bag-mask ventilation to optimize oxygenation before the next attempt. Multiple attempts at intubation may lead to airway and vocal cord edema, which may further compromise ventilation and intubation.

Not all intubation attempts will be successful, and anticipation of a difficult airway is a vital part of the pre-intubation assessment. A history of difficult intubation, obstructive sleep apnea, or frequent snoring should raise concern about the level of difficulty to be expected. Patients with facial abnormalities such as micrognathia, midface hypoplasia, small mouths, large tongues, and morbid obesity often are difficult to intubate. Limited mobility of the temporomandibular joint or the cervical spine, as well as bleeding, masses, or foreign bodies in the upper airway, all present challenges to tracheal intubation.

A backup plan should always be developed prior to intubation. Supplies should be available for multiple attempts, advanced intubation techniques, and cricothyrotomy (discussed in **Table 2-7**). A strategy for management of the "cannot ventilate, cannot intubate" scenario should be developed (**Appendix 8**). If a difficult intubation is anticipated and patient stability permits, it is advisable to have experienced clinicians present before proceeding. Consultation with a pediatric anesthesiologist or otolaryngologist should be considered.

Orotracheal intubation is the most common and preferred method of intubation in emergency situations. The technique is summarized in **Table 2-8** and shown in **Figure 2-10**.

### Table 2-8. Technique for Orotracheal Intubation

- Ensure that the patient is positioned correctly.
- Hold the laryngoscope in your left hand and advance the blade along the right side of the mouth to the base of the tongue.
- Sweep the blade to the midline, thus lifting the tongue out of the visual field and providing an area on the right where the tube can be advanced without losing direct visualization of the laryngeal structures. Ensure that the tongue is properly displaced to ensure optimal visualization and facilitate successful intubation.
- When using a straight blade, position the distal end of the blade just below (posterior to) the epiglottis so it may be used to lift the epiglottis anteriorly. Often, a straight blade will enter the esophagus upon insertion. If the blade tip is in the esophagus, slowly backing out the blade will cause the larynx to fall into view as the blade leaves the esophageal inlet. When a curved blade is used, the end of the blade is placed into the vallecula above (anterior to) the epiglottis. Straight blade and curved blade insertions are illustrated in **Figure 2-10**.

**Figure 2-10.** Insertion of Laryngoscope Blades

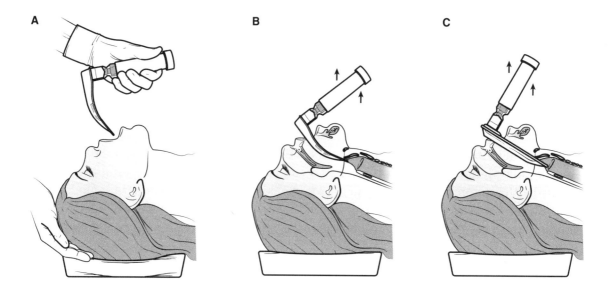

**A**, Insertion of a curved laryngoscope blade. **B**, Insertion of a straight laryngoscope blade. Insertion techniques are summarized in **Table 2-8**.

The anterior placement of the pediatric airway sometimes makes visualization of the epiglottis and larynx difficult. Slight pressure on the cricoid cartilage (Sellick maneuver) may move the larynx and the airway posterior, and improve visualization (**Figure 2-11**).

**Figure 2-11.** Cricoid Pressure (Sellick Maneuver)

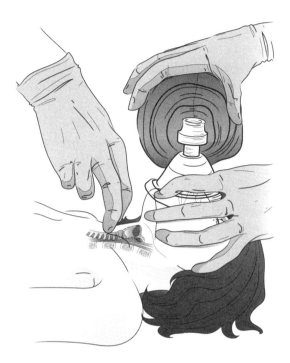

Gentle pressure on the cricoid cartilage by a second person may reduce gastric inflation and decrease the risk of aspiration during bagging. In an infant or child, cricoid pressure can also improve an intubator's view of the larynx.

**Figure 2-12.** Visualization of the Larynx during Laryngoscopy

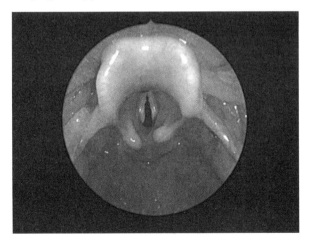

Courtesy of Sanjay Parikh, MD, FACS, University of Washington, Seattle, Washington, USA.

Once either a straight or a curved blade is properly positioned, the laryngoscope handle should be lifted anteriorly along an axis that is approximately 45° from the bed, providing a clearer view of the larynx. Do not lever the blade upwards, as this will result in trauma to the lips, gums, and teeth from the proximal end of the blade and the handle. Remember, even in an edentulous infant, teeth are developing right below the gum line.

Once the larynx is well visualized (**Figure 2-12**), make every effort not to take your eyes off the larynx. To facilitate this, an assistant should place all necessary equipment in the intubator's free hand. Advance the tube from the right corner of the mouth through the vocal cords. Do not advance the tube down the flange of the blade because doing so will obscure the larynx. A good rule of thumb is that if the operator does not see the tube go through the vocal cords, it has not done so.

The tip of the tracheal tube should be placed at the mid-tracheal level. Mid-tracheal placement is facilitated in uncuffed tubes by placing the distal black marker on the tube at the level of the cords. Cuffed tubes should be positioned with the cuff just below the vocal cords.

Once the tube has been inserted, confirm proper tracheal placement. This is initially confirmed by seeing the tube pass through the vocal cords into the trachea. Look for symmetric chest rise and listen for equal breath sounds while delivering positive pressure breaths. If the tube is in the right main-stem bronchus, breath sounds will be more prominent over the right chest, signaling that the tube needs to be repositioned. Slowly pull the tube back while listening to the left chest. When breath sounds become audible on the left, the tube has entered the trachea. Listen over the stomach; if the tube is in the trachea, breath sounds will be absent over the abdomen. Breath sounds are easily transmitted across the chest wall in smaller children, so smaller tidal volumes should be used during auscultation for verification of tube placement. Condensation in the tracheal tube suggests, but does not confirm, tracheal placement.

An end-tidal $CO_2$ detector may also be used to ensure proper placement. During cardiac arrest or when cardiac output is very low, there is minimal to no blood flow to pulmonary capillaries and, consequently, very little to no $CO_2$ delivered to the lungs for exhalation. In such cases, $CO_2$ may not be detected despite proper tube placement, so other methods of confirmation are necessary. Because no single method is completely dependable in all situations, multiple methods of confirmation should always be used. If any question exists, perform laryngoscopy to obtain visual confirmation. A chest radiograph should be acquired as soon as possible to ensure proper position and to evaluate for complications such as pneumothorax.

The tracheal tube should be well secured to the patient's face to avoid unintentional extubation. This can be achieved with adhesive (e.g., tincture of benzoin) and two pieces of tape partially ripped so that each resembles a pair of pants. The "waist" of the tape is placed on the patient's cheek, one leg is placed above the patient's upper lip, and the other is tightly wrapped around the tube. The other piece of tape is placed below the lower lip in the same manner. Commercially manufactured tube holders are also available.

Following intubation, monitoring by electrocardiography, pulse oximetry, and end-tidal $CO_2$ should be continued. Once a patient is connected to a ventilator, an arterial blood gas study should be obtained as soon as possible.

## H. Complications

The physiologic alterations that occur when positive pressure ventilation is initiated can lead to complications that can be anticipated and rapidly treated. As noted earlier, bag-mask ventilation delivers some of the volume from each positive pressure breath to the stomach, leading to distention (which may make it difficult to adequately ventilate the patient) and aspiration. To decrease the likelihood of aspiration, a naso- or orogastric tube may be placed to help decompress the stomach and remove stomach contents.

Stimulation of the airway results in activation of the vagus nerve. When a patient is intubated, this appears clinically as bradycardia. Atropine (0.01 to 0.02 mg/kg; maximum single dose, 1 mg; minimum single dose, 0.1 mg) may be administered to overcome this response. In patients who are bradycardic at baseline, or in whom there is concern for vagal-mediated bradycardia, atropine may be given prior to attempting intubation. Atropine is also used to decrease airway secretions in patients, especially those who receive ketamine for sedation.

Positive pressure ventilation has the potential to cause barotrauma to the alveoli, occasionally resulting in leakage of air into the pleural space (pneumothorax). As air accumulates in the pleural space, the lung becomes compressed, compromising oxygenation and ventilation. If the air leak is ongoing, the pressure in the pleural space rises, causing a tension pneumothorax. This shifts the mediastinum toward the uninvolved side, impairing venous return to the heart and compromising cardiac output. Signs of tension pneumothorax include deviation of the trachea away from the affected side, diminished breath sounds on the affected side, tachycardia, and falling blood pressure. Treatment should be emergent and not be delayed by a chest radiograph. A tension pneumothorax can be decompressed by the sterile passage of an appropriately sized angiocatheter into the pleural space over the top of the third rib in the midclavicular line. A rush of air will be heard as the air under pressure escapes the pleural space. Definitive treatment is with a thoracostomy tube, which should be placed as soon as possible.

Another complication of positive pressure ventilation is decreased cardiac output. The increase in intrathoracic pressure impairs venous return to the right side of the heart, thus decreasing preload. In patients who are dehydrated and have compromised hemodynamic function, this impairment may produce clinically relevant decreases in cardiac output and hypotension. A reduction in tidal volume, along with fluid resuscitation, will often restore preload and improve cardiac output.

## I. Troubleshooting

Acute respiratory deterioration can occur in an intubated patient for a variety of reasons. A commonly used mnemonic in this situation is DOPE: dislodgement of the tube, obstruction of the tube, pneumothorax, and equipment failure. View chest rise and auscultate the chest to ensure proper positioning of the tracheal tube. Asymmetric breath sounds may represent improper tube position or pneumothorax.

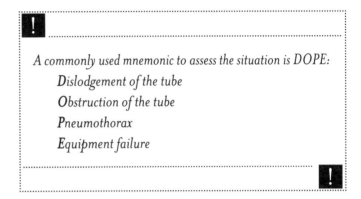

*A commonly used mnemonic to assess the situation is DOPE:*
- *Dislodgement of the tube*
- *Obstruction of the tube*
- *Pneumothorax*
- *Equipment failure*

When asymmetry is present, a chest radiograph can help diagnose the problem. Suction the tube to clear secretions from the lumen. If the patient is on a ventilator, check that it is functioning properly. In cases of uncertainty, it may be helpful to remove the patient from the ventilator and ventilate manually with 100% oxygen.

Respiratory deterioration may be secondary to the patient's underlying condition. Adjustments to the ventilator and other respiratory therapies may be required to improve the child's respiratory status.

# VII. FAILED INTUBATION

When respiratory failure occurs, tracheal intubation is the standard method of controlling the airway and supporting pulmonary function. Sometimes intubation is unachievable due to complete upper airway obstruction, anatomic airway abnormalities, severe facial trauma, or similar circumstances. It is important to have a backup plan in the event that a tracheal tube cannot be placed. First and foremost, bag-mask ventilation may be provided until a definitive airway is established. See **Appendix 5** for additional discussion of airway adjuncts.

## A. Laryngeal Mask Airway

When it is impossible to intubate or manually ventilate a patient by mask, a laryngeal mask airway is a useful adjunct that may provide an open airway and permit gas exchange. A laryngeal mask airway consists of a tube with a cuffed, mask-like projection at the distal end. When properly placed, it sits just above the glottic opening. Laryngeal mask airways now come in sizes appropriate for children. This airway adjunct does not protect against aspiration and should not be used as a definitive airway.

The weight range appropriate for the size of a given laryngeal mask airway is printed on the mask itself. **Appendix 5** shows the insertion technique. The laryngeal mask airway is held like a pencil with the distal opening facing away from the operator (so that it ends up facing anteriorly when placed). The balloon is placed against the hard palate, which is used as a guide as the laryngeal mask airway is inserted. Once definite resistance is felt, the balloon is inflated and bag ventilation can be initiated. Assessment of air entry is the same as for intubated patients, with attention to symmetric lung inflation. Ideally ventilation uses only enough force to move the chest wall adequately, which may be assessed by auscultating the chest for normal respiratory sounds during bagging. Higher ventilation pressures may lead to insufflation of the stomach in addition to the lungs.

A special type of laryngeal mask airway, the intubating laryngeal mask airway, is commercially available for use in larger patients. It has a bar at the distal end that elevates the epiglottis and is wide enough to accommodate a special tracheal tube being passed through the lumen. Once in position, a tracheal tube is passed through the laryngeal mask airway. The epiglottis-elevating bar is forced up, lifting the epiglottis and allowing the tracheal tube to be passed into the trachea. The intubating laryngeal mask airway is then removed over the tracheal tube, which is left in position.

## B. Esophageal-Tracheal Double-Lumen Airway Device

In children over 4 feet tall, it is possible to place an esophageal-tracheal double-lumen airway device. These tubes contain two lumens as well as proximal and distal balloons. They are placed blindly and almost always end up in the esophagus. Both balloons are then inflated to create a seal.

When properly positioned, the distal balloon obstructs the esophagus and the proximal balloon obstructs the distal pharynx. The proximal tube holes are above the distal balloon. Thus, air is forced out of the proximal tube down the trachea. If the tube happens to end up in the trachea, the distal tube may be used to ventilate the patient. A similar device, a laryngeal tube with only one lumen, is available in multiple sizes.

## C. Intubating Stylets

When a patient's vocal cords are well visualized but the tracheal tube cannot be passed, it may be easier to pass an intubating stylet. These stylets are hollow and have a connector at the end that can be attached to an oxygen source or a bag-mask device. Once in place, they can be used to ventilate the patient by hand. A tracheal tube can then be passed over the stylet, and the stylet can be removed, leaving the tracheal tube in place.

## D. Fiberoptic Intubation

Operators familiar with the use of intubating bronchoscopes can provide assistance with a difficult airway. The endotracheal tube is loaded onto the bronchoscope, and the bronchoscope is placed into the trachea through the vocal cords under direct visualization. The endotracheal tube is then slipped off the end of the bronchoscope and left in proper position within the trachea.

## E. Cricothyrotomy

In extreme situations, cricothyrotomy may be performed. With the patient's neck hyperextended, the cricothyroid membrane is located by palpation between the thyroid cartilage and the cricoid cartilage. The area is sterilized, and an intravenous catheter (catheter over needle) is placed through the cartilage into the trachea. Proper completion of this step is confirmed by the patient's aspiration of air, after which the needle is withdrawn while advancing the catheter. The catheter can then be attached to a positive pressure device connected via the Luer-Lok. A 5-mL syringe barrel (with the plunger removed) will accept a standard 15-mm adapter and manual ventilation can be carried out. Commercially available cricothyrotomy kits contain all the necessary supplies. While potentially useful in older children, the unique anatomy of the infant larynx, the small size of the cricothyroid membrane, and the technical difficulty of locating the correct anatomical structures make the use of most of these commercially available cricothyrotomy kits impractical, if not dangerous, in neonates and infants. Consultation with a pediatric otolaryngologist should be considered in situations where a cricothyrotomy or emergency tracheostomy is necessary.

## F. Planning for a Difficult or Failed Intubation

Whenever an airway proves difficult to intubate, or even when difficulty is anticipated, backup personnel with expertise in the management of the pediatric airway should be summoned. Anesthesiologists, otolaryngologists, and pediatric intensivists are considered experts by training in maintaining difficult airways. An algorithm for dealing with difficult intubation is presented in **Appendix 8**.

## Key Points: Airway Management

- Accurate assessment of the work of breathing, airway patency, respiratory drive, and consciousness are crucial first steps in the management of children with breathing difficulty.

- Maintaining a patent airway with manual methods, such as oropharyngeal and nasopharyngeal airways, are important skills in airway management.

- All who care for ill children should be able to supply adequate oxygenation and ventilation with bag-mask ventilation.

- All necessary supplies and personnel must be present before intubation is attempted.

- Expertise with sedatives, analgesics, and neuromuscular blockers is a prerequisite for intubation.

- A backup plan should be developed before a potentially difficult intubation is attempted. The use of airway adjuncts, such as a laryngeal mask airway, and cricothyrotomy may be lifesaving when intubation cannot be achieved.

# Suggested Readings

1. American Heart Association. Respiratory management resources and procedures. In: *Pediatric Advanced Life Support*. Dallas, TX: American Heart Association; 2010.

2. American Society of Anesthesiologists. Practice guidelines for management of the difficult airway: an updated report by the American Society of Anesthesiologists Task Force on Management of the Difficult Airway. *Anesthesiology*. 2003;98:1269-1277.

3. Brain AIJ. *The Intavent Laryngeal Mask: Instruction Manual*. Berkshire, UK: Brain Medical Ltd.; 1992.

4. Cote CJ, Hartnick CJ. Pediatric transtracheal and cricothyrotomy airway devices for emergency use: which are appropriate for infants and children? *Paediatr Anaesth*. 2009;19 Suppl 1:66-76.

5. deCaen A, Duff J, Covadia AH, et al. Airway management. In: Nichols DG, ed. *Rogers' Textbook of Pediatric Intensive Care*. 4th ed. Philadelphia, PA: Lippincott Williams & Wilkins; 208:303-322.

6. Kremer B, Botos-Kremer AI, Eckel HE, Schlöndorff G. Indications, complications, and surgical techniques for pediatric tracheostomies—an update. *J Pediatr Surg*. 2002;37:1556-1562.

7. Mathur NN, Meyers AD. Pediatric tracheostomy. Updated December 2, 2011. Available at: http://emedicine.medscape.com/article/873805. Last accessed February 15, 2012.

8. Thompson AE. Pediatric airway management. In: Fuhrman BP, Zimmerman JJ, eds. *Pediatric Critical Care*. St. Louis, MO: Mosby; 2006:485.

Chapter 3

# PEDIATRIC CARDIAC ARREST

## ✓ Objectives

- Rapidly identify the need for cardiopulmonary resuscitation (CPR) to prevent or treat cardiac arrest.
- Understand the key components of high-quality CPR.
- Understand the physiology of CPR.
- Assess and initiate high-quality, goal-directed post-resuscitation care for infants and children following cardiac arrest.

## 📁 Case Study

A 3-year-old with a 4-day history of progressive upper respiratory congestion and airway obstruction presents to an emergency department in severe respiratory distress with a pulse oximeter saturation of 76% on room air. During your examination, he becomes apneic, bradycardic, and unresponsive to vigorous stimulation. Bag-mask ventilation and chest compressions are initiated.

**Detection**
- What are the key findings in the initial assessment?
- What is the likely diagnosis?

**Intervention**
- With CPR ongoing, what is the most important next step?

**Reassessment**
- What is the appropriate time to reassess the patient's respiratory effort and circulation?

**Effective Communication**
- When the patient's clinical status changes, who needs to know and how will the information be disseminated?
- Where is the best place to care for this patient?

**Teamwork**
- How are you going to implement the treatment strategy?
- Who is to do what and when?

# I. INTRODUCTION

Successful resuscitation from pediatric cardiac arrest depends upon rapid identification and treatment of the cause of the arrest, immediate initiation of high-quality cardiopulmonary resuscitation (CPR), and aggressive post-resuscitation care. Critical factors that influence survival outcomes include the environment in which the arrest occurs, the child's preexisting condition, the duration of no pulsatile flow prior to resuscitation, the initial electrocardiographic (ECG) rhythm detected, the quality of the basic and advanced life support interventions provided during the cardiac arrest, and the meticulous attention to selected post-resuscitation support parameters (e.g., temperature, oxygen, ventilation, blood pressure, glucose, seizure control).

Pediatric in-hospital CPR survival rates are good. Almost two-thirds of in-hospital pediatric arrest patients achieve return of spontaneous circulation (ROSC), more than one-fourth of whom survive to hospital discharge. Most survivors (>75%) have a good neurologic outcome.

Outcomes following pediatric out-of-hospital arrests are not as good; survival to hospital discharge typically occurs in less than 10% of these children, and many have severe neurological sequelae. These poor outcomes are due in part to prolonged periods of no pulsatile flow because many of these cardiac arrests are not witnessed, and only 30% of children receive bystander CPR. In the first year of life, sudden infant death syndrome is the leading cause of out-of-hospital pediatric cardiac arrest, followed by trauma, airway obstruction, and near drowning.

# II. PREVENTION/RECOGNITION

The most common causes of in-hospital cardiac arrest are acute respiratory insufficiency and circulatory shock. Patients often have abnormal physiologic parameters in the hours prior to the event. Mortality and morbidity rates can be decreased in the pre-arrest phase with the utilization of the DIRECT algorithm (**Chapter 1**).

Reassessment and review of vital sign trends is critical. Recognition of end-organ perfusion abnormalities, such as oliguria, altered mental status, and delayed capillary refill, may be hallmarks of impending failure. Gasping, bradycardia, and severe lethargy (e.g., loss of consciousness) are late signs of shock and impending cardiac arrest.

Early warning scores (see PEWS in **Chapter 1**) and rapid response or medical emergency teams are in-hospital emergency systems designed to identify and respond to patients in imminent danger of decompensation, thereby preventing progression to cardiac arrest. The rapid response teams cannot prevent all cardiac arrests, but are able to transfer critically ill children to an intensive care unit for better monitoring and more aggressive interventions to prevent arrest or to provide prompt advanced life support if the arrest occurs. The implication of this paradigm is that any cardiac arrest that occurs outside a monitored unit should be reviewed as a potentially avoidable serious safety event.

# III. DIAGNOSIS OF CARDIAC ARREST

Lack of movement or response to vigorous stimulation, without signs of effective breathing (e.g., no breathing other than an occasional gasp) should be treated as cardiac arrest until proven otherwise. Palpation of a central pulse and other signs are not reliable indicators. If more advanced monitoring is in place at the time of arrest (e.g., pulse oximetry, exhaled $CO_2$, arterial catheter), this can be used to support the diagnosis.

The cause of the arrest should be determined in the early minutes of resuscitation. A focused physical exam should be conducted and a brief medical history obtained. A cardiopulmonary monitor should be placed and the ECG should be examined. A blood gas analysis with electrolytes ($Na^+$, $K^+$, $Ca^{2+}$) should be performed with point-of-care testing if available.

## A. Pulse Check

The triad of pulselessness, apnea, and unresponsiveness defines the clinical state of cardiac arrest. Healthcare providers may spend up to 10 seconds assessing a central pulse, but the empiric provision of chest compressions without a pulse check for the child who "appears dead" (unresponsive to vigorous stimulation, not breathing normally) is appropriate.

## B. Breathing

For decades, guidelines by the International Liaison Committee on Resuscitation used the mnemonic A-B-C (airway-breathing-circulation) for the stepwise assessment and intervention sequence in suspected cardiac arrest. With the change from A-B-C to C-A-B (compressions-airway-breathing), the first steps to evaluation of a collapsed patient no longer involve physically opening the airway and spending up to 10 seconds assessing breathing. Instead, the patient's general appearance, with attention to a lack of effective breathing, must be assessed immediately to determine whether chest compressions are indicated. Irregular or agonal respirations (e.g., gasping) should not be interpreted as a stable respiratory pattern; an unresponsive patient with agonal respirations requires immediate chest compressions.

# IV. MECHANISM OF BLOOD FLOW

## A. Physiology of Coronary Blood Flow

The coronary arteries provide blood flow from the aortic root to the myocardium. The normally beating heart is mainly perfused by coronary blood flow during diastole. When the heart arrests and no blood flows to the aorta, coronary blood flow ceases. During chest compressions, aortic pressure rises at the same time as right atrial pressure. During the decompression phase, the right atrial pressure falls faster and lower than the aortic pressure, generating a pressure gradient that perfuses the heart with oxygenated blood. Coronary perfusion pressure below 15 mm Hg during CPR is a poor prognostic factor for ROSC.

## B. Physiology of Ventilation

The importance of negative intrathoracic pressure on venous return during CPR, and thereby on coronary perfusion pressure and myocardial blood flow during CPR, has been rediscovered. During the decompression phase (chest compression release), negative intrathoracic pressure allows venous return to the heart and improved coronary artery blood flow. This can be experimentally enhanced either by active decompression (suction upwards, manual or automated) or by briefly impeding air flow to the lungs (i.e., with an inspiratory impedance threshold device). Increased negative pressure promotes venous return, cardiac output, and mean aortic pressure.

# V. CARDIOPULMONARY RESUSCITATION

In 2010, the American Heart Association made the recommendation to change the algorithmic sequence of rescue interventions for the arrested patient from A-B-C to C-A-B (compressions-airway-breathing). The change was made because blood flow during cardiac arrest depends on chest compressions, and efforts to address airway and breathing delay the reestablishment of blood flow. The value of this approach is most dramatically demonstrated by the success of compression-only CPR (i.e., without rescue breathing) in adults. Although the C-A-B sequence is the adult recommendation, it is reasonable to use the same approach in children to simplify training for the lay rescuer, especially when the arrest is sudden and witnessed (i.e., higher likelihood of a cardiac etiology). Additionally, starting pediatric resuscitation with compressions instead of ventilation will result in only a brief delay in the first rescue breath. Finally, in a healthcare setting where a team of providers responds to an arrest, multiple tasks are undertaken simultaneously; given that chest compressions can be applied instantaneously and positive-pressure ventilation requires equipment preparation, the C-A-B approach is unlikely to adversely effect results in in-hospital events.

> *The algorithmic sequence of rescue interventions for the arrested patient has changed from A-B-C to C-A-B (compressions—airway—breathing).*

The C-A-B sequence applies to the patient presumed to be in cardiac arrest. In cases of rescue compromise leading to hypoxemia and bradycardia, attention to airway, breathing, and oxygenation pre-arrest can be lifesaving and is recommended.

## A. Circulation

Basic life support with early and effective continuous chest compressions is generally the best way to provide circulation during cardiac arrest. The most critical elements are to **push hard** and **push fast**. Because there is no flow without chest compressions, it is important to **minimize interruptions** in chest compressions. To facilitate good venous return in the decompression phase, **allow full chest recoil** between chest compressions and **avoid overventilation**. The latter can impede venous return because of increased intrathoracic pressure.

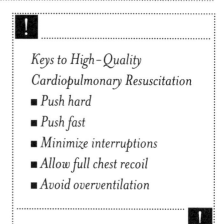

*Keys to High-Quality Cardiopulmonary Resuscitation*
- *Push hard*
- *Push fast*
- *Minimize interruptions*
- *Allow full chest recoil*
- *Avoid overventilation*

Excellent standard closed chest CPR generates approximately 10% to 25% of baseline myocardial blood flow and a cerebral blood flow that is approximately 50% of normal. By contrast, open chest CPR can generate a cerebral blood flow that approaches normal. Although open chest massage improves coronary perfusion pressure and increases the chance of successful defibrillation, surgical thoracotomy is impractical in many situations and increases cost without long-term survival benefit. Early institution of open chest CPR may warrant consideration in select resuscitation circumstances, such as penetrating trauma.

## B. Airway

While securing the airway is important, tracheal intubation requires a care provider with advanced airway skills and often delays or interrupts the initiation of chest compressions. Because effective blood flow is critical to achieving ROSC, compressions or defibrillation must be initiated immediately, along with bag-mask ventilation. Tracheal intubation for ventricular fibrillation (VF) may not be necessary, and defibrillation should be prioritized to ensure the best chance of successful conversion to a perfusing rhythm.

### 1. Why Delayed Intubation With Ventricular Fibrillation Makes Sense

During sudden witnessed collapse (VF cardiac arrest), an oxygen reserve remains in the lungs. Acceptable $Pa_{O_2}$ and $Pa_{CO_2}$ levels persist 4-8 minutes during chest compressions without rescue breathing. Aortic oxygen and carbon dioxide concentrations do not change from pre-arrest levels even without chest compressions because no blood flows and aortic oxygen consumption is minimal. Adequate oxygenation and ventilation can continue without rescue breathing because the lungs serve as a reservoir for oxygen during the low-flow state of CPR. In contrast, during asphyxia, which is the more common etiology of pediatric cardiac arrest, blood continues to flow to tissues; therefore, arterial and venous oxygen saturations decrease while carbon dioxide and lactate levels increase. In addition, continued pulmonary blood flow before the arrest depletes the oxygen reservoir. Therefore, rescue breathing is critical for cardiac arrest preceded by asphyxia because significant arterial hypoxemia and acidemia exists prior to initiation of CPR.

## C. Breathing

### 1. Ventilation and Compression-Ventilation Ratios

Physiologic estimates suggest the amount of ventilation needed during CPR is much less than that needed during a normal perfusing rhythm because the cardiac output during CPR is only 10% to 25% of that during normal sinus rhythm. A chest compression-to-ventilation ratio of 15:2 delivers the same minute ventilation as CPR with a ratio of 5:1, but the number of compressions delivered is 50% higher with the 15:2 ratio (**Table 3-1**).

### Table 3-1  Resuscitation Components: Ratios by Age

| Ventilation Mode | Respirations | Chest Compressions | Notes |
| --- | --- | --- | --- |
| Bag-mask ventilation | • 15 chest compressions<br>• 2 rescue breaths after each<br>• If only 1 rescuer, 2 rescue breaths after each 30 compressions | >100 per minute | Decompress stomach to alleviate gastric inflation. |
| Endotracheal intubation | 8-10 rescue breaths per minute | >100 per minute | • Do not interrupt compressions during ventilation.<br>• Confirm appropriate positioning of the endotracheal tube. |
| Neonates | 3:1 ratio of compressions to rescue breaths | 90 per minute | |

Chest compressions maintain increased aortic pressure and coronary perfusion pressure. When compressions cease, the aortic diastolic pressure rapidly falls, dropping coronary perfusion pressure. Increasing the ratio of compressions to ventilations minimizes these interruptions, thus increasing coronary perfusion pressure (blood flow). The benefits of positive pressure ventilation (increased arterial transport of oxygen and carbon dioxide elimination) must be balanced against the adverse consequence of impeding venous return and cardiac output.

### 2. Rate of Ventilation

The recommended respiratory rate during pediatric CPR is 8-10 breaths per minute in sync with compressions when the patient is not intubated, and 8-10 breaths per minute asynchronously (not coordinated with compressions) in the intubated patient. A common error during the extreme stress of a pediatric cardiac arrest is for providers to deliver ventilation at rates that are substantially higher than recommended. As stated earlier, high ventilation rates increase intrathoracic pressure, impede venous return and coronary artery blood flow, and can result in a lower likelihood of ROSC. Therefore, it is important to monitor the rate of ventilation provided.

## D. Oxygen Management and Monitoring

Pediatric resuscitation for cardiac arrest, beyond the delivery room, should be initiated with 100% oxygen, when available. While studies in neonatal and animal resuscitation have demonstrated evidence of poor neurologic outcomes following resuscitation with 100% oxygen as opposed to room air, similar data do not exist in the pediatric age range. Importantly, the fraction of inspired oxygen ($FIO_2$) administered to a child with ROSC should be actively titrated to avoid hyperoxia in the post-resuscitation period. Current guidelines suggest that the $FIO_2$ be decreased to the lowest possible level while maintaining oxygen saturation levels of between 94% and 99% (i.e., less than 100%). This recommendation is based on the observation that, in the presence of an oxyhemoglobin saturation of 100%, the $PaO_2$ may vary from 50 mm Hg to >600 mm Hg.

# VI. CPR QUALITY

## A. Monitoring

The goal of CPR is to provide near continuous blood flow and perfusion to vital organs. Clinical evidence of good quality CPR during cardiac arrest can include return of movement, persistence of gasping, and eye opening.

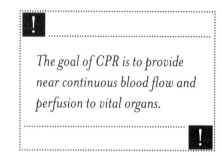

*The goal of CPR is to provide near continuous blood flow and perfusion to vital organs.*

Animal and human studies have demonstrated that changes in cardiac output during resuscitation from shock and cardiac arrest are reliably associated with exhaled or end-tidal carbon dioxide ($ETCO_2$). Continuous monitoring of $ETCO_2$ waveforms has been demonstrated to be useful as a marker of pulmonary blood flow during CPR, and abrupt and sustained marked increase in $ETCO_2$ to >40 mm Hg can be an early indicator of ROSC, without the need to interrupt chest compressions. Multiple studies in adults have shown that an $ETCO_2$ <15 mm Hg during CPR is associated with a decreased likelihood of ROSC.

If CPR is in progress on a patient with continuous $ETCO_2$ capnography waveform monitoring in place, an $ETCO_2$ of <15 mm Hg should prompt the rescuer to increase the quality of chest compressions until $ETCO_2$ is consistently >15 mm Hg. Attention should also be paid to ventilation when $ETCO_2$ <15 mm Hg, as inappropriate hyperventilation during CPR may lower $ETCO_2$.

The utility of $ETCO_2$ for predicting outcomes, or for determining appropriate timing of terminating efforts, is limited by the varied initial $ETCO_2$ values in cardiac arrest patients.

## B. Quality of CPR Monitoring

*The depth, rate, full chest recoil, and ventilation rate should be constantly monitored.*

The depth, rate, full chest recoil, and continuation of chest compressions, as well as the ventilation rate, should be constantly monitored, with or without adjuncts. Because poor-quality CPR is associated with worse outcome and reduces the likelihood of defibrillation success, rescuers should focus on the quality of their efforts. Automated feedback devices to improve CPR quality and compliance with guidelines are available.

## 1. Vascular Access

Rapid vascular access is essential in patients in cardiac arrest or at imminent risk of cardiac arrest. Obtaining intravenous (IV) access can be difficult in the arrested patient. Intraosseous (IO) access has been recognized as safe and quickly effective in children and adults, and the frequency of its complications is negligibly low. Current recommendations state that IO access may be considered as the initial approach to vascular access in the arrested pediatric patient (**Appendix 2**). Multiple mechanical devices designed to assist with IO placement have been shown to be effective and easy to use in pediatric patients.

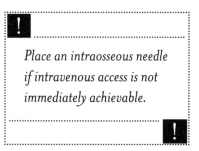
*Place an intraosseous needle if intravenous access is not immediately achievable.*

Although some resuscitation medications (e.g., epinephrine, adrenaline, atropine) have been shown to reach the central circulation when instilled through the endotracheal tube into the tracheobronchial tree, absorption is unreliable. Widespread acceptance of IO access has obviated the need for endotracheal administration, and this approach is no longer routinely recommended.

# VII. PEDIATRIC VENTRICULAR FIBRILLATION AND DEFIBRILLATION

## A. Dosing Recommendations

Defibrillation is necessary for successful resuscitation from VF cardiac arrest (**Appendix 9**). When prompt defibrillation is provided soon after the induction of VF in a cardiac catheterization laboratory, the success and survival rates approach 100%. In general, the mortality rate increases 5% to 10% per minute of delay to defibrillation. Because pediatric cardiac arrests are commonly due to progressive asphyxia or shock (or both), the initial focus of treatment is generally prompt CPR. In sudden VF cardiac arrest in children, prompt defibrillation is the treatment of choice. Thus, the emphasis on early CPR versus early defibrillation must be balanced against the increasing evidence that VF in children is not rare, outcomes from arrhythmogenic VF arrests are superior to those from other types of cardiac arrests, and that early rhythm recognition is necessary for optimal care.

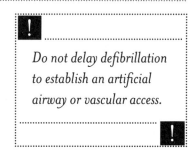
*Do not delay defibrillation to establish an artificial airway or vascular access.*

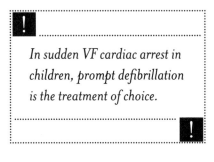
*In sudden VF cardiac arrest in children, prompt defibrillation is the treatment of choice.*

Because of the increasing awareness that "shockable" rhythms are not uncommon in children, greater attention has been focused on the dose for pediatric defibrillation. The recommended shock dose is 2 to 4 J/kg. Because 2 J/kg is often ineffective and higher doses may be needed to terminate VF, recent recommendations suggest an initial dose of 2 to 4 J/kg, followed by 4 J/kg if VF is not terminated; if VF continues, consider increasing the defibrillation dose up to 10 J/kg, not to exceed adult maximum doses.

## B. Automated External Defibrillators

Automated external defibrillators (AEDs) with a dose attenuator (decreases amount of power the patient receives) are recommended for children younger than 8 years (<25 kg). For children <1 year of age, a manual defibrillator is preferred. In the event a dose attenuator (1-8 years) or a manual defibrillator (<1 year) is not available, an AED still may be used, because untreated VF is fatal without a shock.

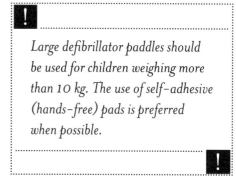

*Large defibrillator paddles should be used for children weighing more than 10 kg. The use of self-adhesive (hands-free) pads is preferred when possible.*

# VIII. MEDICATIONS

## A. Epinephrine (Adrenaline)

During CPR, epinephrine's α-adrenergic effect increases systemic vascular resistance, increasing diastolic blood pressure, which in turn increases the coronary perfusion pressure and blood flow and increases the likelihood of ROSC (**Table 3-2**). Epinephrine also increases cerebral blood flow during CPR because peripheral vasoconstriction directs a greater proportion of flow to the cerebral circulation. The β-adrenergic effect increases myocardial contractility and heart rate and relaxes smooth muscle in the skeletal muscle vascular bed and bronchi,

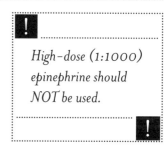

*High-dose (1:1000) epinephrine should NOT be used.*

### Table 3-2  Drug Dosing

| Drug | Dosing |
| --- | --- |
| Epinephrine (adrenaline) | Pulseless arrest<br>• 0.01 mg/kg (0.1 mL/kg) of 1:10,000 IV/IO q 3 to 5 min (maximum 1 mg/dose) |
| Amiodarone | Pulseless arrest<br>• 5 mg/kg IV/IO bolus (maximum 300 mg)<br>• SVT/VT (with pulse)<br>• 5 mg/kg IV/IO over 20-60 min (maximum 300 mg) |
| Lidocaine | VF/pulseless VT<br>• 1 mg/kg IV/IO bolus |
| Vasopressin | Pulseless cardiac arrest<br>• 0.4 to 1 U/kg bolus (maximum 40 units) |
| Atropine | Antidotal therapy |
| Sodium bicarbonate | Hyperkalemia or documented severe metabolic acidosis<br>• 1 mEq/kg IV/IO bolus |
| Calcium chloride | Documented severe hypocalcemia or hyperkalemia with arrest<br>• 20 mg/kg (0.2 mL/kg) IV/IO slow push during arrest |

IV, intravenous; IO, intraosseous; SVT, supraventricular tachycardia; VT, ventricular tachycardia; VF, ventricular fibrillation

although this effect is of less importance. Epinephrine also changes the character of VF (i.e., higher amplitude, more "coarse"), increasing the likelihood of successful defibrillation.

Prospective and retrospective studies indicate that use of high-dose epinephrine in adults or children (0.05-0.2 mg/kg) does not improve survival and may be associated with a worse neurologic outcome. Thus, it is not recommended for routine use during CPR.

## B. Amiodarone and Lidocaine

Amiodarone is recommended as first-line medical therapy for defibrillation-resistant VF/pulseless ventricular tachycardia (pVT) in adults. Data demonstrates improvement in ROSC and survival to hospital admission when amiodarone is compared with lidocaine.

No pediatric data conclusively supports the efficacy of either amiodarone or lidocaine in cardiac arrest due to VF/pVT. Pediatric case reports have demonstrated that amiodarone is effective in terminating life-threatening ventricular dysrhythmias, not cardiac arrest. Pediatric guidelines for antiarrhythmic therapy are extrapolated from adult data, and amiodarone is recommended at 5 mg/kg for cardiac arrest due to VF/pVT; alternatively (e.g., if amiodarone is unavailable) lidocaine at 1 mg/kg may also be used.

## C. Vasopressin

Vasopressin, a non-catecholamine vasopressor, has been shown to be an effective adjunctive and initial vasoactive medication in adult cardiac arrest. Studies on its impact in pediatric cardiac arrest are limited. Data are equivocal, with one retrospective study showing lower rates of ROSC with vasopressin, while multiple case reports have shown that vasopressin resulted in successful ROSC in adult and pediatric cardiac arrests refractory to standard therapy. Published dosing for children is 0.4 to 1 U/kg. Evidence on vasopressin in pediatric cardiac arrest is insufficient to recommend for or against its use.

## D. Other Agents

### 1. Atropine

Evidence is insufficient to support or refute the use of atropine in pediatric cardiac arrest. It may be used for symptomatic bradycardia known to be due to increased vagal tone or drug or environmental intoxications marked by cholinergic excess (e.g., organophosphates, sarin, VX, or other nerve agents). Epinephrine remains the drug of choice as first-line therapy for symptomatic bradycardia in children.

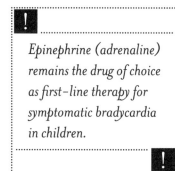

*Epinephrine (adrenaline) remains the drug of choice as first-line therapy for symptomatic bradycardia in children.*

### 2. Bicarbonate

Sodium bicarbonate is not recommended for routine use in pediatric cardiac arrest. Although no randomized trials exist, several studies suggest an association between bicarbonate use and decreased survival, even when controlling for other potentially confounding factors. Exceptions to this recommendation would include cases of cardiac arrest due to special resuscitation circumstances where sodium bicarbonate therapy is part of standard and specific treatment (e.g., tricyclic antidepressant overdose resulting in ventricular dysrhythmia, life-threatening hyperkalemia, severe pulmonary hypertension with acidosis).

### 3. Calcium

Data do not support routine use of calcium salts in cardiac arrest. Two controlled analyses of multihospital data demonstrated significantly decreased survival to hospital discharge among children receiving calcium salts during CPR. Recommendations for their use during CPR are limited to special resuscitation circumstances, such as documented hypocalcemia, hyperkalemia, or known or suspected intoxication with calcium channel blockers.

### 4. Magnesium

Magnesium is the initial drug recommended for torsades de points in adults. No specific recommendations exist for its use in pediatric cardiac arrest. Magnesium should be administered for documented hypomagnesemia. Because magnesium is a vasodilator, hypotension can occur during IV administration.

### 5. Glucose

Routine use of glucose-containing fluids during cardiac arrest resuscitation is not recommended. In cases of documented hypoglycemia, glucose should be administered in doses of 0.5 mg/kg (calculated rapidly by the "rule of 50": 1 mg/kg 50% dextrose, or 2 mg/kg 25% dextrose, or 5 mg/kg 10% dextrose). The empiric administration of glucose for cardiac arrest in children is not recommended.

# IX. SPECIFIC RHYTHMS

 Case Study

A 9-year-old boy is struck in the chest by a baseball. Moments later, he collapses on the field. His coach comes to his side to find him unresponsive and apneic; CPR is begun and the emergency medical service (EMS) phone activation number is called.

**Detection**
– When the ambulance arrives, an AED is applied and a shock is recommended. Following one shock, CPR is resumed and a faint brachial pulse is appreciated two minutes later. He starts to breathe spontaneously and opens his eyes.

**Intervention**
– What is the most appropriate immediate action now?

**Reassessment**
– If the single shock is unsuccessful, what is the next action?
– If the boy continues pulseless, unresponsive, and apneic, what medications are recommended?

**Effective Communication**
- When the patient's clinical status changes, who needs to know and how will the information be disseminated?
- Where is the best place to manage the care of this patient?

**Teamwork**
- How are you going to implement the treatment strategy?
- Who is to do what and when?

This is a case of commotio cordis, where a sudden powerful impact to the chest caused sudden collapse due to ventricular fibrillation

# A. VF/pVT (Shockable Rhythms)

VF is an uncommon, but not rare, electrocardiographic rhythm during out-of-hospital pediatric cardiac arrests (**Appendix 10**). Its incidence varies by setting and age. In special circumstances, such as commotio cordis, tricyclic antidepressant overdose, cardiomyopathy, post-cardiac surgery, and prolonged QT syndromes, VF is a more likely rhythm during cardiac arrest. Commotio cordis or mechanically initiated VF due to relatively low-energy chest wall impact during a narrow window of repolarization (10-30 msec before the T-wave peak in swine models) is reported predominantly in children age 4 to 16 years. Out-of-hospital VF cardiac arrest is uncommon in infants, but occurs more frequently in children and adolescents. Although VF is often associated with underlying heart disease and generally considered the "immediate cause" of cardiac arrest (i.e., an arrhythmogenic arrest), "subsequent" VF can also occur during resuscitation efforts (i.e., after an initial rhythm of asystole or pulseless electrical activity [PEA]). Traditionally, VF and VT have been considered "good" cardiac arrest rhythms, resulting in better outcomes than asystole and PEA. Survival to discharge is much more common among children with an initial shockable rhythm than among those with shockable rhythms occurring later during the resuscitation. Data suggest that outcomes after initial VF/VT are "good," but outcomes after subsequent VF/VT are substantially worse, even compared to initial asystole/PEA without subsequent VF/VT.

Defibrillation (defined as termination of VF) is necessary for successful resuscitation from VF cardiac arrest. The termination of fibrillation can result in asystole, PEA, or a perfusing rhythm. The goal of defibrillation is return of an organized electrical rhythm with pulse. When prompt defibrillation is provided soon after the induction of VF in a cardiac catheterization laboratory, the rates of successful defibrillation and survival approach 100%. When AEDs are used within 3 minutes of adult-witnessed VF, long-term survival can occur in more than 70%. Early and effective, near-continuous chest compressions can attenuate the incremental increase in mortality with delayed defibrillation. Because pediatric cardiac arrests are commonly due to progressive asphyxia and/or shock, the initial treatment of choice is prompt CPR. Therefore, rhythm recognition is emphasized less than in adult cardiac arrests. The earlier that VF can be diagnosed and treated, the higher the success.

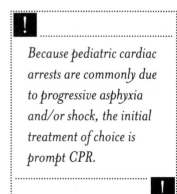

*Because pediatric cardiac arrests are commonly due to progressive asphyxia and/or shock, the initial treatment of choice is prompt CPR.*

## B. Bradycardia: Symptom of Hypoxia and Hypoperfusion

### Case Study

A 16-month-old girl is brought to an emergency department by emergency medical services after a bystander found her unresponsive in a parking lot. En route to the hospital, she is noted to be taking 6 breaths/min and so she receives assisted ventilation.

**Detection**

– On arrival, she has a narrow complex rhythm at a rate of 38 beats/min with faint pulse, and an undetectable blood pressure.

– What are the possible causes of this scenario?

**Intervention**

– What is the most important next step?

**Reassessment**

– After interventions are performed, what is the rhythm?

**Effective Communication**

– When the patient's clinical status changes, who needs to know and how will the information be disseminated?

– Where is the best place to manage the care of this patient?

**Teamwork**

– How are you going to implement the treatment strategy?

– Who is to do what and when?

Neonates, infants, and children are primarily dependent on heart rate for maintenance of cardiac output. They rarely have heart block or a primary cardiac reason for bradycardia. Most frequently bradycardia in infants and children is a manifestation of hypoxia and hypoperfusion. Their ability to augment stroke volume to increase cardiac output is limited, and physiologic or pathophysiologic states leading to an increase in cardiac output have tachycardia as their hallmark. Conversely, illnesses or injuries resulting in negative chronotropy (e.g., heart block, toxicity due to β-blockers or calcium channel blockers) tend to result in more profound shock and hypoperfusion in children than in adults.

Bradycardia with hypoperfusion (without pulselessness) is a common hemodynamic state for critically ill children during the pre-arrest phase. Animal models of asphyxia have demonstrated a predictable hemodynamic progression from tachycardia to bradycardia with hypotension, followed by PEA and asystole. Earlier CPR in this continuum is associated with more favorable outcomes. Given that the majority of children in cardiac arrest were experiencing either respiratory insufficiency and/or circulatory insufficiency prior to the onset of pulselessness, *a bradycardic child in shock should be considered to be in a pre-arrest state.* Multiple reversible causes are possible, but immediate support of cardiovascular status is essential (**Appendix 11**). Neonatal resuscitation algorithms have recommended escalation of respiratory and cardiac support for the neonate whose heart rate is <60 beats/min, including the provision of chest compressions if bradycardia does not resolve with effective ventilation and oxygenation. Multiple studies have shown that CPR is frequently initiated for hospitalized children when they are bradycardic and hypoperfused, and that chest compressions initiated prior to the onset of pulselessness are associated with improved survival. Current American Heart Association guidelines recommend the consideration of immediate chest compressions for a child with a heart rate <60 beats/min with signs and symptoms of hypoperfusion.

## C. Supraventricular Tachycardia

###  Case Study

A 2-month-old infant is brought to the emergency department by a parent who reports that she was well until 1 hour ago. Since then, she has become progressively lethargic, and she is now unresponsive. Initial assessment reveals irregular, gasping respirations, a very weak, rapid, barely palpable pulse, and an electrocardiogram shows a heart rate of 250 beats/min. Bag-mask ventilation is initiated with good chest rise, and chest compressions are begun.

**Detection**
- What are the key aspects of the initial assessment of this infant?
- What is the likely diagnosis?

**Intervention**
- What is the most important next step?

**Reassessment**
- What are the next management steps?

**Effective Communication**
- When the patient's clinical status changes, who needs to know and how will the information be disseminated?
- Where is the best place to manage the care of this patient?

**Teamwork**
- How are you going to implement the treatment strategy?
- Who is to do what and when?

Supraventricular tachycardia, a common arrhythmia in infants and children, may be associated with severe circulatory compromise or even cardiac arrest. Therapy for this arrhythmia should be based on the child's hemodynamic status. In the case of hemodynamically unstable supraventricular tachycardia, immediate cardioversion with 0.5 J/kg should be performed, increasing to 1 J/kg if necessary. Adenosine may also be considered first-line therapy, although IV access is required. In the unstable patient, cardioversion should not be delayed by attempts to achieve vascular access.

The initial dose of adenosine is 0.1 mg/kg given as a rapid IV bolus. Central venous administration is preferable because the drug is rapidly metabolized by red blood cell adenosine deaminase and so has a half-life of less than 10 seconds. When the drug is given, the catheter should be immediately and rapidly flushed with at least 10 mL of saline.

## D. Pulseless Electrical Activity

 Case Study

A 6-year-old girl with necrotizing pneumonia and septic shock is being managed with positive pressure ventilation and dopamine at 10 µg/kg/min. She has an acceptable blood pressure, a pulse oximeter reading in the mid-90% range, and $ETCO_2$ (exhaled) of 40 mm Hg.

**Detection**

- Acutely, her pulse oximetry reading falls to 70% and then loses its waveform, the $ETCO_2$ drops to zero, and the waveform on her arterial catheter becomes flat. She is unresponsive.

**Intervention**

- What is the most important immediate step?
- Assessment of airway and breathing reveals no breath sounds on the right.
- A needle is inserted in the second intercostal space in the mid-clavicular line with prompt return of spontaneous circulation.

**Reassessment**

- What are the next management steps?

**Effective Communication**

- When the patient's clinical status changes, who needs to know and how will the information be disseminated?
- Where is the best place to manage the care of this patient?

**Teamwork**

- How are you going to implement the treatment strategy?
- Who is to do what and when?

PEA is defined as organized ECG activity, excluding ventricular tachycardia and fibrillation, without clinical evidence of a palpable pulse or myocardial contractions. The most common causes of PEA can be remembered as the *6 Hs* and the *6 Ts*, as summarized in **Table 3-3**. All of these causes of PEA are potentially reversible; therefore, prompt efforts should be made to identify and correct them. While such efforts are under way, epinephrine, 10 µg/kg, may be administered every 5 minutes. When the cause of PEA is unknown and the patient does not respond to medications, consider administering a fluid bolus and inserting catheters into the pleural space to rule out pneumothorax and into the pericardial space to rule out cardiac tamponade.

| Table 3-3 | Potentially Reversible Factors in Cardiac Arrest: The 6 Hs and 6 Ts | |
|---|---|---|
| | **The 6 Hs** | **The 6 Ts** |
| | Hypovolemia | Tension pneumothorax |
| | Hypoxia | Tamponade, cardiac |
| | Hydrogen ion (acidosis) | Toxins |
| | Hypoglycemia | Thrombosis, pulmonary |
| | Hypo-/hyperkalemia | Thrombosis, coronary |
| | Hypothermia | Trauma |

# X. SPECIFIC RESUSCITATION CIRCUMSTANCES

## A. Newborn

Worldwide, approximately 4 million newborns suffer from birth asphyxia, resulting in approximately 1 million deaths and another million with neurologic sequelae. Neonatal resuscitation research has focused on how to effectively resuscitate the newborn and decrease the risk of neurologic injury and mortality. The focus is on clearing and opening the airway, initiating the first few breaths effectively to resuscitate the compromised infant, and adding positive pressure or continuous positive airway pressure as needed. If the heart rate drops below 100 beats/min, assisted ventilation should be provided. If the rate is <60 beats/min despite 30 seconds of ventilation with the addition of supplemental oxygen if needed and available, chest compressions should be initiated and intubation should be considered. CPR should be performed utilizing a ratio of 3:1, synchronously targeting 90 compressions and 30 breaths/min. The recent neonatal guidelines focus on using room air resuscitation to avoid hyperoxia. Room air resuscitation has been studied extensively and improves overall mortality rate. Recommendations are that it should be initiated and if bradycardia is <60 beats/min persists for 90 seconds, 100% oxygen should be utilized until recovery of a normal heart rate.

## B. Congenital Heart Disease/Pulmonary Hypertension

Standard pre-arrest and arrest resuscitation should be provided to children with congenital heart disease. Infants in the first few weeks of life who present hypoperfused or in cardiac arrest should be evaluated for the common causes of pediatric arrest, but ductal-dependent congenital heart disease should also be considered.

Patients with single-ventricle physiology and pulmonary blood flow dependent on a systemic-to-pulmonary artery shunt who present with persistent hypoxemia or full arrest may have evolving shunt thrombosis. They may be treatable with systemic heparinization to prevent ongoing thrombosis and increasing systemic vascular resistance (fluid boluses and phenylephrine) to promote pulmonary blood flow. Patients with known pulmonary hypertension and associated right ventricular dysfunction are at high risk for cardiac arrest. Increases in intrathoracic pressure due to positive pressure ventilation can result in inadequate cardiac output and arrest. During cardiac arrest, it may helpful to treat acidosis and administer IV fluids to provide preload to the systemic ventricle. Even in these special circumstances clinicians should follow standard pediatric advanced life support guidelines for pediatric resuscitation (**Figure 3-1**). Consultation with a pediatric cardiologist or cardiac intensivist may be critical to the treatment of these patients.

**Figure 3-1.** American Heart Association Pediatric Cardiac Arrest Algorithm

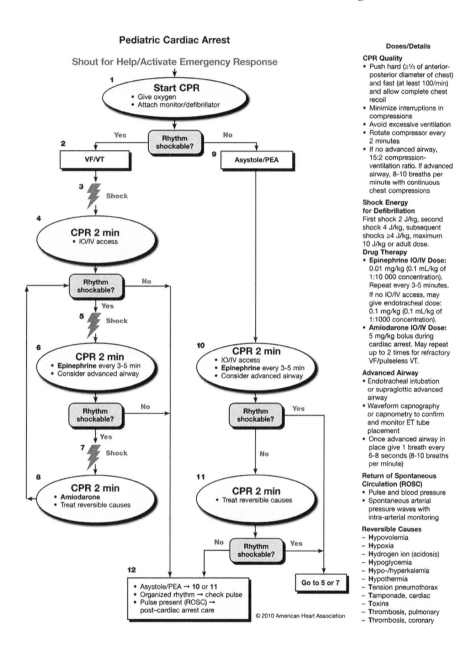

CPR, cardiopulmonary resuscitation; VF, ventricular fibrillation; VT, ventricular tachycardia; PEA, pulseless electrical activity; IO, intraosseous; IV, intravenous; ET, endotracheal
Reprinted with permission. © 2010 American Heart Association, Inc. Kleinman ME, Chameides L, Schexnayder SM, et al. Part 14: Pediatric advanced life support: 2010 American Heart Association Guidelines for Cardiopulmonary Resuscitation and Emergency Cardiovascular Care. *Circulation.* 2010;122(18 Suppl 3):S876-S908.

## C. Anaphylaxis

 ### Case Study

Within minutes of eating a cookie, a 15-year-old girl with a known peanut allergy developed dyspnea, lip swelling, hives, flushing, and dizziness; she complained of an "impending sense of doom." She utilized her epinephrine auto-injector, and emergency medical services was called. When they arrived 10 minutes later, she was cyanotic with severe distress and minimally responsive. Tracheal intubation was performed emergently in the field. While en route to the hospital, she became bradycardic and hypoxic and progressed to cardiopulmonary arrest.

**Detection**

– What is the patient's current clinical condition?

**Intervention**

– What are the most immediate treatment strategies?

**Reassessment**

– What is the patient's response to treatment?
– How does management of this patient differ from that of other cardiac arrest patients?
– What are the next management steps?

**Effective Communication**

– When the patient's clinical status changes, who needs to know and how will the information be disseminated?
– Where is the best place to manage the care of this patient?

**Teamwork**

– How are you going to implement the treatment strategy?
– Who is to do what and when?

Anaphylaxis is a severe systemic allergic reaction which can be reversed with rapid and adequate treatment, but can be fatal without appropriate intervention. Symptoms include tachycardia, flushing, diarrhea, bronchospasm, angioedema, and urticaria; the patient's condition can progress to profound hypotension and cardiovascular collapse. Vasodilation and increased capillary permeability cause relative intravascular depletion and hypotension with systemic hypoperfusion that can progress to cardiac arrest. Standard basic life support and advanced cardiac life support should be utilized for treatment of cardiac arrest, but specific adjunctive medications should be administered for the specific management of anaphylaxis.

A healthcare provider with advanced airway skills may be needed early as lip, pharyngeal, and glottic edema are common and can impede attainment of a secure airway. Intramuscular epinephrine should be administered immediately and can be repeated. Fluid resuscitation should be provided with repeated crystalloid solution boluses of 20 mL/kg to treat hypotension. Persistent hypotension should be managed with continued fluid resuscitation and an epinephrine infusion.

To further treat and abate ongoing symptoms, patients should receive IV steroids, antihistamines (diphenhydramine, $H_2$ blocker), and inhaled β-agonists (racemic epinephrine or albuterol).

## D. Trauma

Cardiac arrest in trauma, particularly blunt trauma, is associated with high mortality, but reversible causes of arrest should be sought and can be treated. Basic and advanced life support should be instituted immediately. Because of the potential for neck injury, a jaw thrust with cervical spine immobilization should be employed to open the airway. For the trauma patient who progresses to cardiac arrest, the most likely causes are hypovolemia from ongoing bleeding, hypothermia from exposure, tamponade from chest trauma, or hemo/pneumothoraces. Aggressive volume resuscitation with crystalloid and/or blood products should be instituted with the goal of achieving normovolemia, and a core temperature should be taken and managed. Breath sounds and radiographs should be evaluated for evidence of hemo/pneumothoraces; if present, chest tube placement should be considered. Cardiac tamponade is another potentially reversible cause of traumatic cardiac arrest that can be treated with pericardiocentesis or emergent thoracotomy. Spinal cord injury can result in hypotensive shock without reflex tachycardia. Specific treatment should focus on increasing vasomotor tone and supplementing chronotropy and vasoconstriction while instituting volume resuscitation.

# XI. POST-RESUSCITATION MANAGEMENT

The goals of post-resuscitation care are to diagnose and treat the underlying cause of the arrest, minimize secondary brain injury, and support end-organ perfusion and function. Aggressive post-resuscitative care may improve survival and neurologic outcomes, and specific attention should be paid to oxygenation, ventilation, temperature control, seizure control, glucose and electrolytes, and hemodynamics with the goal of matching appropriate substrate delivery to critical end-organ tissues demands (**Table 3-4**).

> *The goals of post-resuscitation care are to treat the underlying cause of the arrest, minimize secondary brain injury, and support end-organ perfusion and function.*

### Table 3-4 Cardiac Arrest Treatment Timeline

**First 5 minutes**
- Initiate high quality CPR
- Identify potentially reversible causes

**First 30 minutes**
- If ROSC achieved: determine location of definitive care; check temperature, pulse oximetry, lab results; monitor and treat hypotension
- If resuscitation ongoing: determine if resuscitation should continue based on multiple criteria

**First 3 hours**
- Treat hypotension
- Treat fever
- Maintain normoxia, normal ventilation and electrolyte/glucose levels

**First 48 hours**
- Treat hypotension
- Treat fever
- Monitor for seizures
- Manage temperature, oxygenation, ventilation, electrolytes

CPR, cardiopulmonary resuscitation; ROSC, return of spontaneous circulation

## A. Oxygenation

Following ROSC, both persistent hypoxemia (low $Pao_2$) and hyperoxemia (elevated $Pao_2$) have been associated with poor neurologic outcomes and concerns that hyperoxia may worsen oxidative injury during reperfusion. Therefore, one goal of post-resuscitative care is to deliver adequate oxygen to the patient while minimizing the risk of ongoing oxidative stress. Many patients do not have arterial monitoring early after arrest, but if a patient's saturation is 100%, practitioners should wean the supplemental oxygen to a saturation goal between 94% and 99%.

## B. Ventilation

Arterial $CO_2$ levels directly impact cerebral vascular tone in healthy patients. Following cardiac arrest, cerebral edema may occur and titration of arterial $CO_2$ may impact blood flow. Hyperventilating patients to an arterial $CO_2$ <35 mm Hg can result in cerebral vasoconstriction, hypoperfusion of the already injured brain, and increased intrathoracic pressure thus limiting cardiac output. Likewise, hypoventilation can lead to cerebral vasodilation and increase already elevated intracranial pressure. Although an individual's physiology is variable and intracranial pressure and cerebral blood flow monitoring are not standard after cardiac arrest, clinicians should maintain a normal arterial $CO_2$ between 35 and 45 mm Hg. If an arterial line is not in place, an $ETCO_2$ monitor can be used; however, it should correlate with an arterial blood gas as dead space ventilation is variable among patients and the difference between arterial and $ETCO_2$ also is variable.

## C. Cardiovascular Support

Post-arrest myocardial stunning and hypotensive shock are common after successful resuscitation in children and adults and are generally reversible states among long-term survivors. Post-arrest myocardial stunning is pathophysiologically similar to sepsis-related and post-cardiopulmonary bypass myocardial dysfunctions, including increases in inflammatory mediator and nitric oxide production. While the optimal management of post-cardiac arrest hypotension and myocardial dysfunction has not been established, adult data suggest that early hypotension in the 6 hours after ROSC is associated with increased mortality; therefore, aggressive hemodynamic support may improve outcomes.

Initially, fluid resuscitation should be provided for hypotension. Volume should be titrated to increase the central venous pressure if it is being monitored. Inotropic and/or vasopressor support should be provided for hypotension caused by myocardial dysfunction or vasodilation. Monitoring central venous pressure, central venous oxygen saturations, lactate levels, and urine output may help guide the effectiveness of therapies. General critical care principles suggest that appropriate therapeutic goals are adequate blood pressures; oxygen delivery; and myocardial, cerebral, and systemic blood flows. Reasonable interventions for vasodilatory shock with low central venous pressure include fluid resuscitation and vasoactive infusions. Appropriate considerations for left ventricular myocardial dysfunction include euvolemia, inotropic infusions, and afterload reduction. Echocardiography may contribute adjunctive data to guide therapies.

## D. Temperature

Hyperthermia following cardiac arrest is common in children. Animal and human data show that fever following brain injury is associated with worse outcomes and therefore fever should be aggressively treated following cardiac arrest. Induced hypothermia (89.6°-93.2°F, 32°-34°C) following witnessed adult VF cardiac arrest improves survival and neurologic outcomes and may be considered for children who remain comatose after pediatric cardiac arrest; however, no prospective pediatric data proving efficacy are available.

Following ROSC, clinicians should continuously measure the patient's core temperature (rectal, bladder, or esophageal). It is not uncommon for small children who have had a prolonged resuscitation to be hypothermic. Clinicians should discuss temperature goals with a tertiary care center. At a minimum, hyperthermia (temperature >100.4°F [>38°C]) should be prevented with antipyretics and a cooling blanket. Similarly, hypothermia ≤89.6°F (<32°C) should be corrected as deep hypothermia can lead to arrhythmias and repeat cardiac arrest.

## E. Glucose

Hyperglycemia following adult cardiac arrest is associated with worse neurological outcomes, as is hypoglycemia. Data for evidence-based titration of specific endpoints in children are not available. Therefore, clinicians should frequently monitor blood glucose levels and treat hypoglycemia.

## F. Seizures

Seizures following cardiac arrest are common and often are undetectable without electroencephalography (EEG). Such seizures (clinical and subclinical) are associated with worse neurologic outcomes, although it is unclear whether they are the result of severe brain injury, cause severe brain injury, or both. Clinical convulsions should be aggressively treated and evaluation for correctable causes should be sought (e.g., hypoglycemia, hyponatremia, hypocalcemia, hypomagnesemia). Many patients exhibit electrographic seizures that are undetectable to the clinician even when the patients are not paralyzed. Therefore, clinicians should consider EEG monitoring for the comatose post-arrest patient. If the patient is under neuromuscular blockade, EEG monitoring will be the only means of detecting postischemic seizure.

# XII. EVALUATION OF SUDDEN DEATH

Sudden death in infants, children, and adolescents may be due to underlying cardiac abnormalities such as channelopathies, cardiomyopathies, and coronary artery abnormalities. Genetic mutations leading to channelopathies are relatively common among infants and children with out-of-hospital cardiac arrests. When a child or young adult has an unexplained sudden death, a full past medical history and family history should be obtained, and family members should be referred for evaluation of potential channelopathies. Patients should undergo a full echocardiogram and in the event of death, an autopsy is recommended and, if possible, a genetic tissue evaluation should be performed.

# XIII. ETHICAL ISSUES

## A. Family Presence

Family presence at the bedside during resuscitation has become increasingly common. Those who are present during the resuscitation are able to witness the efforts utilized and, in the event of death, their presence has been shown to help with grieving and may result in less anxiety and depression. While it should not be expected that family members witness resuscitation, the option to be present should be offered when possible. A member of the medical team should be assigned to support the family during the resuscitation and, in the event their presence is disruptive, they should be respectfully asked to leave the room.

## B. Prognosis

Predicting outcome after resuscitation from cardiac arrest is a complex task. Much of the relevant data comes from adult patients who differ in arrest etiology and neurodevelopment. Early prognostication (within 24 hours of arrest) is limited by the fact that no single marker is 100% sensitive for poor outcome. Even fewer data are available to help predict a good outcome. Clinical neurological examination findings of absent pupillary response and motor response predict outcome, but not until 3 days after arrest. Neurophysiological diagnostic studies, such as EEG and somatosensory evoked potentials, may be helpful, but are not standardized in the pediatric population and not available at all centers. Computed tomography scans are not sensitive for early neurological injury, but may be helpful in determining a cause of out-of-hospital arrest including intracranial hemorrhage or intracranial hypertension. Magnetic resonance imaging with diffusion weighting provides valuable information about hypoxic/ischemic injury in the subacute and recovery phases (5-7 days after injury). Thus, comparison to a child's pre-arrest neurological function is difficult and adds another barrier to the assessment and prediction of post-arrest neurological status. All prognostic markers evaluated prior to the use of induced hypothermia need to be reevaluated as they may no longer be reliable. Care providers should take hypothermia into account when making recommendations about withdrawal of care, and neurology consultation should be considered.

## C. Termination of Resuscitative Efforts

No reliable predictor of outcome can determine when to terminate resuscitative efforts. Several factors point to the likelihood of survival after cardiac arrest, including the mechanism of the arrest (e.g., traumatic, asphyxial, progression from circulatory shock), location (e.g., in-hospital or out-of-hospital), response (i.e., witnessed or unwitnessed, with or without bystander CPR), underlying pathophysiology (i.e., cardiomyopathy, congenital defect, drug toxicity, or metabolic derangement), and the potential reversibility of underlying diseases. Patients who have a witnessed arrest, receive bystander CPR, or receive advanced medical care a short time after collapse may have a better chance for a good outcome. When high-quality CPR is provided and rescue extracorporeal membrane oxygenation is available, even CPR lasting an hour may result in a good neurologic outcome. Therefore, it is important to factor in the multiple variables in determining when to terminate efforts.

## Key Points: Pediatric Cardiac Arrest

- Early identification of the decompensating patient is paramount to preventing cardiac arrest.

- Rapid initiation of chest compressions is critical to resumption of blood flow.

- Critical factors in the administration of high-quality CPR are push hard, push fast, minimize interruptions, allow full chest recoil, and avoid overventilation.

- If IV access is difficult to achieve, an intraosseous line should be placed immediately.

- In patients with VF, defibrillation should not be delayed for endotracheal intubation.

- Use of an AED should be considered in efforts to defibrillate children if a manual defibrillator is not available.

- Post-resuscitation assessment and management of temperature, glucose, oxygen saturations, $Pa_{CO_2}$, and blood pressure may improve outcomes from cardiac arrest.

## Suggested Readings

1. Atkins DL, Everson-Stewart S, Sears GK, et al. Epidemiology and outcomes from out-of-hospital cardiac arrest in children: the Resuscitation Outcomes Consortium Epistry-Cardiac Arrest. *Circulation.* 2009;119:1484-1491.

2. Berg MD, Schexnayder SM, Chameides L, et al. Part 13: pediatric basic life support: 2010 American Heart Association Guidelines for Cardiopulmonary Resuscitation and Emergency Cardiovascular Care. *Circulation.* 2010;122(18 Suppl 3):S862-S875.

3. Brilli RJ, Gibson R, Luria JW, et al. Implementation of a medical emergency team in a large pediatric teaching hospital prevents respiratory and cardiopulmonary arrests outside the intensive care unit. *Pediatr Crit Care Med.* 2007;8:236-246.

4. Donoghue AJ, Nadkarni VM, Elliott M, Durbin D. Effect of hospital characteristics on outcomes from pediatric cardiopulmonary resuscitation: a report from the national registry of cardiopulmonary resuscitation. *Pediatrics.* 2006;118:995-1001.

5. Kleinman ME, de Caen AR, Chameides L, et al. Part 14: pediatric advanced life support: 2010 American Heart Association Guidelines for Cardiopulmonary Resuscitation and Emergency Cardiovascular Care. *Circulation.* 2010;122(18 Suppl 3): S876-S908.

6. Meert KL, Donaldson A, Nadkarni V, et al. Multicenter cohort study of in-hospital pediatric cardiac arrest. *Pediatr Crit Care Med.* 2009;10:544-553.

7. Nadkarni VM, Larkin GL, Peberdy MA, et al. First documented rhythm and clinical outcome from in-hospital cardiac arrest among children and adults. *JAMA.* 2006;295:50-57.

8. Perondi MB, Reis AG, Paiva EF, Nadkarni VM, Berg RA. A comparison of high-dose and standard-dose epinephrine in children with cardiac arrest. *N Engl J Med*. 2004;350:1722-1730.

9. Samson RA, Nadkarni VM, Meaney PA, et al. Outcomes of in-hospital ventricular fibrillation in children. *N Engl J Med*. 2006;354:2328-2339.

10. Sanders AB, Kern KB, Otto CW, Milander MM, Ewy GA. End-tidal carbon dioxide monitoring during cardiopulmonary resuscitation. A prognostic indicator for survival. *JAMA*. 1989;262:1347-1351.

11. Tibballs J, Kinney S. Reduction of hospital mortality and of preventable cardiac arrest and death on introduction of a pediatric medical emergency team. *Pediatr Crit Care Med*. 2009;10:306-312.

# Chapter 4

# DIAGNOSIS AND MANAGEMENT OF THE CHILD WITH ACUTE UPPER AND LOWER AIRWAY DISEASE

## ✓ Objectives

- Explain the anatomic and developmental differences that make infants and children prone to disorders of the upper airway.
- Describe how to assess children with upper airway disorders.
- Summarize the diagnosis and treatment of children with upper airway disorders.
- Identify common disorders of the upper airway.
- Outline the pathophysiology of acute lower airway disease.
- Detect respiratory failure with or without accompanying respiratory distress.
- Initiate appropriate diagnostic and therapeutic interventions for the various causes of acute lower airway disease.

## Case Study

You are called to the bedside of a 6-month-old boy who has developed a barky cough and is having difficulty breathing. When you approach the patient, you see deep subcostal retractions. Upon auscultation over the trachea, you hear high-pitched inspiratory noise.

**Detection**
- What problems are in your differential diagnosis?
- What does the high-pitched noise signify?

**Intervention**
- What immediate actions should you take?

**Reassessment**
- How do you know your interventions are effective?
- How do you want to monitor the patient?

**Effective Communication**
- Who needs to know about changes in the patient's clinical condition?
- Where is the best place to manage this patient?

**Teamwork**
- How will you implement your treatment strategy?
- Who is to do what and when?

# I. UPPER AIRWAY DISEASE

Problems related to the upper airway occur frequently in infants and children. These problems range from benign and self-limiting, such as most cases of viral croup, to immediately life-threatening, as in cases of acute upper airway obstruction due to foreign body aspiration. Management strategies for upper airway-related disorders extend from calm reassurance to urgent life-saving intervention. Knowledge of the etiologies of upper airway diseases in children, assessment of their severity, and approaches to treatment is important for treating critically ill hospitalized children.

# II. ANATOMIC DIFFERENCES BETWEEN CHILDREN AND ADULTS

## A. Airway

The airway of a child changes continuously from birth until approximately 8 years of age, when it becomes anatomically similar to an adult's airway. In addition to disorders related to an innately smaller size, congenital abnormalities can affect the airway. Pediatric patients are more susceptible to several illnesses, such as viral croup, that are not as problematic for adults because they have larger airways. After children reach 8 years of age, their upper airway problems become similar to those found in adults.

**Chapter 2** describes many of the developmental differences that exist between newborn, infant, pediatric, and adult airways and the impact of those differences on airway management. **Table 4-1** highlights some differences between the infant and adult airways.

At birth, and for some time afterward, infants are obligate nasal breathers, making them prone to distress from congenital and acquired nasal obstruction. Congenital causes of nasal obstruction include unilateral and bilateral choanal stenosis. Acquired causes of nasal obstruction include mucous plugging and edema from upper respiratory tract infections, such as those due to respiratory syncytial virus (RSV) or other viruses. Suctioning to clear the nasal passages of infants can substantially improve respiratory status. As a child ages, oral breathing becomes possible, but there continues to be a preference for the nose.

# Table 4-1. Anatomic Difference Between Infant, Pediatric, and Adult Airways

| Characteristic | Infant | Pediatric (Age 1 Year) | Adult |
| --- | --- | --- | --- |
| Air entry | Obligate nasal breather | Mouth and nose | Mouth and nose |
| Tracheal diameter | 4 mm | 5-6 mm | 18 mm |
| Laryngeal shape | Funnel | Funnel | Barrel |
| Narrowest portion | Cricoid | Cricoid | Laryngeal inlet |
| Epiglottis | Long, soft, omega-shaped | Long, soft, omega-shaped | Short, firm |
| Laryngeal inlet | C1 | C3-C4 | C5-C6 |
| Proportion of tongue to jaw | Tongue relatively large in proportion to oral cavity (jaw space) | Proportion of tongue to jaw space changes continually up to approximately 8 years of age | Tongue easy to displace into jaw |
| Position of larynx on laryngoscopy | Anterior, cephalad | Transition between infant and adult position | More posterior, caudad |
| Trachea | Soft cartilage | Firmer but still collapsible cartilage | Firm, more rigid tracheal cartilage |

A small chin is developmentally appropriate at birth in that it facilitates both vaginal delivery and breast-feeding. Anatomically, a small chin is manifested by short mandibular rami and short distance from chin to hyoid cartilage. This contributes to a smaller jaw space and is one reason that the tongue is relatively large for the size of the oral cavity around birth. A relatively large tongue-to-mouth ratio facilitates obligate nasal breathing, which, in turn, permits a child to feed without aspirating. The ratio of tongue size to oral cavity size decreases as a child grows. A large tongue in a relatively small mouth, though anatomically normal, makes infants with a decreased level of consciousness more prone to develop upper airway obstruction from the tongue falling back into the pharynx.

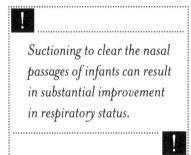

*Suctioning to clear the nasal passages of infants can result in substantial improvement in respiratory status.*

In the Pierre Robin sequence (micrognathia, relative macroglossia, cleft palate), the severe disproportion in size between the tongue and mouth may result in the tongue being pressed back into the pharynx, obstructing the movement of air. A small submental space in infants results in less space into which the tongue can be displaced during laryngoscopy and adds difficulty to intubation. Airway visualization by laryngoscopy is always more difficult in patients with micrognathia, macroglossia, or both.

As a child approaches 8 years of age, the narrowest point of the airway changes from the subglottic space to the laryngeal inlet — the relationship present in adult airways. The airway diameter of newborns, infants, and children increases with growth until the mid-teens, when it reaches adult caliber. The narrower airway diameter of infants and children results in increased resistance to airflow. Resistance to airflow is described mathematically by the Hagen-Poiseuille equation:

$$R = 8\eta l/r^4$$

where $R$ is resistance, $\eta$ is the viscosity of the gas, $l$ is the length of tube that air flows through, and $r$ is the radius of the airway. The equation illustrates that resistance goes up exponentially to the fourth power as airway diameter (2 times the radius) decreases. Therefore, even though the absolute volume of gas flow is less than in adults, resistance to airflow is greater in infants and children (**Chapter 2**).

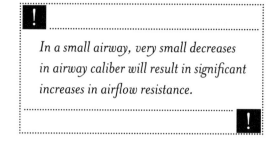

*In a small airway, very small decreases in airway caliber will result in significant increases in airflow resistance.*

**Figure 2-1** in **Chapter 2** illustrates the relative increase in resistance when 1 mm of circumferential airway edema occurs in an infant airway that is 4 mm in diameter, compared to the increase that occurs when the same amount of circumferential edema occurs in the 8-mm diameter airway of an older child or teen. Remembering that 1 mm of circumferential edema results in a 2-mm decrease in diameter and using Poiseuille's law, it is seen that the $1/r^4$ relationship of airway radius to resistance results in a 16-fold increase in airway resistance in the 4-mm airway compared to a 3-fold increase in resistance in the 8-mm airway.

Until a child reaches approximately 8 years of age, the narrowest portion of the airway is in the subglottic space. Infant and pediatric larynges have a funnel shape rather than the barrel shape of an adult larynx. Thus, the adult airway is narrowest at the vocal cords, or laryngeal inlet, whereas the infant and pediatric airways continue to narrow below the vocal cords, reaching their narrowest portion at the level of the cricoid cartilage. With the narrowest portion of the upper airway located in the subglottic space, infants have a susceptibility to significant airflow compromise in response to even a small volume of tissue edema. As the airway diameter increases with growth, the increases in resistance related to airway edema become less significant.

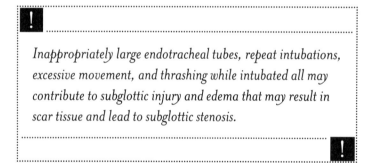

*Inappropriately large endotracheal tubes, repeat intubations, excessive movement, and thrashing while intubated all may contribute to subglottic injury and edema that may result in scar tissue and lead to subglottic stenosis.*

Although passing an endotracheal tube through the vocal cords always places a patient at risk for vocal cord injury, a narrow subglottic space makes infants and children susceptible to subglottic injury.

## B. Epiglottis

The epiglottis of infants and young children differs in shape and consistency from an adult epiglottis. In infants and children, it is longer and softer than in the adult, and assumes an omega-like shape (Ω). The adult epiglottis, in contrast, is shorter, firmer, and squarer than in children. The characteristics of the infant larynx necessitate that the epiglottis be actively displaced from the glottic opening during laryngoscopy for tracheal intubation. The shape of an infant's epiglottis, when exaggerated, contributes to laryngomalacia. In this condition, an infant shows signs of inspiratory upper airway obstruction that are due to the collapse of the epiglottis and laryngeal components over the laryngeal inlet on inspiration.

## C. Larynx

The larynx of infants and young children is anterior and cephalad in position compared with the larynx of an adult. The impact of this relationship on airway visualization during intubation is discussed in **Chapter 2**.

## D. Trachea and Lower Airways

Tracheal cartilage is soft and collapsible in infancy, becoming more rigid with growth. Thus, the walls of the extrathoracic trachea can collapse inward when an infant creates significant negative inspiratory force by inhaling against an obstructed upper airway. **Figure 4-1** illustrates this point.

**Figure 4-1.** Extrathoracic Tracheal Collapse with Forceful Inspiration Against a Subglottic Obstruction

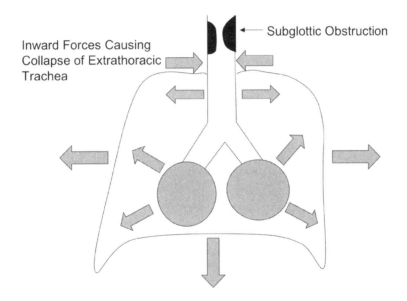

The extrathoracic and intrathoracic portions of the trachea react differently to the forces generated by breathing. The portion of the trachea from the subglottic space to the thoracic inlet is extrathoracic. The trachea from the thoracic inlet to the carina is intrathoracic and sits within the chest, surrounded by lung and pleura, making it subject to the forces generated within the chest during inspiration and expiration. The intrathoracic trachea, as well as the bronchi and all the distal airways, are connected to the surrounding lung parenchyma, which in turn is covered by the visceral pleura. The visceral pleura of the lungs are apposed to the parietal pleura lining the inside of the rib cage by a mechanism known as *viscoelastic coupling*. Natural outward elastic recoil of the rib cage, along with constant tone of the diaphragm, combine to transmit a force to the intrapleural space that results in negative intrapleural pressure at all times. The outward tension of the rib cage, the downward tone of the diaphragm, and a negative intrapleural pressure – all occurring at rest – combine to keep the lungs expanded and, since the airways are connected to the lung parenchyma, the airways as well are held open.

The pleural pressure, which is difficult to measure, is analogous to intrathoracic pressure. During quiet inspiration, the pleural (intrathoracic) pressure becomes more negative when the diaphragm contracts. The negative pleural pressure creates a pressure gradient from the alveoli (where it is most negative) to the mouth (where it is approximately zero). The pressure gradient drives airflow into the lungs. When the diaphragm contracts (and in distress, the accessory muscles of respiration as well), the negative intrathoracic pressure is transmitted to the outside of the trachea, serving as a distending force to keep the intrathoracic airways open. Increased airway resistance during inspiration due to partial or complete airway obstruction causes the diaphragm to contract more forcefully and the accessory muscles of inspiration (external intercostals, scalenes, and sternocleidomastoids) to engage. The negative intrapleural and thus intrathoracic pressures will increase in an effort to move air past the obstruction. Due to the connection of the airways to the lung parenchyma (known as *interdependence*) and the lungs to the pleura, the more negative intrathoracic and intrapleural pressure will tend to keep the intrathoracic airways open while at the same time the extrathoracic trachea, without the surrounding lung parenchyma to pull it open, will tend to close.

Intrathoracic and intrapleural pressures become very positive during forced expiration, as occurs in obstructive diseases such as asthma. When the intrapleural pressure becomes positive, the airway pressure gradient becomes very positive in the alveoli and decreases as it moves toward the mouth, where it is zero. A gradient is necessary for air movement to occur. As the pressure gradient decreases toward the mouth, there may come a point, known as *the equal pressure point*, where the pressure in the airways becomes equal to the intrapleural pressure. At any point closer to the mouth than the equal pressure point, the sum of forces favors closure of the airways.

Thus, the intrathoracic airways, including the intrathoracic trachea, will remain open when inspiratory effort is increased but are prone to closure when expiratory forces are increased. The extrathoracic trachea behaves in a manner opposite to that of the intrathoracic trachea. In the extrathoracic trachea, the outer trachea is not tethered to the lung and pleura to create a distending force to counterbalance the negative intratracheal pressure that occurs during inspiration. During quiet breathing, and when the tracheal cartilage is formed normally, no significant tracheal collapse occurs during inspiration; however, when a patient breathes against a partial upper airway obstruction, as occurs in laryngomalacia or viral croup, the tracheal walls can partially collapse, thus further increasing airway resistance. Collapse of the extrathoracic trachea during inspiration and of the intrathoracic trachea during expiration is much worse in the presence of poor cartilaginous ring development, as is seen in tracheomalacia.

The extrathoracic trachea is not subject to collapse during forced exhalation. The differences between the intrathoracic and extrathoracic airways provide the basis for understanding why problems of the nose, pharynx, larynx, and subglottic trachea have their greatest impact on inspiration, whereas problems of the lower (intrathoracic) airways tend to have greater impact upon exhalation. A tendency for the subglottic, but extrathoracic, trachea to narrow or close when there is very negative intrapleural pressure also explains why patients with upper airway obstruction do worse when they are agitated (**Figure 4-1**).

> **!**
>
> *Changes in Pediatric Airway With Partial Obstruction*
> *Airflow restriction is related to the location of the obstruction.*
> *Extrathoracic obstruction → Inspiratory collapse → Stridor*
> *Intrathoracic obstruction → Expiratory airway collapse →*
> *Wheezing on expiration*
> *In severe cases (e.g., laryngotracheobronchitis), both may be present.*

# III. DISORDERS THAT AFFECT CHILDREN'S AIRWAYS

**Table 4-2** lists some of the disorders that affect the pediatric airway and may present as partial or complete obstruction of the upper airway. The causes are organized by category and will be discussed, along with specific approaches to management. General approaches are discussed in greater detail in a later section.

| Table 4-2 | Causes of Pediatric Airway Disorders |
|---|---|
| **Anatomic Disorders** | **Infectious Disorders** |
| • Altered level of consciousness (airway muscle laxity)<br>• Tonsillar hypertrophy<br>• Subglottic stenosis (acquired or congenital)<br>• Macroglossia<br>• Vocal cord paralysis<br>• Micrognathia<br>• Choanal stenosis<br>• Pierre Robin sequence | • Laryngotracheobronchitis (croup)<br>• Epiglottitis (supraglottitis)<br>• Bacterial tracheitis<br>• Retropharyngeal (parapharyngeal) abscess<br>• Peritonsillar abscess<br>• Infectious mononucleosis |
| **External or Internal Compression Disorders** | **Miscellaneous Disorders** |
| • Tumor<br>• Hemangioma<br>• Hematoma<br>• Cyst<br>• Papilloma<br>• Vascular rings and slings | • Airway trauma<br>• Post-extubation airway obstruction<br>• Angioedema<br>• Spasmodic croup<br>• Foreign body aspiration<br>• Airway trauma<br>• Thermal and chemical burns |

## A. Anatomic Disorders

### 1. Altered Level of Consciousness

An altered level of consciousness is frequently responsible for upper airway obstruction in patients of all ages. For the developmental reasons given earlier, young patients are more prone to upper airway obstruction related to a decreased level of consciousness. For example, the decreased level of consciousness that accompanies the postictal state after a seizure, especially when barbiturates or benzodiazepines have been administered, can lead to upper airway obstruction. Many decreases in oxygen saturation that occur during procedural sedation are related to upper airway obstruction. A child injured in an automobile or bicycle collision and who has decreased level of consciousness is likely to have a partially obstructed airway and may benefit significantly from maneuvers that open and maintain airway patency while protecting the neck's spinal alignment (**Chapter 2** and **Chapter 9**).

### 2. Tonsillar-Adenoidal Hypertrophy

Tonsillar-adenoidal hypertrophy by itself and combined with obesity is responsible for obstructive sleep apnea and acute upper airway obstruction. Though apnea is mostly a chronic problem, there are situations in which such patients develop acute upper airway obstruction. Positive pressure ventilation by continuous positive airway pressure (CPAP) or bilevel positive airway pressure (BiPAP) is often helpful. In an acute emergency, a nasopharyngeal airway may be helpful. Tonsillectomy and adenoidectomy, along with weight loss, are the definitive treatments. Patients may continue to require positive airway pressure for some time after tonsillectomy and adenoidectomy. In acute situations, corticosteroids may be helpful in reducing tonsillar tissue size, especially when the cause is infectious mononucleosis.

### 3. Subglottic Stenosis

Subglottic stenosis (SGS) can be congenital or acquired. Acquired SGS is frequently seen in the neonatal intensive care unit in infants with a history of prematurity and intubation. Sometimes an acute intercurrent viral respiratory infection, especially RSV, can cause SGS to change rapidly from a chronic compensated problem to uncompensated respiratory distress. Racemic epinephrine, dexamethasone, and heliox are all useful interventions for ameliorating a severe event, but a patient with severe SGS ultimately requires airway endoscopy for definitive diagnosis and, potentially, laryngotracheal reconstruction.

### 4. Macroglossia and Micrognathia

Macroglossia (large tongue) and micrognathia (small chin and jaw) are components of several congenital craniofacial anomalies. Their roles in upper airway obstruction were discussed earlier. Severe macroglossia and micrognathia can result in critical airway issues in the perinatal period. These issues become relevant later when a patient either requires procedural sedation or anesthesia with tracheal intubation.

### 5. Vocal Cord Paralysis

Vocal cord paralysis can be either unilateral or bilateral. Unilateral vocal cord paralysis is manifested by weak cry and occasional stridor, and is usually well tolerated. The etiology is often idiopathic, but the condition is occasionally associated with injury to the recurrent laryngeal nerve during thoracic surgery. Bilateral vocal cord paralysis manifests as severe stridor and severe respiratory distress, though often with a normal cry. Bilateral vocal cord paralysis is often associated with central nervous system injury or disease. Children with bilateral vocal cord paralysis often require urgent airway management.

### 6. Choanal Stenosis and Choanal Atresia

Choanal stenosis and choanal atresia may be unilateral or bilateral. Given that infants are obligate nasal breathers, most children with choanal stenosis develop some degree of distress and poor feeding. Bilateral choanal stenosis almost always produces symptoms during the neonatal period. Diagnosis is confirmed by attempting to pass a soft catheter through the nose. Evaluation of the nose and nasopharynx by computed tomographic scanning is helpful in confirming the diagnosis and determining the extent of obstruction. Associated anomalies are common and occur in 20% to 50% of infants with choanal atresia. The syndrome of anomalies, known as the *CHARGE association*, includes coloboma and other ophthalmologic anomalies, heart disease, choanal atresia, growth retardation, genital hypoplasia, and ear anomalies. Choanal stenosis and choanal atresia are treated surgically.

Unilateral choanal stenosis may make it difficult or impossible to pass a nasogastric tube through the stenotic nares. If the tube is instead passed through the unobstructed nostril, an infant will become distressed due to occlusion of the one patent naris.

**7. Pierre Robin Sequence**

Pierre Robin sequence is an example of a congenital syndrome in which upper airway obstruction can occur and can be life-threatening. The primary defect is poor mandibular growth in utero that results in micrognathia, cleft palate, and glossoptosis (posterior displacement or retraction of the tongue). The oral cavity is too small for the tongue, which is usually a normal size. As a result of the mismatch between tongue and jaw sizes, affected infants are very prone to airway obstruction from posterior movement of the tongue against the retropharyngeal wall. Approaches to management include prone positioning to allow the tongue to move forward and away from the pharynx. The placement of a nasopharyngeal (NP) tube made from an appropriately sized endotracheal tube can be lifesaving. The general technique for using NP tubes is presented in **Chapter 2**, but the approach presented in **Figure 4-2** focuses on differences specific to the Pierre Robin sequence.

**Figure 4-2.** Placement of Nasopharyngeal Tube for Airway Obstruction Due to Pierre Robin Sequence

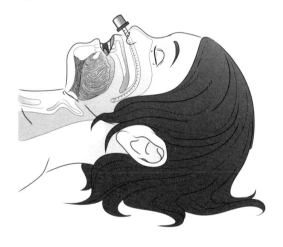

1. Use an uncuffed tracheal tube that fits in a nostril.
2. Match the length of the tube to the approximate distance between the naris and the tragus.
3. Lubricate the tube with surgical lubricant.
4. Insert and advance the tube while listening for air movement.
5. Secure the tube carefully with tape and adhesive.
6. Suction frequently to maintain patency.
7. If air movement through the tube cannot be heard, reposition the tube until airflow is audible.

When air movement through the NP tube is heard and felt, the tube is in the appropriate position; the patient will also be less distressed. The tube should be secured at this position with tape and adhesive in the same way as an endotracheal tube. Though it does not pass through the vocal cords and into the trachea, the NP tube is nonetheless a lifeline through which the patient can move air. The tube should be suctioned as necessary to maintain patency. Should a patient with an NP tube for the Pierre Robin sequence develop distress, suctioning and, if necessary, repositioning of the tube are indicated until air movement is again heard. The tube has a dual purpose in that it not only serves as a conduit for air movement but also pushes the tongue slightly forward off the retropharyngeal wall, thus relieving that level of obstruction.

An additional lifesaving maneuver that has been described for severe cases of obstruction in the Pierre Robin sequence is to pull the tongue forward manually using a towel clamp or similar instrument. Passing a needle with size 0 silk through the tip of the tongue and pulling it forward and out of the mouth may serve a similar purpose. Definitive management for severe cases of the Pierre Robin sequence is surgical, occasionally with a need for tracheostomy.

## B. External or Internal Compression Disorders

###  Case Study

A previously healthy 10-year-old girl is evaluated in the emergency department for gradual new onset wheezing, increased work of breathing, and increased dyspnea in a supine position. Her mother also reports a fever of 102.2°F (39°C), weight loss, and night sweats. The child prefers the sitting position and looks anxious. On exam, her vital signs are as follows: heart rate, 120 beats/min; respiratory rate, 25 breaths/min; blood pressure, 130/75 mm Hg; and pulse oximetry 91% in room air. Inspiratory and expiratory wheezes are found on auscultation with decreased breath sounds in the right upper chest. Despite your recommendation, the patient is placed in a flat supine position. The patient becomes more anxious, her oxygen saturations drops, and the engorgement of her neck veins increases.

**Detection**
- What is happening to this patient?
- What is the differential diagnosis?
- Why did she worsen with being placed supine?
- What tests could be useful to evaluate this patient?

**Intervention**
- What interventions should be made immediately?

**Reassessment**
- How will you know if your interventions are working?
- How should you monitor the patient
- Do you want to do any lab studies?

**Effective Communication**
- Who needs to know about this patient immediately?
- What information needs to be communicated at each stage of movement in the hospital?
- Where is the best place to care for this patient?

**Teamwork**
- How is the work on this patient to be distributed?

**1. Diagnosis of Neoplastic Airway Obstruction**

External or internal compression of the airway can result in upper airway obstruction. Tumors, hemangiomas, hematomas, cysts, papilloma, and vascular rings and slings can all present with signs and symptoms of upper airway obstruction. Lymphoid (Hodgkin and non-Hodgkin lymphoma) and leukemic (acute lymphocytic leukemia) malignancies in children may present with an anterior or middle mediastinal mass. Tumor masses in this location produce superior vena cava obstruction and compression of other mediastinal structures, such as the trachea, main stem bronchus, pulmonary vessels, and aorta. Progressive venous congestion and airway compression will lead to the usual symptoms found in superior vena cava obstruction: facial engorgement, headache, plethora, cyanotic facies, cough, dyspnea, orthopnea, hoarseness, and dysphagia.

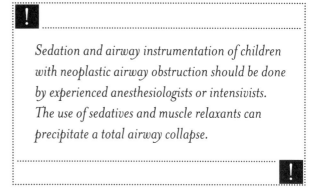

*Sedation and airway instrumentation of children with neoplastic airway obstruction should be done by experienced anesthesiologists or intensivists. The use of sedatives and muscle relaxants can precipitate a total airway collapse.*

Posterior, anterior, and lateral chest radiographs will show a widening of the mediastinum with tracheal deviation or compression.

**2. Management of Neoplastic Airway Obstruction**

Often CPAP and BiPAP can temporarily reduce the degree of airway obstruction and improve airflow. When either is started, it is helpful to auscultate for breath sounds over the lung fields while titrating pressures to find one that results in opening of the airway. Positioning a patient with an anterior mediastinal mass upright, prone, or even on the side can take the pressure of anterior masses off the trachea and relieve obstruction. An experienced anesthesiologist and an ear, nose, and throat surgeon should be available in the event that endotracheal intubation is necessary. The patient's airway is best secured with the patient breathing spontaneously, as catastrophic airway closure can occur with deep sedation or paralysis.

# C. Infectious Causes of Upper Airway Obstruction

Infectious causes of upper airway obstruction are very common in patients of all ages. One significant change over the past 20 years is the reduction in the incidence of epiglottitis due to the addition of the *Haemophilus influenzae* type B (Hib) vaccine in the infant immunization schedule in the United States and developed countries. Prior to vaccine use in the US, the incidence of epiglottitis was 5 cases per 100,000 children 5 years and younger; this incidence decreased to 0.6 to 0.8 cases per 100,000 children after the addition of Hib vaccine to the immunization regimen. *H influenzae* is such a fulminant and life-threatening infection that knowledge of its diagnosis and management remains important. Moreover, the evaluation and care of the patient with epiglottitis often serves as a paradigm of how to approach all problems that can result in severe upper airway obstruction.

**Table 4-3** compares four of the most common infectious causes of upper airway obstruction.

### Table 4-3  Common Infectious Causes of Upper Airway Obstruction

| Characteristic | Croup | Epiglottitis | Bacterial Tracheitis | Retropharyngeal Abscess |
| --- | --- | --- | --- | --- |
| Onset | Gradual, viral prodrome, 1-7 days | Rapid onset, 6-12 hours | Viral prodrome followed by rapid deterioration | Viral prodrome followed by rapid deterioration |
| Typical age at onset | 6 months-4 years | 2-8 years | 6 months-8 years | <5 years |
| Seasonal occurrence | Late fall-winter | Throughout the year | Fall-winter | Throughout the year |
| Causative agents | Parainfluenza, respiratory syncytial virus, influenza A | *Haemophilus influenzae* type B (classically), *Streptococcus pneumoniae*, GABHS | *Staphylococcus aureus* (classically), GABHS, *Streptococcus pneumoniae* | Anaerobic bacteria, GABHS, *Staphylococcus aureus* |
| Pathology | Subglottic edema | Inflammatory edema of supraglottis | Thick, mucopurulent, membranous tracheal secretions | Abscess formation in deep cervical fascia |
| Fever | Low grade | High | High | High |
| Cough | Barking or seal-like | None | Usually absent | Usually absent |
| Sore throat | None | Severe | None | Severe |
| Drooling | None | Frequent | None | Frequent |
| Posture | Any | Sitting forward, mouth open, neck extended (tripod position) | Any | Sitting forward, mouth open, neck extended (tripod position) |
| Voice | Normal or hoarse | Muffled | Normal or hoarse | Muffled |
| Appearance | Nontoxic | Toxic | Toxic | Toxic |

GABHS, group A β-hemolytic streptococci

### 1. Viral Laryngotracheobronchitis (Croup)

Viral laryngotracheobronchitis (croup) is the most common infectious cause of upper airway obstruction in children, primarily affecting children aged 6 months to 4 years, with a peak incidence between 1 and 2 years of age in North America. Cases of croup can be seen throughout the year, with a peak incidence during fall and early winter. It is most commonly caused by parainfluenza virus type 1, though types 2 and 3, *H influenzae* types A and B, RSV, adenovirus, and *Mycoplasma pneumoniae* may all cause croup. Most children are managed as outpatients, but some do require hospitalization, and about 1% of hospitalized children require tracheal intubation and mechanical ventilation. Children with croup usually present after several days of prodromal viral-like symptoms (cough, coryza, rhinorrhea, low-grade fever) with progressively worsening hoarseness, eventually developing a classic seal-like, barky cough and stridor. Stridor is classically inspiratory but may be biphasic, indicating airway edema that extends beyond the subglottic space into the intrathoracic trachea and bronchi. Radiographs of the airway (**Figure 4-3**) may demonstrate a classic steeple sign (narrowing of the subglottic trachea coming to a point at the level of the vocal cords). Lateral neck films in croup may show dilatation of the airway above the level of the vocal cords.

**Figure 4-3.** Laryngotracheobronchitis (Croup)

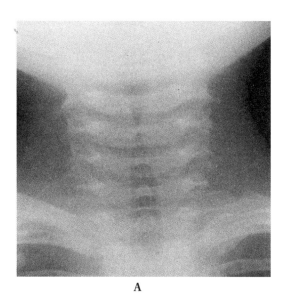 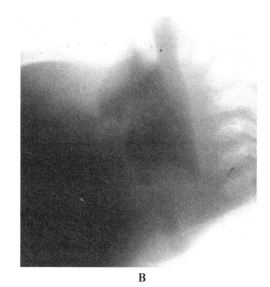

A                                                                                           B

**A**, Anteroposterior radiograph demonstrating narrowing of the airway in a steeple-like manner that is characteristic of viral laryngotracheobronchitis. **B**, A lateral neck radiograph of a patient with viral croup shows a sharp epiglottis, characteristic dilation of the airspace above the level of the vocal cords, and narrowing of the subglottic air column. Courtesy of Terry L. Levin, MD, Children's Hospital at Montefiore Medical Center, New York, New York, USA.

Croup is generally self-limiting and requires only supportive care with cool mist and intravenous (IV) fluids if a patient is unable to drink. Nebulized racemic epinephrine rapidly reduces airway edema and improves symptoms. The reduction in edema is limited by the lifetime of the drug, however, and symptoms usually return within 2 hours. Corticosteroids have been shown to bring about significant improvement and are prescribed routinely. Heliox may be helpful, as described later in this chapter. Nasal CPAP and BiPAP have been used with some success and may hold off tracheal intubation. In the event that intubation is required, a smaller than normal tube size should be used, and the patient should remain intubated until an air leak develops around the tube. The treatment of croup is summarized in **Table 4-4**.

### 2. Epiglottitis (Supraglottitis, Panglottitis)

Epiglottitis is a true emergency. Though it is rare due to widespread use of the Hib vaccine, having knowledge of this life-threatening infection is still very important. The name implies involvement of only the epiglottis, but because all of the supraglottic structures can be involved, the term *supraglottitis* or *panglottitis* is more correct. Historically, epiglottitis was most commonly caused by *H influenzae* type B and was associated with

**Table 4-4** Treatment of Croup

1. Minimize situations that may cause distress in the child, such as separation from parents and unnecessary examination and procedures.
2. Provide blow-by oxygen if desaturation or cyanosis is present.
3. Give oral, intramuscular, or intravenous dexamethasone, 0.6 mg/kg.
4. Administer nebulized racemic epinephrine (adrenaline), 2.25%, 0.5 mL in 2.5 mL saline.
5. If the response is good, observe the patient for 2 hours.
6. If the response is poor or if stridor rapidly recurs, admit the patient to the ICU for observation.
7. Consider heliox 60:40 or 70:30 mixture.
8. Consider nasal continuous positive airway pressure or bilevel positive airway pressure.
9. If intubation is required, select a tube that is smaller than normal for the patient's age.

bacteremia and severe toxicity. However, in the era of widespread Hib vaccination, *Streptococcus pneumoniae*, group A β-hemolytic streptococci (GABHS), and *Staphylococcus aureus* are more common causes.

Children with supraglottitis usually present with rapidly progressive signs and symptoms, including high fever, irritability, drooling, dysphagia, dyspnea, and dysphonia. These children appear toxic and prefer to rest in the tripod position. Stridor occurs late in the course and is usually softer than the loud stridor that occurs with croup. A lateral neck radiograph can be obtained if the suspicion of epiglottitis is relatively low but cannot be totally ruled out; however, it should be deferred if it increases the child's level of anxiety or will delay definitive diagnosis and management. If epiglottitis is present, on lateral view, the epiglottis appears rounded, large, and thumb-shaped in comparison to a normal epiglottis, which is sharp (**Figure 4-4**).

**Figure 4-4.** Radiographs of Healthy Patient and Patient with Epiglottitis

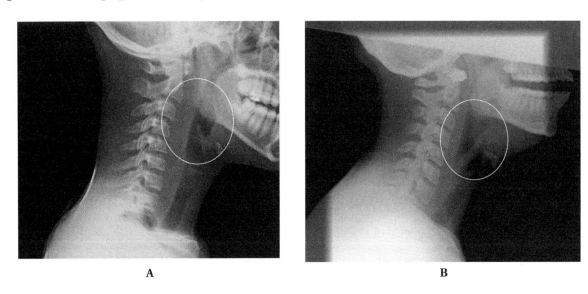

**A**, Healthy patient shows a sharply defined epiglottis (circled). **B**, Patient with epiglottitis demonstrates an edematous, less clearly defined, thumb-like epiglottis (circled), as well as edema of the aryepiglottic folds and other supraglottic tissues consistent with supraglottitis.
Courtesy of Terry L. Levin, MD, Children's Hospital at Montefiore Medical Center, New York, New York, USA.

Even if the likelihood of epiglottitis is low, a healthcare provider trained in airway support and bag-mask ventilation must accompany a child sent to the radiology department for lateral neck radiographs. If epiglottitis is suspected based on history and physical exam, the patient should not be sent to radiology but should instead be brought to the operating room, accompanied by a physician skilled in airway management together and all necessary airway support equipment. The management of suspected epiglottitis is summarized in **Table 4-5**.

| Table 4-5 | Epiglottitis |

- Low suspicion of epiglottitis → Send patient to radiology for lateral neck radiographs
- High suspicion of epiglottitis → Send patient to operating room for direct examination under anesthesia and intubation
- Whether suspicion is low or high, the patient should be:
  - Accompanied by a physician skilled in airway management
  - Kept in a comfortable position
  - Transported with a bag-mask ventilator, with a mask of appropriate size and, if possible, a positive end-expiratory pressure valve

All noxious interventions, such as IV insertion, blood work, and examination of the pharynx, should be deferred until the child is asleep in the operating room and the airway has been secured by tracheal intubation. The child should be permitted to remain in a position of comfort while being transported and during mask induction of anesthesia. Ensure the child is spontaneously breathing under anesthesia before visualizing the larynx via direct laryngoscopy. Tracheal intubation is performed if epiglottitis is confirmed. The endotracheal tube should be secured well before transfer to the intensive care unit. An IV should be inserted and blood work obtained, as well as cultures from the epiglottis, tracheal secretions, and blood. Broad-spectrum antibiotics effective against β-lactamase-producing organisms should be administered. Antibiotic choices include second- and third-generation cephalosporins such as cefuroxime or ceftriaxone or, alternatively, ampicillin-sulbactam. Improvement is usually rapid once antibiotics are started. The patient can be extubated when an audible air leak develops around the tracheal tube.

### 3. Bacterial Tracheitis

Bacterial tracheitis, a relatively rare but potentially life-threatening cause of upper airway obstruction in children, is one of the most common causes of pediatric airway emergencies requiring admission to the intensive care unit. In bacterial tracheitis, thick mucopurulent membranous secretions obstruct the airway and cannot be cleared by cough. Hence, tracheal intubation is usually required. Children typically present with a viral prodrome of several days duration that develops into a croup-like illness with low-grade fever, cough, and stridor. This illness then worsens rapidly, and the patient develops high fever, signs of increasing respiratory distress, inability to clear secretions, and a toxic appearance. Radiographic imaging shows a croup-associated steeple sign. The similarity of the prodromes of croup and bacterial tracheitis has led to an impression that bacterial tracheitis is a bacterial superinfection of viral croup. Data from the U.S., Australia, and Great Britain confirm that bacterial tracheitis affects children aged 6 months to 8 years, with a peak incidence during the fall and winter, corresponding to the viral respiratory season.

Children who present to an emergency department with bacterial tracheitis may be indistinguishable from those with epiglottitis and therefore should be managed according to a suspected epiglottitis protocol. Direct inspection of the airway usually reveals subglottic edema with ulcerations, erythema, and pseudomembrane formation in the trachea. Historically, *S aureus* is the most common causative agent, but *S pneumoniae*, GABHS, and viruses have also been identified. On occasion, a patient who has been in an intensive care unit with croup-like symptoms will acutely worsen and require tracheal intubation, resulting in copious thick secretions that come up through the tracheal tube and lend support to a diagnosis of bacterial tracheitis.

Pulmonary and tracheal toilet, tracheal intubation, and broad-spectrum antibiotics directed against *Staphylococcus* and *Streptococcus* species are the basics of treatment. A second-generation cephalosporin, such as cefuroxime, is a reasonable choice of antibiotic. Extubation may be attempted following clinical improvement and development of an air leak around the tracheal tube. This may take 3 to 5 days.

### 4. Retropharyngeal Abscess (Parapharyngeal Abscess)

Retropharyngeal abscess is an infection of the soft tissues of the posterior pharyngeal wall. The retropharyngeal space consists of a loose network of connective tissue and lymph nodes that drain the nasopharynx, paranasal sinuses, middle ear, teeth, and facial bones. Infection and abscess formation in this area usually result from lymphatic spread of infection or direct spread from the nasopharynx, paranasal sinuses, or middle ear. These lymph nodes atrophy during early childhood, thus decreasing the risk of disease in older children and adolescents. For this reason, direct trauma to the posterior pharynx from a pencil or stick in the mouth and ingestion of foreign bodies account for the majority of cases in older children and adolescents. Most cases occur in children younger than 5 years, thereby overlapping the most common ages for epiglottitis and bacterial tracheitis.

Children with retropharyngeal abscesses have a nonspecific collection of symptoms that eventually coalesce as high fever, sore throat, and stiff neck. Symptoms are similar to those of epiglottitis, and physical exam may reveal a bulging unilateral neck mass. Neck stiffness may mimic that seen in meningitis. Diagnosis may be confirmed by the presence of an increased prevertebral soft tissue space on lateral neck radiograph (**Figure 4-5**). The radiograph may also show the presence of gas or air fluid levels in the retropharyngeal space as well as loss of the normal cervical lordosis. Retropharyngeal abscess is usually a polymicrobial infection. The cultures often yield anaerobic organisms such as *Prevotella, Porphyromonas, Fusobacterium,* and *Peptostreptococcus*. Additionally, *S aureus*, GABHS, and *H influenzae* may be identified.

**Figure 4-5.** Retropharyngeal Abscess

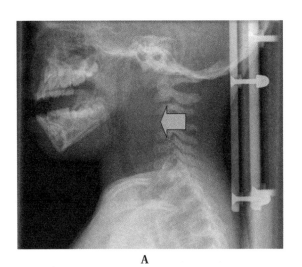 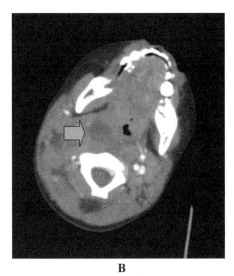

A                                                                                                B

**A**, Arrow on radiograph points to a widened distance between the air column and the anterior aspect of the spinal column (prevertebral space). **B**, Arrow on computed tomography image points to a retropharyngeal abscess.
Courtesy of Terry L. Levin, MD, Children's Hospital at Montefiore Medical Center, New York, New York, USA.

Management of retropharyngeal abscess includes close observation and broad-spectrum antibiotics that have anaerobic coverage. Abscess drainage is recommended for cases refractory to antibiotics. Complications are rare with early recognition and appropriate antibiotic treatment, but serious complications include rupture of the abscess into the posterior pharynx (resulting in aspiration of infectious material), lateral spread of infection, and dissection into the posterior mediastinum through fascial planes. Deaths have been reported.

### 5. Peritonsillar Abscess (Quinsy)

Peritonsillar abscess (quinsy) is the most common deep-space infection of the head and neck tissues in children. It results from direct contiguous spread of infection from the tonsils. Older children and adolescents are most commonly affected without seasonal preference. Children with peritonsillar abscess have sore throat, neck pain, pain with swallowing or dysphagia, and fever. Physical exam reveals enlargement of the cervical lymph nodes, uvular deviation, and muffled ("hot potato") voice. Treatment options include broad-spectrum antibiotics, needle aspiration with opening of the abscess, incision and drainage, and tonsillectomy. Complications include extension of the infection, rarely acute upper airway obstruction, and rupture of the abscess with aspiration of purulent material.

### 6. Infectious Mononucleosis

Infectious mononucleosis is a triad of fever, lymphadenopathy, and tonsillar pharyngitis. It may lead to acute upper airway obstruction due to the enlargement of tonsils and adenoids. Fortunately, this complication, which tends to occur in younger children, is rare. Oral or parenteral corticosteroids may be helpful. Tracheal intubation or noninvasive positive-pressure ventilation (NPPV) by CPAP or BiPAP may be required.

### 7. Miscellaneous Disorders

#### a. Airway Trauma

Traumatic injury to the upper airway may be caused by foreign bodies, thermal or chemical injury, or direct blunt or penetrating trauma. Foreign body aspiration is a leading cause of accidental death and severe neurologic impairment in young children. Infants are at significant risk of foreign body aspiration due to their tendency to put any and all objects into their mouths. Many aspirated foreign bodies pass through the vocal cords and become lodged in the distal airways. Any foreign body that becomes lodged in the larynx is life-threatening. A high index of suspicion is always necessary in that an actual aspiration event is frequently not identified. Children with a history of choking and respiratory distress should undergo immediate rigid bronchoscopy for diagnosis and treatment.

Life-threatening airway obstruction may develop as a result of inhalation injury, laryngeal burns, or caustic ingestions. Any child with a scald injury to the face or neck should be evaluated by bronchoscopy for potential inhalational injury. Inhalation injury should be suspected in children with evidence of soot in sputum or vomitus, singed nasal hairs, facial burns, lip burns, wheezing, stridor, or extensive surface burns. Early endoscopic evaluation is helpful for determining the presence and extent of airway injury. Management of the airway includes early tracheal intubation because airway burns tend to worsen with edema for several days before they begin to resolve (**Chapter 10**).

Blunt injury to the neck can cause edema and hematoma formation that can result in acute upper airway obstruction. Penetrating injury is less common in children. Imaging and surgical consultation are necessary.

### b. Post-extubation Airway Obstruction

Patients who are intubated sometimes develop signs and symptoms of airway obstruction upon extubation, referred to as *post-extubation stridor*. This condition is related to several factors, including preexisting tracheal irritation from gastroesophageal reflux disease, an inappropriately sized tracheal tube, traumatic intubation, the duration of intubation, global body edema, and a loosely secured endotracheal tube. Post-extubation stridor is often self-limited, resolving over 12 to 24 hours, but may also require interventions as described later in this chapter. Reintubation is necessary on some occasions. Assessment and treatment is similar to that of viral croup. Dexamethasone may be administered both as treatment and as pre-extubation prophylaxis if there is suspicion that post-extubation airway obstruction may occur. Repeated episodes of post-extubation airway obstruction requiring reintubation and prolonged stridor after extubation are indications for bronchoscopy.

### c. Angioedema

Angioedema is an immunologically mediated acute edema that may result in acute upper airway obstruction. It may affect the larynx; tissues of the head, neck, face, and lips; tongue; and pharynx. Angioedema most often occurs as an allergic reaction to food or medication, upper respiratory infection, or insect sting. IV corticosteroids, antihistamines, and intramuscular (IM) epinephrine (adrenaline) usually will bring about rapid improvement in symptoms. In the event that medical interventions do not result in improvement or are not working rapidly enough, the airway should be secured in a child who demonstrates progressive signs and symptoms of acute upper airway obstruction.

### d. Spasmodic Croup

Spasmodic croup is probably an allergic disease, not caused by infection. The infant typically wakes with sudden onset of respiratory distress, inspiratory stridor, and a loud, croupy cough. There may be a mild intercurrent upper respiratory illness, and there is often a family history of asthma or allergies. The episodes may recur on successive nights. By the time the patient reaches the hospital, symptoms have usually resolved. The family often reports that symptoms abated in the cool night air. Dysphagia, drooling, high fever, and a toxic appearance are all absent in spasmodic croup.

# IV. PHYSICAL FINDINGS AND ASSESSMENT

## A. History

A brief history and careful physical exam will provide much of the information necessary to reach a diagnosis. Emergent intervention must take precedence when a child appears in severe distress from airway obstruction.

The duration of symptoms and their rapidity of onset are key areas on which to focus. Children with viral croup often have symptoms of upper respiratory infection for ≥1 days prior to the onset of stridor. Airway obstruction due to foreign body aspiration has an almost instantaneous onset. Epiglottitis has an acute onset, with fever and distress appearing without prodrome. Retropharyngeal and parapharyngeal abscesses typically cause upper airway obstruction after several days of sore throat and related symptoms. A history of intubation in the neonatal intensive care unit may precede a presentation of subglottic stenosis.

Additional points to cover in a history include: whether distress is stable or worsening; whether symptoms are intermittent or persistent; whether positional changes affect symptoms; presence or absence of fever; history of trauma or exposure to allergen, smoke, chemical vapors, or steam; changes in voice quality; report of choking episode or possible foreign body aspiration.

## B. Observation and Appearance

The degree of distress and severity of airway obstruction can often be ascertained by observation. Audible stridor indicates turbulent airflow through narrowed passages, but airflow is nonetheless present. Infants and young children with partial upper airway problems may appear calm, whereas older children and adults with partial airway obstruction will be agitated and extremely fearful. Some children, especially those with chronic airway obstruction, appear surprisingly at ease considering the difficulty they have breathing. Observe for accessory muscle use. Children who have been breathing against partially obstructed airways for several years often develop visible hypertrophy of accessory muscles of inspiration.

> *The degree of distress and severity of airway obstruction can often be ascertained by observation.*

> *Children with acute airway-related processes often adopt a position of comfort in order to maximize airway patency and airflow.*

Children with acute airway-related processes often adopt a position of comfort in order to maximize airway patency and airflow. It is important to appreciate this positioning and attempt to maintain it. For example, a child who seems most comfortable in a caregiver's arms should not be removed. The most comfortable position is usually upright, and a patient may vigorously resist being moved out of this position. Moving children out of the position of comfort may induce unnecessary fear and worsen the degree of airway obstruction. As discussed earlier, increasing respiratory effort against an upper airway obstruction will result in tracheal collapse and worsening of obstruction. Thus, a patient with signs and symptoms of upper airway obstruction should be kept as calm as possible. Sedating a child with partial upper airway obstruction before intubation or positioning a patient to facilitate laryngoscopy may also result in complete airway obstruction.

> *Sedating a child with partial upper airway obstruction before intubation or positioning a patient to facilitate laryngoscopy may result in complete airway obstruction.*

A tripod position, in which a child sits upright and leans forward on outstretched arms, is a sign of upper airway obstruction. By leaning forward, the patient tries to relieve upper airway obstruction by using gravity to move enlarged tonsils, redundant pharyngeal tissue, or an edematous epiglottis forward and away from the airway, thus opening an air passage. A component of the tripod posture is the forward jutting of the jaw, which is an attempt by the patient to perform a jaw-thrust maneuver that will move pharyngeal contents anteriorly.

In laryngomalacia, the epiglottis is long and soft and closes in over the laryngeal inlet with inspiration. Given that the epiglottis is an anterior component of the larynx, placing an infant in a prone position permits gravity to move the epiglottis out of the airway. Frequently an infant with laryngomalacia breathes more easily when placed in a prone position rather than a supine position.

A listless appearance may indicate fatigue and signify impending respiratory or cardiac arrest. Observe for cyanosis. Listen for the quality of cough or voice, as it can guide the diagnosis.

## C. Physical Examination

The physical exam should focus on the quantity and quality of airflow. Inspiration and expiration are normally quiet. Noise, accessory muscle use, and an appearance of unease indicate the presence of a pathologic situation. Inspiratory noise that emanates from the nose or pharynx is called *stertor*. Partial nasal obstruction, tonsillar-adenoidal hypertrophy (infectious and noninfectious), and peritonsillar and parapharyngeal abscesses may all cause this sound. Noise cannot occur without air movement. The absence or disappearance of respiratory noise may indicate resolution of the abnormality or conversion to complete upper airway obstruction.

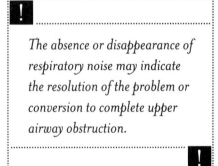

*The absence or disappearance of respiratory noise may indicate the resolution of the problem or conversion to complete upper airway obstruction.*

### 1. Inspiratory and Expiratory Noises

Inspiratory noise is characteristic of airway disorders from the nose to the subglottic, but extrathoracic, space. The presence of an expiratory component indicates that the process extends to the airways of the chest as well. For example, viral laryngotracheobronchitis may affect the airway from the level of the subglottic space (extrathoracic) to the bronchi (intrathoracic). The edema and mucous accumulation associated with severe croup may thus cause both inspiratory stridor from involvement of the extrathoracic airway and an expiratory component from involvement of the intrathoracic airways. Laryngomalacia involving the epiglottis, arytenoid cartilages, and laryngeal structures is extrathoracic and causes inspiratory noise. Tracheomalacia, in which the tracheal tissue is prone to collapse, may involve both intrathoracic and extrathoracic parts of the trachea. The extrathoracic trachea is prone to collapse with inspiration, whereas involved intrathoracic areas are prone to collapse with expiration, thus accounting for a characteristic biphasic stridor seen in severe tracheomalacia.

Stridor is a raspy, higher-pitched noise that is caused by air moving through narrowed passages of the supraglottic, glottic, and subglottic spaces. Stridor occurs most commonly with inspiration but may occur during expiration. It is most often associated with viral croup, subglottic stenosis, epiglottitis, and post-extubation airway edema. Stridor may be present at rest or during agitation.

When airway edema is treated with nebulized racemic epinephrine (adrenaline), stridor may disappear and then return when the medication wears off.

Children and infants who are large enough to move sufficient amounts of air often manifest a characteristic barky or seal-like cough with viral croup. Sufficient airflow is required for a cough to be present, and thus absence of cough is not necessarily reassuring. Small infants with viral croup may not manifest a classical croupy cough.

Peritonsillar abscess is associated with a "hot potato voice," which occurs due to pain and edema in the peritonsillar tissues that make it difficult to enunciate clearly.

Noisy stertorous sounds are usually associated with obstruction in the nose or retropharynx. In patients who can open their mouths, it may be possible to see obstructing tonsillar tissue or an exudative pharyngitis associated with infectious mononucleosis. It is unwise to persist at trying to open the mouth of a child who resists doing so. A tongue blade should not be used to examine the pharynx of a child with suspected epiglottitis because of the risk of converting a partial upper airway obstruction into a complete obstruction.

Auscultation over the nares can determine the presence or absence of airflow. High-pitched sounds over the throat indicate narrowing of the air passage. During auscultation of the chest, careful attention should be paid to whether adventitious sounds are inspiratory, expiratory, or both, and to which component is louder. Sounds related to the trachea and bronchi will be louder centrally, whereas small, distal airway-related sounds will be more prominent in the peripheral chest.

### 2. Fever

The presence of fever depends on the etiology of the airway disease. Congenital and acquired disorders, such as laryngomalacia and subglottic stenosis, are not associated with fever. Viral laryngotracheobronchitis is infectious in etiology, and a low-grade fever may be present. High fevers are usually associated with bacterial infections of the airway, such as parapharyngeal abscess, epiglottitis, and bacterial tracheitis.

## D. Measurements and Imaging

Pulse oximetry is neither threatening nor painful and is useful in assessing a patient with acute upper airway disease. Acceptable oxygen saturation indicates that even in the presence of clinically visible distress, gas exchange is sufficient to provide an adequate amount of oxygen to the bloodstream. A drop in oxygen saturation may suggest a worsening of obstruction or the development of muscle fatigue and impending respiratory arrest.

Upper airway diseases do not usually affect the regions of the lungs responsible for gas exchange, but if airway obstruction limits gas flow to the extent that inadequate oxygen reaches the alveoli, the patient will manifest desaturation. Another mechanism of desaturation is ventilation-perfusion mismatch from atelectasis that develops

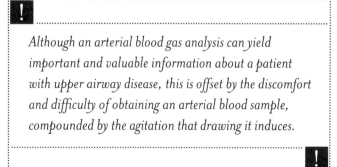

*Although an arterial blood gas analysis can yield important and valuable information about a patient with upper airway disease, this is offset by the discomfort and difficulty of obtaining an arterial blood sample, compounded by the agitation that drawing it induces.*

when unrelieved inspiratory effort against an obstruction leads to respiratory muscle fatigue. The work of breathing and the oxygen consumption necessary to support the diaphragm and accessory muscles of inspiration can be tremendous when a patient breathes against a partially obstructed airway. The inability to meet the demand for oxygen in the face of inadequate gas flow ultimately results in anaerobic metabolism and lactic acidosis.

Although an arterial blood gas analysis can yield important and valuable information about a patient with upper airway disease, this is offset by the discomfort and difficulty of obtaining an arterial blood sample, compounded by the agitation that drawing it induces. One of the prime directives of managing a patient with upper airway obstruction is to limit noxious stimuli, and blood gas measurement in the absence of an indwelling arterial line is noxious.

Sidestream end-tidal $CO_2$ sampled via nasal cannula can be helpful in assessing ventilation adequacy in a patient with upper airway obstruction. However, the necessary devices are not widely available.

Radiographic imaging, when safe for a patient with a compromised airway, can yield helpful information. Anteroposterior and lateral neck views with filtering to gain increased soft tissue resolution may potentially show:

- Narrowing in the subglottic space consistent with viral croup (steeple sign) (**Figure 4-3**)
- Radio-opaque foreign bodies
- Enlarged, edematous epiglottis (thumb-print sign) consistent with epiglottitis (**Figure 4-4**)
- Hypertrophied adenoidal and tonsillar tissue
- Abnormally wide retropharyngeal or prevertebral tissues consistent with mass or with retropharyngeal or parapharyngeal abscess (**Figure 4-5**)

For comparison, films of a patient with normal airway anatomy are shown in **Figure 4-6**. Plain view radiographs of the chest can show a deviated or narrowed tracheal air column, compressed or narrowed bronchi, or the presence of atelectasis or pneumonia. More advanced imaging of the airways by techniques such as fluoroscopy and computerized tomographic scanning with 3D reconstruction can also yield important information. The stability of the patient and the maintenance of the airway must be given top priority in planning all radiographic imaging.

> *For distressed patients of all ages with upper airway problems, the safest and most effective approach to diagnosis begins with monitored transfer to an operating room or intensive care unit.*

The safest and most effective approach to diagnosis begins with monitored transfer to an operating room or intensive care unit for a distressed patient with an upper airway obstruction. Skilled personnel in these locations can perform a careful examination of the airway by direct laryngoscopy or bronchoscopy. A multidisciplinary approach to management of upper airway obstruction should be the standard operating procedure in any facility that cares for children.

**Figure 4-6.** Normal Airway

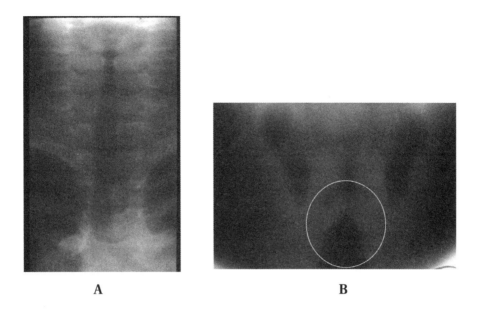

**A**, An anteroposterior radiograph of a normal tracheal airway shows a widely patent air column with some narrowing at the level of the vocal cords. **B**, An airway tomogram demonstrates a widely patent tracheal air column to the level of the vocal cords (circled), showing the typical "shoulders" seen in a normal airway.
Courtesy of Terry L. Levin, MD, Children's Hospital at Montefiore Medical Center, New York, New York, USA.

Several clinical scoring tools are available to assist in assessing the severity of croup. The Westley croup scoring system has been extensively studied and validated. The scoring rubric (**Table 4-6**) is based on the presence and extent of inspiratory stridor, retractions, air entry, and cyanosis, and on the patient's mental status. A Westley croup score lower than 3 suggests mild disease, a score of 3 to 6 indicates moderate disease, and a score higher than 6 represents severe disease.

### Table 4-6  Westley Croup Score

| Finding | 0 | 1 | 2 | 3 | 4 | 5 |
|---|---|---|---|---|---|---|
| Stridor | None | With agitation | At rest | | | |
| Retractions | None | Mild | Moderate | Severe | | |
| Air Entry | Normal | Mild decrease | Marked decrease | | | |
| Cyanosis | None | | | | With agitation | At rest |
| Level of Consciousness | Normal | | | | | Depressed |

**3 points: Mild disease**
**4-6 points: Moderate disease**
**>6 points: Severe disease**

# V. MANAGEMENT OF ACUTE UPPER AIRWAY DISEASE

Patients with upper airway obstruction will appear frightened, anxious, and very uncomfortable. The degree of interventions should be proportional to the level of distress and severity of the patient's clinical condition. For example, an infant with mild to moderate viral croup is comfortable in the caregiver's arms with blow-by humidified oxygen and can tolerate oral intake; arterial blood gas analysis, extensive blood testing, or an IV or fluid is not needed. In upper airway disorders, anxiety and agitation may worsen a patient's clinical condition. Interventions should be carried out in progressive steps from least to most invasive. In general, it is best to do the least, keeping in mind that definitive action may be required in some circumstances and cannot be delayed.

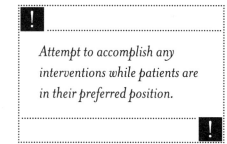

*Attempt to accomplish any interventions while patients are in their preferred position.*

Children should be allowed to find a position of comfort that maximizes their ability to maintain a patent airway. Attempt to accomplish any interventions while patients are in their preferred position. Children with epiglottitis are often in their caregivers' arms, positioned with their chins up and jutted forward in a spontaneous jaw-thrust position. This will maintain a patent airway in the presence of a swollen epiglottis. One general approach to such patients is to keep them in their caregivers' arms until they are brought to the operating room for mask induction and intubation.

Find a position that maximizes airflow and minimizes obstruction in a patient with a decreased level of consciousness. An infant with disorders of the chin and tongue, such as Pierre Robin sequence, may have a completely obstructed airway when lying supine, but may be able to breathe easily in a prone position. Align the oral, pharyngeal, and tracheal axes in a spontaneously breathing patient to maintain airway patency. As described in **Chapter 2**, the airway axes can be lined up by placing a small roll under the shoulders of an infant or under the occiput of an older child, followed by careful neck flexion to place the patient in the sniffing position. Monitor the changes in airflow through the nose and mouth or watch the oxygen saturation to evaluate the efficiency of these maneuvers. Patients with severe tonsillar-adenoidal hypertrophy are usually able to move air more easily in an upright position.

Partial upper airway obstruction due to backward movement of the tongue and reduced hypopharyngeal tone occurs frequently in children with a decreased level of consciousness. It may be seen, for example, in a child who has sustained a closed head injury, is recovering from surgical anesthesia, or is undergoing procedural sedation. In the latter situation, administration of supplemental oxygen will delay desaturation by replacing the patient's functional residual capacity with oxygen, but oxygen alone will not be effective in the presence of airway obstruction. In sedation-induced airway obstruction, open the patient's airway by a chin-lift or jaw-thrust maneuver, which is more effective in improving oxygen saturation than supplemental oxygen. After the

*In sedation-induced airway obstruction, opening the airway by means of chin lift, jaw thrust, or a combination of both will be more effective than supplemental oxygen in reversing oxygen desaturation.*

airway is opened, oxygen saturation will usually rise quickly provided the patient is not apneic. Maintaining airway patency by means of chin-lift and jaw-thrust maneuvers is a skill that all healthcare providers involved with caring for seriously ill children should possess. These maneuvers are discussed in detail in **Chapter 2**.

## A. Medical Interventions

### 1. Heliox

Helium-oxygen mixtures, known as heliox, are extremely useful when any form of obstruction limits airflow. Heliox comes in 60:40, 70:30, and 80:20 helium-oxygen percentage mixtures. It can be administered by non-rebreather face mask or nasal cannula. A significant improvement in comfort is often seen upon initiation of heliox therapy. The oxygen concentration is not high; with an 80:20 mixture, it is actually below the oxygen concentration of room air. Thus, heliox alone may not be adequate if a patient has a significant oxygen requirement due to parenchymal lung disease.

Heliox is effective because it is less dense than either oxygen or air and has a more laminar flow. When airways become narrowed by edema, compression, or anatomic abnormality, the gas flow becomes turbulent due to abrupt changes in velocity. In croup, airflow becomes turbulent due to constriction in the subglottic space.

Heliox is a very light, leaky gas owing to the same properties that make it work for airway problems. The use of a tight-fitting face mask and secure connections will ensure adequate delivery.

### 2. Racemic Epinephrine (Adrenaline)

Racemic epinephrine (adrenaline) (2.25% by nebulizer), frequently used as a topical vasoconstrictor in the management of stridor, is usually effective in post-extubation stridor. For children younger than 4 years, the dose is 0.05 mL/kg mixed with 3 mL normal saline and administered by nebulizer every 2 to 4 hours. For children >4 years, the dose is 0.5 mL mixed with 3 mL normal saline administered every 2 to 3 hours. The maximum dose is 0.5 mL every 1 to 2 hours. Onset of action can be expected in 1 to 5 minutes, and the effect may last 1 to 3 hours. Although racemic epinephrine is usually prescribed for croup, it can be used for any upper airway disorder in which tissue edema may be a contributing factor. Rebound stridor may occur in 2 to 3 hours and has been reported as a reason for hospital admission in children who receive racemic epinephrine in the emergency department. The subglottic narrowing of viral croup is of longer duration than the half-life of racemic epinephrine.

There is little information about the use of continuous nebulized racemic epinephrine, but if a patient with a complicated airway is showing some clinical response, continuous nebulized treatments may be helpful.

### 3. Dexamethasone

Dexamethasone administered orally or parenterally has been shown to be effective in viral laryngotracheobronchitis. The literature provides a dose of 0.6 mg/kg given once. For post-extubation airway edema, the dosing is 0.5 to 2 mg/kg/day IM or IV divided every 6 hours. Dexamethasone can be used to prevent post-extubation stridor by administering it 24 hours before extubation and continuing for 4 to 6 doses after extubation.

### 4. Noninvasive Positive-Pressure Ventilation

NPPV by either CPAP or BiPAP may be useful in cases of upper airway obstruction. The addition of positive pressure to the airways can decrease the amount of extrathoracic tracheal collapse that occurs when a patient attempts to inhale against a partial obstruction. Those with upper airway obstruction due to tonsillar-adenoidal hypertrophy can experience significant relief through the use of NPPV. Although NPPV may be beneficial, it may also force secretions down into the trachea and inhibit their clearance.

In cases of severe inspiratory difficulty, complete airway obstruction, or respiratory arrest, it is usually possible to support a patient by means of bag-mask ventilation. Effective ventilation may be difficult to achieve with obstruction. Healthcare providers must maintain an open airway. It may be more effective to perform 2-person bag-mask ventilation (**Chapter 2**); one person can ensure the mask is tightly sealed on the patient's face while the other can compress the bag to ensure adequate chest rise. The addition of a positive end-expiratory pressure valve to the bag-mask ventilator provides a means to prevent end-exhalation airway collapse and may facilitate ventilation.

Direct laryngoscopy should be considered in a patient suspected of foreign body aspiration who has not responded to basic life support.

> *Racemic Epinephrine*
> 2.25% administered by nebulizer
> <4 years old: 0.05 mL/kg mixed with 3 mL normal saline every 2–4 hours
> ≥4 years old: 0.5 mL mixed with 3 mL normal saline every 2–4 hours
> Maximum dose: 0.5 mL every 1–2 hours
> Onset of action: 1–5 minutes
> Duration of action: 1–3 hours
> Possible rebound: 2–3 hours
>
> *Dexamethasone*
> Viral croup → 0.6 mg/kg (PO, IM, IV) once
> Post-extubation stridor → 0.5–2 mg/kg/day IM or IV divided every 6 hours; start 24 hours before extubation and continue for 4–6 doses after extubation

# VI. ACUTE LOWER AIRWAY DISEASE

### Case Study

A 5-year-old girl with a history of asthma since she was 2 years old is brought to the emergency department with worsening tachypnea and wheezing despite frequent albuterol inhalation treatments at home. Her vital signs are as follows: heart rate, 135 beats/min; respiratory rate, 40 breaths/min; and pulse oximetry, 89% on room air. She appears anxious. On auscultation she has bilateral inspiratory and expiratory wheezes with intercostal retractions. She is given an albuterol nebulizer treatment followed by oxygen by face mask. You are asked to assist in her management.

**Detection**
- What is the diagnosis?
- What is her physiologic state?
- Is she in respiratory distress or respiratory failure?

**Intervention**
- What are the next interventions?

**Reassessment**
- How do you assess her response to therapy?
- How should she be monitored?

**Effective Communication**
- What will be your instructions to the primary care team with respect to signs of worsening clinical condition?
- For what should they call you back to reassess the patient?

**Teamwork**
- How are you going to implement the treatment strategy?
- Who is to do what and when?

Respiratory failure is the inability of the pulmonary system to meet the metabolic needs of the body. The pulmonary system is involved in two crucial metabolic roles: elimination of $CO_2$ and oxygenation of the blood. There are three forms of respiratory failure: hypoxemic, hypercapnic, and mixed. Hypoxemic respiratory failure is defined by a room air $Pao_2$ ≤60 mm Hg (≤8.0 kPa). It may be caused by:

- Ventilation-perfusion mismatch
- Decreased diffusion of oxygen across the alveolocapillary membrane
- Alveolar hypoventilation
- High altitude or other causes of low inspired oxygen tension

Hypercapnic respiratory failure is defined by $Paco_2$ ≥50 mm Hg (>6.7kPa) with an accompanying acidosis (pH <7.35). It may be caused by:

- Decreased tidal volume
- Decreased respiratory rate
- Increased physiologic dead space
- Increased $CO_2$ production, which rarely produces significant hypercapnia

In both of these types of respiratory failure, hypoxemia is present to some degree. The diagnosis of respiratory failure by arterial blood gas analysis may not be readily available at the first encounter with the ill child, so the clinician may need to rely on the clinical indicators (**Table 4-7**).

| Table 4-7 | Clinical Indicators of Respiratory Failure |
|---|---|

- Marked tachypnea (respiratory rate >60 breaths/min abnormal at any age)
- Bradypnea and/or apnea
- Cyanosis
- Worsening oxygen saturations despite intervention
- Tachycardia or bradycardia
- Poor or absent distal air movement
- Lethargy, stupor, and coma

# VII. MANAGEMENT OF RESPIRATORY FAILURE

The initial goal of the management of respiratory failure is the restoration and stabilization of ventilation and oxygenation. The interventions should focus on a rapid assessment of the type and severity of respiratory compromise rather than on the precise etiology. An action plan with direct management should follow, emphasizing the need for frequent reassessment of the response to treatment and the planning of further interventions as needed.

The most vital aspect of management is securing the patient's airway. While attempting to establish an airway, it may be necessary to assist ventilation with a bag-mask device (**Chapter 2**). Oxygen saturation, end-tidal $CO_2$, and cardiovascular monitoring should be implemented.

# VIII. CAUSES OF ACUTE RESPIRATORY FAILURE

Acute respiratory failure develops in a variety of clinical settings. In children, it typically results from diseases affecting the upper airway, lower airway, and lung parenchyma. All etiologies of upper and lower respiratory disease discussed in this chapter can result in respiratory failure. Diseases affecting other organ systems, including the cardiovascular and central nervous systems, may result in acute respiratory failure without respiratory distress.

## A. Asthma

### 1. Pathophysiology of Asthma

Asthma is an inflammatory disease that is manifested by air flow obstruction. This obstruction results from narrowing of the small and intermediate airways as a result of both bronchospasm (due to airway hyperresponsiveness) and mucosal edema with mucous plugging. Asthma is the most common chronic disease of childhood, is a leading cause of school absence, and accounts for a growing number of hospitalizations each year. Asthma exacerbations can be triggered by inhaled irritants (cigarette smoke), exercise, gastroesophageal reflux, allergen exposure, respiratory viral infections, and psychological stress. Airway obstruction results from the triad of smooth muscle spasm, mucosal inflammation, and mucous plugging. The obstruction and increased airway resistance due to bronchoconstriction and airway edema impede airflow (expiratory greater than inspiratory), resulting in air trapping, hyperinflation, and ventilation-perfusion (V/Q) mismatch. Pulmonary mechanics are further hampered by hyperinflation and flattening of the diaphragms. Expiration becomes an active process, requiring the use of accessory muscles. The increased work of breathing increases tissue oxygen demand which can't be satisfied in the face of hypoxemia from V/Q mismatch. These factors combine to result in tissue hypoxia, respiratory muscle fatigue, and respiratory failure.

## 2. Clinical Findings and Diagnosis of Asthma

Cough, dyspnea, and wheezing are the major clinical features in asthma, but the presentation varies with age. In some children, the presentation is persistent cough at night and during exercise. In others, shortness of breath may be the predominant symptom. In infants, the first asthmatic episode is frequently associated with viral infection. In older children, episodes are usually preceded by symptoms of upper respiratory tract infection (i.e., rhinorrhea and coughing followed by wheezing). During acute exacerbation, the cough usually sounds tight and is generally not productive. The degree of wheezing does not correlate well with the severity, but the relative absence of wheezing in the presence of respiratory distress and poor air entry on lung auscultation is indicative of severe airflow obstruction. The use of accessory muscles of respiration and the presence of pulsus paradoxus signify severe compromise of respiratory function.

Children with severe acute asthma usually present with tachypnea, hyperpnea, retractions, and nasal flaring. These patients appear anxious; they may prefer a tripod sitting position, remain undistracted from just breathing, and are typically unable to speak in full sentences.

### a. Laboratory Tests

The routine complete blood count is usually normal and rarely useful in the assessment of acute asthma. Elevated blood counts usually show eosinophilia and leukocytosis; the latter may be induced by stress or corticosteroid administration. Therefore, an elevated white blood cell count does not always signify the presence of infection.

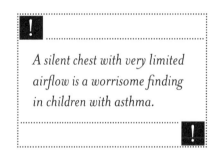

*A silent chest with very limited airflow is a worrisome finding in children with asthma.*

A chest radiograph is indicated when the patient demonstrates poor response to bronchodilators. The radiograph can define the extent of any associated parenchymal disease, complications (e.g., pneumothorax), and foreign bodies. The chest radiograph of a patient with asthma frequently shows hyperinflation and peribronchial thickening. Small segmental areas of atelectasis are frequently observed during the acute exacerbation and may be misinterpreted as pneumonia.

Typical blood gas findings in an acute uncomplicated asthma attack reveal low $Pa_{O_2}$, low $Pa_{CO_2}$, and respiratory alkalosis. Hypoxemia is due to V/Q mismatch, and low $Pa_{CO_2}$ is due to hyperventilation. Normalization of the $Pa_{CO_2}$ in a patient with worsening airway obstruction should be interpreted as a sign of respiratory muscle fatigue and impending respiratory failure. Hypoxemia is a more ominous finding in acute asthma and requires rapid intervention. Patients with respiratory acidosis with or without metabolic acidosis should be monitored closely in an intensive care unit. Hypercapnia by itself is not an indication for intubation if a patient is responding to therapy and remains conscious and hemodynamically stable.

Conversely, normocapnic patients who exhibit hypoxemia, unconsciousness, or hemodynamic instability require immediate intubation and ventilator support.

### b. Differential Diagnosis of Asthma

*Congenital Malformations.* Anomalies of respiratory, cardiovascular, and gastrointestinal systems can cause varying degrees of airway obstruction that may mimic asthma. Among the most common are laryngotracheomalacia, vocal cord paralysis, tracheal or bronchial stenosis, lobar emphysema, lung cysts, vascular rings, and gastroesophageal reflux.

*Foreign Bodies.* Sudden onset of dyspnea, cough, and respiratory distress in previously healthy children without a history of recurrent episodes is suggestive of a foreign body in either the trachea or bronchial tree. Aids to diagnosis include a high degree of suspicion, differential sounds on chest auscultation, and a chest radiograph in inspiratory, expiratory, and lateral decubitus positions.

*Croup.* The prevalence rate of recurrent croup is increased in children with asthma, as well as the incidence of persistent airway hyperreactivity of both the upper and the lower respiratory tract in children with recurrent croup.

*Acute Bronchiolitis.* Syndromes caused by RSV and other respiratory viruses occur in infants and young children in the first 2 years of life. Clinical signs include cough, coryza, wheezing, and progressive dyspnea. The condition may progress to respiratory failure or a child may present in respiratory failure. These syndromes are difficult to differentiate from asthma. Chest radiographs often show evidence of hyperinflation resulting from generalized bronchiolar obstruction, patchy pulmonary infiltrates, and atelectasis.

## 3. Management of Asthma

Critically ill children with status asthmaticus are often dehydrated as a result of decreased oral intake prior to admission and increased insensible fluid losses from increased minute ventilation (tachypnea). Providing appropriate fluid resuscitation and ongoing maintenance fluid is essential.

### a. Corticosteroids

Corticosteroids are a mainstay in the management of acute and chronic asthma. Glucocorticoids suppress cytokine production, granulocyte-macrophage colony-stimulating factor, and inducible nitric oxide synthase activation, all of which are components of the inflammatory processes of asthma. Methylprednisolone is the most common corticosteroid used in critically ill asthmatics. An initial dose of 2 mg/kg is followed by 0.5 to 1 mg/kg/dose IV every 6 hours. Corticosteroids begin to exert their effect in 1 to 3 hours and reach a maximal effect in 4 to 8 hours. The duration of therapy is dictated by the clinical response. Consider gradually tapering the corticosteroids in patients requiring more than 5 to 7 days of steroid therapy.

### b. Inhaled Beta-Agonists

Beta-agonists cause direct bronchial smooth muscle relaxation and are key components of acute and chronic asthma therapy. Albuterol (salbutamol) is recommended at a dose of 0.05 to 0.15 mg/kg every 20 minutes for 3 doses. Continuous albuterol nebulization is effective and should be considered in patients failing to respond to intermittent treatments. The recommended dose for continuous albuterol is 0.15 to 0.45 mg/kg/h, with a maximum dose of

20 mg/h. The recommended levalbuterol dose is 0.075 mg/kg (minimum dose of 1.25 mg) every 20 minutes for 3 doses followed by 0.075 to 0.15 mg/kg (not to exceed 5 mg) every 1 to 4 hours as needed. It is important to monitor serum potassium levels in patients undergoing continuous inhalational therapy due to intracellular potassium shifts that can result in hypokalemia. Frequent administration of high-dose inhaled beta-agonists in patients who are dehydrated often results in severe tachycardia that can be ameliorated by judicious fluid boluses.

### c. Intravenous and Subcutaneous Beta-Agonists

Intravenous and subcutaneous administration of beta-agonists is beneficial in children with severe status asthmaticus, in whom reduced respiratory air flow may limit distribution of inhaled medications. Terbutaline is a relatively selective $beta_2$-agonist. Subcutaneous administration is primarily used for patients without IV access and as a rapidly available adjunct to an inhaled beta-agonist. The subcutaneous dosing for terbutaline is 0.01 mg/kg/dose with a maximum dose of 0.3 mg. The dose may be repeated every 15 or 20 minutes for up to 3 doses. IV terbutaline is also useful in severe status asthmaticus and is started with a loading dose of 10 µg/kg over 10 minutes, followed by a continuous infusion of 0.1 to 1 µg/kg/min. It is rare that a dose higher than 4 µg/kg/min is needed.

### d. Anticholinergic

Ipratropium is the most frequently used anticholinergic agent in the treatment of asthma. It promotes bronchodilation without inhibiting mucociliary clearance. It can be delivered either by aerosol or metered-dose inhaler. Dose range is 125 to 500 µg (nebulized) or 4 to 8 puffs administered every 20 minutes for up to three doses. Subsequent recommended dosing interval is every 4 to 6 hours.

### e. Magnesium Sulfate

Magnesium acts as a bronchodilator primarily through its activity as a calcium channel blocker and its role in activation of adenylate cyclase in smooth muscle cells. As a result, magnesium inhibits calcium-mediated smooth muscle contraction and facilitates bronchodilation. The usual dosing of magnesium is 25 to 50 mg/kg/dose IV over 30 minutes, administered every 4 hours. It can also be given by continuous infusion at a rate of 10 to 20 mg/kg/h. Signs of hypermagnesemia include hypotension, nausea, and flushing. Serious toxicity involving cardiac arrhythmias, muscle weakness, loss of deep tendon reflexes, and respiratory depression may occur at higher doses (levels usually over 10 or 12 mg/dL). Serum magnesium levels should be monitored regularly.

### f. Methylxanthines

Methylxanthines promote relaxation of bronchial smooth muscle. The exact mechanism remains controversial, although suggested mechanisms include increasing intracellular cyclic adenosine monophosphate levels by blocking phosphodiesterase 4, control of calcium influx, inhibition of endogenous calcium release, and prostaglandin antagonism. Though not recommended in the National Heart, Lung, and Blood Institute acute asthma management guidelines, theophylline therapy can be helpful in critically ill children with an inadequate response to steroids and beta-agonist therapy. Aminophylline and theophylline, though often effective in very sick patients, have complicated pharmacokinetics and serious side-effect profiles. They should be used with careful attention to the complexities of their pharmacology.

Aminophylline is administered by continuous IV infusion following a loading dose of 5 to 7 mg/kg infused over 20 minutes. Continuous infusion should begin immediately after the loading dose at a rate of 0.5 to 0.9 mg/kg/h. Serum theophylline levels should be measured 2 to 4 hours after the loading dose and then about 6 to 8 hours after initiation of continuous infusion. The pharmacokinetics of aminophylline is usually consistent and an average volume of distribution of 0.5 L/kg can often be reliably used to predict serum levels from dosing. However, at serum levels greater than 20 to 25 µg/mL (20 to 25 mg/L), pharmacokinetics can become zero order and thus levels are not in a fixed relationship to dose. For maximal therapeutic benefit, the serum level goal of theophylline level is 10 to 20 µg/mL (10 to 20 mg/L). All patients on continuous IV infusions of beta-agonists or aminophylline should be monitored by continuous cardiac monitoring.

### g. Heliox

Heliox in helium-oxygen concentrations of 80:20 and 70:30 may be useful as adjuvant therapy in severe asthma. Due to its low density, heliox can potentially improve the work of breathing by facilitating laminar gas flow in areas of high airway resistance and help in the delivery of albuterol. The use of heliox is recommended in non-hypoxemic patients who fail to respond to conventional treatments. The low $F_{IO_2}$ in heliox mixtures may limit use in hypoxemic patients.

### h. Noninvasive Positive-Pressure Ventilation

NPPV (CPAP and BiPAP) has been shown to decrease the work of breathing and improve air movement in adults and children with asthma. By stenting open edematous narrowed airways and limiting expiratory airway collapse, NPPV can reduce work of breathing, reduce distress, and improve hypoxemia. It may reduce the need for intubation and mechanical ventilation in some patients. It is a reasonable intervention for patients who have dyspnea and signs of increased work of breathing (intercostal and subcostal retractions). NPPV provides almost instant reduction in the work of breathing, which results in it being generally well tolerated by children. Both intermittent and continuous nebulized medications can be administered while the patient is receiving NPPV.

A nasal or full face mask that fits well is absolutely necessary. Patients who are not severely distressed may feel better even with a nasal mask. Initial settings with a peak pressure of around 10 to 12 cm $H_2O$ and PEEP of 5 to 6 cm $H_2O$ are reasonable for initiation of therapy.

### i. Invasive Mechanical Ventilation

Though efforts are always made to minimize tracheal intubation in pediatric asthma patients, there are times when intubation is absolutely indicated and should not be delayed. Tracheal intubation is indicated for children following cardiorespiratory arrest, those with refractory hypoxemia and hypercarbia (not responsive to BiPAP or NPPV), severe respiratory and metabolic acidosis, and depressed mental status. Mechanical ventilation is intended to provide a stable airway, oxygen delivery, and ventilation adequate to reduce severe acidosis while the underlying pathology resolves. Most importantly, mechanical ventilation helps alleviate the extreme work of breathing that occurs in status asthmaticus.

The goals of ventilatory support in status asthmaticus should be to maintain adequate oxygenation and allow for permissive hypercarbia (moderate respiratory acidosis) by adjusting minute ventilation (peak pressure, tidal volume, and rate) to maintain pH >7.2.

Ventilator management strategies should minimize dynamic hyperinflation from air trapping. Utilizing a low breath rate with a long expiratory phase and short inspiratory time (a low inspiratory-expiratory ratio) will ensure that expiratory airflow returns to zero before initiation of the next inspiration, thus minimizing air trapping. Using ventilator graphics in addition to physical exam to insure termination of exhalation prior to initiation of the next breath can help minimize dynamic hyperinflation.

> *Careful attention to dynamic hyperinflation is required during the intubation process. Overzealous bag-valve-mask ventilation of a patient in status asthmaticus before and after endotracheal intubation can result in severe hyperinflation, significant reduction in cardiac output with hypotension, pneumothorax, and even cardiac arrest.*

Judicious use of PEEP (5 to 10 cm $H_2O$) can facilitate expiratory airflow by limiting expiratory airway collapse. Efforts to normalize $P_{CO_2}$ by increasing ventilator rates usually result in even higher $P_{CO_2}$ values and intrathoracic pressures.

Once intubated and on a ventilator, efforts should be made to minimize the use of non-depolarizing neuromuscular blockade agents. These agents greatly increase the risk of severe and prolonged myopathy that can occur when the muscle relaxants are used simultaneously with high-dose corticosteroids.

## B. Bronchiolitis

### Case Study

A previously healthy 1-month-old boy, born at 34 weeks' gestation, is brought to the emergency department by his mother. She reports that about 1 week ago the infant developed a runny nose and some cough. His symptoms have not improved despite nebulized albuterol treatments every 6 hours. During the last 12 hours, he has begun grunting, flaring, and retracting. He appears less active and has been feeding poorly. The mother is concerned because the infant stops breathing intermittently.

**Detection**
- What is the likely diagnosis?
- What else is in the differential diagnosis?
- What tests would be useful to evaluate the severity of his condition?

**Intervention**
- What pharmacologic treatment should be initiated?

**Reassessment**
- How should the patient be monitored and in what setting?
- Intermittent apneas continue; are there other interventions to try?

**Effective Communication**

- What do you want to be called back to the patient for?
- What do you want to tell the nursing team about the patient?

**Teamwork**

- Who is going to do what and when?
- How will you implement the treatment plan?

### 1. Pathophysiology of Bronchiolitis

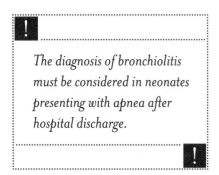

*The diagnosis of bronchiolitis must be considered in neonates presenting with apnea after hospital discharge.*

Bronchiolitis is an acute inflammatory disease of the lower respiratory tract that results in obstruction of small airways. It is the most frequent cause of apnea after hospital discharge in patients younger than 2 months. RSV, human metapneumovirus, rhinovirus, and coronavirus are the most common causes and tend to occur in epidemics during winter and spring. Bronchiolitis may also occur with other viruses, including adenovirus, influenza, and parainfluenza.

Preterm infants, those with cyanotic and non-cyanotic congenital heart disease, infants with bronchopulmonary dysplasia, and children with immunodeficiency or immunosuppression are more susceptible to bronchiolitis and tend to have more severe manifestations of the illness.

### 2. Clinical Manifestations of Bronchiolitis

The infant is typically exposed to an adult or another child with an upper respiratory tract infection. Initial symptoms include cough, sneezing, rhinorrhea, and often low-grade fever. Subsequently, patients develop tachypnea, nasal flaring, retractions, wheezing, and irritability. Cyanosis may be reported. Thoracoabdominal asynchrony correlates with the degree of airflow obstruction. Lung examination reveals diffuse wheezes, prolonged expiration, and rales. Apnea occurs both as a presenting symptom and later in the illness.

### 3. Diagnosis of Bronchiolitis

Appropriate laboratory tests for patients with severe bronchiolitis include a chest radiograph, complete blood count, rapid fluorescent antibody test for RSV and influenza, and polymerase chain reaction for common viruses, if available. In most infants with bronchiolitis, the chest radiograph demonstrates hyperinflation due to air trapping, and patchy infiltrates are common. Often, the radiograph reveals new atelectasis in an infant with bronchiolitis who has a sudden decompensation. The complete blood count is usually normal.

### 4. Management of Bronchiolitis

#### a. Hydration and Oxygen

Hydration and oxygen are the backbone of care for an infant with bronchiolitis. Oral hydration should be attempted, but if the patient is unable to tolerate this because of respiratory distress, nasogastric feeding or IV fluids can be considered. Thickening infant formula

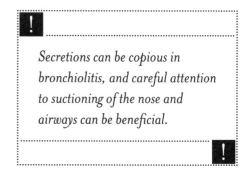

*Secretions can be copious in bronchiolitis, and careful attention to suctioning of the nose and airways can be beneficial.*

with rice cereal may make it more tolerable for infants in respiratory distress. Supplemental oxygen in various forms (i.e., nasal cannula or face mask) should be used to maintain oxygen saturations above 92%. Humidification of supplemental oxygen is mandatory to prevent desiccation of airway secretions.

### b. Beta$_2$-Agonists

There is no proven benefit to inhaled beta-agonists in bronchiolitis. However, in a clinical setting, it remains common practice to administer a beta-agonist by nebulizer at least on a trial basis. If clinical improvement is not noted or if worsening is observed, these agents should be discontinued.

### c. Racemic Epinephrine (Adrenaline)

Racemic epinephrine (adrenaline) has been studied, and a trial of racemic epinephrine (2.25% solution: 0.05 mL/kg/dose diluted in 3 mL of saline via nebulizer) may be warranted. Discontinue if no improvement is observed. Rebound may occur in 2 to 3 hours and is cited as a reason for the hospital admission of children who receive racemic epinephrine in the emergency department.

### d. Inhaled and Systemic Steroids

The use of inhaled and systemic steroids is controversial, as these agents have not been proven to have any effect in acute bronchiolitis. When the distinction between viral bronchiolitis and recurrent wheezing due to asthma is difficult to discern, steroids may be tried as a therapeutic intervention.

## C. Pneumonia

### 1. Pathophysiology and Classification of Pneumonia

Pneumonia is an inflammation of the lung parenchyma caused by bacterial or viral infection and is characterized by a reduction in total lung capacity that is associated with a decrease in compliance. Expiratory flow rates are usually preserved, and major obstructive defects are rare. Progressive alveolar involvement and deterioration of gas exchange lead to respiratory distress and failure.

Pneumonia can be classified by the anatomic location (lobar, lobular, alveolar, or interstitial), environment where it was acquired (community or nosocomial), or causative organism. Although a universal definition is lacking, community-acquired pneumonia is usually defined as a lung infection with acute symptoms (fever, cough, dyspnea), associated with altered pulmonary auscultation (crackles) or the presence of an acute infiltrate on the chest radiograph of a previously healthy child. Pneumonias acquired after 48 to 72 hours of hospitalization are considered nosocomial.

When a child presents with recurrent pneumonia, the possibility of an underlying disease (e.g., acquired or congenital lung anatomic abnormalities, immunodeficiency, tracheoesophageal fistula, foreign body, cystic fibrosis, heart failure, untreated asthma, bronchiectasis, ciliary dyskinesia, neutropenia, and increased pulmonary blood flow) should be considered.

## 2. Diagnosis of Pneumonia

The diagnosis of parenchymal lung disease is challenging. Auscultative findings may be completely normal unless significant consolidation or small airway disease (fine crackles late in inspiration) exist. A chest radiograph is critical for both the diagnosis and the management of pneumonia.

Fever and cough are frequently present, and clinical signs of accessory muscle retractions and altered pulmonary auscultation tend to be the most specific indicators of lower airway compromise. Usual signs and symptoms of pneumonia are fever, lethargy, poor appetite, pallor or cyanosis, toxemia or toxic appearance, and abdominal distension. Right lower lobe pneumonia has been mistaken for appendicitis. Signs of lung compromise include intercostal and subcostal retractions, nasal flaring, and thoracic pain. Findings on auscultation vary and may include alterations in breath sounds, such as bronchophony and crackles.

## 3. Management of Pneumonia

### a. Supportive Therapy

Supportive therapy includes maintenance of nutritional state; fluid, electrolyte, and acid base balance; humidified oxygen therapy; thinning of secretions; and physiotherapy. Tracheal and mechanical ventilation is necessary in severe cases with respiratory failure.

### b. Antibiotic Therapy

Group B streptococci and Gram-negative bacteria prevail among newborns until the age of 3 weeks; in most of the cases, IV ampicillin and gentamicin should be used. In severe disease, a third-generation cephalosporin (cefotaxime) should be used, along with ampicillin to provide coverage for potential *Listeria monocytogenes*. In children between 4 months and 4 years of age, ampicillin at 200 mg/kg/day every 6 hours should be administered. Ceftriaxone should be used in severe cases. In selecting antibiotics, careful attention must be given to local bacterial resistance patterns.

In children older than 5 years, a 5-day course of azithromycin can be used for routine treatment of atypical bacteria, particularly *M pneumoniae*. Recommended dosing is 10 mg/kg on day 1, followed by 5 mg/kg/day for 4 subsequent days. Ceftriaxone, with or without macrolides, may be used in more acutely ill children. At all ages, if the clinical manifestations suggest the presence of *S aureus*, oxacillin or vancomycin should be used, depending on the prevalence of methicillin-resistant staphylococcus in the community.

### c. Positive Pressure Ventilation

NPPV with CPAP or BiPAP should be utilized for patients who remain hypoxemic despite high oxygen concentrations. Indications for intubation in pneumonia are respiratory failure with severe hypoxemia, worsening muscle fatigue, and altered mental status. If endotracheal intubation is necessary, consider adding a PEEP valve to the bag-valve-mask prior to intubating, as PEEP will improve oxygenation and recruit collapsed alveoli.

## 4. Complications

Complications of pneumonia include pleural effusions, empyema, extrapulmonary infections and sepsis, acute respiratory distress syndrome, shock, lung abscess, pneumothorax, atelectasis, and multiple organ system dysfunctions. Pleural effusion and empyema are the most frequent complications.

Pleural effusions often accompany bacterial pneumonia in pediatric patients. *Streptococcus pneumoniae* is the most commonly associated organism, accounting for 22% of cases in the United States. *S aureus* and *S pyogenenes* are also associated with high incidence of pleural effusion and empyema. Parenchymal necrosis appears to be an increasingly common complication of pediatric bacterial pneumonia.

Chest radiographs, sometimes with right and left lateral decubitus views, are used to diagnose pleural effusions, assess their size, and determine if they are free flowing. Increasingly, ultrasound of the chest is used to assess specific locations of effusions and whether or not they contain fibrinous strands, which contribute to loculations that make thoracentesis drainage difficult. Empyema is distinguished from a parapneumonic effusion in that it is purulent with a high white blood cell count and a low pH. Empyemas also tend to be less free flowing with a greater incidence of loculation.

Treatment options for effusions and empyema include provision of supplemental oxygen and/or antibiotics, supportive therapy plus pleural drainage via thoracostomy tube with or without intrapleural thrombolysis, or supportive therapy plus more aggressive pleural drainage using techniques such as video-assisted thoracoscopic surgery. The decision to perform thoracostomy drainage in pediatric patients with a parapneumonic effusion may depend on the clinical context in which it occurs. In cases of significant pleural fluid organization, some favor the administration of intrapleural thrombolytics to facilitate evacuation of fluid through the chest drain; studies assessing the efficacy of this practice have produced conflicting results. Video-assisted thoracoscopic surgery recently has gained popularity as a way to facilitate chest drainage through direct visual inspection of the pleural space, mechanical disruption of adhesions, and placement of chest drains in strategic locations.

## D. Cystic Fibrosis

 ## Case Study

A 17-year-old girl with cystic fibrosis comes to the emergency department with a 1-week history of increased cough, wheezing, and changes in the quantity and quality of her sputum. She has had chest pain and increased work of breathing since this morning. Her current oxygen saturations of 89% are considerably lower than her baseline.

**Detection**
- What are possible explanations for her clinical condition?
- What diagnostic studies should be obtained?
- What tests would be useful to evaluate the severity of the patient's condition?

**Intervention**
- What treatment interventions should be instituted?

**Reassessment**
- With what frequency should her condition be reassessed?
- What clinical indicators should be followed?

**Effective Communication**
- Who should be informed of this patient's condition?
- What should the inpatient staff be told about this patient?

**Teamwork**
- How are you going to implement the treatment strategy?
- Who is doing what and when?

### 1. Pathophysiology of Cystic Fibrosis

Cystic fibrosis (CF) is an autosomal recessive disorder involving a mutation on the long arm of chromosome 7 that causes abnormal chloride and sodium ion transport across epithelial surfaces, resulting in viscid secretions that lead to the blockage of airways. The lower airway is normal at birth but over time will develop obstructive pulmonary disease as a result of recurrent airway inflammation, chronic mucus production, and recurrent infections. Children usually present with recurrent coughing and wheezing, bronchiolitis, asthma, and pneumonia. They eventually develop hyperinflation with chronic diffuse bronchiectasis. Pneumothorax occurs in about 10% of the patients and can be a common cause of chest pain and respiratory failure.

### 2. Diagnosis of Cystic Fibrosis

Patients with CF tend to have upper airway involvement with pansinusitis and nasal polyps. Bacteria responsible for exacerbations early in the disease process may include *S aureus*, *H influenzae*, and *Klebsiella* species. *Pseudomonas aeruginosa* (mucoid strain), *Aspergillus fumigatus*, *Burkholderia cepacia*, and *Stenotrophomonas maltophilia* become the predominant responsible organisms later in the process.

Sweat testing should be considered in patients with:

- History of meconium ileus with prolonged jaundice in the neonatal period
- Rectal prolapse, chronic diarrhea with steatorrhea
- Nasal polyps and pansinusitis
- Chronic coughing and wheezing
- Documented *S aureus* pneumonia or documented *Pseudomonas* in sputum culture
- Failure to thrive
- Digital clubbing
- Family history of CF

### 3. Management of Cystic Fibrosis

Respiratory failure is relatively uncommon in children with CF. It may, however, occur in undiagnosed children presenting with viral or bacterial pneumonia, in patients with advanced CF presenting with pneumonia or an acute pneumothorax, or in terminally ill CF patients presenting with right heart failure.

A patient with CF may benefit from:

- Chest physical therapy and postural drainage
- Inhalation therapy with bronchodilators
- Mucolytic agents (*N*-acetylcysteine, 3-5 mL of 20% solution via nebulizer 3 times daily)
- Recombinant human DNase
- Vasoconstrictors

Antibiotic treatment may vary from a short course of one antibiotic for uncomplicated cases to a longer term course of multiple antibiotics in more complex cases. Treatment should be initially directed against *Pseudomonas* species. Recommended IV therapy includes cefepime, 150 mg/kg/day; or ceftazidime, 150 mg/kg/day; in combination with tobramycin, 7.5 mg/kg/day. Vancomycin, 45 mg/kg/day IV, should be considered in patients with suspected staphylococcal infections.

## E. Acute Respiratory Distress Syndrome

### 1. Definition and Pathophysiology of Acute Respiratory Distress Syndrome

The acute respiratory distress syndrome (ARDS) is manifested as acute non-cardiogenic pulmonary edema with bilateral pulmonary infiltrates on a chest radiograph and is associated with significant hypoxemia. In 2012, an international consensus conference issued new diagnostic criteria (**Table 4-8**). In the absence of arterial blood gas measurements, the oxygenation deficit for mild ARDS can be fulfilled by a ratio of oxygen saturation ($Sao_2$) to $Fio_2$ of ≤263. Moderate ARDS can be diagnosed with a ratio of ≤201 along with the required PEEP or CPAP requirement.

**Table 4-8. Diagnostic Criteria for Acute Respiratory Distress Syndrome, 2012 Berlin Consensus Conference**

| | |
|---|---|
| Timing | Occurs within 1 week of known clinical insult or new or worsening respiratory symptoms |
| Chest imaging | Bilateral opacities not explained by effusions, lobar and lung collapse or nodules |
| Origin of edema | Respiratory failure not explained by cardiac failure or fluid overload |
| Oxygenation deficit | **Mild:** 200 ≤$Pao_2/Fio_2$ ≤300 with PEEP or continuous PEEP ≥5 cm $H_2O$ <br> **Moderate:** 100 <$Pao_2/Fio_2$ ≤200 with PEEP ≥5 cm $H_2O$ <br> **Severe:** $Pao_2/Fio_2$ ≤100 with PEEP ≥5 cm $H_2O$ |

ARDS can develop following either direct or indirect lung injury. Pneumonia and pulmonary aspiration commonly cause direct lung injury and can result in ARDS, but traumatic pulmonary contusion, fat embolism, submersion injury, and inhalation injury are relatively common causes as well. The most common forms of indirect lung injury include systemic conditions such as sepsis, shock, cardiopulmonary bypass, and transfusion-related lung injury. Direct injury is suspected of causing regional

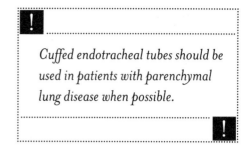

*Cuffed endotracheal tubes should be used in patients with parenchymal lung disease when possible.*

consolidation from destruction of the alveolar architecture, while indirect injury is believed to be associated with pulmonary vascular congestion, interstitial edema, and less severe alveolar involvement. ARDS progresses through states defined by associated clinical, radiographic, and histopathological features. The first, or exudative, phase is characterized by the acute development of decreased pulmonary compliance and hypoxemia. The alterations in pulmonary mechanics lead to tachypnea. Arterial blood gas analysis typically reveals hypercarbia, and the chest radiograph reveals diffuse alveolar infiltrates from pulmonary edema. The pro-inflammatory events that occur in the exudative phase create the setting for transition into the fibroproliferative stage, during which increased alveolar dead space and refractory pulmonary hypertension may develop as a result of chronic inflammation and scarring of the alveolar capillary unit. The fibroproliferative phase gives way to a recovery phase, with restoration of the alveolar epithelial barrier, gradual improvement in pulmonary compliance, resolution of arterial hypoxemia, and eventual return to premorbid pulmonary function in many patients.

## 2. Management of Acute Respiratory Distress Syndrome

The mainstay of therapy for ARDS is supportive care, of which a critically important component is positive pressure ventilation. The breakdown of the alveolar capillary barrier in ARDS, as well as surfactant dysfunction, lead to a severe decline in pulmonary compliance and lung volume, leading to ventilation and perfusion mismatch. This explains why hypoxemia in ARDS is usually refractory to supplemental oxygen alone and requires the application of positive pressure ventilation. A trial of BiPAP is warranted; however, in severe hypoxemia, invasive mechanical ventilation may be required as the initial mode of support. Strategies for mechanical ventilation in ARDS include aggressive efforts to reduce ventilator-associated lung injury by using low tidal volumes (as low as 4 to 6 mL/kg) to maintain ventilator plateau pressures ≤30 cm $H_2O$ and reduction of administered oxygen by using PEEP aggressively to recruit and maintain patency of alveolar lung units. The ARDSNet study demonstrated improved outcomes in adult patients with ARDS who were treated with these strategies; no similar studies have been done in pediatric patients.

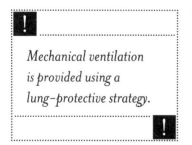

*Mechanical ventilation is provided using a lung-protective strategy.*

Adjuvant therapies include prone positioning and use of surfactant and corticosteroids. Alveolar consolidation occurs along the gravitational axis in acute lung injury and ARDS, and pulmonary blood flow is distributed preferentially to dorsal (dependent) lung regions. It is logical to speculate that the ventilation-perfusion ratio in the injured lung can be improved by changing body position. Studies have failed to show a decrease in mortality with prone positioning. Occasionally improvements in gas exchange may be substantial enough to allow the patient to wean from potentially injurious inflation pressure or high oxygen concentrations.

Surfactant was identified as a potential therapy when alterations in the lipid-protein ratio of endogenous surfactant was noted in postmortem bronchoalveolar lavage fluid and lung specimens of adult patients. Randomized controlled trials in adult patients failed to show a mortality benefit with surfactant administration in ARDS, but one pediatric study did show a significant reduction in mortality with the administration of surfactant.

Corticosteroids limit transudation of plasma across the capillary endothelium and exert anti-inflammatory effects. Studies evaluating a short course of high-dose corticosteroids administered in early ARDS did not demonstrate an outcome benefit.

## F. Pulmonary Edema

### 1. Pathophysiology of Pulmonary Edema

There are 2 types of pulmonary edema: high-pressure pulmonary edema and permeability pulmonary edema. The former is frequently cardiogenic in origin, whereas the latter is typically caused by a disruption of the alveolocapillary membrane. The increase in capillary pressure associated with high-pressure pulmonary edema is caused by conditions that result in obstruction of blood flow into the left atrium (pulmonary venous obstruction) or through the left heart (impaired left ventricular function or mitral valve stenosis). Rising left atrial pressure due to impaired mitral valve function or poor left ventricular function is transmitted in a retrograde fashion through the pulmonary veins to the pulmonary capillary bed and increases the rate of fluid flux into the interstitial space surrounding the alveoli. This net flow overwhelms the lymphatic system's ability to clear the fluid. Edema fluid can break through the tight walls of the alveolar epithelium and cause flooding in the alveolar air space, producing hypoxemia and a decrease in alveolar compliance. Peribronchial edema leads to small airway closing, decreasing pulmonary compliance further and increasing the work of breathing. Increased hydrostatic pressure is the primary mechanism by which interstitial and alveolar flooding occurs in cardiogenic pulmonary edema. Patients with low plasma protein are more likely to develop pulmonary edema at lower levels of left atrial pressure than those with normal oncotic pressure.

Permeability or non-cardiogenic pulmonary edema occurs when the alveolar capillary membrane is damaged directly by an inhaled toxin or when pulmonary surfactant is inadequate in quantity or does not function adequately.

Postobstructive pulmonary edema sometimes occurs in patients whose severe upper airway obstruction has been relieved. It is seen in patients with severe obstructive sleep apnea who undergo tonsillectomy and adenoidectomy and who suddenly become hypoxemic postoperatively, as well as in patients with acute upper airway obstruction who are intubated and pink frothy fluid is subsequently suctioned from their tracheal tube.

### 2. Diagnosis of Pulmonary Edema

Children might present with only mild dyspnea and failure to thrive. With worsening symptoms, chest radiographs show cephalization of fluid, pulmonary congestion, and clearly evident Kerley B lines. The presence of frank pulmonary edema may become known only when a patient is intubated and pink frothy fluid is suctioned.

### 3. Management of Pulmonary Edema

Patients with pulmonary edema may benefit from:

- A timely cardiology consultation if a cardiogenic, high-pressure etiology is suspected.

- Furosemide (1 to 2 mg/kg/day in divided doses every 6 to 12 hours) to reduce extracellular volume and decrease systemic venous return, by lowering atrial filling pressure and improving cardiac function. The acute relief in pulmonary congestion is probably related to a venodilatory effect. The drug also promotes transcapillary refill from the interstitial space.

- Bed rest in a semi-sitting position, with the head of the bed at 30° to 45°.

- Reduction of pulmonary venous return (preload) and systemic vascular resistance (afterload).

- Morphine (0.1-0.2 mg/kg/dose) to reduce preload by increasing venous capacitance. Morphine decreases venous return and reduces total peripheral resistance.

- Reduction of myocardial metabolic demand by treating hyperthermia.

- Positive pressure ventilation, either NPPV or invasive, in pulmonary edema. This will be more effective in easing the increased work of breathing and hypoxemia than supplemental oxygen.

Care should be used in administering large amounts of supplemental oxygen to patients with cardiogenic or high-pressure pulmonary edema because the reduction in pulmonary vascular resistance may worsen pulmonary edema by dilating the pulmonary venous system.

Endotracheal intubation should be considered in patients with persistent hypoxemia and respiratory failure despite maximum noninvasive supplementary oxygen support and in patients with hemodynamic compromise. The cardiovascular collapse noted in some patients after endotracheal intubation and hand bag-valve ventilation may be the result of a decrease in venous return with positive pressure ventilation.

Additionally, measures designed to minimize the increase in intrathoracic pressure, such as decreasing inspiratory time, decreasing tidal volume, and minimizing the amount of PEEP, should be considered. Cardiopulmonary resuscitation may be necessary, and healthcare providers must always be prepared for this possibility.

# G. Acute Chest Syndrome in Sickle Cell Disease

Acute chest syndrome (ACS) is an acute lung injury syndrome that occurs frequently in patients with sickle cell disease. This lung injury syndrome is defined as a new pulmonary infiltrate on a chest radiograph consistent with alveolar consolidation but not atelectasis, involving at least one complete lung segment. The radiographic findings are usually accompanied by chest pain, fever, tachypnea, wheezing, cough, or hypoxemia. Although often self-limited, some episodes progress rapidly to acute respiratory failure, causing high rates of morbidity and death.

The 3 mechanisms usually postulated to cause ACS are pneumonia or systemic infection, fat embolism, and direct pulmonary infarction from sickle hemoglobin-containing erythrocytes. Though patients with sickle cell disease are at increased risk of pulmonary thromboembolism, the role of pulmonary emboli in ACS has not been clarified. The systemic hypoxemia associated with a pulmonary process in sickle cell disease may serve to worsen sickling overall and especially in the affected lung areas. ACS may develop 1 to 3 days after hospitalization for sickle cell veno-occlusive disease or may be the cause for admission.

Therapeutic interventions that are useful in ACS include:

1. Hydration with IV fluids

2. Oxygen for hypoxia

3. Antibiotics to treat the usual causes of bacterial pneumonia, as well as macrolide therapy

4. Analgesia sufficient to permit deep breathing and incentive spirometry

5. Simple red blood cell transfusion if hemoglobin is <10 g/dL

6. Partial or full volume exchange transfusion if severe symptoms persist when the hemoglobin is >10 g/dL

7. NPPV to improve hypoxia

On most occasions, a substantial improvement in oxygenation and comfort is achieved with simple or exchange transfusion.

# Diagnosis and Management of the Child With Acute Upper and Lower Airway Disease

**Key Points**

- Airway maneuvers such as jaw thrust and chin lift can reverse hypoxemia due to upper airway obstruction caused by decreased levels of consciousness.

- A nasopharyngeal tube can be lifesaving in patients with severe airway obstruction due to Pierre Robin sequence.

- Children should be allowed to remain in their position of comfort as long as possible.

- A multidisciplinary team with expertise in medical and surgical airway management should be assembled for cases of suspected epiglottitis and other severe cases of upper airway obstruction.

- Direct examination of the airway in the operating room by skilled anesthesiologists and otolaryngologists is the correct way to diagnose severe upper airway obstruction. Radiographic examination should be reserved for children who are relatively stable and whose diagnosis is in question.

- Bag-mask ventilation can provide lifesaving oxygenation and ventilation even in cases of complete airway obstruction duc to epiglottitis.

- Heliox is useful in all varieties of upper airway obstruction.

- Any intervention should focus on a rapid assessment of the type and severity of respiratory compromise rather than the precise etiology.

- Frequent reassessment of the response to treatment is vital for good outcome.

- Respiratory failure can exist with or without respiratory distress.

- In patients with asthma, the degree of wheezing is unrelated to the severity of the disease. A silent chest with very limited airflow is a worrisome finding.

- Chest radiography should be repeated between 6 and 24 hours after the initiation of therapy to ensure there is no progression of disease or unsuspected pathology.

- Cuffed endotracheal tubes should be used when a significant change in compliance is anticipated.

Suggested Readings

1. Backofen JE, Rogers MC. Upper airway disease. In: Rogers MC, ed. *Textbook of Pediatric Intensive Care*. 2nd ed. Baltimore, MD: Williams & Wilkins; 1992:231-257.

2. Cherry JD. Clinical practice. Croup. *N Engl J Med*. 2008;358:384-391.

3. Cote CJ, Todres ID, Ryan JF, Goudsouzian NG. *A Practice of Anesthesia for Infants and Children*. 3rd ed. Philadelphia, PA: Saunders; 2001.

4. deCaen A, Duff J, Couvadia AH, et al. Airway management. In: Nichols DG, ed. *Rogers' Textbook of Pediatric Intensive Care*. 4th ed. Philadelphia, PA: Lippincott Williams & Wilkins; 2008:303-322.

5. Fraser RS. Histology and gross anatomy of the respiratory tract. In: Martin JG, Hamid Q, Shannon J, eds. *Physiologic Basis of Respiratory Disease*. Ontario, BC, Canada: Decker; 2005:1-14.

6. Gupta VK, Cheifetz IM. Heliox administration in the pediatric intensive care unit: an evidence-based review. *Pediatr Crit Care Med*. 2005;6:204-211.

7. Khemani RG, Patel NR, Bart RD, Newth CJL. Comparison of the pulse oximetric saturation/fraction of inspired oxygen ratio and the $PaO_2$/fraction of inspired oxygen ratio in children. *Chest*. 2009;135:662-668.

8. McBride TP, Davis HW, Reilly JS. Otolaryngology. In: Zitelli BJ, Davis HW, eds. *Atlas of Pediatric Physical Diagnosis*. 3rd ed. St. Louis, MO: Mosby; 1997:683-728.

9. Mercier J, Dauger S, Durand P, et al. Acute respiratory syndrome in children. In: Fuhrman BP, Zimmerman JJ, eds. *Pediatric Critical Care*. 3rd ed. Philadelphia, PA: Mosby; 2006:731-743.

10. Miller AC, Gladwin MT. Pulmonary complications of sickle cell disease. *Am J Respir Crit Care Med*. 2012;185:1154-1165.

11. Ralston M, Hazinski MF, Zaritsky AL. Management of respiratory distress and failure. In: Ralston M, Hazinski MF, Zaritsky AL, eds. *Pediatric Advanced Life Support*. Dallas, TX: American Heart Association; 2006:45-59.

12. Ralston M, Hazinski MF, Zaritsky AL. Recognition of respiratory distress and failure. In: Ralston M, Hazinski MF, Zaritsky AL, eds. *Pediatric Advanced Life Support*. Wheeling, IL: World Point; 2006:33-43.

13. Rotta A. Asthma. In: Fuhrman BP, Zimmerman JJ, eds. *Pediatric Critical Care*. 3rd ed. Philadelphia, PA: Mosby; 2006:588-607.

14. Scharf S. Mechanical cardiopulmonary interactions in critical care. In: Dantzker DR, Scharf SM, eds. *Cardiopulmonary Critical Care*. 3rd ed. Philadelphia, PA: Saunders; 1998:75-91.

15. Shah RK, Roberson DW, Jones DT. Epiglottitis in the Hemophilus influenza type B vaccine era: changing trends. *Laryngoscope*. 2004;114:557-560.

16. Soroksky A, Stav D, Shpirer I. A pilot prospective randomized placebo-controlled trial of bilevel positive airway pressure in acute asthma attack. *Chest*. 2003;123:1018-1025.

17. Teague WG. Noninvasive ventilation in the pediatric intensive care unit for children with acute respiratory failure. *Pediatr Pulmonol*. 2003;35:418-426.

18. The Acute Respiratory Distress Syndrome Network. Ventilation with lower tidal volumes as compared with traditional tidal volumes for acute lung injury and the acute respiratory distress syndrome. *N Engl J Med*. 2000;342:1301-1308.

19. Thill PJ, McGuire JK, Baden HP, Green TP, Checchia PA. Noninvasive positive-pressure ventilation in children with lower airway obstruction. *Pediatr Crit Care Med.* 2004;5:337-342 (published erratum appears in *Pediatr Crit Care Med.* 2004;5:590).

20. Ventre KM, Wolf GK, Arnold JH. Pediatric respiratory diseases: 2011 updated for the Rogers' Textbook of Pediatric Intensive Care. *Pediatr Crit Care Med.* 2011;12:325-338.

21. Ware LB, Matthay MA. The acute respiratory distress syndrome. *N Engl J Med.* 2000;342:1334-1349.

22. Westley CR, Ross EK, Brooks JG. Nebulized racemic epinephrine by IPPB for the treatment of croup. *Am J Dis Child.* 1978;132:484-487.

23. Wheeler DS. The pediatric airway. In: Conway EE, Relvas MS, eds. *Pediatric Multiprofessional Critical Care Review.* Chicago, IL: Society of Critical Care Medicine; 2006:37-51.

24. Woods CR. Clinical features, evaluation, and diagnosis of croup. www.UpToDate.com. Updated November 6, 2012. Accessed April 18, 2013.

# Chapter 5

# Mechanical Ventilation

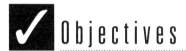Objectives

- Identify the indications, advantages, and disadvantages of noninvasive positive-pressure ventilation.

- Describe the distinguishing characteristics of the different mechanical ventilators and their modes.

- Select the appropriate mode of ventilation, ventilator settings, and monitoring parameters to initiate mechanical ventilation.

- Explain the relationship between parameters of mechanical ventilation and modifications needed to avoid its harmful effects.

- Briefly discuss approaches to weaning from mechanical ventilation.

- Outline the use of lung-protective strategies in patients with acute respiratory insufficiency and acute respiratory distress syndrome.

 Case Study

A 6-year-old boy underwent thoracotomy and drainage of a pleural abscess 2 days ago. A left thoracostomy tube was left in place. The operative course was uneventful, and he was extubated on postoperative day 1 without difficulty. This morning, he is noted to have increased work of breathing and saturations of 92% on 5 L of oxygen via face mask. A chest radiograph shows complete atelectasis of the left lung. He is started on noninvasive positive-pressure ventilation (NPPV) with the following settings: peak inspiratory pressure, 12 cm $H_2O$; positive end-expiratory pressure (PEEP), 6 cm $H_2O$; and $F_{IO_2}$, 0.5 with a backup rate of 20. A repeat chest radiograph 4 hours later shows near-complete re-expansion of the left lung.

**Detection**

– What was the most likely reason for the radiographic findings prior to the initiation of NPPV?

– What are the advantages and disadvantages of NPPV therapy in this setting?

**Intervention**

– How will you manage the noninvasive ventilator settings, and what tests or assessments are appropriate at this time?

### Reassessment
- Is the current treatment strategy effective?
- Are there any other interventions that might be helpful to this patient?
- If the repeat chest radiograph did not show any improvement, what steps might have been taken to promote lung re-expansion?

### Effective Communication
- What is the best clinical setting in which to manage the care of this patient?
- How will you communicate a change in status? Who needs to know the care plan? How will that information be disseminated?

### Teamwork
- How will you implement the treatment plan?
- Who is responsible for implementing ventilation changes?

# I. INTRODUCTION

The recognition of and response to respiratory failure continues to be a top priority in the management of critically ill children. The anatomic considerations unique to the respiratory tracts of infants and children and the inherent lack of respiratory reserve during times of stress pose special challenges to the caretaker confronted with this urgent situation. Regardless, the goal is always the same: to restore and maintain adequate oxygenation and ventilation while optimizing patient comfort and avoiding further injury. Failure to accomplish this goal can lead to devastating consequences, including cardiopulmonary arrest and death.

This chapter briefly outlines the general approach to the management of the child requiring mechanical ventilation, with a focus on the use of mechanical ventilation in specific clinical settings in the child with normal lungs or mild respiratory disease. We both review conventional ventilation techniques and introduce more recent advances in respiratory support.

Escalating to pediatric critical care is essential in children with more severe lung disease who require ongoing care.

# II. NONINVASIVE POSITIVE-PRESSURE VENTILATION

NPPV can augment oxygenation and ventilation without insertion of an artificial airway. One form of NPPV, bilevel positive airway pressure, augments ventilation by delivering pressurized air through a facial or nasal mask, or a mouthpiece. Both the nasal mask and the face mask must be tight fitting to avoid leakage. A helmet-like apparatus may improve patient tolerance, but is not commonly used in pediatrics (**Figure 5-1**).

**Figure 5-1.** Devices for Delivery of Noninvasive Positive-Pressure Ventilation

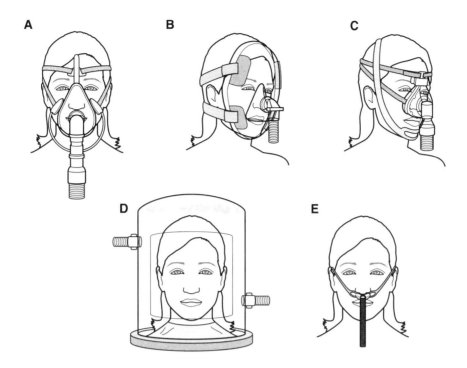

**A)** face mask, **B)** total face mask, **C)** nasal mask with chin strap, **D)** helmet, **E)** nasal pillows

The delivery of positive inspiratory pressure has been found helpful in patients with chronic obstructive lung disease, neuromuscular disorders, obstructive sleep apnea, cystic fibrosis, upper airway obstruction, and thoracic dysplasia. It has also been used as a means to avoid intubation in patients with mild to moderate acute respiratory insufficiency. NPPV can significantly improve the respiratory rate, heart rate, work of breathing, and dyspnea score in the acute setting, and it has been especially useful in previously healthy children with respiratory embarrassment due to muscle deconditioning following prolonged intubation.

NPPV is contraindicated in patients with:

- Rapidly progressive respiratory failure
- Hemodynamic instability
- Significant risk of aspiration
- Loss of protective airway reflexes or inability to clear copious oropharyngeal secretions
- Inability to properly fit the mask

NPPV respiratory support requires the patient's cooperation, including a willingness to tolerate little or no sedation. Initial settings are presented in **Table 5-1**.

| Table 5-1 | Initial Settings for Noninvasive Positive-Pressure Ventilation[a] |

| Age | Initial Setting |
| --- | --- |
| Infants <12 months | Nasal CPAP should be attempted first. If CPAP does not provide adequate support, tracheal intubation is indicated. |
| Toddlers 1-2 years | Ppeak, 8 cm $H_2O$; PEEP, 4 cm $H_2O$; $F_{IO_2}$, 1.0; ± backup rate appropriate for age and disease. |
| Children >2 years | Ppeak, 10 cm $H_2O$; PEEP, 5 cm $H_2O$; $F_{IO_2}$, 1.0; ± backup rate appropriate for age and disease. |

CPAP, continuous positive airway pressure; Ppeak, peak inspiratory pressure; PEEP, positive end-expiratory pressure
[a]*Note:* Maximum settings are dependent on patient and age, and effective delivery relies at least in part on the adequacy of the seal rather than the settings. If a Ppeak >18-20 cm $H_2O$ and PEEP >12-15 cm $H_2O$ can be tolerated but does not decrease work of breathing or improve oxygenation sufficiently, or if respiratory insufficiency is not improved, tracheal intubation is indicated.

Machines designed to deliver NPPV offer a variety of modes:

1. **Spontaneous:** The patient triggers the inspiratory and expiratory pressure cycles and the rate and depth of breathing.

2. **Spontaneous/timed:** Similar to the spontaneous mode, but machine breaths are delivered at a set frequency for patients who may be intermittently apneic.

3. **Timed positive pressure:** Breaths are delivered at a set frequency, but the patient can still breathe spontaneously.

4. **Continuous positive airway pressure (CPAP):** A baseline system pressure is provided (usually 4 to 8 cm $H_2O$ for children), but respiratory drive and effort must be maintained by the patient.

Appropriate settings are based on the nature and severity of the patient's respiratory insufficiency. A word of caution: machines are often insufficiently sensitive to the respiratory efforts of small patients. Careful observation is required to prevent counterproductive or poorly timed mechanical breaths (i.e., dyssynchrony).

## A. Advantages and Disadvantages

The advantages of NPPV include decreased laryngeal trauma, risk of ventilator-associated pneumonia, tracheitis, and the need for sedation and analgesia. In addition, if a nasal mask is utilized, the patient can talk, cough, cooperate with pulmonary toilet, and sip clear liquids.

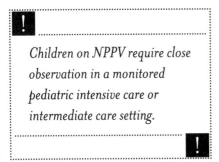

*Children on NPPV require close observation in a monitored pediatric intensive care or intermediate care setting.*

The disadvantages of NPPV in children include the risk of skin breakdown over the nasal bridge and an increased risk of aspiration due to gastric distension. Masks may not fit tightly and may not provide effective ventilation, particularly in small patients. Restriction of activity is often needed to maintain optimal mask placement. Tracheal suctioning requires mask removal, which can lead to respiratory decompensation.

## B. Continuous Positive Airway Pressure

CPAP increases the baseline system pressure (higher than atmospheric pressure) during spontaneous breathing, thus preventing collapse of distal small airways and alveoli. It can be delivered via nasal cannula, mask, tracheostomy, or endotracheal tubes. CPAP is not a true mode of mechanical ventilation because no additional positive pressure is applied above end-expiratory airway pressure during inspiration. Therefore, CPAP allows application of PEEP in a spontaneously breathing patient. The respiratory rate and tidal volume ($V_T$) are dependent on the patient's inspiratory effort.

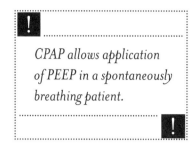

*CPAP allows application of PEEP in a spontaneously breathing patient.*

# III. MECHANICAL VENTILATORY SUPPORT

## A. Indications

Indications for endotracheal intubation are addressed in **Chapter 2**. When hypoxemic or hypercapnic respiratory failure cannot be treated by other means, the generally accepted indications for initiating mechanical ventilatory support may apply (**Table 5-2**).

### Table 5-2  Indications for Mechanical Ventilatory Support

| | |
|---|---|
| Ventilation abnormalities | Respiratory muscle dysfunction<br>• Respiratory muscle fatigue<br>• Chest wall abnormalities<br>• Neuromuscular disease |
| | Decreased ventilatory drive |
| | Increased airway resistance and/or obstruction |
| Oxygenation abnormalities | Refractory hypoxemia |
| | Need for positive end-expiratory pressure, as in pulmonary edema or pulmonary hemorrhage |
| | Excessive work of breathing |

Mechanical ventilation is also indicated for the following purposes:

- To permit heavy sedation and/or neuromuscular blockade
- To decrease systemic and myocardial oxygen consumption
- To allow transient hyperventilation for critically elevated intracranial pressure
- To facilitate alveolar recruitment and prevent atelectasis
- To improve oxygen delivery in conditions associated with inadequate oxygen supply/demand states (shock, sepsis, cardiopulmonary arrest)
- To prevent aspiration in patients with abnormal airway protective reflexes

## B. Ventilator Variables

### 1. Phase Variables

Mechanical ventilators and their modes can be distinguished by the phase variables—trigger, limit, and cycle—that govern the characteristics of the inspiratory phase of each breath. The trigger regulates the start of each breath. The limit sustains inspiration. The cycling controls the termination of inspiration.

Early positive-pressure ventilators had no mechanism to detect patient effort; this sometimes resulted in asynchrony and poor tolerance. Newer ventilators can detect changes in flow as the patient inhales.

> *For the purposes of the Pediatric Fundamental Critical Care Support course, volume-preset ventilation is generally preferred over pressure-preset ventilation to assure appropriate tidal volume is maintained.*

### 2. Volume and Pressure

Common ventilator modes are limited by either volume or pressure. Targeting $V_T$ with volume-preset ventilation is generally preferred over pressure-preset ventilation. In the past, infants were ventilated primarily with pressure-preset modes due to limitations in flow delivery and imprecise tidal-volume measurement in older ventilators. With newer machines, nearly all patients, including premature infants, can be managed using a volume-control mode.

### 3. Time Cycling, Flow Cycling, and Other Variables

Ventilator modes are typically time cycled; in other words, inspiration is terminated after a specified time. Flow cycling is used in specialized modes of ventilation, such as pressure support.

# IV. MODES OF MECHANICAL VENTILATION

The choice of ventilator mode depends on how much of the function of gas exchange can be contributed by the patient and how much must be done by the machine. A trial of NPPV may be considered in some circumstances (detailed earlier in this chapter). Frequently used ventilation modes include controlled mechanical ventilation, assist-control ventilation, synchronized intermittent mandatory ventilation, and pressure-support ventilation (**Figure 5-2**). Each has advantages and disadvantages, as summarized in **Table 5-3**. When choosing a mode of ventilation, it is important to consider the goals: (1) to provide adequate ventilation and oxygenation, (2) to reduce the work of breathing, and (3) to ensure patient comfort and synchrony with the ventilator.

## A. Controlled Mechanical Ventilation

Controlled mechanical ventilation delivers ventilator breaths at a preset rate. Each breath is time cycled and either volume limited or pressure limited. A preset $V_T$ (volume-control ventilation) or a preset applied pressure and time (pressure-control ventilation) is delivered at a preset rate. Controlled mechanical ventilation is used effectively only in patients who are heavily sedated and often pharmacologically paralyzed.

**Figure 5-2.** Airway Pressure and Flow Tracings

### A. Spontaneous Breathing

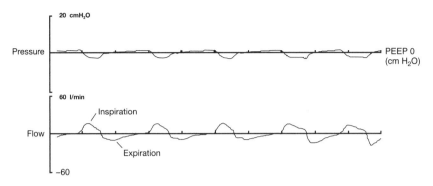

### B. Continuous Positive Airway Pressure

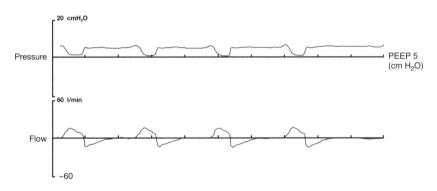

### C. Volume Assist-Control Ventilation

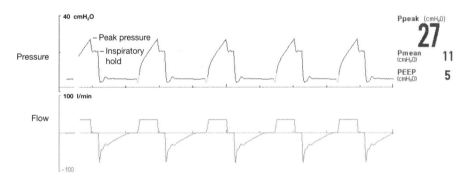

### D. Pressure Assist-Control Ventilation

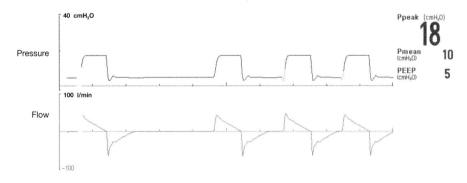

**Figure 5-2.** Airway Pressure and Flow Tracings (continued)

### E. Pressure Support Ventilation

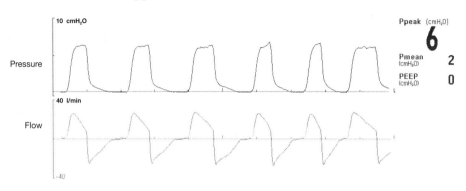

### F. Synchronized Intermittent Mandatory Ventilation Without Pressure Support

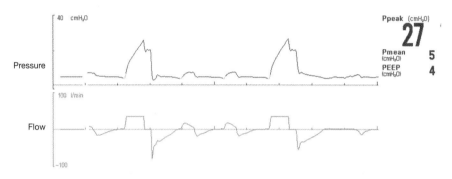

### G. Synchronized Intermittent Mandatory Ventilation With Pressure Support

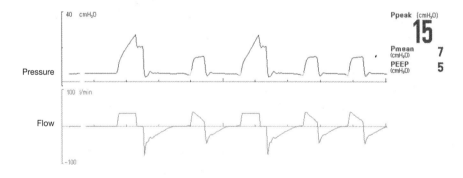

Ppeak, peak inspiratory pressure; PEEP, positive end-expiratory pressure
Time is represented on the horizontal axis and pressure or flow on the vertical axis.
Tracings provided courtesy of Paul Ouellet, PhD(c), RRT, FCCM.

## Table 5-3. Potential Advantages and Disadvantages of Selected Modes of Mechanical Ventilation

| Mode | Advantages | Disadvantages |
| --- | --- | --- |
| Controlled mechanical ventilation | Rests muscles of respiration | Requires use of sedation/neuromuscular blockade; potential adverse hemodynamic effects |
| AC ventilation | Patient can increase ventilatory support; reduced work of breathing compared to spontaneous breathing | Potential adverse hemodynamic effects; delivery of full breath with each patient effort may lead to inappropriate hyperventilation, breath stacking, and inadvertent positive end-expiratory pressure |
| AC volume-control ventilation | Guarantees delivery of set tidal volume (unless peak pressure limit is exceeded) | May lead to excessive inspiratory pressures |
| AC pressure-control ventilation | Allows limitation of peak inspiratory pressures | Potential hyper- or hypoventilation with lung resistance/compliance changes |
| Synchronized intermittent mandatory ventilation | Less interference with normal cardiovascular function | Increased work of breathing compared to AC ventilation; added patient-ventilator synchrony |
| Pressure support ventilation | Patient comfort; improved patient-ventilator interaction; decreased work of breathing | Apnea alarm is only backup; variable patient tolerance |

AC, assist-control

## B. Assist-Control Ventilation

Assist-control (AC) ventilation is controlled mechanical ventilation with a triggering mechanism that allows synchronization with the patient's respiratory effort. A preset volume or pressure is delivered at a preset minimum rate. A full ventilator breath is delivered with each spontaneous inspiratory effort; therefore, patients who are tachypneic due to their illness or agitation are likely to hyperventilate in this mode. AC ventilation is commonly used when mechanical ventilation is initiated in patients with acute respiratory failure when pulmonary compliance is not significantly abnormal.

With proper use of AC ventilatory support, the work of breathing may be significantly decreased. However, if the ventilator and the patient are not in synchrony or if the ventilator flow rates are not matched with patient demand, this mode of support may actually lead to an increase in the work of breathing.

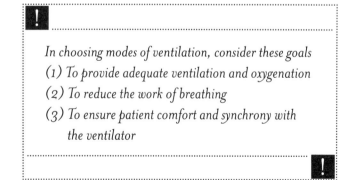

*In choosing modes of ventilation, consider these goals*
*(1) To provide adequate ventilation and oxygenation*
*(2) To reduce the work of breathing*
*(3) To ensure patient comfort and synchrony with the ventilator*

Decreasing the work of breathing may be important for clinical situations in which there is inadequate cardiac output. Resting the diaphragm and respiratory muscles may allow redistribution of blood flow and better delivery of oxygen to vital organ systems.

## C. Synchronized Intermittent Mandatory Ventilation

Synchronized intermittent mandatory ventilation (SIMV) delivers either volume-preset or pressure-preset breaths at a preset rate. Most frequently, it is used with breaths in a volume-cycled mode. Unlike AC ventilation, no additional ventilator breaths are delivered above the preset rate. Spontaneous breathing above that rate is possible, but the $V_T$ is limited to that which the patient can generate. The use of synchronization allows for enhanced patient-ventilator interaction by delivering the preset machine breaths in conjunction with the patient's inspiratory effort. When no effort is sensed, the ventilator delivers the preset $V_T$ at the set rate. SIMV is often combined with pressure-support ventilation (discussed later) to augment the $V_T$ during spontaneous breathing. Pressure support should be set to deliver an appropriate $V_T$, and offset endotracheal tube (ETT) resistance, usually 5 to 10 cm $H_2O$.

One advantage of the SIMV mode is that it allows the patient to contribute to the minute ventilation requirement with spontaneous, negative-pressure breaths. The negative inspiratory pressure (relative to PEEP, not atmospheric pressure) leads to an increased venous return to the right side of the heart, which may improve cardiac output and cardiovascular function.

## D. Pressure-Support Ventilation

Pressure-support ventilation (PSV) provides a preset level of inspiratory pressure with each spontaneous breath. All breaths are flow cycled and pressure limited. This inspiratory assistance is generally selected to overcome the increased work of breathing imposed by the disease process, the ETT, the ventilator inspiratory valves, and other mechanical aspects of ventilatory support. The pressure support augments each patient-generated, spontaneous breath. The patient controls the respiratory rate and exerts a strong influence on the duration of inspiration, inspiratory flow rate, and $V_T$. The delivered $V_T$ is influenced by pulmonary compliance and resistance. Rapid changes in these parameters may alter the minute ventilation and respiratory work. PSV can also be coupled with SIMV, primarily as a means to diminish work of breathing during spontaneous breaths.

The amount of pressure support set during mechanical ventilation is titrated to the patient's exhaled $V_T$. It should be set to achieve adequate gas exchange and optimize patient comfort. PSV only supports spontaneous breathing; when used alone, it will not provide ventilation during periods of apnea. Therefore, a backup, mandatory ventilation setting is required and is standard on many ventilators. Potential benefits of PSV include improved comfort and tolerance for awake, spontaneously breathing patients and reduced work of breathing due to enhanced patient-ventilator interaction. Typically, as pressure support is increased in patients with lung disease, the patient's work of breathing and respiratory rate decrease and $V_T$ increases. Alternatively, patients recovering from severe lung disease who were initially placed on high levels of pressure support can be effectively weaned from mechanical ventilation by gradually decreasing the pressure support, thus requiring progressively more work from deconditioned respiratory muscles. The presence of a bronchopleural fistula or an ETT cuff leak may interfere with appropriate cycling in this mode due to the escaping gas.

# V. INITIAL VENTILATOR SETTINGS

When initiating ventilatory support, an $F_{IO_2}$ of 1.0 is generally used to maximize the oxygen available during the transition to positive pressure ventilation and to compensate for any periods of respiratory or hemodynamic instability (but not in some children with congenital heart defects and parallel circulation). $V_T$ levels are set between 6 and 8 mL/kg in patients with reasonably normal lung compliance. Lower levels are considered when lung compliance is reduced (discussed later) or for the neonate (**Chapter 1**); higher levels are generally avoided to decrease the risk of lung trauma. The choice of the initial respiratory rate in children is usually based on age and disease process and is subsequently titrated by measurement of pH and, to a lesser extent, $Paco_2$ in arterial blood. Guidelines for initiation of mechanical ventilation are listed in **Table 5-4**.

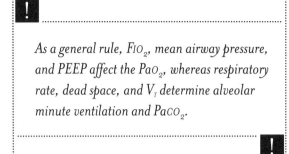

*As a general rule, $F_{IO_2}$, mean airway pressure, and PEEP affect the $Pao_2$, whereas respiratory rate, dead space, and $V_T$ determine alveolar minute ventilation and $Paco_2$.*

### Table 5-4  Guidelines for Initiation of Mechanical Ventilation

1. Choose a ventilator mode with which you are familiar. The primary goals of ventilatory support are adequate oxygenation/ventilation, reduced work of breathing, synchrony between the patient and ventilator, and avoidance of high end-inspiration alveolar pressures (maintain plateau pressure <30 cm $H_2O$).

2. Use initial $F_{IO_2}$ level of 1.0; thereafter it can be titrated downward to maintain an $Spo_2$ of 92% to 94%. In severe ARDS, $Spo_2$ ≥88% may be acceptable, lowering the therapeutic goal in favor of minimizing ventilator-associated lung injury.

3. Set initial $V_T$ between 6-8 mL/kg and adjust according to blood gas analysis results. Patients with neuromuscular disease often require $V_T$ levels of 10-12 mL/kg to satisfy air hunger. In some patients with ARDS, a $V_T$ level of 4-6 mL/kg is recommended to avoid high inspiratory plateau pressures (>30 cm $H_2O$).

4. Choose a respiratory rate and minute ventilation appropriate for the particular clinical requirements. Rate is dependent upon age and disease process, generally 12 breaths/min (adolescents) to 24 breaths/min (neonates). Target pH primarily and $Paco_2$ secondarily.

5. Set TI for each breath according to the patient's age and disease process. Neonates with normal lung function require TI of 0.35-0.6 sec, whereas the TI for children older than 2 years is generally 0.85-1.0 sec. In addition, I:E ratio should be set with the patient's specific needs in mind. Start with an I:E ratio of 1:2 in patients with healthy lungs. Patients with respiratory illnesses marked by difficulty with oxygenation (ARDS) may require a TI >1 and I:E ratio >1:1, whereas patients with obstruction to outflow (as in asthma and bronchopulmonary dysplasia) will require ample expiratory time and I:E ratios of 1:3.5 to 1:4 to avoid auto-PEEP (see below). Parameters for inspiration and exhalation are somewhat rate dependent.

6. Use PEEP to achieve and maintain optimal alveolar recruitment. In diffuse lung injury, PEEP will improve oxygenation and reduce the $F_{IO_2}$ (**Table 5-5**). If volume is held constant, PEEP increases mean airway pressure, but it may also increase peak inspiratory airway pressure, depending on ventilator mode, and this may result in potentially undesirable consequences in ARDS. Set PEEP to 5 cm $H_2O$ when initiating mechanical ventilation in children with healthy lungs. PEEP levels >15 cm $H_2O$ are rarely necessary.

7. Set the trigger sensitivity to allow minimal patient effort to initiate inspiration. Beware of autocycling if trigger setting is too sensitive.

8. Consider sedation, analgesia, and/or neuromuscular blockade when poor oxygenation, inadequate ventilation, or excessively high peak inspiratory pressures are thought to be related to patient intolerance of ventilator settings and cannot be corrected by ventilator adjustments.

9. Call a pediatric critical care consultant or other specialist in respiratory care for assistance.

$Spo_2$, peripheral oxyhemoglobin saturation; ARDS, acute respiratory distress syndrome; $V_T$, tidal volume; TI, inspiratory time; I:E ratio, ratio of inspiratory to expiratory time; PEEP, positive end-expiratory pressure
The exception to this recommendation is the patient with congenital heart disease, whose condition will be exacerbated by oxygen-driven decreases in pulmonary vascular resistance.

### Table 5-5   Use of Positive End-Expiratory Pressure in ALI/ARDS

**Initiation of PEEP in ARDS**
- PEEP at 5 cm $H_2O$ and titration in increments of 2-3 cm $H_2O$
- Full recruitment effect may not be apparent for several hours
- Monitoring of blood pressure, heart rate, and $Pao_2$ during PEEP titration and at intervals while the patient is receiving PEEP therapy
- Optimal PEEP settings are typically 8-15 cm $H_2O$

**Adverse Effects of PEEP**
- Barotrauma
- Decreased venous return, decreased preload, decreased cardiac output, and hypotension
- Increase in $Paco_2$ (increase in dead space)
- Worsening oxygenation (especially with asymmetric ALI) as healthy lung is overdistended

ALI, acute lung injury; ARDS, acute respiratory distress syndrome; PEEP, positive end-expiratory pressure

# VI. CONTINUING CARE DURING MECHANICAL VENTILATION

After mechanical ventilation has been initiated, the parameters listed below should be assessed frequently to guide changes in the ventilator settings. Care should be taken when any change is made because adjusting one parameter is likely to affect the others. This interdependency may cause a change that is beneficial in one respect to be harmful in another. In complex situations, such as those discussed later in this chapter, a critical care consultation should be obtained.

## A. Fraction of Inspired Oxygen

Inspired oxygen may be harmful to the lung parenchyma after prolonged exposure due to the production of toxic oxygen-derived radicals. Although the precise threshold for concern is not known, it is desirable to reduce the $Fio_2$ to 0.5 (50% oxygen) or below as soon as possible, ideally within the first 24 hours. Except in the premature neonate, to whom oxygen toxicity may be equally damaging, hypoxemia is usually considered a greater risk to the patient than high $Fio_2$ levels.

The primary determinants of oxygenation during mechanical ventilation are $Fio_2$ and mean airway pressure ($P\overline{aw}$). In the patient with acute lung injury or acute respiratory distress syndrome, PEEP becomes an additional independent determinant. $V_T$, the relationship of inspiratory time to expiratory time (I:E ratio), PEEP, and several other factors beyond the scope of this chapter, all interact to affect $P\overline{aw}$. The interrelationships of those factors, as already discussed, must be considered when formulating the plan for mechanical ventilation.

## B. Humidification

Gases delivered by mechanical ventilators are typically dry, and the upper airways are bypassed by artificial airways. These circumstances result in loss of heat and moisture from the respiratory tract. Gases are routinely heated and humidified during mechanical ventilation to prevent mucosal damage and minimize inspissation of secretions. Available systems include passive humidifiers (artificial nose) or active, microprocessor-controlled heat and humidifying systems (heated humidifiers). The passive humidifiers are contraindicated in the presence of copious secretions, minute ventilation >12 L/min, or blood in the airway.

## C. Inspiratory Pressure

During positive-pressure ventilation, airway pressure rises progressively to a peak inspiratory pressure (Ppeak), which is reached at end inspiration. Ppeak may also be abbreviated as *PIP* or referred to as *peak pressure* or *peak airway pressure*. Ppeak is the sum of 2 pressures: the pressure required to overcome airway resistance and that required to overcome the elastic properties of the lung and chest wall. If a pause is set at the end of inspiration (zero gas flow with the airway closed), the pressure drops slightly below the Ppeak to the inspiratory plateau pressure (Pplat) (**Figure 5-3**). Pplat reflects the pressure required to overcome elastic recoil and is the best estimate of peak alveolar pressure, which is an important indicator of alveolar distension. Accurate measurement of Ppeak requires the absence of any patient effort during inspiration or exhalation.

Potential adverse effects from high inspiratory pressure include barotrauma, volutrauma, and reduced cardiac output. Barotrauma (pneumothorax, pneumomediastinum) and volutrauma (lung parenchymal injury due to overinflation), although linked to high Ppeak, correlate best with Pplat, a better measurement of alveolar pressure. An example of the relationship of Ppeak and Pplat to alveolar distension is demonstrated by the effect of ETT size on Ppeak and Pplat. As the internal diameter of the ETT is decreased in a patient receiving volume ventilation, the same $V_T$ will result in higher Ppeak, yet Pplat and alveolar distension remain unchanged as the pressure is dissipated across the ETT. The

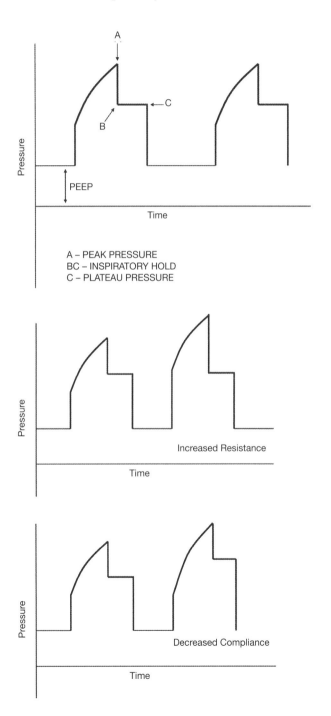

**Figure 5-3.** Relationship of Peak Inspiratory Pressure and Inspiratory Plateau Pressure

A – PEAK PRESSURE
BC – INSPIRATORY HOLD
C – PLATEAU PRESSURE

same $V_T$, regardless of the type of breath, produces the same alveolar distension at end inspiration. Inspiratory plateau pressure should ideally be <30 cm $H_2O$.

> ! *Pplat should ideally be <30 cm $H_2O$.* !

Elevated Pplat may be reduced by decreasing PEEP, which may also decrease oxygenation, or by decreasing $V_T$, which may lead to a reduction in minute ventilation. Permissive hypercapnia and a controlled reduction in pH may be accepted when high Pplat must be reduced. Permissive hypercapnia should not be used in patients with elevated intracranial pressure because $Paco_2$ >35 to 40 mm Hg (>4.7 to 5.3 kPa) may increase cerebral blood flow and cerebral blood volume and further elevate the intracranial pressure.

## D. Relationship of Inspiratory Time to Expiratory Time and Auto-PEEP

The total respiratory cycle time is calculated by dividing 60 seconds by the respiratory rate.

$$\text{Total Respiratory Cycle} = \frac{60 \text{ seconds}}{\text{Respiratory rate}}$$

The times for inhalation (inspiratory time) and exhalation (expiratory time) occur within the total cycle time and are termed the *I:E ratio*. During spontaneous breathing, the normal I:E ratio is ~1:2, indicating that for normal patients, the exhalation time is about twice as long as inhalation time. In chronic lung disease and other conditions associated with obstruction to expiratory flow, such as asthma, the exhalation time becomes prolonged, and the I:E ratio changes (e.g., 1:2.5 or 1:3). Such changes reflect the pathophysiology of the lung disease and directly influence techniques used during mechanical ventilation.

The inspiratory time during volume breaths (AC or SIMV modes) is often determined by the $V_T$ and inspiratory gas flow rate (flow × inspiratory time = $V_T$). A greater $V_T$ takes longer to deliver if the flow rate remains constant, and the same $V_T$ takes longer to deliver if the flow rate is reduced. In both cases, the inspiratory time is longer. However, given that the respiratory rate is constant, the total cycle time remains the same, and thus the time available for exhalation (the expiratory time) must be shortened to fit into the cycle time. In this situation, the inspiratory time is actively set by adjusting $V_T$ and the inspiratory flow rate or by the use of inspiratory pauses on the ventilator. The expiratory time, however, is passively determined (i.e., what is left over in the cycle time before the next inspiratory cycle of the mechanical ventilator or spontaneous breath) and varies inversely with the respiratory rate set on the ventilator.

If the expiratory time is too short to allow full exhalation, the next lung inflation is superimposed upon the residual gas in the lung and breath stacking occurs. This process will result in hyperinflation of the lung and the development of PEEP that exceeds the level of PEEP preset on the ventilator. This increase in end-expiratory pressure is auto-PEEP, or intrinsic, inadvertent, or occult PEEP. Auto-PEEP can be quantified by using manual methods or through electronic programs available in some ventilators. It is most easily diagnosed qualitatively by the flow-over-time graphic waveform tracing available on most mechanical ventilators (**Figure 5-4**). The potentially harmful physiologic effects of auto-PEEP on Ppeak, Pplat, and P$\overline{\text{aw}}$ and on lung and cardiovascular function are the same as those of preset PEEP (**Table 5-5**). Auto-PEEP may also increase work of breathing because the difference between the set PEEP and auto-PEEP must be overcome on inspiration to allow for fresh gas flow.

Reduction in auto-PEEP can be accomplished by:

- Shortening the inspiratory time. This extends the expiratory time to allow full exhalation of the $V_T$; however, it may cause alveoli with longer time constants to fill incompletely.
- Decreasing the respiratory rate. This is the most effective way to decrease auto-PEEP.
- Decreasing $V_T$. Increasing the inspiratory flow rate (volume breaths) is typically less effective unless flow rates are set inappropriately low. The influence of a decreased respiratory rate and $V_T$ on the $Pa_{CO_2}$, pH, and minute ventilation must be considered.

**Figure 5-4.** Flow-Versus-Time Waveform Demonstrating Auto-PEEP

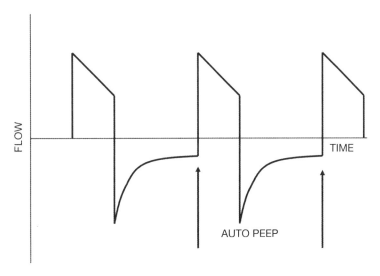

PEEP, positive end-expiratory pressure

## E. Minute Ventilation

The primary determinant of $CO_2$ exchange during mechanical ventilation is alveolar minute ventilation ($V_A$), calculated as:

$$V_A = (V_T - V_D) \times f$$

where $V_D$ is dead space and $f$ is respiratory rate. The $V_T$, the respiratory rate, and their interrelationships with other ventilatory parameters have already been discussed. Physiologic $V_D$ represents, in general, lung units that are relatively well ventilated but underperfused. The physiologic effect of increased $V_D$ is hypercapnia. Increased physiologic $V_D$ may result from the pathologic process in the lung, high airway pressures associated with mechanical ventilation, low intravascular volume, or low cardiac output. If hypercapnia persists during mechanical ventilation despite use of appropriate $V_T$ and rates, consultation with a pediatric intensivist should be sought.

It may be necessary to tolerate a higher $Pa_{CO_2}$ to avoid high airway pressure and auto-PEEP. This permissive hypercapnia technique should be initiated only with the support of an appropriate pediatric critical care consultant.

As previously discussed, adequate ventilation is assessed by consideration of both $Pa_{CO_2}$ and pH. Hyperventilation resulting in a low $Pa_{CO_2}$ may be an appropriate short-term compensatory goal during metabolic acidosis until the primary problem can be corrected. Similarly, a patient with chronic hypercapnia and increased $Pa_{CO_2}$ at baseline, who maintains a near-normal pH by renal compensation (retention of bicarbonate), should receive only enough minute ventilation to maintain a normal pH. Driving $Pa_{CO_2}$ to normal levels in the patient with chronic $CO_2$ retention will lead to severe alkalemia and loss of retained bicarbonate and may blunt the patient's respiratory drive.

# VII. SEDATION, ANALGESIA, AND NEUROMUSCULAR BLOCKADE

Endotracheal intubation and mechanical ventilation can be painful, frightening, and anxiety provoking. To improve patient comfort, relieve anxiety, and lessen the work of breathing, anxiolytics, sedatives, analgesics, and neuromuscular blocking agents are frequently administered. Guidelines for the use of these agents are outlined in **Chapter 20** and **Appendix 7**.

# VIII. VENTILATORY GUIDELINES FOR SPECIFIC CLINICAL SITUATIONS

## A. Acute Lung Injury/Acute Respiratory Distress Syndrome

 ### Case Study

A 16-year-old boy who underwent splenectomy 2 months ago presents to the emergency room with a 3-day history of fevers (101.8°F [38.8°C]), shaking, chills, and increasing shortness of breath. Oxygen saturations are 86% while breathing room air and increase to 90% on 100% non-rebreather facemask. On exam, his respiratory rate is 24 breaths/min, and coarse crackles can be heard throughout both lungs. All extremities are pale and cool, with a capillary refill of approximately 4 seconds. He is drowsy and disoriented. Analysis of an arterial blood gas drawn while on the non-rebreather mask shows: pH 7.26; $Pa_{CO_2}$, 54 mm Hg (7.1 kPa); $Pa_{O_2}$, 62 mm Hg (8.1 kPa); base excess, -5 mEq/L; saturation, 88%. The chest radiograph shows bilateral patchy infiltrates.

**Detection**

– What is the most likely diagnosis in this patient?

– What is the significance of his history of splenectomy?

### Intervention
- What is the best next intervention in the management of this patient?
- Is this patient a good candidate for NPPV? Why or why not?

### Reassessment
- Is the current oxygenation and ventilation strategy effective?
- What assessments need to be done?
- What changes would you make at this time?

### Effective Communication
- When changes are made or the patient's status changes, how will the information be communicated and to whom?
- Where is the best place to manage this patient?

### Teamwork
- Who is involved in the patient's care?
- How are you going to implement treatment for this patient?

Compromised or inadequate oxygenation is the hallmark of acute respiratory distress syndrome (ARDS), thus its alternative name, *acute hypoxemic respiratory failure*. Infection and/or inflammation in the lungs triggers the release of chemical mediators that disturb normal lung function, cause capillary leak, and increase intrapulmonary shunting, thereby worsening ventilation-perfusion mismatch. Poor lung compliance and increased airway resistance require the use of high pressures during mechanical ventilation to restore adequate gas exchange, and the challenge lies in how best to support respiration while causing the least amount of trauma to the lungs. The landmark ARDS Network study, published in 2000, showed that the use of low $V_T$ (6 mL/kg) compared to standard $V_T$ (12 mL/kg) resulted in decreased mortality rates and more ventilator-free days for adults with acute lung injury and ARDS. A similar strategy has been widely adopted in pediatric intensive care units throughout the world. Strategies borrowed from the neonatal experience with hyaline membrane disease – such as high-frequency oscillatory ventilation, surfactant instillation, and inhaled nitric oxide – have also been employed in pediatric patients with ARDS, but none has been shown to improve outcomes in large prospective randomized clinical trials.

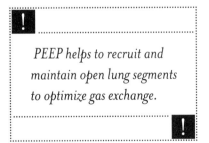

*PEEP helps to recruit and maintain open lung segments to optimize gas exchange.*

Although the strategy for mechanical ventilation in patients with ARDS focuses on optimizing oxygenation, care must be taken to avoid breath stacking and inadvertent auto-PEEP that may result from the use of prolonged inspiratory time and inverse I:E ratios.

## B. Obstructive Airway Disease

### Case Study

An 11-year-old, 50-kg girl with a history of mild intermittent asthma presents to the emergency department complaining of chest pain and shortness of breath that has worsened over the past 2 days. Her respiratory rate is 36 breaths/min, and oxygen saturations are 92% on room air. Examination reveals mild suprasternal retractions, and only minimal air entry is appreciated on auscultation. Continuous inhaled bronchodilators and methylprednisolone are given without improvement, and she is rapidly transferred to the pediatric intensive care unit, where a terbutaline infusion is started, but her heart rate increases to 180 beats/min with S-T wave elevations. Soon after arrival, the patient becomes drowsy and disoriented. As she is being prepared for intubation, an arterial blood gas analysis shows the following values: pH 7.14; $Paco_2$, 80 mm Hg (10.7 kPa); $Pao_2$, 76 mm Hg (10.1 kPa); base excess, -8 mEq/L; and saturation, 88%. She is emergently intubated, and positive-pressure ventilation is initiated in SIMV–volume-control mode with the following settings: respiratory rate, 12 breaths/min; $V_T$, 350 mL; $Fio_2$, 1.0; PEEP, 5 cm $H_2O$; inspiratory time, 1 second; I:E ratio, 1:4.

#### Detection
– What are the potential risks and benefits of endotracheal intubation and mechanical ventilation in this patient with severe status asthmaticus?

#### Intervention
– What are important considerations when setting the ventilator parameters in this patient?

– What is the indication for PEEP in a patient with obstructive lung disease whose lungs are already hyperinflated?

#### Reassessment
– What would you monitor in a patient with severe status asthmaticus?

– What changes are necessary if auto-PEEP is detected?

#### Effective Communication
– What clinical changes occur requiring communication?

– What level of care does this patient require?

#### Teamwork
– What team members need to be involved?

– How will you implement the treatment plan?

Intubation and mechanical ventilation of the patient with status asthmaticus should be an intervention of last resort, utilized only after all other measures have been exhausted. Laryngoscopy can trigger profound bronchospasm and should be performed by the most capable and experienced healthcare provider available. The lungs of patients with respiratory failure due to asthma are generally hyperinflated, and the risk of pneumothorax and pneumomediastinum is high.

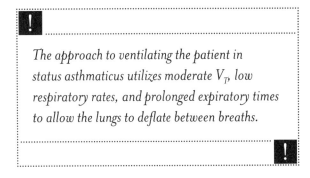

*The approach to ventilating the patient in status asthmaticus utilizes moderate $V_T$, low respiratory rates, and prolonged expiratory times to allow the lungs to deflate between breaths.*

The use of PEEP in these patients is controversial and stylistic. Large randomized controlled studies comparing the use of physiologic PEEP to no PEEP in the management of children receiving mechanical ventilation for severe asthma have not been done. When the patient with asthma is intubated for hypercarbic respiratory failure, it is likely due to air trapping rather than hypoventilation, and setting a high respiratory rate on the ventilator to blow off $CO_2$ will not result in the desired outcome. Bronchospasm and small airway obstruction should be treated aggressively with parenteral or inhaled bronchodilators and corticosteroids to relieve the obstruction and reverse the acute process. Patients intubated for status asthmaticus should be extubated as soon as the bronchospasm is under control and they meet clinical criteria for extubation.

Recent published cases describe pediatric patients who have developed cerebral edema in the setting of profound respiratory acidosis (with $Pa_{CO_2}$ >100 mm Hg [13.3 kPa]) associated with status asthmaticus. Patients requiring intubation for hypercarbic respiratory failure should be monitored closely for signs of increased intracranial pressure.

## C. Asymmetric Lung Disease

Asymmetric lung disease or injury that occurs after aspiration, contusion, localized pneumonia, or hemorrhage may cause abnormal distribution of ventilation and gas exchange during mechanical ventilation. Because the conditioned gas from the ventilator follows the path of least resistance along the bronchi, the $V_T$ is distributed primarily to the less-affected (more compliant) lung and may overexpand it. Overdistension of the less-affected lung and poor expansion of the diseased or injured lung worsen ventilation-perfusion relationships in both lungs, and hypoxemia and hypercapnia may occur, persist, or worsen. Standard settings and principles of ventilatory support should be initiated. If this attempt is unsuccessful, expert consultation should be obtained regarding further patient management. Positioning the patient so that the healthier, better-ventilated lung is in the gravitationally dependent position (sick side up) is a simple strategy for improving ventilation-perfusion matching and should result in improved oxygenation. Other techniques, such as differential lung ventilation, may be required.

## D. Heart Disease

###  Case Study

A 3-month-old male infant with trisomy 21 (Down syndrome) and a complete atrioventricular canal defect is brought to his cardiologist 3 weeks after digoxin and furosemide have been initiated. His mother reports he still requires 45 minutes to take 30 mL of formula and then is too exhausted to take any more. He has gained only 150 grams since birth and has fallen off his growth curve. On exam he is breathing at 72 breaths/min with deep suprasternal retractions. His liver edge is firm and palpable 4 cm below the right costal margin. Extremities are pale and cool, and pulses are diminished.

**Detection**

- What respiratory signs or symptoms do you find?
- What is the likely cause of this patient's respiratory distress?

**Intervention**

- Would this patient be a good candidate for NPPV? Why or why not?
- If the patient is placed on conventional ventilation, what settings would be appropriate?
- What other interventions are appropriate?

**Reassessment**

- When managing this patient, what additional assessments must be completed?
- What is the best range for the pH?
- How would the initiation of positive-pressure ventilation impact this child's circulatory status?

**Effective Communication**

- Where is the best place to manage this patient?
- If the patient's clinical status deteriorates, who needs to be contacted?

**Teamwork**

- Who should implement the treatment strategy?
- How should the responsibilities be divided?

The primary goal of ventilatory support in patients with myocardial ischemia or heart failure is to decrease the work of breathing and thereby ensure adequate oxygen delivery to the myocardium. Decreasing work of breathing reduces consumption of oxygen by respiratory muscles and increases the amount of oxygen available to the heart and end organs. Patients with cardiogenic pulmonary edema may also benefit from the increased thoracic pressure with positive pressure ventilation, which decreases biventricular filling (lowering pulmonary capillary pressure) and unloads the left ventricle (increasing stroke volume).

High $P\overline{aw}$ during mechanical ventilation may adversely affect cardiac performance by increasing right ventricular afterload and reducing venous return. Therefore, the parameters that affect $P\overline{aw}$ should be monitored and adjusted to maintain adequate cardiac function.

## E. Neuromuscular Disease

 ### Case Study

A 9-year-old boy is admitted to the pediatric intensive care unit for observation after falling down a flight of stairs. His parents report that his knees "just gave out from under him." His review of systems is significant only for a bout of "walking pneumonia" 2 weeks ago, from which he recovered uneventfully. On examination, you note tenderness in both lower extremities, absent patellar reflexes, and decreased muscle tone. On the night of admission, he develops difficulty swallowing, followed by respiratory distress requiring emergent intubation and positive-pressure ventilation.

**Detection**
- What unique considerations must be addressed when ventilating the child with neuromuscular disease?

**Intervention**
- Would this patient be a good candidate for NPPV? Why or why not?
- If the patient is placed on conventional ventilation, what settings would be appropriate?

**Reassessment**
- What additional assessments must be completed?
- What is the best target range for the pH?

**Effective Communication**
- Where is the best place to manage this patient?
- If the patient's clinical status deteriorates, who needs to be contacted?

**Teamwork**
- Who should implement the treatment strategy?
- How should the responsibilities be divided?

Patients with peripheral neuromuscular disease typically have an intact respiratory drive and normal lungs. These patients may require a higher $V_T$ to avoid the sensation of dyspnea. Adjustments may need to be made in other ventilatory parameters to ensure a normal arterial pH. Whenever possible, supported spontaneous breathing should be encouraged to prevent further deterioration in respiratory muscle function.

# IX. MONITORING MECHANICAL VENTILATORY SUPPORT

Patients who receive mechanical ventilatory support require continuous monitoring to assess the effects of treatment (**Table 5-6**). Arterial blood gas measurement provides valuable information about the adequacy of oxygenation, ventilation, and acid-base balance (**Appendix 3**). This information is mandatory during initiation of ventilator support, periods of patient instability, and weaning from mechanical ventilation.

Ventilators are equipped with sophisticated alarms and monitors to assist with patient management and the detection of adverse events. When initiating ventilator support, the respiratory care practitioner usually establishes alarm parameters for low and high minute ventilation, high inspiratory pressures, and low exhaled volumes and pressures. In addition, many ventilators allow for the measurement of auto-PEEP.

The low-pressure alarm is intended to alert the clinician to a leak in the circuit or ventilator disconnection. A high-pressure alarm alerts the clinician that the set maximum Ppeak has been exceeded. This alarm is usually set 5 to 10 cm $H_2O$ above the patient's baseline Ppeak. A high-pressure alarm for a patient receiving volume ventilation may indicate the presence of a mucous plug, a sudden change in airway or lung compliance due to an accumulation of secretions, or a change in ETT position. The patient may not receive the entire set $V_T$, because inspiration ends when the pressure limit is exceeded. For this reason, the frequent sounding of ventilator alarms should not be attributed to machine malfunction and should never be ignored or disabled.

### Table 5-6. Recommendations for Monitoring Mechanical Ventilatory Support

1. Obtain a chest radiograph after intubation and intermittently as needed to evaluate placement of the endotracheal tube and deterioration in status.
2. Obtain arterial blood gas measurements after initiation of mechanical ventilation and intermittently based upon patient status.
3. Measure vital signs intermittently; frequently observe the patient directly (including evaluation of patient-ventilator interaction).
4. Measure inspiratory plateau pressure as clinically appropriate.
5. Use continuous pulse oximetry to measure oxygenation.
6. Use ventilator alarms to monitor key physiologic and ventilator parameters.

# X. HYPOTENSION WITH INITIATION OF MECHANICAL VENTILATION

## A. Tension Pneumothorax

When hypotension occurs immediately after initiation of mechanical ventilation, a tension pneumothorax is possible. Diagnosis of this condition is based on a physical examination that finds decreased or absent breath sounds and tympani to percussion on the side of the pneumothorax. Changes in vital signs may include decreased oxygen saturation, tachycardia, and an increased respiratory rate if the patient is breathing spontaneously. Tracheal deviation away from the side of the pneumothorax may be observed, although such a finding is uncommon after placement of an ETT.

Treatment involves emergent decompression by insertion of a large-bore catheter or needle into the second or third intercostal space in the midclavicular line (**Appendix 12**). This should not be delayed to await radiographic confirmation. Decompression is both diagnostic and therapeutic and will restore blood pressure and vital signs to normal. The insertion of the catheter or needle must be followed by placement of a thoracostomy tube to prevent recurrence of the pneumothorax.

## B. Conversion from Negative to Positive Intrathoracic Pressure

Normal intrathoracic pressure is slightly negative in relation to the atmosphere. When positive pressure ventilation is initiated, intrathoracic pressure becomes positive. As intrathoracic pressure rises, right atrial pressure rises, and the intravascular pressure gradient for return of blood from the large extrathoracic veins into the right heart decreases. As a result, systemic venous return to the heart is reduced. Left ventricular preload, stroke volume, cardiac output, and blood pressure may then decrease in sequence. The deleterious effects on cardiac output and blood pressure are exacerbated by underlying intravascular volume depletion.

Treatment of this common complication involves volume resuscitation using rapidly infused fluid boluses, in aliquots of 10 or 20 mL/kg, to raise extrathoracic venous pressure and increase venous return to the right heart until the blood pressure increases. Oxygen saturation should be monitored to avoid overly aggressive fluid resuscitation. Use of ventilation techniques that incorporate high $P\overline{aw}$ may exacerbate the deleterious hemodynamic consequences of positive-pressure ventilation.

## C. Auto-PEEP

Auto-PEEP occurs when the lungs do not empty completely before the initiation of a subsequent breath. Due to either obstruction to outflow of gas or a need for an excessively long inspiratory time, the combination of ventilator settings and patient physiology results in an inadequate expiratory time (**Figure 5-4**). Excessive auto-PEEP may increase intrathoracic pressure and cause hypotension because of decreased venous return to the heart. Although auto-PEEP may occur in any patient, those with obstructive airway disease are particularly predisposed to this condition. Assessment and treatment of auto-PEEP is performed as previously described.

## D. Acute Myocardial Ischemia/Infarction

Factors that can increase myocardial oxygen demand include: stress from acute respiratory failure, intubation, and the transition to positive-pressure ventilation, β-adrenergic medications (i.e., epinephrine [adrenaline], dobutamine), and some anesthetic agents (ketamine). In older children and adults with inadequate cardiac reserve, this may lead to acute myocardial ischemia and subsequent hypotension.

# XI. WEANING FROM MECHANICAL VENTILATION

Although beyond the scope of this fundamental course, no discussion of mechanical ventilation would be complete without a short review of current approaches to weaning the patient from the ventilator. This process should be considered as soon as pulmonary function begins to improve. Decisions concerning weaning are separate and apart from decisions concerning extubation.

During weaning from mechanical ventilation, a patient gradually takes on more of the function of gas exchange while the ventilator contributes less to the patient's minute ventilation. The circumstances that required mechanical ventilation support must be resolving. In addition, the patient must actively participate in the process, and objective and subjective criteria must be set to monitor the success or failure of the process. Factors that influence weaning from mechanical ventilation include the patient's level of alertness, need for sedative medication, respiratory drive, and the time elapsed since the patient's most recent episode of respiratory or hemodynamic decompensation.

Several approaches to weaning have been proposed for adults and children. They include the demonstration of the patient's readiness for further weaning and ultimately for extubation, and almost universally include a spontaneous breathing trial. The conditions under which the trial takes place may vary, but an important component is the use of pressure support to prevent the patient's work of breathing from being hampered by the resistance of the ventilator circuit. In small children with an ETT of <3.5 mm, unsupported spontaneous breathing may be akin to breathing through a straw. If respiratory muscles are deconditioned, the child's effort may be insufficient to overcome tube resistance. Fatigue and respiratory distress may ensue unless pressure support is added.

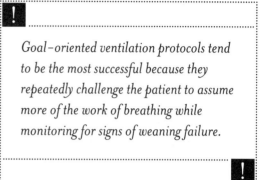

*Goal-oriented ventilation protocols tend to be the most successful because they repeatedly challenge the patient to assume more of the work of breathing while monitoring for signs of weaning failure.*

The rate at which a patient is weaned from mechanical ventilation is based on a number of factors, including the patient's physical condition and the duration of mechanical ventilation. A patient with normal lungs who is placed on mechanical ventilation for general anesthesia during an elective surgical procedure can be weaned and extubated rapidly, which anesthesiologists often do in the operating room. This is in contradistinction to the patient who is intubated for several days or weeks for severe systemic illness, who requires a more gradual, closely monitored weaning regimen. Conditions should be optimized prior to initiating weaning; this includes adjusting sedatives and discontinuing neuromuscular blocking medications, optimizing nutrition and ensuring a positive nitrogen balance, and optimizing fluid and acid-base status. Patients with severe metabolic alkalosis (often the result of aggressive diuretic therapy) should have their acid-base status normalized to ensure optimal respiratory drive.

Once weaning has begun, a change in vital signs – such as an increase in heart rate or respiratory rate, and an increase or decrease in blood pressure – may indicate a patient's inability to tolerate the process. Clinical signs of fatigue, including paradoxical breathing or use of accessory muscles of respiration, diaphoresis, or agitation, suggest that the patient is not ready to be weaned further. Patients who become air hungry are easily recognized by their inability to attend to anything other than their next breath. The patient who becomes more tachypneic, develops retractions, and requires more oxygen to maintain the same saturations is failing to wean and should be placed back on a higher level of support. Arterial blood gases are a good objective indicator of how well a patient is tolerating weaning from mechanical ventilation. A need for more than 50% $F_{IO_2}$ to achieve $Pa_{O_2}$ >60 mm Hg (>8.0 kPa) or a $Pa_{CO_2}$ >50 mm Hg (>6.7 kPa) usually indicates that the patient is not a candidate for further weaning. A chest radiograph should be obtained during the final stages of weaning to ensure there are no significant contraindications to extubation, such as atelectasis or pneumothorax.

## Mechanical Ventilation

**Key Points**

- Mechanical ventilation is indicated when less-invasive interventions for hypoxic or hypercapnic respiratory failure are unsuccessful.

- The primary goals of mechanical ventilation are to support ventilation and oxygenation and to reduce the work of breathing while ensuring patient comfort.

- Various types of breaths and modes of ventilation are available to facilitate synchrony between the patient and the ventilator.

- The following guidelines may be used when initiating volume control ventilation: $F_{IO_2}$ of 1.0; an age-appropriate rate, usually between 12 and 24 breaths/min; $V_T$ of 6 to 8 mL/kg that results in adequate chest rise ($V_T$ of 4 to 6 mL/kg for lungs with low compliance); and PEEP between 2 and 5 cm $H_2O$. The inspiratory time, usually 0.5 to 1 second, is based on patient age and disease process.

- The complex interactions between inspiratory pressures, I:E ratio, $F_{IO_2}$, and PEEP must be appreciated to predict the potential beneficial and harmful effects in each patient.

- The primary determinants of oxygenation are $F_{IO_2}$ and $P\overline{aw}$, whereas minute alveolar ventilation (respiratory rate and $V_T$) primarily affects $CO_2$ exchange. In the patient with acute lung injury or ARDS, PEEP becomes an additional independent determinant of oxygenation.

- The importance of closely monitoring the patient during mechanical ventilation cannot be overstressed. This includes appropriate setting of and attention to ventilator alarm functions, continuous pulse oximetry, frequent bedside assessment of the patient, and obtaining arterial blood gases and chest radiographs as needed.

- Weaning from mechanical ventilation is an active process that should be started as soon as the indications for ventilation have begun to resolve. Close monitoring during the weaning process is required to avoid any additional stress and to ensure patient comfort.

## Suggested Readings

1. Acute Respiratory Distress System Network. Ventilation with lower tidal volumes as compared with traditional tidal volumes for acute lung injury and the acute respiratory distress syndrome. *N Engl J Med*. 2000;342:1301-1308.

2. Arnold JH, Anas NG, Luckett P, et al. High-frequency oscillatory ventilation in pediatric respiratory failure: a multicenter experience. *Crit Care Med*. 2000;28:3913-3919.

3. Cheifetz I. Invasive and noninvasive pediatric mechanical ventilation. *Respir Care*. 2003;48: 453-458.

4. Dekel B, Segal E, Perel A. Pressure support ventilation. *Arch Intern Med*. 1996;156:369-373.

5. Dick CR, Sassoon CSH. Patient-ventilator interactions. *Clin Chest Med*. 1996;17:423-438.

6. Fortenberry JD, Del Toro J, Jefferson LS, Evey L, Haase D. Management of pediatric acute hypoxemic respiratory insufficiency with bilevel positive pressure (BiPAP) nasal mask ventilation. *Chest.* 1995;108:1059-1064.

7. Habashi NM. Other approaches to open-lung ventilation: airway pressure release ventilation. *Crit Care Med.* 2005;33(3 suppl):S228-S240.

8. Jubran A, Tobin MJ. Monitoring during mechanical ventilation. *Clin Chest Med.* 1996;17:453-473.

9. Kaplan LJ, Bailey H, Formosa V. Airway pressure release ventilation increases cardiac performance in patients with acute lung injury/acute respiratory distress syndrome. *Crit Care.* 2001;5:221-226.

10. Keith RL, Pierson DJ. Complications of mechanical ventilation: a bedside approach. *Clin Chest Med.* 1996;17:439-451.

11. Padman R, Lawless ST, Kettrick R. Noninvasive ventilation via bilevel positive airway pressure support in pediatric practice. *Crit Care Med.* 1998;26:169-173.

12. Schultz TR, Costarino AT, Durning SM, et al. Airway pressure release ventilation in pediatrics. *Pediatr Crit Care Med.* 2001;2:243-246.

13. Venkataraman ST. Mechanical ventilation and respiratory care. In: Fuhrman BP, Zimmerman J, eds. *Pediatric Critical Care.* 3rd ed. Philadelphia, PA: Mosby; 2006:683-718.

# Chapter 6

# Diagnosis and Management of Shock

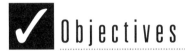

## Objectives

- Define shock.
- Identify the 5 major categories of shock and their typical presentation.
- Determine the initial steps in the evaluation and management of a child in shock.
- Discuss the goals of fluid resuscitation for pediatric patients in shock.
- Describe the physiologic effects of vasopressors and inotropic agents.

## I. INTRODUCTION

Shock, which may be simply described as inadequate provision of oxygen and other essential substrates to vital organs, is a common problem in acute care settings. Oxygen delivery ($Do_2$) is compromised in shock states. It is directly related to the arterial oxygen content ($Cao_2$) and cardiac output (CO), a function of the heart rate and stroke volume, the amount of blood ejected from the left ventricle with each beat. $Cao_2$ represents the amount of oxygen bound to hemoglobin plus the very small amount of oxygen dissolved in arterial blood.

$$Do_2 = Cao_2 \times CO$$

$$Cao_2 = (\text{Hemoglobin} \times 1.34 \times Sao_2) + (0.003 \times Pao_2)$$

$$CO = \text{Heart Rate} \times \text{Stroke Volume}$$

Stroke volume is a function of preload, defined as the volume of blood in the ventricular cavities at the end of diastole, the afterload or resistance to ventricular ejection, and myocardial contractility, the force exerted by the myocardium. Inadequate cardiac output can be corrected by ensuring optimal preload, afterload, and contractility and, in some cases, increases in heart rate. In addition, $Do_2$ can be increased by optimizing hemoglobin oxygen saturation and raising the circulating hemoglobin concentration with packed red blood cell transfusion.

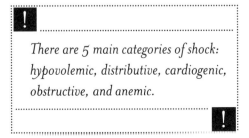

*There are 5 main categories of shock: hypovolemic, distributive, cardiogenic, obstructive, and anemic.*

Shock-related mortality has decreased dramatically over the last few years largely due to prompt diagnosis and management according to established guidelines, which emphasize the importance of prompt diagnosis and rapid, serial goal-directed interventions designed to reverse the signs of shock and restore vital signs to threshold values. Han et al demonstrated that the reversal of shock within the first hour of a patient's presentation to a community hospital was associated with dramatic improvements in mortality and functional outcome (**Figure 6-1**).

Developmental differences between pediatric and adult patients strongly influence management decisions. Although cardiac rate and contractility usually increase in acutely ill adult patients, ventricular function is relatively fixed in babies, so that any decrease in heart rate critically diminishes cardiac output. Infants and children also have higher baseline heart rates, which limits their ability to improve cardiac output by increasing that rate. Systemic vascular resistance can increase significantly in the acutely ill child, so blood pressure may remain in a falsely reassuring range until the onset of decompensated shock. Elevated systemic vascular resistance also compromises cardiac output in the presence of hypovolemia or decreased myocardial function.

**Figure 6-1.** Survival Rates of Pediatric Patients with Shock Reversal Versus Persistent Shock

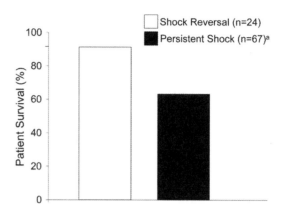

[a]p <0.05.
Shock reversal from resuscitative efforts by community hospital physicians resulted in 96% survival versus 63% survival among patients who remained in a persistent state of shock.
Data were derived from Han YY, Carcillo JA, Dragotta MA, et al. Early reversal of pediatric-neonatal septic shock by community physicians is associated with improved outcome. *Pediatrics*. 2003;112:793-799.

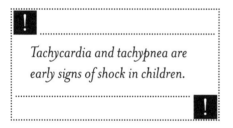

*Tachycardia and tachypnea are early signs of shock in children.*

Early shock in pediatric patients often has subtle presentations. Tachycardia and tachypnea may be the only abnormalities. Failure to detect and reverse these phenomena may allow a compensated, easily manageable shock state to progress to irreversible organ dysfunction.

## II. TYPES OF SHOCK

### A. Hypovolemic Shock

###  Case Study

A previously healthy 2-year-old boy is brought to the emergency department. His family reports that he has had copious diarrhea and vomiting with an inability to tolerate any oral fluids. The child's heart rate is 172 beats/min, and his blood pressure is 92/70 mm Hg. He is cool and mottled, and has thready pulses. His capillary refill is severely delayed, and he barely reacts when intravenous access is attempted.

**Detection**

- What does this toddler have?

**Intervention**

- Which mechanisms are in place in this situation?
- How should this child's shock be addressed?

**Reassessment**

- The child is able to sit up and interact appropriately with caregivers after receiving isotonic crystalloid, 40 mL/kg.
- Is the current treatment strategy effective?
- Does he need more fluid resuscitation and/or other therapeutic interventions?

**Effective Communication**

- When the patient's clinical status changes, who needs to know and how will the information be disseminated?
- Where is the best place to manage the care of this patient?

**Teamwork**

- How are you going to implement the treatment strategy?
- Who is to do what and when?

Hypovolemic shock, the most common type of shock seen in children, occurs when circulating intravascular blood volume decreases until adequate tissue perfusion can no longer be maintained. Hypovolemia causes a decrease in preload, adversely affecting cardiac output. The initial response to hypovolemia is the activation of peripheral and central baroreceptors, in turn promoting catecholamine-mediated vasoconstriction and tachycardia. These mechanisms can maintain adequate circulation and blood pressure even after acute loss of as much as 30% of the circulating blood volume. However, acute losses in excess of 30% of the circulating blood volume result in a much more clinically obvious state that may cause life-threatening organ compromise.

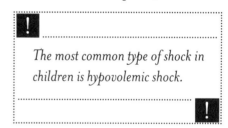

*The most common type of shock in children is hypovolemic shock.*

The most common cause of hypovolemia is diarrhea, which may occur rapidly in patients unable to replenish ongoing losses due to concurrent vomiting. Patients with other disease processes, such as traumatic injuries with significant or ongoing blood losses, are also encountered in the emergency setting. These patients typically present with tachycardia, a narrowed pulse pressure, delayed capillary refill, orthostatic changes, and in late stages, frank hypotension. They commonly show signs of decreased end-organ perfusion, such as altered mentation and decreased urine output in the absence of an osmotic load.

## B. Cardiogenic Shock

### Case Study

An 8-month-old boy is being treated for presumed bronchiolitis. The nurses caring for him in the emergency department report that he appears to be getting sicker rather than better. His wheezing has not responded to several hours of continuous albuterol, and he is poorly responsive to his environment. A physician is called to the bedside when a wide-complex tachycardia is seen on the monitor.

**Detection**

- The child has barely perceptible pulses, markedly delayed capillary refill, and a gallop. Rales and hepatomegaly are noted.
- What physical exam findings suggest the correct diagnosis?

**Intervention**

- Further evaluation demonstrates cardiomegaly, ventricular tachycardia, and evidence of end-organ ischemia. The child arrests shortly after admission to the pediatric intensive care unit (PICU).
- What are the immediate interventions needed?
- What are the general management principles for pediatric shock?

**Reassessment**

- Is the current treatment strategy effective?
- What else does the boy need? Other therapeutic interventions?

**Effective Communication**

- When the patient's clinical status changes, who needs to know and how will the information be disseminated?
- Where is the best place to manage the care of this patient?

**Teamwork**

- How are you going to implement the treatment strategy?
- Who is to do what and when?

Cardiogenic shock is characterized by significant decrease in cardiac output. Myocardial dysfunction is the most common cause of cardiogenic shock. Among the many causes of myocardial dysfunction are primary or familial cardiomyopathies, infectious myocarditis, and systemic inflammatory processes such as sepsis, autoimmune diseases, impaired coronary perfusion, exposure to cardiopulmonary bypass, acidosis, and hypoxic-ischemic events. Abnormalities in heart rate, such as profound bradycardia in patients with complete heart block or severe tachycardia in patients with ventricular or supraventricular dysrhythmias, also may cause cardiogenic shock.

Cardiogenic shock must be in the differential diagnosis when acute illness is encountered in young infants. Babies may develop cardiac failure very quickly as a complication of supraventricular tachycardia or other tachydysrhythmias. Likewise, infants with ductal dependent lesions may also present with cardiogenic shock within the first 2 months of life. A significant gradient in the blood pressure measured in the upper extremities compared to the lower extremities is typical of left-sided, ductus-dependent congenital cardiac lesions, which may rapidly cause life-threatening shock and organ dysfunction. An infusion of prostaglandin $E_1$ should be started immediately and continued until echocardiography definitively excludes a ductus-dependent lesion.

Patients with cardiogenic shock are usually – but not always – tachycardic, with cool extremities, a narrow pulse pressure, and respiratory distress. Rales or gallop rhythm may be audible, and an enlarged liver may be felt. Jugular venous distention may be difficult to visualize in children. Cardiomegaly is usually evident on chest radiograph.

Treatment of cardiogenic shock centers on optimizing intravascular volume, improving myocardial contractility with inotropic agents, and reducing afterload with the use of vasodilators. General supportive measures of are of paramount importance. The provider should pay close attention to fluid management as overzealous fluid resuscitation in a child already in congestive heart failure can worsen the clinical condition.

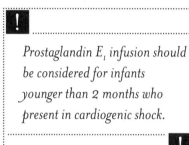

*Prostaglandin $E_1$ infusion should be considered for infants younger than 2 months who present in cardiogenic shock.*

## C. Distributive Shock

 Case Study

A 13-year-old girl ingests several medications, including tricyclic antidepressants, after an argument with her parents. She is very sleepy, hypotensive (70/35 mm Hg), and flushed in appearance. Her capillary refill is brisk. She has mildly broadened QRS complexes and a prolonged QT interval.

**Detection**

- What are the important clues to this child's underlying physiology?
- What are common causes of distributive shock?

**Intervention**

- What are the immediate interventions needed?
- How should this child be stabilized?
- What are the general management principles for pediatric shock?

**Reassessment**

- She improves rapidly after appropriate volume resuscitation, sodium bicarbonate, and vasoactive support are given.
- Is the current treatment strategy effective?
- What else does she need? Other therapeutic interventions?

**Effective Communication**
- When the patient's clinical status changes, who needs to know and how will the information be disseminated?
- Where is the best place to manage the care of this patient?

**Teamwork**
- How are you going to implement the treatment strategy?
- Who is to do what and when?

Distributive shock is a state of inadequate substrate delivery precipitated by inappropriately decreased systemic vascular resistance with redistribution of blood flow away from vital organs. This type of shock may be observed in patients with early septic shock, anaphylaxis, toxic ingestions, spinal or epidural anesthesia, and spinal cord injuries. Those with distributive shock typically have a flushed appearance, warm extremities with bounding pulses, and tachycardia with a wide pulse pressure. Capillary refill may be instantaneous. Distributive shock due to spinal cord injury may occur without significant compensatory rises in heart rate. Treatment should focus on reversal of the underlying etiology (whenever possible), rapid expansion of intravascular volume, and infusion of vasopressor medications with predominantly α-adrenergic activity, such as norepinephrine (noradrenaline) or phenylephrine.

# D. Obstructive Shock

 ## Case Study

An 8-month-old infant with pneumococcal sepsis is deteriorating rapidly. She has extremely poor perfusion, a narrow pulse pressure, and is hypotensive. She continues to worsen during transport to a tertiary PICU despite vigorous fluid administration and vasoactive support.

**Detection**
- What are the important clues to this child's underlying physiology?
- Physical exam reveals somewhat distant heart tones, and she is noted to have marked cardiomegaly when her most recent chest radiograph is compared to the previous day's film.
- What are common causes of obstructive shock?
- What are the clinical findings that suggest pericardial effusion?

**Intervention**
- What are the immediate interventions needed?
- How should this child be stabilized?
- What are the general management principles for pediatric shock?

**Reassessment**
- A fibrinous pericardial effusion is urgently decompressed under echocardiographic guidance and the patient improves rapidly.
- What general management principles must be observed?
- Is the current treatment strategy effective?

**Effective Communication**
- When the patient's clinical status changes, who needs to know and how will the information be disseminated?
- Where is the best place to manage the care of this patient?

**Teamwork**
- How are you going to implement the treatment strategy?
- Who is to do what and when?

Obstructive shock is relatively uncommon in pediatrics, thus requiring a high index of suspicion. It is the result of the influence of extrinsic forces on intrathoracic great vessels or cardiac chambers. Limitation of cardiac output occurs despite normal intravascular volume and myocardial contractility. Common causes of obstructive shock include pleural collections such as pneumothoraces. Pulmonary embolism is a rare cause that should be considered in children at risk, including those with hypercoagulable states or long bone fractures. Tamponade physiology may occur when pericardial effusions form rapidly and limit ventricular filling.

Clinical clues to the diagnosis of obstructive shock include tachycardia, cool extremities with delayed capillary refill, a narrow pulse pressure, distended neck veins, distant heart tones, and asymmetric breath sounds. Treatment centers on the prompt reversal of the underlying cause. Dramatic improvement usually follows evacuation of a tension pneumothorax or drainage of a pericardial effusion. Volume resuscitation with isotonic crystalloids or colloids is an essential temporizing measure. Drugs capable of decreasing systemic vascular resistance, such as benzodiazepines, opioids, or propofol, should be used with extreme caution until the cause of the obstructive shock is reversed.

# E. Anemic Shock

Children with chronic severe anemia have high cardiac output failure. Research done in the malaria belt of Africa shows that these children are harmed by fluid boluses but benefit from intravenous fluids administered at a maintenance infusion rate and from blood transfusion for hemoglobin <5 g/dL. Acute anemic shock that occurs without trauma responds better to blood transfusion than to fluid boluses.

# III. EVALUATION OF SHOCK

The evaluation of any illness or injury in all patients must include thorough initial and serial assessments of the airway, breathing, and circulation, with complete sets of vital signs, including blood pressure measurements. Fluctuations in levels of consciousness are important clinical clues to be followed using the conventional or modified Glasgow Coma Scale.

## A. ABCs: Assessment of Airway, Breathing, and Circulation

Airway patency, respiratory rate, pattern, and work of breathing should be noted. All children with suspected shock should receive supplemental oxygen, regardless of their baseline oxygen saturations. Positioning should be optimized to ensure airway patency and minimize work of breathing. Continuous pulse oximetry is usually well tolerated, even by irritable children, and is mandatory in the evaluation and monitoring of any sick patient. Hypoxemia or the presence of poor pulse oximeter signal must be considered ominous signs. Children displaying severe respiratory distress may require immediate assisted ventilation. Any patient with a rapidly declining Glasgow Coma Scale (**Chapter 15**) or a score of 8 or less is at risk for respiratory arrest, severe hypoxemia, and severe hypercarbia; these patients should have the airway secured as soon as possible by the most experienced practitioner available. Ventilation can be assisted with careful bag-mask ventilation until preparations have been made for endotracheal intubation.

> *Oxygen should be provided to all children with suspected shock, regardless of the oxygen saturation reading.*

Severe bradycardia (heart rate <90 beats/min in an infant) or severe tachycardia (heart rate >180 beats/min in ill-appearing children younger than 1 year or >140 beats/min in older children and adolescents) are markers of the severe systemic compromise that may precede circulatory collapse. Severe tachycardia in an obviously ill child may be quickly followed by hypotension and cardiac arrest. Any abnormality in heart rate should be confirmed with a rhythm strip or an electrocardiogram to define the underlying rhythm. A pediatric intensivist or cardiologist should be contacted for optimal management of dysrhythmias in children.

> *Hypotension is a late finding in pediatric shock.*

Hypotension is a late finding in pediatric shock, given children's capacity to increase systemic vascular resistance during the initial phase of decreased cardiac output. Children may be normotensive or even hypertensive in the presence of established shock, but blood pressure may fall precipitously in these patients. Failure to diagnose shock in a timely manner—before the onset of hypotension—may allow progression to an uncompensated and possibly irreversible state (**Table 6-1**).

### Table 6-1 Minimum Acceptable Blood Pressure Values for Ill-Appearing Children

| Age Group | Systolic/Diastolic Values (mm Hg) |
| --- | --- |
| Term neonate | 60/30 |
| Infant | 80/40 |
| Child | 90/60 |
| Adolescent | 100/70 |

Classified using US Department of Health and Human Services. *The Fourth Report on Diagnosis, Evaluation and Treatment of Hypertension in Children and Adolescents.* Bethesda, MD: National Institutes of Health; 2005. NIH Publication 05-5267.

Fever is common but not universal in pediatric patients with serious infections. In fact, hypothermia may be noted in infants and in septic patients of any age, making core temperature monitoring extremely important. Infants commonly react to a cold environment with apnea and bradycardia. Surface temperatures and capillary refill, easily reproducible indicators of perfusion, should be assessed in a central location and in an extremity that has not been exposed to a cold environment. Significant difference in the temperatures of the torso and the toes suggests impaired perfusion. Capillary refill is complete within 2 to 3 seconds under normal conditions. Abnormalities in refill time give important clues about the etiology of the circulatory derangement and can help assess response to interventions. These measures, along with the quality of central and peripheral pulses, are markers that must be followed closely as resuscitation progresses.

## B. Blood Glucose

A bedside assessment of blood glucose is essential on presentation and at appropriate intervals in all acutely ill children. Infants are particularly vulnerable to hypoglycemia given their high metabolic rates and limited glycogen reserves. Failure to promptly diagnose and treat hypoglycemia may result in permanent neurologic disability (**Chapter 8**).

## C. History and Physical Examination

A patient's history and physical examination will reveal important clues to the etiology of shock. Utilizing the DIRECT algorithm (**Chapter 1**), serial assessments of a child's vital signs, mentation, and perfusion are essential. The lung fields should be auscultated to detect new rales. A gallop rhythm may indicate underlying heart disease or hypervolemia due to overzealous fluid resuscitation. Palpation of the liver edge below the costal margin can indicate hypervolemia or cardiac failure. Rapidly evolving purpuric or petechial rashes may suggest an infectious origin. A careful secondary survey can demonstrate previously missed injuries in children with unclear or unknown histories.

# IV. MANAGEMENT OF SHOCK

All patients presenting with shock should be placed on high-flow oxygen while their initial evaluation is performed. Vascular access, control of the airway, fluid resuscitation, provision of appropriate vasoactive infusions, and appropriate antibiotic therapy are priorities to be addressed within the first few minutes of presentation.

## A. Vascular Access

Vascular access must be obtained as soon as possible. Intravenous cannulas may be difficult to place in acutely ill children with poor peripheral perfusion. Common sites for catheter placement include the dorsum of the hands, the saphenous vein just anterior to the medial malleolus, and the veins in the antecubital fossae. Initial volume resuscitation may be readily accomplished using scalp veins in babies. Care should be taken to avoid cannulation of the temporal artery when these veins are utilized. Umbilical venous access is an option for neonates if a skilled provider is available to perform the insertion.

> *Vascular access should be established early in children presenting with signs of shock.*

The external jugular vein may be accessible to cannulation; however, care should be used in the presence of respiratory distress or increased intracranial pressure to avoid further compromise with positioning. The site must be monitored for infiltration and removed as soon as more secure access is obtained, as the potential for infiltration with movement increases the risk for embolism and thrombosis.

Professionals caring for sick children should have a low threshold for placing intraosseous needles for initial or supplemental vascular access. Intraosseous access is a simple, safe, and effective measure to be considered early in the care of children with inadequate vascular access. Alternative sites, such as the distal femur, should be considered when indicated (**Appendix 2**).

Central venous catheters are helpful in complex resuscitations and should be placed by healthcare providers with expertise in this procedure when transfer to a tertiary center may be delayed. Proper control of the airway, correct positioning, adequate analgesia, local anesthesia, and strict sterile technique with full barrier precautions are required (**Appendix 13**).

Subclavian venous access is more treacherous in children than in adults, and a pneumothorax or vascular injury may be rapidly fatal in patients with preexisting hypovolemia. Therefore, subclavian cannulation should generally be avoided in children with shock, particularly in those with suspected coagulopathy.

The right internal jugular vein can be cannulated blindly using the posterior approach, which entails entering the vein as it courses beneath the sternocleidomastoid muscle. This is most easily performed by piercing the skin at the lateral border of the muscle immediately above the external jugular vein. The needle is advanced under the muscle towards an imaginary line that connects the point of entry with the sternal notch and the left nipple, with the head turned to the left and the neck slightly extended with a roll under the shoulders. Other approaches to the internal jugular vein, such as the central or anterior, are facilitated by ultrasonography. Although the left internal jugular vein may also be accessed with these techniques, this approach carries the added risk of injury to the thoracic duct.

Cannulation of the femoral vein is relatively easy and safe, although life-threatening retroperitoneal hematoma or injury to the femoral artery may occur rarely. Babies are at higher risk for vascular injury, particularly if the provider is inexperienced. The vein is readily accessed medially to the femoral pulse. Ultrasound guidance is recommended for central vascular access in all patients when available.

Central venous pressure monitoring is recommended for all acutely ill children, either on a continuous basis or as a trend every few hours if the lumen is required for infusion. Low central venous pressures are indicative of absolute hypovolemia in the ill, supine patient. High venous pressures suggest the opposite, with the caveat that they may be increased by high intrathoracic pressures, pneumothorax, or pericardial effusion, underscoring the importance of clinical correlation. Some patients with underlying cardiac disease require higher filling pressures; subspecialty consultation is helpful in such cases.

Arterial cannulation with continuous monitoring is recommended for critically ill children. Peripheral access is preferred, as injury to the femoral artery may occur. Important information that is afforded by this intervention includes the continuous display of heart rate, blood pressure, and pulse pressure, trends that inform patient management. The presence of a sloped upstroke suggests myocardial dysfunction with poor contractility (**Appendix 16**).

## B. Fluid Resuscitation

Large amounts of fluids are commonly required for resuscitation in children, due to their higher surface area to volume ratios and potential for ongoing losses. Children are less likely to have underlying comorbidities than adults and are generally better able to handle the large amounts of fluids administered during the course of resuscitation.

> *Start early fluid resuscitation with 20 mL/kg 0.9% saline solution as quickly as possible (<20 minutes). Continuous monitoring and frequent reassessment are recommended. Smaller and slower boluses are appropriate for neonatal patients, in severely anemic children, or if cardiogenic shock is a consideration.*

Only isotonic solutions should be used in the rapid intravascular volume expansion of children in shock. Normal saline (0.9% NaCl) is readily available and should be administered in aliquots of 20 mL/kg as quickly as possible (preferably <20 minutes) using peripheral intravenous or intraosseous access. Smaller fluid boluses should be used for neonates or if cardiogenic shock is suspected. Resistance to flow is significant when small central venous catheters are utilized, underscoring the value of peripheral and intraosseous access.

Although vigorous fluid resuscitation does not correlate with adverse pulmonary or neurologic outcomes in children, there are some concerns when normal saline is used for resuscitation. One is that the resuscitation fluid begins to redistribute to the extravascular space in as little as 1 hour. Hyperchloremic metabolic acidosis is common but transient. Dilution of plasma proteins with development of ascites, pleural effusions, and anasarca is commonly observed as well. Lactated

Ringer solution (Hartmann solution) is used extensively in some countries and can be effective in the management of moderate to severe shock, particularly if albumin solutions are unavailable. It is less likely to produce hyperchloremic acidosis but must be used with caution in patients at high risk for hyperkalemia.

Some experts advocate the use of 5% albumin, which remains in the intravascular space longer, as a strategy to possibly mitigate such problems. A reasonable approach is to use isotonic crystalloid initially and to continue volume resuscitation using 5% albumin if more than 40 to 60 mL/kg are required to normalize perfusion. One meta-analysis suggested that volume expansion with crystalloids may be advantageous for pediatric patients with gastroenteritis and injuries, including burns and traumatic brain injury. Volume expansion with colloids may be preferable in severe sepsis.

Smaller aliquots of resuscitation fluid (5-10 mL/kg) should be considered for neonates and children with known or suspected myocardial dysfunction or heart disease. Frequent reassessment is mandatory in this situation, so that adequate resuscitation is not delayed. Children, particularly those with septic shock or significant ongoing losses, may require very large amounts of fluid. Improved outcomes have been observed when at least 60 mL/kg of rapid intravascular fluid expansion is given within the first hour of treatment to children with septic shock (**Figure 6-2**).

**Figure 6-2.** Effects of Early Fluid Resuscitation on Pediatric Patients With Septic Shock

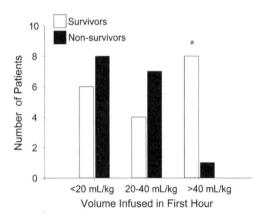

[a]Increased survival compared to all other groups.
Number of survivors and nonsurvivors among pediatric patients with septic shock stratified in groups according to the volume of fluid resuscitation received within the first hour of presentation to the emergency department.
Data were derived from Carcillo JA, Davis AL, Zaritsky A. Role of early fluid resuscitation in pediatric septic shock. *JAMA*. 1991;266:1242-1245.

A common but dangerous error is to infuse fluid boluses over 1 hour. The infusion pumps routinely used for medication and intravenous fluids are not effective for rapid resuscitation. The simplest measure is to interpose a 3-way stopcock (tap) into the intravenous line, so that fluids may be pulled from the bottle or bag (taking care not to aspirate and inject an air bolus, which could be fatal) and then administered to the patient via the peripheral or central venous line or intraosseous needle. Serial reassessment is extremely important to help guide the initial fluid resuscitation, which should be continued until adequate perfusion is achieved, the child's vital signs have returned to target values, and general appearance has improved. Use of the DIRECT algorithm is recommended.

Hemodilution associated with crystalloid or colloid boluses may compromise oxygen delivery in the presence of severe anemia, underscoring the need for red blood cell transfusion in these circumstances. Anemic children with severe malaria, respiratory distress, or neurologic dysfunction who are receiving care for shock in resource-limited settings, such as sub-Saharan Africa, appear to benefit from early transfusion of packed red blood cells as opposed to boluses of isotonic crystalloid or colloid.

Blood products may also be required in special circumstances, including traumatic injury or surgical losses in critically ill patients. The risk of hypotension precludes the rapid infusion of fresh frozen plasma. Platelets and cryoprecipitate may be indicated in the presence of thrombocytopenia and hypofibrinogenemia, which underscores the importance of obtaining appropriate laboratory studies as soon as possible during the resuscitation.

Hypoglycemia diagnosed on presentation should be managed with boluses of a 10% dextrose solution (5 mL/kg). For older children, 25% glucose can be used as required to achieve a serum glucose level >100 mg/dL, rather than with large volumes of dextrose-containing crystalloids, which may be relatively hypotonic and also carry the risk of inducing osmotic diuresis.

Fluid resuscitation should be continued until clinical improvement is clear or clinical evidence of a hypervolemic state is seen, suggested by new rales, a gallop rhythm, or hepatomegaly. Continued bolus administration of fluids at this point will cause excessive myocardial wall forces and depress function. Diuretic therapy with small doses of furosemide (0.3-0.5 mg/kg) may be considered if hypervolemia is suspected in an otherwise stabilizing child. This strategy may result in improved myocardial performance, enhanced urine output, and the possible mitigation of oliguric renal failure if acute tubular necrosis has developed. Higher doses of diuretics may be required in certain children, but it is prudent to administer a small dose first, particularly in the presence of hemodynamic instability.

Children who required resuscitation and are felt to be close to a normovolemic state (neither "wet" nor "dry") may be placed on maintenance fluids, with additional boluses of normal saline or 5% albumin as required. Infants are at high risk of developing hypoglycemia and therefore should receive dextrose-containing fluids, such as 5% to 10% dextrose with appropriate sodium and potassium supplementation and hourly bedside glucose monitoring.

A useful formula for calculating the infusion rate of maintenance fluids is to provide 4 mL/kg/h for the first 10 kg of body weight, plus 2 mL/kg/h for each additional kilogram up to 20 kg, with 1 mL/kg/h for each additional kilogram of body weight thereafter. Adult-sized children can be managed with maintenance infusions of 125 to 150 mL/h. An alternative is to calculate the body surface area and provide 1500 mL/m$^2$ as a 24-hour infusion, to be supplemented with isotonic or colloid boluses as required.

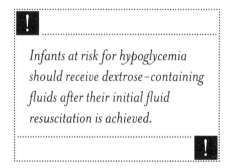

*Infants at risk for hypoglycemia should receive dextrose-containing fluids after their initial fluid resuscitation is achieved.*

Patients at risk for neurologic injury due to trauma or a hypoxic-ischemic insult are best managed with isotonic intravenous fluids. Although normal saline is commonly used, hypoglycemia is possible and may cause severe permanent injury. Hyperglycemia is commonly observed in acute stress and usually resolves during resuscitation without specific intervention. Aggressive treatment of hyperglycemia is treacherous during patient transfers. Regular insulin infusions must be used with great caution when absolutely indicated, started at low rates, and monitored closely at the bedside, at no more than hourly intervals, for appropriate management of hypo- or hyperglycemia.

## C. Vasoactive and Inotropic Support

Although shock in adults, particularly septic shock, displays typical and relatively static hemodynamic patterns, these are less predictable and can change rapidly in children. Invasive hemodynamic monitoring with an arterial catheter and a central venous catheter should be used to provide continuous measurements and establish trends in cardiovascular performance. Serial assessments of venous saturation at the superior vena cava are useful in guiding management and have been shown to reduce mortality in children with septic shock. Vasoactive and inotropic infusions are extremely helpful in stabilizing the child in shock, but their use in those who have not yet received adequate volume resuscitation has been associated with a poor outcome.

**1. Dopamine**

Dopamine, with its varied physiologic actions, is considered by most clinicians to be the first-line vasoactive medication for treatment of shock. It has dose-related clinical effects. Renal vasodilation is thought to occur at low infusion rates, although its significance in clinical practice is probably irrelevant. At intermediate doses, $\beta_1$ and $\beta_2$ effects predominate, resulting in inotropy, chronotropy, and vasodilatation, which may be advantageous in some situations. Higher infusion rates, typically in excess of 10 µg/kg/min, result in $\alpha_1$-receptor activation, with increases in systemic and pulmonary vascular resistance.

Relatively small doses of dopamine, such as 5 µg/kg/min, may be all that is needed to provide inotropic support for some children. The drug should always be started at higher doses, typically 10 µg/kg/min in children who are hypotensive, to avoid possible β-receptor–mediated vasodilation. Increasing the dose of dopamine beyond 20 µg/kg/min is not beneficial. Infants may be relatively insensitive to dopamine, requiring a directly acting catecholamine such as epinephrine (adrenaline) or norepinephrine (noradrenaline). Clinically significant increases in pulmonary vascular resistance have been described in some neonates when dopamine and other vasopressor medications are used (**Table 6-2**).

**2. Dobutamine**

Dobutamine has significant inotropic effects due to its preferential activation of β-receptors. Although it may have a role in the management of infants with mild hypoperfusion, typically in doses of 5 µg/kg/min, higher doses may be associated with unacceptable tachycardia. This agent is not as helpful in older children, particularly in adolescents with septic shock, in whom a decrease in systemic vascular resistance and an increase in heart rate may compromise coronary perfusion. However, dobutamine is a useful agent when ventricular dysfunction is suspected or documented. This drug is commonly used following cardiac transplantation, surgery to repair congenital heart defects, myocardial revascularization, and when myocardial function is significantly depressed, but it has a limited role in the contemporary management of pediatric septic shock.

### Table 6-2. Hemodynamic Effects of Commonly Used Vasoactive and Inotropic Agents

| Agent | α₁ | β₁ | β₂ | D₁ | V₁ |
|---|---|---|---|---|---|
| Dopamine[a] | Vasoconstriction; ↑ SVR, PVR | Inotropy; chronotropy | Vasodilatation | Vasodilatation (renal) | |
| Dobutamine | | Inotropy | | | |
| Epinephrine[b] (adrenaline) | Vasoconstriction; ↑ SVR, PVR | Inotropy; chronotropy | | | |
| Norepinephrine (noradrenaline) | Vasoconstriction; ↑ SVR, PVR | Inotropy (minor) | | | |
| Vasopressin | Potentiates | Potentiates | | | Vasoconstriction |
| **Non-receptor-mediated** | | | | | |
| Milrinone | | Inotropy, lusitropy, vasodilatation | | | |

D₁, dopamine receptor; PVR, pulmonary vascular resistance; SVR, systemic vascular resistance.
[a]Dose-related effects: at low dose, D₁-receptor effects might predominate; at intermediate doses, β₁ and β₁-receptor effects predominate; and at high doses, α₁-receptor effects predominate.
[b]Dose-related effects: at low doses β₁ and β₂-receptor effects predominate; at high doses, α₁-receptor effects predominate on peripheral vasculature.
Adapted with permission. © 2006 Elsevier. Smith L, Hernan L. Shock states. In: Fuhrman BP, Zimmerman J, eds. *Pediatric Critical Care*. 3rd ed. Philadelphia, PA: Mosby; 2006:394-410.

### 3. Epinephrine (Adrenaline)

Epinephrine (adrenaline) has many important physiologic effects from the activation of α- and β-receptors, including clinically relevant chronotropy, increased cardiac contractility, and increased systemic vascular resistance, making it a very useful agent in the management of children with shock.

Epinephrine should be administered as a continuous infusion into a reliable peripheral vein until a central venous catheter is in place. Nebulized racemic epinephrine can be used in the initial stabilization while vascular access is secured for volume resuscitation and vasoactive support. Epinephrine may increase myocardial oxygen consumption and cause a decrease in splanchnic perfusion. Because epinephrine also has the potential to decrease systemic vascular resistance under some circumstances, it may decrease coronary perfusion pressures, particularly in the presence of hypovolemia or severe tachycardia. These are important considerations in older children, who may be at greater risk for myocardial ischemia and dysrhythmias. A typical starting dose for epinephrine is 0.05 to 0.1 µg/kg/min, titrated to clinical effect (**Table 6-3**). Epinephrine is the drug of choice for cold septic shock, anaphylactic shock, and cardiogenic shock in patients with hypotension.

### Table 6-3  Suggested Infusion Doses for Commonly Used Vasoactive and Inotropic Agents

| Agent | Inotropic | Pressor |
| --- | --- | --- |
| Dopamine | 2-15 μg/kg/min | >12 μg/kg/min |
| Dobutamine | 2.5-20 μg/kg/min | |
| Epinephrine (adrenaline) | 0.05-0.5 μg/kg/min | 0.1-1 μg/kg/min |
| Norepinephrine (noradrenaline) | | 0.05-1 μg/kg/min |
| Vasopressin | | 0.5 mU |
| **Non-receptor-mediated** | | |
| Milrinone | 0.25-0.75 μg/kg/min | |

Adapted with permission. © Elsevier 1986. Park MK. Use of digoxin in infants and children, with specific emphasis on dosage. *J Pediatr*. 1986;108:871.

### 4. Norepinephrine (Noradrenaline)

Norepinephrine (noradrenaline) differs from epinephrine (adrenaline) in its strong α-receptor selectivity, resulting in increased vascular tone with minimal effect on the heart rate. This, in turn, translates into higher coronary and splanchnic perfusion pressures and, possibly, decreased end-organ dysfunction. The typical starting dose is 0.05 to 0.1 μg/kg/min and is quickly titrated to the desired effect. Norepinephrine is the drug of choice in warm septic shock and is a good choice for spinal cord shock.

### 5. Milrinone

Milrinone is commonly utilized in pediatric critical care for its inotropic and lusitropic effects in patients with myocardial dysfunction in the presence of a high systemic vascular resistance and low cardiac output. Milrinone has a long elimination half-life and duration of action, and requires dose adjustment in patients with renal and hepatic failure. Significant and prolonged hypotension may be observed, particularly when a loading dose or doses in excess of 0.3 μg/kg/min are employed or in the presence of renal or hepatic dysfunction. Milrinone is thus best initiated after admission to the PICU, with continuous intravascular monitoring.

### 6. Nitroprusside and Nitroglycerin

Nitroprusside and nitroglycerin have vasodilator effects and much shorter half-lives than milrinone, making these agents more appropriate for short-term use if a vasodilator is considered essential before transfer to a tertiary center. These agents can be utilized at very low doses, such as 0.05 μg/kg/min, to achieve desired decreases in systemic vascular resistance. Adequate volume loading with isotonic crystalloids or colloids, and the immediate availability of a vasopressor (such as epinephrine [adrenaline] or norepinephrine [noradrenaline]) are required for use.

### 7. Vasopressin

Vasopressin is a potent vasoconstrictor, useful in the management of shock with decreased systemic vascular resistance. It exerts its hemodynamic effects via the $V_{1a}$-receptor, promoting an increase in intracellular calcium, thus restoring systemic vascular tone. Vasopressin has been associated with improved blood pressure and urine output in patients with catecholamine-refractory vasodilatory shock and often allows weaning of catecholamines. Although a pediatric dose has not been established, some experts recommend starting with 0.5 mU/kg/min (0.0005 U/kg/min) for children. The standard adult dose of 0.03 or 0.04 U/min should not be exceeded.

## D. Endotracheal Intubation and Mechanical Ventilation

Mechanical ventilation, with careful preparation for intubation and meticulous attention to tidal volumes and pressures, may reduce or obviate the work of breathing, optimize oxygen transport, and improve hemodynamic performance by reducing left ventricular afterload. Subsequent planned and emergent procedures are significantly facilitated by a secure airway.

Due to the potential for deterioration during intubation in patients with shock, the most experienced person available should perform this procedure, preferably after volume resuscitation is well under way. A vasopressor infusion should be mixed and either be started or available for immediate use.

Preoxygenation via a non-rebreathing face mask or an anesthesia circuit is extremely important. A rapid-sequence intubation that includes cricoid pressure should be utilized in patients with recent oral intake or those at risk for delayed gastric emptying. Care must be taken not to distort anatomical landmarks if cricoid pressure is applied. Gastrostomies may be present in chronically ill children and should be open to air or gravity drainage. A nasogastric tube may be placed if excessive gastric distention has already occurred, but is best placed after the airway has been secured to prevent aspiration during intubation.

Given infants' fixed myocardial contractility and their dependence on heart rate for adequate cardiac output, drug premedication should include atropine to prevent vagally mediated bradycardia. Atropine improves intubating conditions in patients of all ages by minimizing airway secretions and possibly decreasing airway tone. There are no contraindications to using atropine in appropriate doses, even in the presence of tachycardia. Therefore, it may be helpful for all children requiring emergent intubation.

Drugs that may decrease systemic vascular resistance, such as large doses of midazolam or morphine, should be avoided in children with shock. Although many sources cite midazolam doses of 0.1 mg/kg, that amount may have significant deleterious hemodynamic effects in tenuous patients. Midazolam should be titrated carefully in small aliquots of 0.05 mg/kg or less, with the intention of using it as an adjuvant rather than the primary agent for intubation. Small doses of fentanyl (1-2 µg/kg) are preferred to morphine, which has substantially more hemodynamic effects.

Ketamine, with its dissociative anesthetic properties and its minimal adverse effects on hemodynamics, is the drug of choice for intubating patients in shock. A dose of 1 to 2 mg/kg is usually effective and enables ventilating the patient before administering neuromuscular blocking agents. Ketamine is usually avoided in patients known to have significant intracranial pathology and, by some practitioners, in patients suspected of having pulmonary hypertension. Ketamine is generally safe and effective in emergencies. It may be given intramuscularly at a dose of 3 mg/kg with atropine in patients who do not have vascular access. The use of small doses of benzodiazepines may decrease the incidence of emergence phenomena such as hallucinations following ketamine administration. Atropine or glycopyrrolate should always be given with ketamine to mitigate the sialorrhea invariably associated with this drug.

Etomidate can cause adrenal insufficiency and has been associated with increased risk of mortality in recent studies. This drug should not be used routinely unless there is a specific and compelling contraindication to the previously mentioned agents, such as known or strongly suspected intracranial pathology in a hemodynamically unstable patient requiring urgent intubation.

Rocuronium and vecuronium are neuromuscular blocking agents frequently utilized in securing the airway. Atracurium and cisatracurium may have a relatively higher propensity to cause histamine release with consequent hypotension and bronchospasm. They are best used in the PICU for specific indications.

Most patients with shock but normal pulmonary mechanics can be ventilated with standard tidal volumes of 6 to 8 mL/kg. For more information, please see **Chapter 5** on mechanical ventilation. Specific problems, such as the presence of congenital heart disease or persistent pulmonary hypertension in the newborn, may call for advanced mechanical ventilation strategies. These, however, should be attempted only in consultation with the tertiary center.

## E. Control of Acidosis

Metabolic acidosis, frequently offset by respiratory alkalosis in the initial stages of shock, may become evident as a child's condition worsens. Optimal management includes addressing underlying causes, such as hypovolemia and abnormal organ perfusion, using volume resuscitation, and vasoactive infusions as required. Adequate ventilation and oxygenation should be ensured by using cautious doses of sedation and analgesia, with neuromuscular blockade added only if absolutely necessary.

Sodium bicarbonate is indicated primarily for patients with hyperkalemia or intoxication with sodium channel-blocking drugs, but it may also be considered in the management of selected profoundly acidemic (pH <7), adequately ventilated patients. Because the use of sodium bicarbonate may increase intracellular acidosis, this treatment is no longer routinely recommended. Agents such as tromethamine given slowly, generally at 3 to 5 mL/kg over an hour, may be helpful in extreme situations, with the caveat that they can worsen hypokalemia, hyperkalemia, and hypoglycemia; they should be avoided in the presence of established renal failure.

## F. Laboratory Evaluation

A bedside glucose assay should be performed at presentation for any child who is acutely ill because significant time may elapse between sampling and report of the laboratory results. The initial laboratory evaluation should also include a complete blood count, a complete chemistry profile, ionized calcium, blood gas analysis, and coagulation testing as warranted by the child's condition and a presumed cause of shock. A blood sample should be sent for blood typing and cross-matching as soon as possible to expedite the availability of blood products that may be required for ongoing resuscitation.

Although blood and urine cultures are important in determining the cause of infections, antibiotics should not be delayed by difficulty in securing appropriate samples. Lumbar puncture should be deferred until a child has stabilized, because its findings will not affect the initial management; in fact, it may instead result in significant deterioration and cardiopulmonary arrest, particularly in the presence of increased intracranial pressure, coagulopathy, or limited reserve, as may be found in patients who remain in shock without a secure airway.

Additional laboratory studies, such as an ammonia level, serum amino acids, and urine organic acids, may be indicated in patients suspected of having inborn metabolic errors. These problems are usually detected in early infancy but may present in older infants and children. Toxicology screens are important for any child presenting with shock and encephalopathy. Assays for endocrine dysfunction, including cortisol levels and thyroid function tests, should be considered in specific circumstances, although they should not delay the administration of hydrocortisone (1 mg/kg, up to 50 mg intravenously every 6 hours) in children with suspected adrenal insufficiency.

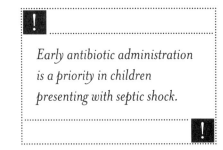

*Early antibiotic administration is a priority in children presenting with septic shock.*

## G. Radiographic Studies

A chest radiograph is essential to the complete evaluation of any child presenting with shock. Heart size provides important clues: most children with hypovolemia have a small or normal-appearing heart. A generous cardiac silhouette suggests myocardial dysfunction, hypervolemia, or pericardial effusion. The position of all tubes and lines should be noted. A more extensive survey that includes the lateral cervical spine and pelvis is required in patients who have sustained traumatic injuries. Careful consideration should be given to securing and maintaining the airway of a child requiring transfer out of the emergency department for imaging, because deterioration may occur rapidly in these situations.

## V. GENERAL CARE

The shock treatment goals for the first hour of care include complete initial and serial assessment of airway, breathing, and circulation, which can be guided by utilizing the DIRECT algorithm. Adequate vascular access must be secured within the first few minutes of presentation. It may be necessary to control the airway to ensure adequate oxygenation and ventilation, normalize perfusion, and restore vital signs to the threshold values for age.

Appropriate monitoring includes continuous pulse oximetry, electrocardiography, frequent (every 5 min) blood pressure measurements, hourly temperature and urine output measurement via an indwelling urinary catheter, and frequent assessments of glucose and ionized calcium. Once arterial and central venous pressure monitoring catheters have been placed, which may not be possible at the primary hospital, perfusion pressures and optimizing oxygen delivery are monitored continuously. A bedside glucose level should be measured hourly in patients at high risk of hypoglycemia, especially infants. Laboratory data that would be indicators of end-organ dysfunction, coagulation, and gas exchange should be evaluated at least every 6 hours.

A systematic, head-to-toe approach should be employed. Appropriate analgesia, sedation, and neuromuscular blockade decrease oxygen consumption. Sedation and analgesia can be safely and effectively accomplished using small, intermittent doses of benzodiazepines and fentanyl or ketamine (**Chapter 20**).

Although propofol is used widely in adult medicine, it commonly causes hypotension in children, particularly in the presence of hypovolemia or myocardial dysfunction. Therefore, it is not recommended in the management of shock in pediatric patients, particularly if transport is required. Neuromuscular blockade may be necessary to ensure patient safety and ventilator synchrony, but it should be utilized only with adequate sedation and analgesia by individuals with excellent airway management skills. Soft restraints should be considered for all children.

Continued meticulous attention to maintaining optimal preload, afterload, and contractility is essential. An adequate hemoglobin concentration and oxygen saturation should be maintained with a judicious transfusion strategy, inspired supplemental oxygen, and positive end-expiratory pressure. Lactate concentration, a surrogate marker of energy delivery to tissues and substrate utilization, should be followed at frequent intervals until shock has resolved.

Targeted antibiotic therapy should be given to children of all ages within an hour of presentation when infection is suspected, even if suitable culture samples cannot be obtained in a timely fashion. Maintaining the glucose level below 200 mg/dL may help mitigate any ongoing fluid losses due to osmotic diuresis. Glucose levels must be measured hourly when insulin therapy is used.

Enteral nutrition should be delayed until the shock state has resolved. A nasogastric/orogastric tube should be placed to gravity drainage unless there is a specific indication for continuous or intermittent suction, such as abdominal distention. Gastric protection with an $H_2$ blocker or proton pump inhibitor should be considered for every patient. If a child is oliguric or has evidence of renal dysfunction, pertinent adjustments to drug doses should be made based on creatinine clearance, and the trough levels of potentially nephrotoxic agents, such as aminoglycosides, should be monitored closely.

# VI. ADDITIONAL CONSIDERATIONS

## A. Management of Neonates and Young Infants

Very young infants with pulmonary and systemic circulations that are transitioning from the fetal to adult pattern are at risk for rapidly developing acute right ventricular failure, manifested as shock with hepatomegaly and other indicators of worsening cardiac output and increased pulmonary and systemic vascular resistances. Echocardiography demonstrates tricuspid regurgitation. In these infants, patency of the ductus arteriosus may result in pulmonary edema during volume resuscitation, mandating careful serial reevaluation and the use of discrete boluses of isotonic fluids.

While the cause of shock in the older child is generally easy to discover, the differential diagnosis is much more diverse in neonates. One of the most important causes is congenital heart disease, specifically ductus-dependent left-sided obstructive lesions that may have gone undetected until ductal closure and the onset of obvious shock. Any clinical suspicion of congenital heart disease should be addressed with appropriate support of ventilation and circulation, expansion of the intravascular space with isotonic fluids, and administration of inotropic and vasoactive infusions.

An infusion of prostaglandin $E_1$ must be started immediately at 0.05 to 0.1 µg/kg/min in neonates presenting with shock and should be continued with close attention to possible adverse effects, including apnea, hypotension, and fever. The infusion should be continued until echocardiography definitively excludes a lesion, such as coarctation of the aorta, interrupted aortic arch, critical aortic stenosis, or the constellation of malformations known as hypoplastic left heart syndrome.

Inborn errors of metabolism and congenital adrenal hyperplasia may present with hypoglycemia, metabolic acidosis, and evidence of end-organ dysfunction. These abnormalities must be treated aggressively. Appropriate management before PICU admission includes close monitoring of glucose (at least hourly) and ionized calcium in addition to other general supportive measures. Antibiotics must be initiated immediately, as a variety of pathogens may be rapidly fatal in neonatal sepsis.

## B. Shock in the Injured Child

A careful secondary trauma survey is essential as soon as fluid resuscitation is begun and the airway has been secured. Scalp lacerations may cause hypovolemia in patients of all sizes. Infants and toddlers with compliant skulls may develop hypovolemic shock from intracranial hemorrhage. Pelvic fractures may cause profuse internal hemorrhage; these fractures must be stabilized mechanically. Embolization of lacerated pelvic vessels may be lifesaving. Computed tomography scanning of suspected sites of injury (head, chest, abdomen, and pelvis) can complement the initial basic trauma imaging obtained in the emergency department. Administration of packed red blood cells, including O-negative blood that has not been cross-matched, may be lifesaving, especially in the presence of ongoing blood losses.

## C. Septic Shock

 ### Case Study

A previously healthy adolescent complains of severe malaise and shortness of breath. He describes the onset of an influenza-like illness and left knee swelling 2 days before his arrival in the emergency department. He is alert but clearly ill and severely tachycardic, with a heart rate of 160 beats/min.

**Detection**

- What are the important clues to this patient's underlying physiology?
- He has brisk capillary refill, bounding pulses, and a blood pressure of 86/30 mm Hg.
- What is the cause for this septic shock?

**Intervention**

- What are the immediate interventions needed?
- He receives 500 mL of normal saline over 1 hour and is then transferred to the PICU. Is this an appropriate volume for fluid resuscitation?

- What is the correct period of time over which to administer the fluid bolus?
- How should this boy be stabilized?
- What are the management priorities for pediatric shock?

**Reassessment**
- On arrival, he is noted to be obtunded, with extremely poor perfusion and undetectable blood pressure.
- What general management principles must be observed?
- What are common pitfalls in the management of pediatric shock?
- Why is "cold shock" difficult to reverse?

**Effective Communication**
- When the patient's clinical status changes, who needs to know and how will this information be disseminated?

**Teamwork**
- How are you going to implement the treatment strategy?
- Who is to do what and when?

Patients with septic shock often manifest elements typical of hypovolemic, distributive, and cardiogenic shock. They can have relative or absolute hypovolemia, abnormal vascular tone, maldistribution of blood flow, and myocardial dysfunction along with refractory acidosis, coagulopathy, and metabolic and endocrine derangements culminating in abnormalities in energy utilization at the subcellular level. Capillary leak syndromes develop quickly and may further complicate patient management (**Table 6-4**).

> *Hypotension may or may not be part of the initial presentation of "cold" or "warm" shock, and its absence should never be reassuring to the clinician.*

Many children with dopamine-resistant shock have: clinical features of low cardiac output, including tachycardia; altered mental status; poor peripheral pulses; mottled skin; and prolonged capillary refill. This presentation has often been referred to as *cold shock*. Adults and some children with septic shock may display a hyperdynamic, high cardiac output state characterized by vasodilatation, tachycardia, bounding pulses, brisk capillary refill, and flushed appearance, a pattern commonly called *warm shock*. Cardiac output can change from high to low rapidly as septic shock progresses. These patients go from a flushed, warm, hyperdynamic state to one marked by hypoperfusion with tachypnea, tachycardia, hypotension, prolonged capillary refill, weak pulses, and metabolic (lactic) acidosis.

Treatment goals include prompt identification of shock, rapid reversal of the cardiovascular dysfunction with adequate intravascular volume expansion, early intubation, vasoactive and inotropic support, and control of the infectious organism (antimicrobials or surgical debridement, if indicated).

### Table 6-4  Possible Etiologies of Shock

**Hypovolemic Shock**

- Fluid losses: gastrointestinal disorders (acute gastroenteritis, pancreatitis), renal dysfunction
- Blood loss: hemorrhage resulting from trauma or coagulopathy
- Capillary leak: burns, intestinal ischemia caused by volvulus, intussusception, or necrotizing enterocolitis

**Distributive Shock**

- Neurogenic shock: head injury, spinal cord injury
- Anaphylaxis
- Drug toxicity
- Adrenal insufficiency: congenital adrenal hyperplasia

**Cardiogenic Shock**

- Congenital heart lesions
- Myocardial dysfunction (systolic or diastolic): ischemic heart disease (Kawasaki disease), cardiomyopathies
- Dysrhythmia: supraventricular tachycardia
- Metabolic disorders
- Drug poisoning

**Septic Shock**

- Bacterial
- Viral
- Fungal
- Rickettsial
- Parasitic

**Obstructive Shock**

- Aortic stenosis, coarctation of the aorta or other left-heart obstructive lesion (infants <6 mo)
- Unrecognized pneumothorax
- Cardiac tamponade
- Pulmonary embolism

Triage tools, flow sheets, order sets, and management protocols, targeting previously healthy children and those whose comorbidities place them at risk for sepsis, expedite care while facilitating communication between healthcare providers. Measures that ensure optimal care – including fluid resuscitation, prompt antibiotic administration, and titrated vasoactive infusions to achieve normalization of vital signs and central venous saturations >70% – translate into significant decreases in patient morbidity and mortality.

## D. Adrenal Insufficiency

Young infants are at increased risk of adrenal insufficiency, particularly if they have hypoglycemia, hyponatremia, and hyperkalemia on their initial laboratory screen. Also at risk are previously healthy children with profound shock refractory to conventional management and children with rapidly evolving rashes (especially if they are purpuric or petechial in nature), any exposure to etomidate, a history of systemic steroid use within the last year, severe head or abdominal injury, or a history of panhypopituitarism. Patients with known or suspected adrenal insufficiency should be treated with hydrocortisone, which will provide both mineralocorticoid and glucocorticoid support at stress doses of at least 1 mg/kg as a bolus and 1 mg/kg every 6 hours. Higher doses are recommended by some experts. Enteral fludrocortisone may be required in children with congenital adrenal hyperplasia.

## E. Shock in Children with Diabetes

Children with new-onset diabetes presenting with diabetic ketoacidosis may have severe hypovolemia and hypoperfusion. Hemodynamic instability in these children is appropriately addressed with volume resuscitation as in any child with hypovolemic shock. However, once hemodynamic stability has been attained with normal saline or 5% albumin, most intensivists and endocrinologists recommend repleting the intravascular space more gingerly than when correcting hypovolemia stemming from other causes. Gradual control of the hyperglycemia is essential to correction of the catabolic state and ongoing fluid losses (**Chapter 8**). Bedside glucose assays must be performed frequently to avoid excessive decreases, particularly when the child must be transported.

## F. Refractory Shock

Shock that is refractory to initial treatment should raise suspicions of alternative diagnoses, such as congenital cardiac disease, acquired cardiac disease (including blunt trauma to the heart), pericardial tamponade, pneumothorax, hemothorax, pulmonary hypertension, toxins, occult ongoing blood loss, inborn metabolic errors or adrenal insufficiency, abdominal catastrophe with evolving abdominal hypertension or compartment syndrome, and persistent infectious nidus.

## G. Pediatric Shock in Developing Countries

Management of pediatric shock may be particularly challenging in settings with limited resources. Educational strategies targeted at the lay public and healthcare providers may increase awareness, early intervention, and close observation. The importance of early use of enteral rehydration (avoiding centrally acting antiemetics such as promethazine) or parenteral fluid therapy using intraosseous or peripheral access cannot be overemphasized. Antibiotics should be administered as soon as possible. Children known to have severe anemia appear to benefit from early blood transfusion rather than vigorous crystalloid or colloid infusion. Frequent reassessment using simple clinical tools may help prevent pulmonary edema and other manifestations of hypervolemia in critically ill children.

## Key Points

## Diagnosis and Management of Shock

- Complete initial and serial assessment of airway patency, breathing, and circulation are essential for successful management of any seriously ill or injured patient. A bedside glucose assay should be performed along with a comprehensive laboratory panel.

- Oxygen should be administered to all patients at risk for shock, regardless of their initial saturation readings.

- Vascular access should be secured within the first few minutes of presentation, with prompt consideration of intraosseous needle placement.

- Fluid resuscitation should begin with isotonic crystalloid, such as 0.9% normal saline given in rapid boluses titrated to clinical response.

- Ketamine and atropine are the drugs of choice for airway control in the presence of shock.

- Antibiotics must be given within an hour of presentation.

- Careful physical examination will reveal clues to the underlying cause of shock.

- Hypotension is a late finding in pediatric shock of any etiology and may precede full arrest.

## Suggested Readings

1. Aneja RK, Carcillo JA. Differences between adult and pediatric septic shock. *Minerva Anestesiol.* 2011;77:986-992.

2. Brierley J, Carcillo JA, Choong K, et al. Clinical practice parameters for hemodynamic support of pediatric and neonatal septic shock: 2007 update from the American College of Critical Care Medicine. *Crit Care Med.* 2009;37:666-688.

3. Carcillo JA, Davis AL, Zaritsky A. Role of early fluid resuscitation in pediatric septic shock. *JAMA.* 1991;266:1242-1245.

4. Carcillo JA, Piva JP, Thomas NJ, Han YY, Lin JC, Orr RA. Shock and shock syndromes. In: Slonim AD, Pollack MM, eds. *Pediatric Critical Care Medicine.* Philadelphia, PA: Lippincott Williams & Wilkins; 2006:438-471.

5. Carcillo JA, Tasker RC. Fluid resuscitation of hypovolemic shock: acute medicine's great triumph for children. *Intensive Care Med.* 2006;32:958-961.

6. Colletti JE, Homme JL, Woodridge DP. Unsuspected neonatal killers in emergency medicine. *Emerg Med Clin North Am.* 2004;22:929-960.

7. Cruz AT, Perry AM, Williams EA, Graf JM, Wuestner ER, Patel B. Implementation of goal-directed therapy for children with suspected sepsis in the emergency department. *Pediatrics.* 2011;127:e758-e766.

8. Han YY, Carcillo JA, Dragotta MA, et al. Early reversal of pediatric-neonatal septic shock by community physicians is associated with improved outcome. *Pediatrics.* 2003;112:793-799.

9. Larsen GY, Mecham N, Greenberg R: An emergency department septic shock protocol and care guideline for children initiated at triage. *Pediatrics.* 2011;127:e1585-e1592.

10. Maitland K, Kiguli S, Opoka RO, et al. Mortality after fluid bolus in African children with severe infection. *N Engl J Med.* 2011;364:2483-2495.

11. Melendez E, Bachur R. Advances in the emergency management of pediatric sepsis. *Curr Opin Pediatr.* 2006;18:245-253.

12. Oliveira CF, Nogueira de Sa FR, Oliveira DS, et al. Time- and fluid-sensitive resuscitation for hemodynamic support of children in septic shock. *Pediatr Emerg Care.* 2008;24:810-815.

13. Parker MM, Hazelzet JA, Carcillo JA. Pediatric considerations. *Crit Care Med.* 2004;32:S591-S594.

14. Pizarro CF, Troster EJ, Damiani D, Carcillo JA. Absolute and relative adrenal insufficiency in children with septic shock. *Crit Care Med.* 2005;33:855-859.

15. Smith L, Hernan L. Shock states. In: Fuhrman BP, Zimmerman JP, eds. *Pediatric Critical Care.* 3rd ed. Philadelphia, PA: Mosby Elsevier; 2006:394-410.

Chapter 7

# Acute Infections

## ✓ Objectives

- Recognize severe, life-threatening infections.
- Initiate timely, goal-directed management.
- Identify possible pathogens or pathology (including noninfectious) based on clinical findings and epidemiology.
- Select adequate initial antimicrobial treatment.
- Recognize and manage severe infections endemic in developing countries.

## 📁 Case Study

An 11-year-old girl is admitted with a 2-day history of fever, abdominal pain, vomiting, and irritability. On physical exam, she is tachycardic (154 beats/min) and tachypneic (28 breaths/min); her abdomen is tender with guarding, rebound tenderness, and rigidity. Her white blood cell (WBC) count is 18,500/mm³. You suspect she is septic and initiate aggressive fluid resuscitation and antibiotic therapy.

**Detection**

- What physiologic parameters concern you about this patient?
- What site of infection would you suspect, and how would you investigate it?
- What diagnoses should you consider?

**Intervention**

- What additional tests are needed to confirm the diagnosis?
- What are the most immediate treatment strategies?

**Reassessment**

- Is the current treatment strategy effective?
- Are there any adjunctive therapies you should consider?

**Effective Communication**

- When the patient's clinical status changes, who needs to know and how will the information be disseminated?
- Where is the best place to manage the care of this patient?

**Teamwork**

- How are you going to implement the treatment strategy?
- Who is to do what and when?

# I. INTRODUCTION

Acute infections are very common in the pediatric population and are often a component of acute illness faced by clinicians caring for children. These infections may present with life-threatening symptoms, or may be more subtle and progress to severe conditions if undetected. Despite advances in the management of critically ill children, morbidity and mortality rates remain high in children with severe infections. This is related to the increase in high-risk pediatric populations encountered in clinical care, such as children with chronic systemic disorders (e.g., congenital heart disease, chronic pulmonary disorders) and conditions with immunosuppression (e.g., congenital immune deficiencies, malignancies, and organ or stem cell transplants).

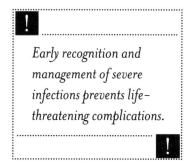

*Early recognition and management of severe infections prevents life-threatening complications.*

The outcome of acute infections in pediatric patients is directly related to the timely recognition of infections and the prompt initiation of appropriate therapy. Delayed diagnosis may result in significant organ dysfunction, shock, multiple organ failure, and death. Because the signs and symptoms of serious infections may be subtle, healthcare providers caring for these children must have a high index of suspicion. Close monitoring and frequent, thorough physical examinations must be made due to the dynamic process of disease progression. Age-dependent variations in vital signs must be recognized to detect physiologic derangements associated with acute infections (**Table 7-1**). Definitions of terms related to pediatric sepsis are presented in **Tables 7-2** and **7-3**.

# II. DIAGNOSIS

Illnesses caused by infections have a wide variety of signs and symptoms, some of which are clear and easy to detect, while others are often subtle and nonspecific. A thorough and meticulous physical exam, and an understanding of age-related differences in anatomy and physiology, are vitally important in identifying an infectious cause of illness. A high index of suspicion for an infectious etiology should always be maintained. The earlier a severe infection is diagnosed, the better the outcome the patient generally will have. Prompt recognition of a severe infection is based on a clear understanding of the risk factors, epidemiology, and the findings on the physical exam. The diagnostic process can also be aided by laboratory and radiologic examinations. Properly performed microbiologic testing can be an invaluable tool to making the correct diagnosis.

### Table 7-1: Age-Specific Upper Values (95th Percentile) for Heart Rate and Respiratory Rate, and Lower Values (5th Percentile) for Systolic Blood Pressure and Heart Rate

| Age Group | Tachycardia (beats/min) | Bradycardia (beats/min) | Tachypnea (breaths/min) | Leukocyte Count (x $10^3$/mm$^3$) | Systolic Blood Pressure (mm Hg) |
|---|---|---|---|---|---|
| 0 days-1 week | >180 | <100 | >50 | >34 | <65 |
| 1 week-1 month | >180 | <100 | >40 | >19.5 or <5 | <75 |
| 1 month-1 year | >180 | <90 | >34 | >17.5 or <5 | <100 |
| 2-5 years | >140 | NA | >22 | >15.5 or <6 | <94 |
| 6-12 years | >130 | NA | >180 | >13.5 or <4.5 | <105 |
| 13 to <18 years | >110 | NA | >14 | >11 or <4.5 | <117 |

NA, not applicable
Adapted with permission. © 2005 Wolters Kluwer Health. Goldstein B, Giroir B, Randolph A, et al. International pediatric sepsis consensus conference: Definitions for sepsis and organ dysfunction in pediatrics. *Pediatr Crit Care Med*. 2005;6:2-8.

### Table 7-2: Criteria for Systemic Inflammatory Response Syndrome, Infection, Sepsis, Severe Sepsis, and Septic Shock

**Systemic Inflammatory Response Syndrome**
SIRS is characterized by the presence of at least 2 of the following 4 criteria, 1 of which must be abnormal temperature or abnormal leukocyte count:
- Core temperature (measured by rectal, bladder, oral, or central catheter probe) of >101.3°F (>38.5°C) or <96.8°F (<36°C).
- Tachycardia, defined as a mean heart rate >2 SD above the normal for age in the absence of external stimulus, chronic drug use, or painful stimuli or otherwise unexplained persistent elevation over a 30-min to 4-h period OR for children <1 year, bradycardia, defined as a mean heart rate <10th percentile for age in the absence of external vagal stimulus, ß-blocker drugs, or congenital heart disease, or otherwise unexplained persistent depression over a 30-min period.
- Mean respiratory rate >2 SD above normal for age or mechanical ventilation for an acute process unrelated to underlying neuromuscular disease or the receipt of general anesthesia.
- Leukocyte count elevated or depressed for the patient's age (not secondary to chemotherapy-induced leukopenia) or >10% immature neutrophils.

**Infection**
A suspected or proven (by positive culture, tissue stain, or polymerase chain reaction test) infection caused by any pathogen OR a clinical syndrome associated with a high probability of infection. Evidence of infection includes positive findings on clinical examination, imaging, or laboratory tests (e.g., white blood cells in a normally sterile body fluid, perforated viscus, chest radiograph consistent with pneumonia, petechial or purpuric rash, or purpura fulminans).

**Sepsis**
SIRS in the presence of, or as a result of, suspected or proven infection.

**Severe Sepsis**
Sepsis with cardiovascular organ dysfunction before treatment or corrected by fluid resuscitation of <40 mL/kg/h OR acute respiratory distress syndrome OR 2 or more other organ dysfunctions. Organ dysfunctions are defined in **Table 7-3**.

**Septic Shock**
Sepsis with cardiovascular organ dysfunction as defined in **Table 7-3**.

SIRS, systemic inflammatory response syndrome; SD, standard deviation
Adapted with permission. © 2005 Wolters Kluwer Health. Goldstein B, Giroir B, Randolph A, et al. International pediatric sepsis consensus conference: Definitions for sepsis and organ dysfunction in pediatrics. *Pediatr Crit Care Med*. 2005;6:2-8.

### Table 7-3  Organ Dysfunction Criteria

**Cardiovascular Dysfunction**

Despite administration of isotonic fluid bolus ≥40 mL/kg in 1 h:

- Decrease in BP (hypotension) <5th percentile for age or systolic BP <2 SD below normal for age

OR

- Need for vasoactive drugs to maintain BP in normal range

OR

- 2 of the following:
  - Unexplained metabolic acidosis: base deficit >5 mmol/L
  - Increased arterial lactate >2 times upper limit of normal
  - Oliguria: urine output <0.5 mL/kg/h
  - Prolonged capillary refill: >5 s
  - Core to peripheral temperature gap >37.4°F (>3°C)

**Respiratory**[a]

- $Pao_2/Fio_2$ <300 in absence of cyanotic heart disease or preexisting lung disease

OR

- $Paco_2$ >20 mm Hg over baseline reading

OR

- Proven need for >50% $Fio_2$ to maintain saturation ≥92%

OR

- Need for nonelective invasive or noninvasive mechanical ventilation

**Neurologic Dysfunction**

- Glasgow Coma Scale score ≤11

OR

- Acute change in mental status with a decrease in Glasgow Coma Scale score ≥3 points from abnormal baseline

**Hematologic Dysfunction**

- Platelet count <80,000/mm$^3$ or a decline of 50% in platelet count from highest value recorded over the past 3 days (for chronic hematology/oncology patients)

OR

- International normalized ratio >2

**Renal Dysfunction**

- Serum creatinine ≥2 times upper limit of normal for age or a 2-fold increase in baseline creatinine

**Hepatic Dysfunction**

- Total bilirubin ≥4 mg/dL (not applicable for newborn)

OR

- ALT 2 times upper limit of normal for age

BP, blood pressure; SD, standard deviation; ALT, alanine transaminase
[a]Acute respiratory distress syndrome must include a $Pao_2/Fio_2$ ratio ≤200 mm Hg, bilateral infiltrates, acute onset, and no evidence of left heart failure. Acute lung injury is defined identically, except the $Pao_2/Fio_2$ ratio must be ≤300 mm Hg. Proven need assumes oxygen requirement was tested by decreasing flow, subsequently increasing flow if required. In postoperative patients, this requirement can be met if the patient has developed an acute inflammatory or infectious lung process that prevents extubation.
Adapted with permission. © 2005 Wolters Kluwer Health. Goldstein B, Giroir B, Randolph A, et al. International pediatric sepsis consensus conference: Definitions for sepsis and organ dysfunction in pediatrics. *Pediatr Crit Care Med.* 2005;6:2-8.

## A. General Signs of Infection

The host responds to an invading organism with a cascade of immune-mediated events. These lead to the activation of numerous physiologic systems, resulting in responses that should alert the clinician to the possibility of an infection.

Fever is the most common sign of infection. The best estimate of the core temperature is taken rectally, but an oral or bladder temperature reading is acceptable. A core temperature above 100.4°F (38°C) is usually considered a fever, but a temperature of 101.3°F (38.5°C) improves the specificity and is a commonly used threshold in clinical practice. Patients who are immunocompromised have a significantly higher risk of acquiring life-threatening infections, and a temperature of 100.4°F (38°C) should lead to further investigation. Most infections in children present with fever; however, some patients (especially neonates) with severe infections may present with hypothermia (temperature less than 96.8°F [36°C]). Fever, however, may be caused by a wide variety of noninfectious etiologies as well, such as inflammatory diseases, drugs, blood products, neoplasms, endocrine disorders, central nervous system bleeding, thrombosis, recent surgery, or iatrogenic causes such as excessive patient bundling. Temperatures above 105.8°F (41°C) are seldom associated with an infectious cause.

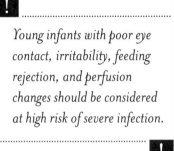

*Young infants with poor eye contact, irritability, feeding rejection, and perfusion changes should be considered at high risk of severe infection.*

**Table 7-4** outlines signs of infection specific to organ systems. Symptoms may be specific to a primary site of infection, or may reflect the systemic effect of a remote infection.

Skin manifestations (rashes) are common in the clinical presentation of a variety of infectious organisms. A basic understanding of the various types of skin manifestations is essential in making an accurate assessment and determining the severity and acuteness of the patient's illness. Common skin lesions are given in **Table 7-5**. Maculopapular rashes are most commonly seen in viral illnesses, immune-mediated syndromes, and some bacterial infections. Location of the rash on the body (i.e., peripheral or central distribution) may be helpful in narrowing the differential diagnosis. Petechial rashes deserve immediate attention and evaluation to rule out severe illness. Most commonly, petechiae that are isolated to the portion of the body above (cephalad) the nipple line are not due to a severe infection.

## B. Laboratory Findings

A complete blood count is routinely performed in a patient suspected of having a severe infection. Leukocytosis (WBC count >12,000/mm$^3$) may be a reaction to an infectious or an inflammatory process, among other causes. Most bacterial infections cause leukocytosis with neutrophilia (neutrophil count ≥8,000/mm$^3$ in adults and children older than 1 year); however, severe infections may present with leukopenia (leukocyte count <4,000/mm$^3$), especially in young infants. The presence of leukocytosis or neutrophilia alone cannot accurately predict the presence or absence of bacterial infection. Platelets are acute phase reactants, so thrombocytosis (platelet count >450,000/mm$^3$) can be an indirect sign of infection; however, thrombocytopenia (platelet count <150,000/mm$^3$) and other clotting abnormalities are well-known complications of sepsis.

### Table 7-4  General Signs of Infection Based on Organ System Involved

| Organ System | Clinical Finding |
| --- | --- |
| Cardiovascular | Tachycardia<br>Diminished or bounding peripheral pulses<br>Gallop rhythm<br>Murmur or rub |
| Respiratory | Tachypnea<br>Cough<br>Dyspnea<br>Chest pain<br>Nasal flaring<br>Grunting<br>Retractions<br>Cyanosis<br>*Auscultation*: crackles, decreased breath sounds, abnormal vocal resonance |
| Central nervous system | *Infants*: fever, lethargy, irritability, bulging anterior fontanelle, apnea, seizure, poor eye contact<br>*Children*: fever, headache, vomiting, irritability, mental status changes, nuchal rigidity, focal neurologic signs |
| Urinary tract infection | *Infants*: fever, irritability, vomiting, poor feeding, hyperbilirubinemia, failure to thrive<br>*Children*: dysuria, urgency, increased frequency of voiding |
| Cutaneous infection | Pain<br>Erythema<br>Induration<br>Warmth<br>+/- fever<br>Systemic involvement possible |
| Abdominal Infection | Fever<br>Diffuse abdominal pain<br>Vomiting<br>Tenderness +/- rebound tenderness<br>Rigid abdominal wall |
| Septic arthritis or osteomyelitis | Fever<br>Pain<br>Swelling<br>Erythema<br>Movement limitation |
| Nonspecific | *Children*: chills, myalgia, fatigue, anorexia<br>*Neonates*: irritability, poor feeding, mottled skin |

Alterations in the prothrombin time and activated partial thromboplastin time can be suggestive of disseminated intravascular coagulation during severe sepsis. Elevated D-dimers and fibrin degradation products in association with low fibrinogen confirm the diagnosis, although confirming the diagnosis must take into consideration other clinical entities that may yield similar laboratory results, such as thrombotic thrombocytopenic purpura, which often require further laboratory or clinical findings to help discern them from disseminated intravascular coagulation. Other acute phase reactant biomarkers that may indicate the presence of an acute infection, although not specific, are an elevation of C-reactive protein, erythrocyte sedimentation rate, and procalcitonin. In the acute setting, when used together with other markers of inflammation and with clinical criteria, these may help in identifying the presence of an infectious etiology. Trending the levels of these biomarkers may also aid in determining the efficacy of treatment.

| Table 7-5 | Common Primary Skin Lesions |
|---|---|
| **Lesion Type** | **Description** |
| Macule | Circumscribed area of change in normal skin color, with no skin elevation or depression; may be any size |
| Papule | Solid, raised lesion <0.5 cm in greatest diameter |
| Nodule | Similar to papule but located deeper in dermis or subcutaneous tissue; differentiated from papule by palpability and depth, rather than size |
| Plaque | Elevation of skin occupying a relatively large area in relation to height; often formed by confluence of papules |
| Pustule | Circumscribed elevation of skin containing purulent fluid of variable character (i.e., fluid may be white, yellow, greenish, or hemorrhagic) |
| Vesicle | Circumscribed, elevated, fluid-containing lesion <0.5 cm in greatest diameter; may be intraepidermal or subepidermal in origin |
| Bulla | Same as vesicle, except lesion >0.5 cm in greatest diameter |

Classified using Fitzpatrick TB, Johnson RA, Polano MK, et al. *Color Atlas and Synopsis of Clinical Dermatology: Common and Serious Diseases*. 3rd ed. New York, NY: McGraw-Hill; 1997. Habif TP, ed. *Clinical Dermatology: A Color Guide to Diagnosis and Therapy*. 3rd ed. St. Louis, MO: Mosby; 1996.

To assess the adequacy of oxygen delivery, a blood gas measurement (arterial or capillary) is useful. A metabolic acidosis accompanied by high lactate levels or low bicarbonate levels indicates an imbalance in the delivery of oxygen compared to patient demand. Differences in arterial and central venous contents of oxygen can also assess the adequacy of oxygenation, with a difference of more than 25% to 30% indicating inadequate delivery. The $Pao_2$ or pulse oximetry ($Spo_2$) may be used to confirm oxygenation and help in the diagnosis of conditions such as acute lung injury or acute respiratory distress syndrome. The $Paco_2$ can be low during respiratory compensation (<35 mm Hg [4.6 kPa]) or elevated (>45 mm Hg [5.9 kPa]) during a disease with ventilation impairment. Also, blood samples from a central venous catheter (preferably from the superior vena cava) for mixed venous oxygen saturation ($Svo_2$), when measured by co-oximetry, are useful to guide treatment during severe sepsis (**Chapter 6**).

Inadequate oxygen delivery may also be recognized clinically. In particular, alterations in central nervous system and renal function are early signs of impending cardiovascular compromise. The brain and kidneys receive 20% of cardiac output; if compromised by the effect of a severe infection, alterations in organ function occur. These alterations may appear subtle, such as agitation, anxiety, lethargy, somnolence, or more profound, such as encephalopathy. Further, normal urine output and mental status generally suggest adequate cardiac output.

Severe infections may affect renal function directly (by nephrotoxins, as in the hemolysis of malaria) or indirectly (by decreased renal blood flow, by shock); therefore, blood urea nitrogen (BUN) and serum creatinine should always be measured. During acute kidney injury, doses of renally excreted drugs (e.g., antibiotics) should be adjusted to creatinine clearance.

Hypoglycemia (in neonates and young infants) or hyperglycemia may be present during severe infections. Hyperglycemia has been associated with increased mortality in critically ill adults, and the use of insulin to achieve normoglycemia (while assiduously avoiding hypoglycemia) seems to improve mortality and morbidity in surgical intensive care units. Evidence for the use of insulin therapy is controversial in pediatrics; however, hyperglycemia is commonly treated in children when glucose values are persistently >180 to 200 mg/dL (9.98-11.1 mmol/L). More recent data also suggest that large variations in blood glucose levels may be associated with poor outcomes. Blood glucose should be routinely measured at the bedside as part of the initial stabilization and followed through the course of illness. Most recently, however, maintaining strict euglycemia with insulin therapy did not show any benefit in pediatric patients undergoing cardiopulmonary bypass for correction of congenital heart lesions, again throwing doubt on the utility of glycemic control in critically ill children.

Lastly, as all organ systems can be primarily or secondarily affected by an acute infection, measures of serum electrolytes (sodium, potassium, calcium, phosphorus, magnesium, or serum bicarbonate) and liver enzyme and renal function tests need to be followed (**Chapter 8**). Further, various infectious syndromes are defined by derangements in certain of these laboratory values.

## C. Microbiology Tests

Microbiology tests are essential in helping establish the final etiology. Healthcare providers must choose the correct laboratory tools to improve the diagnostic sensitivity and specificity.

Meticulously obtained routine cultures of any fluid collection, infected tissue, or fluid should be obtained. Gram stain can quickly provide important information that can be applied immediately to patient care. It is particularly useful in the diagnostic confirmation of bacterial meningitis, urinary tract infection, or other infected fluid collections, such as abscesses, empyema, and peritonitis. Specimens obtained via biopsy or bronchoscopy should be sent routinely for Gram stain. Other stains should be considered (acid-fast bacilli, silver stain [pneumocystis], fungal, etc.), depending on the type of infection that is suspected. The growth of microorganisms in specific growth mediums (aerobic, anaerobic, fungal, mycobacterial) will determine the microbiologic diagnosis and facilitate testing for antimicrobial susceptibility. Any material appropriately obtained can be sent for culture. A minimum of 2 mL of blood should be drawn whenever possible for optimizing the chances of isolating a blood pathogen. For patients 45 kg or larger, a 2-bottle adult blood culture system should be inoculated with 10 mL per bottle. If possible, one set of blood cultures should be taken from ≥2 separate sites (i.e., ≥2 sets) to increase specificity. Malaria is still routinely identified on blood films: a thick film to identify parasites and a thin film to speciate the organism. Also available are rapid diagnostic tests which provide quick, point-of-care information about the involved species. Antigen-detection tests using direct immunofluorescence, enzyme immunoassay, or latex agglutination techniques for rapid detection of bacterial antigens can be performed in diverse specimens such as urine, sputum, or throat swab, among others. Antigen-detection tests can give useful information; however, because the sensitivity of that information can be low, initial antibiotic management of severe infections should not be based solely on the results of these tests.

Polymerase chain reaction (PCR) for the detection of microbial DNA or RNA can be a useful technique for the detection of diverse microorganisms. It is now the standard and preferred methodology to detect herpes viruses and enterovirus in cerebrospinal fluid (CSF).

Serologic testing for the detection of antibodies is the test of choice for some infections, such as Epstein-Barr virus infection, Rocky Mountain spotted fever, and dengue, and for some fungal infections.

# III. INFECTIOUS SYNDROMES

## A. Sepsis

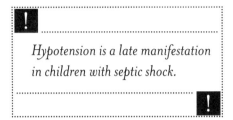

*Hypotension is a late manifestation in children with septic shock.*

Sepsis is the result of activation of the systemic inflammatory response syndrome (SIRS) (**Table 7-2**) caused by an identified or presumed infection. This syndrome can lead to high mortality if not treated adequately. The use of intensive care and goal-directed therapies has been shown to improve outcome.

The clinical definition of SIRS (and therefore sepsis) in children differs slightly from the adult definition. In children, temperature or leukocyte abnormalities must be present, in addition to abnormalities of the heart rate or respiratory rate. Bradycardia may be a sign of SIRS in the newborn age group, but not in older children (in whom it is a near-terminal event).

Early clinical suspicion should be based on the presence of hyperthermia or hypothermia, changes in mental status, and alterations in peripheral perfusion. Evaluation of children with suspected sepsis is based on a meticulous and repeated physical assessment. Heart rate, capillary refill, respiratory rate, mental status, urinary output, and alteration in the skin's appearance should be evaluated carefully.

*Rapid initiation of adequate empirical antibiotic therapy is imperative for lowering mortality during severe infections.*

Management should be started as soon as sepsis is suspected. The goal of therapy is to avoid or to correct abnormalities that arise due to inadequate oxygen delivery at the cellular level by maintaining adequate oxygenation of hemoglobin, adequate hemoglobin levels, and sufficient cardiac output to deliver it where it is needed.

As with all critically ill patients, assessment of the airway, proper ventilation, the establishment of adequate circulation, and prompt administration of appropriate antibiotics are the main priorities. Fluid and inotropic management of the septic patient is discussed at length in **Chapter 6**.

Early recognition of the septic patient and early, aggressive therapy are crucial for an optimal outcome. After cultures have been obtained, administering appropriate antibiotics within the first hour of disease recognition is recommended. If appropriate cultures cannot be obtained in a timely manner, broad-spectrum empiric antibiotics should not be delayed. Goal-directed initial fluid resuscitation is also fundamental in managing these patients. After rapidly obtaining intravenous or intraosseous access, initial resuscitation should begin with 20 mL/kg isotonic crystalloid boluses over 5-10 minutes. Patients usually require 40-60 mL/kg, but significantly higher volumes may be needed. Fluid resuscitation should be targeted to improvement in physiologic parameters: normalization of heart rate, urine output >1 mL/kg/h, capillary refill <2 seconds, and normal mental status. Blood pressure by itself is not a reliable end-point for assessing the adequacy of resuscitation (**Chapter 6** and **Chapter 8**). Hepatomegaly occurs in fluid overload, and so when present, it represents adequacy of fluid resuscitation.

If hemodynamic goals have not been achieved despite appropriate fluid resuscitation, vasopressors or inotropes should be given. Dopamine is the first medication recommended. In cases of dopamine-resistant shock, a second agent must be added. The choice of medications should be determined by the clinical exam: direct vasopressors or vasodilators may be needed in the presence of low cardiac output with low or high systemic vascular resistance, respectively.

Therapeutic goals for patients in septic shock include the clinical findings previously described as well as other measures of oxygen delivery. Targeting a decrease in serum lactate or $S_{CVO_2}$ >70% can aid in management and lead to improved outcomes (**Figure 7-1**).

**Figure 7-1.** Approach to Pediatric Shock

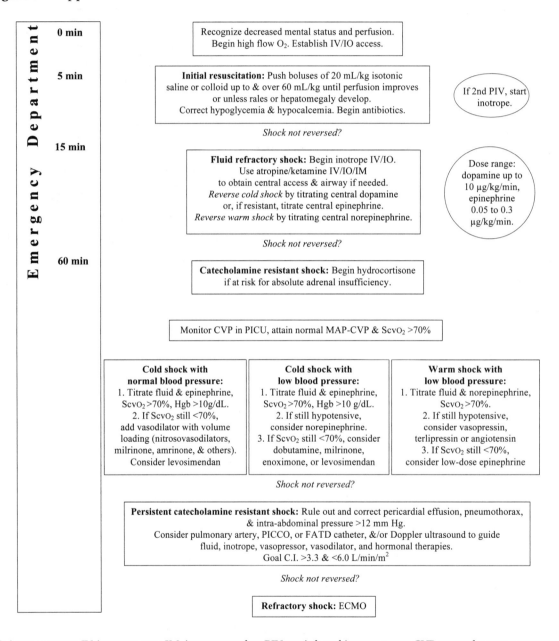

IO, intraosseous; IV, intravenous; IM, intramuscular; PIV, peripheral intravenous; CVP, central venous pressure; PICU, pediatric intensive care unit; MAP-CVP, mean arterial pressure-central venous pressure; $S_{CVO_2}$, central venous oxygen saturation; Hgb, hemoglobin; PICCO, pulse-induced contour cardiac output; FATD, femoral arterial thermodilution technique; ECMO, extracorporeal membrane oxygenation; CI, cardiac index

Reproduced with permission. © 2009 Wolters Kluwer Health. Brierley J, Carcillo JA, Choong K, et al. Clinical practice parameters for hemodynamic support of pediatric and neonatal septic shock: 2007 update from the American College of Critical Care Medicine. *Crit Care Med.* 2009;37:666-688.

### 1. Steroids

There is continuous debate regarding the use of steroids in pediatric sepsis. Current guidelines recommend the use of hydrocortisone in the presence of catecholamine-resistant shock and risk of adrenal insufficiency. Risk factors for adrenal insufficiency include meningococcemia, chronic use of steroids, and pituitary or adrenal abnormalities. Recommended doses of hydrocortisone may vary from 1 to 2 mg/kg/day for stress coverage to 50 mg/kg for treatment of refractory shock followed by the same dose as a 24-hour infusion. When possible, blood cortisol concentrations should be obtained before the first dose of hydrocortisone.

### 2. Antibiotic Therapy

Antibiotics should be administered within the first hour of treatment, immediately after cultures have been obtained. However, if microbiology samples are difficult to obtain, treatment should be started without delay.

Broad-spectrum antibiotics should be given empirically with the choice of agent dependent on the patient's clinical, laboratory, and imaging characteristics. Considerations vary depending on the patient's age, physical findings, immunological status, previous hospitalizations, previous antibiotic treatment, and presence of central catheters or other medical devices. Knowledge of local microbe resistance patterns may also help guide antimicrobial selection. Possible pathogens of sepsis are summarized in **Table 7-6**.

**Table 7-6  Possible Sepsis Pathogens**

| Age Group | Pathogens |
| --- | --- |
| 0-30 days | Group B streptococci, *Escherichia coli* and other Enterobacteriaceae, *Staphylococcus aureus*, and *Listeria monocytogenes* |
| 1-3 months | *Streptococcus pneumoniae, Neisseria meningitidis, Haemophilus influenzae*, and *E coli* and other Enterobacteriaceae |
| 3 months-5 years | *S pneumoniae, N meningitidis, H influenzae*, and *S aureus* |
| >5 years | *S pneumoniae, N meningitidis*, group A β-streptococcus, *S aureus*, and *Fusobacterium necrophorum* |
| Immunocompromised or hospitalized children | *S aureus, Staphylococcus epidermidis* and other coagulase-negative rods, *Streptococcus mitis*, and *Candida* |

Antibiotic treatment depends on the suspected infection. In community-acquired sepsis in immunocompetent patients, cefotaxime or ceftriaxone with vancomycin provides adequate initial empiric coverage in most nontropical areas. In certain areas of the world, organisms such as *Rickettsia, Burkholderia*, and malaria are prevalent, and antimicrobials directed at these organisms should also be considered as initial empiric therapy. In patients with risk factors or in hospitalized children, Gram-negative coverage should be expanded with an aminoglycoside in combination with an extended spectrum β-lactam (e.g., piperacillin-tazobactam, or meropenem). If a central venous catheter is present, vancomycin should be added. Further, infections associated with indwelling central venous catheters should result in the prompt removal of the catheter when possible, although some practitioners may attempt to treat through an infected catheter if the patient's condition is stable. Empiric antibiotic choices for severe infections acquired outside of hospital settings are summarized in **Table 7-7**. Antibiotic doses are described in **Table 7-8**.

When a removable source of infection is present, such as an infected foreign body or an abscess, it should be removed if feasible and the abscess drained.

### Table 7-7. Empiric Antibiotic Choices for Community-Acquired Sepsis[a]

| Age | Suspected Bacteremia | Sepsis Syndrome and/or Severe Infection |
|---|---|---|
| <4 weeks | Ampicillin **AND** cefotaxime or gentamicin | Ampicillin **AND** vancomycin **AND** cefotaxime or gentamicin |
| 4-7 weeks | Ampicillin **AND** ceftriaxone or cefotaxime | Ampicillin **AND** vancomycin **AND** ceftriaxone or cefotaxime |
| 8 weeks-adolescence | Ceftriaxone or cefotaxime | Vancomycin **AND** clindamycin **AND** ceftriaxone or cefotaxime |

[a]Local resistance patterns need to be considered when selecting empiric antibiotics for community-acquired sepsis.

### 3. Other Considerations

Useful blood tests during initial stabilization include blood gas, lactate, electrolytes, BUN, creatinine, glucose, complete blood count, and coagulation parameters (prothrombin time, activated partial thromboplastin time, fibrinogen, and D-dimer). Maintaining a hemoglobin level of approximately 10 g/dL has been recommended to optimize oxygen delivery in a patient who is clinically septic or in septic shock. Hypoglycemia and electrolyte abnormalities should be corrected.

Lastly, in patients with refractory septic shock and/or respiratory failure despite maximal conventional therapies, the use of extracorporeal membrane oxygenation can be considered.

| Table 7-8 | Antimicrobial Treatment of Sepsis |

| Age Group | Treatment[a] |
|---|---|
| Neonates ≤7 days | • Ampicillin 50-100 mg/kg/dose every 12 h<br>　The higher doses are for meningitis or group B streptococcal sepsis.<br>• Gentamicin<br>　– <29 wk: 5 mg/kg/dose every 48 h<br>　– 30-34 wk: 4.5 mg/kg/dose every 36 h<br>　– >35 wk: 4 mg/kg/dose every 24 h (depending on gestational age)<br>• Cefotaxime 50 mg/kg/dose every 12 h |
| Neonates >7 days | • Ampicillin 50-75 mg/kg/dose every 6-8 h, depending on gestational age<br>　The higher doses are for meningitis or group B streptococcal sepsis.<br>• Gentamicin 4 mg/kg/dose every 24 h (if >30 wk); interval depends on plasma levels<br>• Cefotaxime 50 mg/kg/dose every 8-12 h, depending on gestational age<br>• Vancomycin 15 mg/kg/dose every 6-12 h, depending on gestational age<br>• Metronidazole 7.5 mg/kg/dose every 12-48 h, depending on gestational age |
| Previously healthy infants and children | • Ceftriaxone 50 mg/kg/dose every 24 h; if dose >2 g, divide and administer every 12 h<br>• Vancomycin 15 mg/kg/dose every 6 h for CNS infection or 15 mg/kg/dose every 8 h for non-CNS infections<br>• Metronidazole 7.5 mg/kg/dose every 6 h |
| Hospitalized or immunosuppressed children | • Ceftriaxone 75-100 mg/kg/day every 24 h; if dose >2 g, divide and administer every 12 h. (Use higher dose for meningitis.)<br>• Gentamicin 2-2.5 mg/kg/dose every 8 h<br>• Amikacin 7.5-10 mg/kg/dose every 8 h<br>• Ceftazidime 50 mg/kg/dose every 8 h<br>• Metronidazole 7.5 mg/kg/dose every 6 h<br>• Vancomycin 15 mg/kg/dose every 6 h for CNS infection or 15 mg/kg/dose every 8 h for non-CNS infections<br>• Meropenem 20 mg/kg/dose every 8 h; 40 mg/kg/dose every 8 h for meningitis |

CNS, central nervous system
[a]Local resistance patterns need to be considered when selecting empiric antibiotics for community-acquired sepsis.

## B. Toxic Shock Syndrome

 Case Study

A 16-year-old girl presents to the emergency department with a fever of 104°F (40°C), malaise, headache, confusion, diarrhea, and skin rash. She is not sexually active and started her menstrual period 2 days ago. Her pulse rate is 130 beats/min and blood pressure is 98/50 mm Hg. She has a diffuse erythroderma and mild abdominal tenderness. You are concerned about this patient's condition and immediately initiate therapy.

**Detection**

– What is the likely etiology of this illness?

– How would you describe her physiologic condition?

**Intervention**

– What therapy should be initiated?

**Reassessment**
- After fluid resuscitation, what other therapies should be considered?

**Effective Communication**
- When the patient's clinical status changes, who needs this information and how will it be disseminated?
- Where is the best place to manage the care of this patient?

**Teamwork**
- How are you going to implement the treatment strategy?

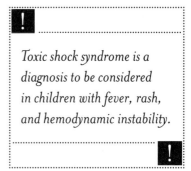

*Toxic shock syndrome is a diagnosis to be considered in children with fever, rash, and hemodynamic instability.*

Toxic shock syndrome (TSS) is a life-threatening syndrome that should be considered in ill patients with fever and erythroderma, with or without hypotension. The syndrome, caused by *Staphylococcus aureus*, was first described in children with postoperative wounds, but an epidemic was recognized in young women in the 1980s due to use of highly absorbent tampons during menstruation. Since then, the incidence of TSS with tampons has sharply declined, but cases continue to occur in the absence of tampon use. Nonmenstrual TSS has been associated with *S aureus* infections in surgical and postpartum wounds, mastitis, sinusitis, respiratory illness (especially following influenza), osteomyelitis, arthritis, burns, and other skin and soft tissue infections. Most of the cases are due to methicillin-susceptible *S aureus*, but cases with methicillin-resistant strains have been reported. TSS is caused by the action of the toxin, namely TSST-1 or staphylococcal enterotoxin B, that acts as a superantigen and binds to and stimulates certain T cells independent of major histocompatibility complex presentation. Stimulated T cells release tumor necrosis factor and other chemokines that cause fever, rash, and capillary leakage, resulting in hypotension and organ damage.

Patients often present with acute onset of fever, sore throat, intense myalgia, profuse diarrhea, and sometimes vomiting. The rash in TSS, which is an early finding, is described as erythroderma and has sometimes been mistaken for a sunburn rash, which it closely resembles. A scarlatiniform rash can also been seen. Patients may present with listlessness or confusion. A nonpurulent conjunctival hyperemia, pharyngeal inflammation, or strawberry tongue can also be seen. TSS affects multiple organ systems, and patients can present with signs of acute respiratory distress syndrome, renal failure, or other signs of gastrointestinal and hematologic involvement. Progression to fulminant shock can occur rapidly. Desquamation of digits, palms, and soles occurs typically in convalescence.

The specific criteria for diagnosing TSS due to *S aureus* are shown in **Table 7-9**. Blood cultures are rarely positive as the organism need not spread systemically; this is an exotoxin-mediated syndrome. *S aureus* can be isolated from wound, respiratory, or other mucosal sites, although its isolation is not required for the diagnosis of staphylococcal TSST-1. Other abnormalities in laboratory results reflect the degree of organ involvement, such as transaminitis, coagulopathy, and elevated creatinine.

TSS can also be caused by *Streptococcus pyogenes* (group A β-hemolytic *Streptococcus*, or GABHS) and is seen in children with focal infections such as myositis, pneumonia, necrotizing fasciitis, or during varicella infection. The clinical features and lab abnormalities are similar to those caused by *S aureus*.

| Table 7-9 | Definition of Toxic Shock Syndrome Due to *Staphylococcus aureus*[a] |
|---|---|

**1. Fever**
Temperature >102.0°F (>38.9°C)

**2. Hypotension**
Systolic blood pressure: ≤90 mm Hg for adults or <5th percentile by age for children <16 years of age
Orthostatic drop in diastolic blood pressure ≥15 mm Hg
Orthostatic syncope or dizziness

**3. Rash**
Diffuse macular erythroderma

**4. Desquamation**
1-2 weeks after onset of illness, particularly involving palms and soles

**5. Multisystem involvement (3 or more of the following organ systems)**
**Gastrointestinal:** Vomiting or diarrhea at onset of illness
**Muscular:** Severe myalgia or creatine phosphokinase elevation >2 times normal upper limit
**Mucous membranes:** Vaginal, oropharyngeal, or conjunctival hyperemia
**Renal:** Blood urea nitrogen or serum creatinine >2 times normal upper limit, or pyuria (>5 white blood cells per high-powered field)
**Hepatic:** Bilirubin or transaminases >2 times the normal upper limit
**Hematologic:** Platelets <100,000/μL
**Central nervous system:** Disorientation or alterations in consciousness without focal neurologic signs in the absence of fever and hypotension

**Laboratory criteria: negative results on the following tests, if obtained**
Blood, throat, or cerebrospinal fluid cultures for another pathogen (blood cultures may be positive for *S aureus*)
Serologic tests for Rocky Mountain spotted fever, leptospirosis, or measles

[a]Case definition of toxic shock syndrome due to *S aureus* from the Centers for Disease Control and Prevention. Requires meeting laboratory criteria plus 5 clinical findings including desquamation (unless the patient dies before desquamation occurs) for a confirmed case, and meets laboratory criteria plus 4 of 5 clinical findings for a probable case.

Patients with suspected TSS should receive clindamycin in addition to vancomycin. Nafcillin can also be started initially and continued or stopped once the susceptibility of *S aureus* is available. Surgical drainage of any identified collections should be undertaken, in addition to removal of any tampon present. Administration of intravenous immune globulin (IVIG) can be considered in *S aureus* TSS, particularly in patients who are severely ill and have not responded to the initial supportive measures and antibiotics; however, no controlled data support the use of IVIG.

## C. Meningococcemia

 Case Study

A 15-year-old boy is admitted with sudden onset of high fever, shaking chills, vomiting, and diffuse non-blanching skin lesions. Vital signs show he is tachycardic and hypotensive.

**Detection**
- What physiologic parameters concern you about this patient?
- What is the most likely diagnosis? The worst possible diagnoses?

### Intervention

- What are the most immediate treatment strategies?

### Reassessment

- Is the current treatment strategy effective?
- Are there any adjunctive therapies you should consider?

### Effective Communication

- When the patient's clinical status changes, who needs the information and how will it be disseminated?
- Where is the best place to manage the care of this patient?

### Teamwork

- How are you going to implement the treatment strategy?
- Who is to do what and when?

*Neisseria meningitidis* is a Gram-negative diplococcus that causes meningococcemia and meningitis, as well as other localized infections such as pneumonia, pericarditis, arthritis, peritonitis, and occult bacteremia. The main serogroups that cause the disease are A, B, C, Y, and W135. The two age groups at highest risk are infants younger than 2 years and adolescents aged 15 to 18 years. Crowded living environments with a high number of adolescents and young adults increases the rate of disease.

> *Children with fever and petechiae should be suspected of having meningococcemia until proven otherwise.*
>
> *When meningococcal disease is suspected, management must be started rapidly without waiting for laboratory results.*

Meningococcemia is a severe illness that progresses to septic shock within 12 to 24 hours in most cases. Initial symptoms can be nonspecific and mimic a common viral illness, including fever, headache, vomiting, abdominal pain, and myalgia. The classic rash of petechiae, purpura, and ecchymosis may appear later in the disease, but the rash can take any form (e.g., vesicular, blanching macules) or may be absent. Other signs of shock can occur, such as tachycardia, poor peripheral perfusion, tachypnea, oliguria, confusion, decreased consciousness, and evidence of multiorgan failure. Poor prognostic signs include coma, hypothermia, hypotension, leukopenia, and thrombocytopenia. Patients may also have meningitis. *N meningitidis* can be isolated from the blood and CSF. Therefore, appropriate cultures should be obtained in any patient presenting with signs of fever, petechial rash, and systemic illness. Samples for Gram stain and culture can also be taken from petechial skin lesions, sputum, synovial fluid, and other body fluids.

Because of the fulminant progress of infection, serological testing is unreliable. Meningococcal capsular antigen for capsular types A, C, Y, and W135 sampled from the CSF, blood, and even urine is useful, especially in those who have received antibiotics before the samples were obtained; the yield for type B, the predominant subtype in the United States, Europe, and Australia-Pacific, is lower. PCR for bacterial DNA is useful in those who have received antibiotics as it does not rely upon living organisms and requires only small amounts of DNA to provide a result.

Meningococcemia requires early, aggressive fluid resuscitation and hemodynamic and respiratory support as in other causes of septic shock. If patients are hypotensive despite adequate fluid resuscitation and inotropic and vasopressor support, administration of corticosteroids can be considered because of the concern for adrenal insufficiency. *N meningitidis* currently is susceptible to antibiotics. Third-generation cephalosporins (i.e., cefotaxime or ceftriaxone) are appropriate initial antibiotics choices, but therapy may be narrowed to penicillin G if the organism is susceptible. Surgical management of ischemic tissue is occasionally required.

Chemoprophylaxis should be given to household contacts, childcare or nursery school contacts who had contact in the 7 days before onset of illness, or those exposed directly to the patient's oral secretions through kissing, sharing utensils, or during close unprotected physical examination. Antibiotics used for chemoprophylaxis are rifampin, ciprofloxacin, or ceftriaxone (**Table 7-10**).

### Table 7-10 Chemoprophylaxis for High-Risk Contacts of Invasive Meningococcal Disease

| Age | Dose | Duration |
| --- | --- | --- |
| **Rifampin**[a] | | |
| <1 mo | 5 mg/kg, orally, every 12 h | 2 days |
| ≥1 mo | 10 mg/kg (maximum 600 mg), orally, every 12 h | 2 days |
| Adults | 600 mg, orally, every 12 h | 2 days |
| **Ceftriaxone** | | |
| <15 y | 125 mg, intramuscularly | Single dose |
| ≥15 y | 250 mg, intramuscularly | Single dose |
| **Ciprofloxacin**[a] | | |
| ≥1 mo | 20 mg/kg (maximum 500 mg), orally | Single dose |
| Adults | 500 mg, orally | Single dose |
| **Azithromycin** | 10 mg/kg (maximum 500 mg) | Single dose |

[a]Not recommended for use in pregnant women.
Classified using Bilukha OO, Rosenstein N. Prevention and control of meningococcal disease. *MMWR*. 2005;54:1-21. Centers for Disease Control and Prevention Web site. http://www.cdc.gov/mmwr/indrr_2005.html. Accessed April 17, 2013.

## D. Rocky Mountain Spotted Fever

### Case Study

A 9-year-old girl presents in September with a 3-day history of fever to 102.2°F (39°C), severe headache, and a rash. She is not sexually active, and her last menstrual period was 2 weeks ago. She denies dysuria. Her pulse rate is 103 beats/min and blood pressure is 125/75 mm Hg. On exam, a maculopapular rash is noted on her extremities, trunk, and palms and soles, some of which is non-blanching. She also has conjunctival injection and tender muscles.

### Detection
 – What physiologic parameters concern you about this patient?
 – What are the possible etiologies for this patient?

**Intervention**

- What are the most immediate treatment strategies?

**Reassessment**

- Is the current treatment strategy effective?
- Are there any adjunctive therapies you should consider?

**Effective Communication**

- When the patient's clinical status changes, who needs to know and how will the information be disseminated?
- Where is the best place to manage the care of this patient?

**Teamwork**

- How are you going to implement the treatment strategy?
- Who is to do what and when?

Rocky Mountain spotted fever (RMSF) is a result of infection by an obligate intracellular coccobacillus, *Rickettsia rickettsii*, transmitted by the American dog tick. Most cases occur between April and September in the United States. This bacterium infects endothelial cells of small vessels of all major tissues and results in a systemic vasculitis. The classic clinical tetrad of RMSF is fever, severe headache, muscle tenderness, and rash. The initial rash is a blanching macular-papular rash on the ankles and wrist that spreads centripetally to involve the trunk and spreads to the palms and soles. The rash evolves into a non-blanching petechial rash. Other clinical features seen are nausea, vomiting, abdominal pain, conjunctivitis, stupor, edema, meningismus, and coma. Laboratory features suggestive of RMSF include hyponatremia, hypoalbuminemia, anemia, and thrombocytopenia. The WBC count can be normal or elevated. If CSF is obtained, an elevated WBC count with monocyte predominance may be seen. The diagnosis is confirmed with rickettsial serological tests, but empiric antimicrobial treatment of a suspected case should not await these results because they are typically not available rapidly and initial serology may be negative.

RMSF can be a very serious infection, and treatment should be initiated based on clinical suspicion. Early treatment yields very good outcomes. The drug of choice is doxycycline or tetracycline; alternatively, chloramphenicol can also be used. Although staining of teeth by tetracycline is a concern, this is a dose- and duration-related complication, less likely with doxycycline than with tetracycline, and therefore unlikely to occur when the drug is administered for a short course. In light of the potential severity of this infection, administration of doxycycline should not be delayed.

## E. Necrotizing Fasciitis

 Case Study

A 15-year-old girl presents to the emergency department with marked pain in the left ankle, erythema, and swelling. She has a temperature of 102°F (39.4°C), is tachypneic, has an elevated heart rate, and the $Spo_2$ is 88% on room air. You are concerned that an apparent localized infection is presenting with systemic symptoms.

**Detection**
- What physiologic parameters concern you about this patient?
- What diagnosis are you most likely considering?
- What infectious etiologies are you concerned about with these findings?

**Intervention**
- What are the most immediate treatment strategies?

**Reassessment**
- Is the current treatment strategy effective?
- Are there any adjunctive therapies you should consider?

**Effective Communication**
- When the patient's clinical status changes, who needs to know and how will the information be disseminated?

**Teamwork**
- How are you going to implement the treatment strategy?
- Who is to do what and when?

Soft tissue infections consist of a spectrum of diseases, ranging from superficial (and more benign) infections (erysipelas, impetigo, or cellulitis) to the most life-threatening deep infections (necrotizing fasciitis and myonecrosis). Although necrotizing fasciitis is an uncommon disease, early recognition and treatment is critical for patient survival. GABHS is the most common individual bacterial species, but the feared microbe responsible for gas gangrene, *Clostridium perfringens*, is well described; community-acquired methicillin-resistant *S aureus* is also increasingly common, but most infections are polymicrobial. There is no difference in outcomes whether single-organism or polymicrobial infection. The necrosis of skin, underlying fat, and fascial layers leads to the clinical presentation of erythema, warmth, swelling, fever, and exquisite tenderness out of proportion to the rest of the physical exam. The overlying skin may develop crepitance as well as serous or hemorrhagic bullae. Patients may present in septic shock or multiple organ failure. Untreated, necrotizing fasciitis is invariably fatal; therefore, a high index of suspicion must be maintained and treatment rapidly instituted. Diagnosis relies primarily on the clinical exam, but may be supported by either computed tomography (CT) or magnetic resonance imaging (MRI), and laboratory values such as increased C-reactive protein, WBC count, serum creatinine, and serum glucose, and decreased hemoglobin or serum sodium. Biopsy may be confirmatory.

Early aggressive treatment, including surgical debridement, is necessary for patient survival. Initial antibiotic therapy should include broad-spectrum coverage of aerobic Gram-positive and Gram-negative organisms and anaerobes, such as is achieved with carbapenem. For GABHS, high-dose parenteral clindamycin is optimal, with the addition of high-dose penicillin recommended by some, particularly in the presence of gas-forming organisms. If methicillin-resistant *S aureus* is suspected, then vancomycin or daptomycin should be used.

Additional therapies, such as high-dose IVIG, has proven beneficial in many cases. Hyperbaric oxygen may be considered as it both speeds healing and limits tissue loss.

## F. Bacterial Meningitis

### Case Study

A 7-month-old boy is admitted to the pediatric ward with a 3-day history of an upper respiratory infection and a 1-day history of high fever, vomiting, and inconsolable irritability. He has not been feeding well and has had decreased urine output over the previous day. His heart rate is 148 beats/min, and his respiratory rate is 24 breaths/min.

**Detection**
- What physiologic parameters concern you about this patient?
- What diagnoses should you consider?

**Intervention**
- What additional tests are needed to confirm the diagnosis?
- What are the most immediate treatment strategies?

**Reassessment**
- Is the current treatment strategy effective?
- Are there any adjunctive therapies you should consider?

**Effective Communication**
- When the patient's clinical status changes, who needs to know and how will the information be disseminated?
- Where is the best place to manage the care of this patient?

**Teamwork**
- How are you going to implement the treatment strategy?
- Who is to do what and when?

Fever and vomiting without diarrhea can occur early in the course of a common infection, like acute gastroenteritis, but may be a sign of an intracranial infection, such as meningitis. Immediate identification of acute infections of the central nervous system (CNS) is very important due to the life-threatening or life-altering nature of untreated infections, although this task may prove difficult due to the varied presentations. Bacterial or viral meningitis, viral meningoencephalitis, or viral encephalitis account for most CNS infections in children. Typical symptoms of CNS infection are:

- Acute onset of fever
- Altered consciousness
- Headache
- Stiff neck

- Photophobia
- Nausea and vomiting
- Anorexia
- Seizures
- Bulging fontanelle

Often a child will have an antecedent upper respiratory tract infection. Children younger than 18 months with meningitis may not have signs of meningeal irritation (i.e., neck stiffness, Kernig sign, Brudzinski sign), making it important to keep a high index of suspicion for meningitis or another CNS infection.

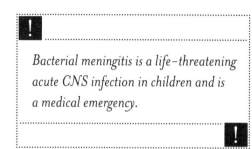

*Bacterial meningitis is a life-threatening acute CNS infection in children and is a medical emergency.*

Bacterial meningitis is the most common life-threatening acute CNS infection in children and is a medical emergency. Common pathogens based on patient age are summarized in **Table 7-11**. Diagnosis of bacterial meningitis is made on the basis of clinical presentation and confirmed by the culture of pathogenic organisms in the CSF obtained by lumbar puncture. Circumstances in which a lumbar puncture may place the patient at risk and may be contraindicated are in a patient with cardiorespiratory instability, bleeding disorders, signs of raised intracranial pressure (irregular pupils, abnormal breathing pattern, hypertension, bradycardia, decerebrate or decorticate posturing), evidence of a soft tissue infection over the lumbar puncture site, recent (<30 minutes) or prolonged (>30 minutes) seizure, Glasgow Coma Scale (GCS) score <13, the presence of papilledema, localized neurologic signs, and intracranial mass or hydrocephalus. A normal CT scan does not rule out the possibility of cerebral herniation; CT of the head is not a prerequisite for performing a lumbar puncture. Also, the presence of an open anterior fontanelle does not protect infants from cerebral herniation. If a lumbar puncture is deferred, antibiotic therapy appropriate for bacterial meningitis should be administered immediately. The CSF analysis consistent with bacterial meningitis, compared to other types of CNS infections, is described in **Table 7-12**. Blood cultures should also be obtained, as they are often positive for the offending organism.

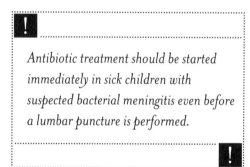

*Antibiotic treatment should be started immediately in sick children with suspected bacterial meningitis even before a lumbar puncture is performed.*

### Table 7-11 Common Pathogens Causing Bacterial Meningitis

| | |
|---|---|
| Neonates | Group B streptococci<br>*Escherichia coli*<br>Other Gram-negative bacilli<br>*Listeria monocytogenes* |
| Older infants and children | *Streptococcus pneumoniae*<br>*Neisseria meningitidis*<br>*Haemophilus influenzae* type b (in those not immunized) |

### Table 7-12  Cerebrospinal Fluid Findings in Meningitis and Encephalitis

| Type of Meningitis | Opening Pressure | Leukocytes (mm³) | Glucose | Proteins (mg/dL) |
|---|---|---|---|---|
| Bacterial meningitis | Elevated | 100-10,000 (usually >1000); usually PMNs | Low (less than two-thirds normal serum glucose) | >40 (usually >200) |
| Viral meningitis | Normal to elevated | 10-1000 (usually 100-500); usually lymphocytes | Usually normal | 50-100 |
| Tuberculous meningitis | Usually elevated | 5-500; usually mononuclear cells | Normal to low | >500 |
| Fungal meningitis | Usually elevated | 5-500 | Normal to low | 100-500 |
| Viral encephalitis | Normal to elevated | Normal to mild pleocytosis; either PMNs or mononuclear cells | Normal to mildly low | Normal to 100 |

PMN, polymorphonuclear leukocytes

Prompt administration of appropriate antibiotics in appropriate doses is the basis of curative therapy. Empiric antibiotic choices are based on the patient's age and risk factors. In neonates, ampicillin combined with gentamicin or cefotaxime is the appropriate empiric therapy. In older infants and children, a third-generation cephalosporin (cefotaxime or ceftriaxone) combined with vancomycin should be started until bacterial identification and susceptibility have been established.

Although controversial, the administration of steroids (dexamethasone) early in the course of bacterial meningitis should be considered in children older than 8 weeks; it has been shown to decrease the incidence of hearing loss in patients with *Haemophilus influenzae* and *Streptococcus pneumoniae* meningitis. If prescribed, a dose of 0.15 mg/kg/dose, given every 6 hours, should be administered for a total of 2 to 4 days, with the first dose given before or at the time of the first antibiotic dose. Chemoprophylaxis in cases of *H influenzae* type b (HIB) should be given to all household contacts with at least 1 susceptible contact in the home (i.e., child <4 years of age who is incompletely immunized against HIB, child <12 months of age, or child who is immunocompromised). Chemoprophylaxis should also be given to nursery contacts in the presence of at least 2 cases of invasive disease within 2 months. Rifampin 20 mg/kg once daily for 4 days (maximum dose, 600 mg) or 10 mg/kg/day in infants younger than 2 months is recommended. Pregnant women should receive ceftriaxone 125 to 250 mg intramuscularly as a single dose. Chemoprophylaxis for contacts of persons with meningococcal meningitis is the same as for meningococcemia.

## G. Aseptic and Viral Meningitis

Viruses are the causative agent in the majority of cases of "aseptic meningitis." Other etiologies are: *Mycoplasma pneumoniae*, Lyme disease, *Mycobacterium tuberculosis*, and RMSF. Parasitic causes (i.e., *Angiostrongylus, Gnathostoma, Schistosoma, Toxocara, Echinococcus*) should also be considered in relevant geographic areas and returned travelers as they have a very different prognosis and are generally treatable. Rare noninfectious cases may represent malignancy, autoimmune disease, drug reaction, collagen vascular disease, or sarcoidosis (among other causes). Enteroviruses are the most common viral cause (especially echovirus and Coxsackie virus). Generally, the CSF cell count, differential, glucose concentration, protein concentration, and Gram stain results will help differentiate between viral and bacterial causes, as the clinical presentations overlap. Although lymphocytes are the predominant cell type found in the CSF of patients with viral meningitis, a neutrophil predominance may be seen early in the course. Treatment is largely supportive, placing focus on airway, breathing, and circulation, as well as symptomatic therapy, such as control of temperature, seizures, and hydration status.

## H. Encephalitis

Acute encephalitis is characterized by changes in mental status. It is frequently caused by a virus such as enterovirus, herpes simplex virus (HSV), or another virus (i.e., Epstein-Barr, cytomegalovirus, varicella-zoster virus, or an arbovirus). *M pneumoniae* and other etiologic agents may also be implicated. In many cases, the etiology remains unknown despite investigations.

Results of CSF studies usually show a mild pleocytosis, but may be normal. PCR in CSF should be used to detect enterovirus and HSV infections. CNS imaging with MRI is more sensitive than CT and may detect areas of inflammation or help rule out noninfectious causes. For instance, during HSV encephalitis, the MRI may show alterations in the medial temporal lobe and/or frontal lobes, and the electroencephalogram may show typical periodic lateralized epileptiform discharges. In patients with suspected HSV encephalitis, urgent treatment with intravenous acyclovir should be initiated until this etiology can be ruled out. There is insufficient data to determine if the use of antibiotics in *M pneumoniae* encephalitis improves the clinical course or outcome.

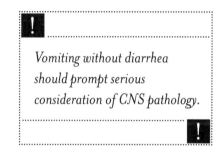

*Vomiting without diarrhea should prompt serious consideration of CNS pathology.*

## Case Study

A 16-year-old girl presents to the emergency department with a 1-day history of a temperature to 104°F (40°C), abdominal and back pain, and 1 episode of vomiting. She is not sexually active and denies dysuria or discharge. On physical examination you note diffuse abdominal tenderness more pronounced on her left side. Her heart rate is 124 beats/min, and her respiratory rate is 22 breaths/min.

**Detection**

– What physiologic parameters concern you about this patient?

– What are the most likely, and most serious, diagnoses you must consider?

**Intervention**

– What are the most immediate treatment strategies?

– What further investigation is needed to identify the etiology?

**Reassessment**
- Is the current treatment strategy effective?
- Are there any adjunctive therapies you should consider?

**Effective Communication**
- When the patient's clinical status changes, who needs to know and how will the information be disseminated?
- Where is the best place to manage the care of this patient?

**Teamwork**
- How are you going to implement the treatment strategy?
- Who is to do what and when?

The differential diagnosis of acute abdominal pain is extensive and involves many diagnoses that are not emergent. Both infectious and noninfectious illnesses within the abdominal compartment may need immediate attention due to their serious nature. The following noninfectious disorders can be acutely life-threatening and, among others, should be considered:

- Malrotation with volvulus
- Acute small or large bowel obstruction
- Intestinal perforation
- Acute kidney injury due to obstructive uropathy
- Viscus injury due to trauma
- Peptic ulcerative disease
- Acute pancreatitis
- Ectopic pregnancy
- Ovarian/testicular torsion

# I. Urinary Tract Infection

Acute infections of the urinary tract can involve the bladder (cystitis) or the kidneys (pyelonephritis), and the latter may lead to systemic bacteremia and sepsis (urosepsis). In children experiencing their first urinary tract infection (UTI), the most frequent pathogen is *Escherichia coli*. Other organisms, such as *Klebsiella, Proteus, Enterococcus faecalis, Staphylococcus saprophyticus*, or *Pseudomonas aeruginosa*, may be present, particularly in children who have urinary tract obstruction or a urinary catheter.

The diagnosis of UTI is usually established with urinalysis and urine culture. A urinalysis that shows pyuria and a Gram stain that reveals bacteria can provide rapid evidence of the presence of a UTI. The "gold standard" diagnostic technique for obtaining urine is a suprapubic aspiration; when this technique is used, any bacterial growth is indicative of infection. However, urine for a culture is most frequently obtained using the midstream, clean-catch technique, intermittent catheterization, or a Foley catheter already in place.

It can be difficult to differentiate upper from lower UTI. Fever, leukocytosis, and flank tenderness may be present in patients with acute pyelonephritis. Urgency, frequency, and dysuria are classic symptoms of cystitis.

Children with a toxic appearance should always be treated with parenteral antibiotics. Cefotaxime or ceftriaxone is a good empiric choice in children and adolescents, while ampicillin and gentamicin are often prescribed for neonates. Extended spectrum β-lactamase- and metallo-β-lactamase-producing Gram-negative organisms are rapidly becoming the major cause of UTIs in Asia. They require treatment with aztreonam, tigecycline, or polymyxin. Neonates with UTIs should receive parenteral treatment because of the high prevalence of concomitant bacteremia.

## J. Peritonitis

Depending on the source of infection, peritoneal infections can be classified as primary or secondary peritonitis. Peritonitis is considered primary when the peritoneal cavity is infected via hematogenous or lymphatic dissemination and the cause is a single organism. The bacterial organisms that most frequently cause primary peritonitis are *Streptococcus pneumoniae*, GABHS, and *E coli* or other enteric bacteria. The most frequent predisposing factor for primary peritonitis is the presence of ascites caused by cirrhosis, portal hypertension, or nephrotic syndrome.

Secondary peritonitis results from the rupture or extension of an intra-abdominal viscus or abscess; therefore, it is usually polymicrobial. The most frequent pathogens are enteric Gram-negative bacteria, such as *E coli*, *Klebsiella*, or *Enterobacter*, plus anaerobes and, at times, *Enterococcus*.

A patient suspected of having peritonitis should be managed with the aid of a pediatric surgeon. Diagnostic techniques, such as ultrasound and CT scan, can help localize the source and extent of the infection. Empiric antibiotic treatment for primary peritonitis is usually cefotaxime or ceftriaxone in combination with an aminoglycoside. Antibiotic treatment for secondary peritonitis should be aimed at treating anaerobic and Gram-negative organisms. Extended spectrum β-lactams like piperacillin/tazobactam, carbapenems like meropenem, ampicillin/sulbactam or ampicillin in combination with gentamicin and metronidazole or clindamycin are used frequently. Where vancomycin-resistant enterococci are prevalent, medications such as linezolid/daptomycin/tigecycline/colistin should be considered.

## K. Acute Hepatic Failure

Acute or "fulminant" hepatic failure refers to the metabolic and systemic consequences of hepatic cellular dysfunction and necrosis, specifically including the hepatic encephalopathy and coagulopathy that develops within 8 weeks of onset of liver disease in a patient without preexisting liver disease.

Approximately 6% of cases of acute hepatic failure in the United States are due to primary viral infections, the second most common identifiable source of liver failure after acetaminophen toxicity. Responsible viruses are adenovirus, cytomegalovirus, Epstein-Barr virus, enterovirus, hepatitis A and hepatitis C viruses, and HSV. Worldwide, other organisms known to cause diffuse hepatic dysfunction are hepatitis B and hepatitis D viruses, echovirus, and leptospira.

Most patients with fulminant hepatic failure present with hepatic dysfunction, hypoglycemia, coagulopathy, and encephalopathy. Jaundice may be a late finding. Most have no history of other chronic medical problems or known exposure to hepatitis.

Management of fulminant hepatic failure is primarily supportive as no specific therapy exists other than liver transplant. Hepatic support, treatment of acquired infections, and prevention and treatment of complications are indicated while the patient awaits recovery of liver function. Extracorporeal hepatic support is often used as a bridge to liver transplant. Rapid referral to a transplant center, if an available option, is crucial, as patients may deteriorate rapidly, making them unsuitable for stable transfer. Broad-spectrum antibiotics are only indicated if sepsis is suspected or liver transplantation is anticipated.

## L. Myocarditis and Pericarditis

 ### Case Study

A 7-year-old boy presents to the emergency department with a 1-day history of increased work of breathing and worsening cough. One week prior, he had been diagnosed with an upper respiratory infection consisting of a temperature to 101.2°F (38.4°C), cough, and nasal discharge. On presentation, his respiratory rate is 42 breaths/min, heart rate is 184 beats/min, and $SpO_2$ is 88% on room air. You hear crackles bilaterally on chest auscultation and feel a liver edge palpable 2 cm below the costal margin.

**Detection**
- What physiologic parameters concern you about this patient?
- What are the most likely, and most serious, diagnoses you must consider?

**Intervention**
- What are the most immediate treatment strategies?
- What further investigation is needed to identify the etiology?

**Reassessment**
- Is the current treatment strategy effective?
- Are there any adjunctive therapies you should consider?

**Effective Communication**
- When the patient's clinical status changes, who needs to know and how will the information be disseminated?
- Where is the best place to manage the care of this patient?

**Teamwork**
- How are you going to implement the treatment strategy?
- Who is to do what and when?

Respiratory distress or failure is not always due to primary pathology within the lungs. Primary myocardial failure (i.e., cardiomyopathy) or inflammatory heart disease often presents with respiratory symptoms. Inflammatory heart disease encompasses a wide array of clinical entities, many of which are a result of acute infections of the pericardium and/or myocardium. Pericarditis may be caused by viral, bacterial, mycobacterial, or fungal infections. Viruses are the main cause of myocarditis. **Table 7-13** lists many of the infectious etiologies of pericarditis and myocarditis. Rheumatic fever, an immune-mediated illness that follows group A β-hemolytic streptococcal pharyngitis, may present with fever and carditis.

### Table 7-13 Infectious Causes of Myocarditis and/or Pericarditis[a]

| Viruses | Bacteria | Parasites | Fungi |
|---|---|---|---|
| • **Adenovirus** | • ***Borrelia burgdorferi*** | • Echinococcosis | • *Candida* |
| • **Coxsackie virus A, B** | • *Chlamydia psittaci* | • *Plasmodium falciparum* | • *Coccidioides* |
| • **Echovirus** | • *Corynebacterium diphtheriae* | • Schistosomes | • *Histoplasma* |
| • **Parvovirus B19** | • *Leptospira* | • Toxoplasmosis | • *Aspergillus* |
| • **Epstein-Barr virus** | • Meningococcus | • *Trichinella spiralis* | • *Cryptococcus* |
| • Hepatitis B virus | • ***Mycoplasma pneumoniae*** | • *Trypanosoma cruzi* | • *Blastomyces* |
| • Herpes simplex virus | • ***Staphylococcus aureus*** | | |
| • **Human immunodeficiency virus (HIV)** | • *Streptococcus sp* | | |
| • Influenza virus A, B | • *Treponema pallidum* | | |
| • Mumps virus | • *Actinomyces* | | |
| • Poliovirus | • *Haemophilus influenzae* type b | | |
| | • *Mycobacterium tuberculosis* | | |

[a]Some common etiologies of myocarditis or pericarditis are indicated in bold.

Patients with pericarditis may present with chest pain and fever. The pain is often substernal and may radiate to the middle of the back, increase with inspiration, and be relieved by leaning forward. If the effusion that develops within the pericardial space becomes sufficiently large, patients may also have dyspnea, shortness of breath, shock, or respiratory failure. A friction rub may be heard on auscultation, but may be absent in the presence of a large effusion. A chest radiograph revealing an enlarged cardiac silhouette, an electrocardiogram showing ST- and T-wave changes or diminished QRS amplitudes supports the diagnosis, and an echocardiogram can confirm the diagnosis. Laboratory findings are nonspecific.

Myocarditis occurs when the myocardium is directly affected by an invading organism, often leading to inflammatory changes and myocyte necrosis. The spectrum of infectious etiologies is similar to that of pericarditis, but is most commonly viral in etiology. The range of presentations varies from an asymptomatic patient to a one with obvious signs of congestive heart failure. Many children will have a febrile illness preceding the episode of myocarditis. They may present with chest pain or syncope, but commonly the multisystem effects and symptoms of the underlying viral illness overshadow the symptoms related to the cardiovascular system. Infants may present with irritability and poor feeding. Dysrhythmias such as ventricular ectopy, atrioventricular block, ST- and T-wave abnormalities, or tachycardia out of proportion to the fever at presentation, may suggest the presence of myocarditis. Sudden death is possible in a patient with severe acute myocarditis. The majority of laboratory and electrocardiographic findings are nonspecific. Elevation of troponin I is the most sensitive diagnostic marker other than myocardial biopsy results. Laboratory evidence of poor oxygen delivery due to poor cardiac output (i.e., serum lactate) or myocardial stretch due to volume overload (i.e., B-type natriuretic peptide) is often sought. The diagnosis is often difficult to establish and is generally made on circumstantial evidence, such as a recent viral infection and the sudden onset of cardiac dysfunction. Isolation of the infectious etiology should be pursued, but is often elusive; use of PCR may increase the likelihood of success.

Myocarditis and pericarditis therapies include treating the infecting pathogen (if possible), as well as providing medical support of myocardial function with a combination of afterload reduction (i.e., milrinone), inotropy (i.e., dopamine or epinephrine [adrenaline]), and diuretics (i.e., furosemide). Severe myocardial dysfunction may also necessitate mechanical ventilation, either noninvasively with bilevel positive airway pressure or invasively with intubation. If a large pericardial effusion is present and impinging on cardiac function or if purulent pericarditis is present, drainage is indicated. IVIG is indicated in the treatment of viral myocarditis.

## M. Neonatal Herpes Simplex Virus Infections

###  Case Study

A 4-day-old, full-term healthy infant is admitted to the hospital with a history of a temperature to 104°F (40°C). Her physical examination appears normal, including the skin. The infant was born via normal spontaneous vaginal delivery after 18 hours of ruptured membranes. The maternal history revealed no known risk factors. A full sepsis workup is done, and the infant is started on ampicillin and cefotaxime. Despite antibiotics, she developed respiratory distress and hypotension.

**Detection**
- What physiologic parameters concern you about this patient?
- What are the most likely, and most serious, diagnoses you must consider?

**Intervention**
- What are the most immediate treatment strategies?
- What further investigation is needed to identify the etiology?

**Reassessment**
- Is the current treatment strategy effective?
- Are there any adjunctive therapies you should consider?

**Effective Communication**
- When the patient's clinical status changes, who needs to know and how will the information be disseminated?
- Where is the best place to manage the care of this patient?

**Teamwork**
- How are you going to implement the treatment strategy?
- Who is to do what and when?

In addition to bacterial infection, two viral etiologies should be entertained in a newborn presenting with multisystem involvement with or without hypotension: HSV infection and enterovirus sepsis.

Neonatal HSV is most commonly acquired in the peripartum period. Approximately 50% of cases are due to HSV-1 and the remaining to HSV-2. Of the affected infants, 50% to 70% are born to women who were asymptomatic at delivery. The highest risk of acquisition (50%) is in infants born to women with primary infection during pregnancy.

Neonatal HSV can present in 3 forms:

1. Disseminated disease accounts for approximately 25% of these infections. It usually presents in the first 2 weeks of life with multisystem involvement, including the lungs, liver, adrenal glands, skin, eye, and/or brain. Mortality is >80% without treatment and is usually due to severe coagulopathy, liver failure, and/or respiratory failure.

2. CNS disease without skin lesions presents later than 2 weeks and manifests as fever, irritability, poor feeding, and seizures, which can be either focal or generalized. Such cases account for approximately 25% of neonatal HSV cases.

3. Disease limited to the skin, eye, and/or mouth (SEM) occurs in 50% of neonatal HSV infections. These babies should have a CSF evaluation as one-third have CNS involvement.

Typical vesicular skin lesions can occur at anytime in the course of illness, but 10% to 20% of infants with either disseminated infection or CNS involvement do not develop lesions. This makes the initial diagnosis difficult as the signs and symptoms of sepsis due to other etiologies are similar and nonspecific. A high index of suspicion should be maintained in a neonate with either sepsis or seizures. To make the correct diagnosis, swabs for viral culture using appropriate transport media should be collected from any suspicious lesions, as well as surface cultures from the mouth, nasopharynx, conjunctivae, and rectum. Routine CSF evaluation should include PCR for HSV. Blood also should be tested by PCR, if available.

Treatment consists of high-dose acyclovir at 60 mg/kg/day divided every 8 hours. The duration of disseminated and CNS disease is 21 days, and 14 days for skin, eye, and/or mouth disease without CNS involvement.

## N. Lemierre Disease (Necrobacillosis)

 **Case Study**

You are caring for a 16-year-old previously healthy boy who developed a sore throat and malaise about 5 days before admission. After 2 days, he began having pain in the right side of his neck and had difficulty turning his head from side to side. He also reports chills with fever, pleuritic chest pain, and abdominal pain. He appears ill, is tachypneic, and febrile to 102.2°F (39°C). His pharynx appears normal, and he has a tender, ill-defined mass in the right sternocleidomastoid muscle. His lung and heart exams are normal. Multiple bilateral nodular infiltrates are seen on chest radiograph.

### Detection
- What physiologic parameters concern you about this patient?
- What are the most likely, and most serious, diagnoses you must consider?

### Intervention
- What are the most immediate treatment strategies?
- What further investigation is needed to identify the etiology?

### Reassessment
- Is the current treatment strategy effective?
- Are there any adjunctive therapies you should consider?

### Effective Communication
- When the patient's clinical status changes, who needs to know and how will the information be disseminated?
- Where is the best place to manage the care of this patient?

### Teamwork
- How are you going to implement the treatment strategy?
- Who is to do what and when?

The most likely causative organism is the anaerobe *Fusobacterium necrophorum* or another *Fusobacterium* sp. Other organisms have also been reported with this illness, such as anaerobic streptococci, *S aureus*, and *Bacteroides* sp. This illness typically affects adolescents and young adults. Originally described in the early 20th century and also referred as to as *post-anginal sepsis* or *necrobacillosis*, Lemierre disease is thought to be caused by the spread of infection from the oropharynx into the parapharyngeal space, resulting in septic thrombophlebitis of the internal jugular vein, bacteremia, septic emboli, and at times septicemia. Most patients present with fever and a sore throat, followed by neck pain that can be associated with neck swelling, trismus, and dysphagia. Septic emboli most often spread to the lungs, and these patients present with pneumonia with empyema. Chest radiographs can show bilateral nodular infiltrates, cavitary lesions, effusions, or pneumatoceles. Dissemination can also occur to other organs, such as the musculoskeletal system, causing septic arthritis and osteomyelitis, or to the liver, spleen, and kidneys. Occasionally retrograde spread to the brain can cause cerebral venous sinus thrombosis, meningitis, or brain abscess.

Both anaerobic and aerobic blood cultures should be obtained in adolescents older than 11 years with a febrile illness and a suspicion for Lemierre disease. Imaging of the neck also should be performed to detect thrombophlebitis of the internal jugular vein. Ultrasound is useful if positive but is not very sensitive; therefore, either a CT or MRI scan may be performed to establish the diagnosis.

Patients with Lemierre disease should receive a penicillin/β-lactamase inhibitor agent (such as piperacillin/tazobactam) or a combination of ceftriaxone and clindamycin to treat both *Fusobacterium* and streptococci that might be present. Metronidazole is active against all *Fusobacterium* and is often used with a β-lactam. The duration of antibiotic treatment is usually 4 to 6 weeks. Anticoagulation therapy has been used in both adults and children with jugular vein thrombosis and cavernous sinus thrombosis. This may decrease the risk of clot extension and shorten recovery time, although its use is still controversial due to a lack of definitive data. Surgical intervention involving debridement or incision and drainage is occasionally necessary.

## O. Malaria

### Case Study

A 12-year-old boy presents to the emergency department with a fever of 7 days' duration; it developed shortly after his return from a 3-week trip to Ghana. For the last 3 days, he has had vomiting and diarrhea, with progressive confusion and the development of delusions on the day of admission. His temperature is 102.7°F (39.3°C), pulse is 129 beats/min, blood pressure is 112/73 mm Hg, and respiratory rate is 32 breaths/min. Physical examination reveals hepatosplenomegaly, jaundice, slurring of speech, disorientation, and an inability to follow commands. His laboratory results include the following: WBC, 10.7 mm$^3$ (65% neutrophils, 20% bands); hemoglobin, 9.4 g/dL; and platelets, 47,000 mm$^3$.

**Detection**
- What physiologic parameters concern you about this patient?
- What are the most likely, and most serious, diagnoses you must consider?

**Intervention**
- What are the most immediate treatment strategies?
- What further investigation is needed to identify the etiology?

**Reassessment**
- Is the current treatment strategy effective?
- Are there any adjunctive therapies you should consider?

**Effective Communication**
- When the patient's clinical status changes, who needs to know, and how will the information be disseminated?
- Where is the best place to manage the care of this patient?

**Teamwork**
- How are you going to implement the treatment strategy?

In any patient with a significant travel history it is necessary to consider and recognize certain infections endemic to specific regions of the world, as morbidity and mortality may be high.

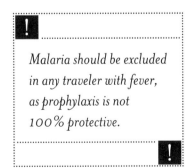
*Malaria should be excluded in any traveler with fever, as prophylaxis is not 100% protective.*

Malaria is transmitted by the bite of the female Anopheles mosquito. Of the 5 *Plasmodium* species that cause malaria in humans, *P falciparum* is the most severe. Infection with *P falciparum* is potentially fatal and is responsible for 40% to 60% of the world's cases of malaria and for 95% of deaths from malaria. Complications include severe anemia, cerebral malaria, and pulmonary edema. *P vivax* and *P ovale* can be dormant in the liver, and illness can occur as long as several years after initial infection or can relapse. *P malariae* can lead to chronic, long-term illness. The newly described *P knowlesi* is largely confined to Indonesia and Malaysia, presents in a manner similar to *P falciparum* malaria, and may be fatal. Knowledge of travel destinations and distribution of *Plasmodium* species are important in the selection of antimalarial drugs. Dual infection is possible and, in fact, common in some areas.

The initial presentation of malaria is nonspecific and can include fever, chills, headache, vomiting, diarrhea, myalgias, weakness, dizziness, and splenomegaly. The classic cyclic fever every second day (*P falciparum, P vivax,* and *P ovale*) and every third day (tertian fever) is infrequent in children. The physical exam may include hepatosplenomegaly, jaundice, diaphoresis, and pallor.

The diagnosis is based on demonstration of parasites in thick and thin blood smears. A single negative smear does not rule out malaria, and multiple smears should be done several hours apart if the index of suspicion is high. PCR for the malaria parasite is highly sensitive and specific, and can diagnose both the presence of the parasites and the species involved. Other laboratory abnormalities are low hemoglobin, low platelet count, hyperbilirubinemia, and increased hepatic enzymes. Severe malaria (altered conscious state, seizures, anemia, oligoanuria/acute kidney injury, acidosis, hypoglycemia) is a medical emergency. The choice of antimicrobial therapy depends on several factors, including type of *Plasmodium* species, drug susceptibility of the infecting parasite, severity of illness, and availability of medications. Oral medications include artemether and artemisinin combination therapy, chloroquine, atovaquone-proguanil, mefloquine, and quinine sulfate plus doxycycline, tetracycline, or clindamycin. When the species of *Plasmodium* is unknown, it is prudent to assume that the parasite is *P falciparum* and to treat accordingly. Chloroquine can be used in patients from areas where drug resistance has not been reported. Details of treatment are available at http://www.who.int/malaria and http://www.cdc.gov/malaria/.

Severe malaria in everyone other than women in their first trimester of pregnancy should be treated with the usual resuscitative measures in conjunction with intravenous artesunate, 2.4 mg/kg immediately, repeated at 12 and 24 hours, then once daily until oral therapy is available. Oral therapy is usually lumefantrine, amodiaquine, sulfadoxine-pyrimethamine, or mefloquine. Oral artemisinin combination therapies are available (i.e., artemether-lumefantrine). Rectal administration is also an option in the comatose patient in whom intravenous and intraosseous access is not possible. Artemisinin compounds must not be given alone due to the high risk of inducing resistance. Those women in their first trimester should receive intravenous quinine or quinidine, which requires admission to the intensive care unit for cardiac monitoring. Exchange transfusion should be considered in the most severe cases (i.e., *P falciparum* with >10% parasitemia and end-organ damage) as a means of removing parasitized red blood cells.

## P. Dengue Fever

The dengue virus is transmitted by the female *Aedes aegypti* and *A albopictus* mosquitoes. The typical incubation period is 4 to 7 days. Patients can present with a subclinical mild febrile illness or the classic dengue fever (breakbone fever). Signs consist of fever and headache; severe muscle, joint, bone (back) pain; nausea and vomiting; rash; and mild bleeding. The rash can be macular, scarlatiniform, or petechial, sparing the palms and soles. Dengue is a self-limited illness, lasting 3 to 10 days. The most severe form of illness, dengue hemorrhagic fever/dengue shock syndrome, can be a life-threatening condition. Warning symptoms of severe disease are recrudescence after initial improvement, severe abdominal pain, persistent vomiting, and development of hypothermia, hemorrhage, or change in mental status. Diagnosis of a dengue viral infection requires PCR or serial immunoglobulin M antibody titers, although the latter are notoriously difficult to interpret due to significant cross-reactivity with other flaviviruses.

The treatment of dengue fever is mainly supportive, with fluid resuscitation and hemodynamic support paralleling that of septic shock, and includes close monitoring of blood tests.

## Key Points: Acute Infections

- Signs and symptoms of infection are multiple and vary with age. Detection of potentially severe infections is based on a meticulous clinical examination.

- Adequate cultures should be obtained before starting antibiotic treatment unless there are specific contraindications.

- The choice of antibiotics depends on the patient's age, the type of infection suspected, risk factors (such as immunosuppression, presence of invasive medical devices, or recent hospitalization), and knowledge of local antimicrobial resistance patterns.

- Severe infections and localizing signs of infection can be difficult to detect in young children, infants, and neonates. Management is based on risk factors, toxic appearance criteria, and laboratory findings.

- Suspicion of sepsis requires rapid management with goal-directed therapy. Antibiotic treatment should be started within the first hour.

- *S aureus* and *S pyogenes* can produce toxin-mediated diseases, such as toxic shock syndrome.

- Meningococcemia should be considered in all children with fever and petechiae.

- Meningitis should always be treated urgently. Lumbar puncture can be diagnostic, but there are contraindications for this procedure. Acyclovir treatment for HSV encephalitis should be considered in patients with fever and disturbances of consciousness.

- Hospitalized children with fever should be suspected of having nosocomial infections. The most frequent bacteria involved in nosocomial infections include coagulase-negative staphylococci and Gram-negative enteric rods.

- Infected lines or medical devices should be removed.

- Endemic infections, such as dengue and malaria, produce high mortality when not treated adequately. These infections should always be considered in patients traveling in regions where such infections are prevalent.

## Suggested Readings

1. American College of Emergency Physicians Clinical Policies Committee; American College of Emergency Physicians Clinical Policies Subcommittee on Pediatric Fever. Clinical policy for children younger than three years presenting to the emergency department with fever. *Ann Emerg Med*. 2003;42:530-545.

2. Brierley J, Carcillo JA, Choong K, et al. Clinical practice parameters for hemodynamic support of pediatric and neonatal septic shock: 2007 update from the American College of Critical Care Medicine. *Crit Care Med*. 2009;37:666-688.

3. Carcillo JA. Pediatric septic shock and multiple organ failure. *Crit Care Clin*. 2003;19:413-440.

4. Carcillo JA, Field AI, American College of Critical Care Medicine Task Force Committee Members. Clinical practice parameters for hemodynamic support of pediatric and neonatal patients in septic shock. *Crit Care Med*. 2002;30:1365-1378.

5. Goldstein B, Giroir B, Randolph A, International Consensus Conference on Pediatric Sepsis. International Pediatric Sepsis Consensus Conference: definitions for sepsis and organ dysfunction in pediatrics. *Pediatr Crit Care Med*. 2005;6:2-8.

6. Hart CA, Thomson AP. Meningococcal disease and its management in children. *BMJ*. 2006;333:685-690.

7. Isturiz R, Torres J, Besso J. Global distribution of infectious diseases requiring intensive care. *Crit Care Clin*. 2006;22:469-488.

8. McIntosh K. Community-acquired pneumonia in children. *N Engl J Med*. 2002;346:429-437.

9. Melendez E, Bachur R. Advances in the emergency management of pediatric sepsis. *Curr Opin Pediatr*. 2006;18:245-253.

10. Pickering LK, Baker CJ, Long SS, McMillan JA, eds. *Red Book: 2006 Report of the Committee on Infectious Diseases*. 27th ed. Elk Grove Village, IL: American Academy of Pediatrics; 2006.

11. Pollard AJ, Britto J, Nadel S, DeMunter C, Habibi P, Levin M. Emergency management of meningococcal disease. *Arch Dis Child*. 1999;80:290-296.

# Chapter 8

# Fluids, Electrolytes, and Neuroendocrine Metabolic Derangements

## ✓ Objectives

- Summarize basic concepts in the maintenance of intravascular fluid homeostasis.
- Discuss the common electrolyte disturbances, their recognition, and management.
- Describe common neuroendocrine emergencies, including those related to glucose metabolism, and discuss their management.

## Case Study

A 12-month-old infant presents to the emergency department, via emergency medical service, with a 3-day history of vomiting, diarrhea, and a temperature of 104°F (40°C). The patient is lethargic and has cracked lips and a sunken fontanel. Laboratory results are as follows: $Na^+$, 125 mEq/L (125 mmol/L); $K^+$, 4.8 mEq/L (4.8 mmol/L); $Cl^-$, 89 mEq/L (89 mmol/L); glucose, 89 mg/dL (4.9 mmol/L); $CO_2$, 7 mEq/L (7 mmol/L); blood urea nitrogen (BUN), 50 mg/dL; creatinine, 1.2 mg/dL (106.08 µmol/L).

### Detection
- What are the most important clinical signs?
- What are the most likely diagnoses?

### Intervention
- After initial fluid boluses with isotonic saline, what is your plan for ongoing fluid management?
- If the sodium level drops to 117 mEq/L and the patient begins to seize, how will you respond?

### Reassessment
- Check the patient's response to the intervention.
- Is the current treatment strategy effective?
- Therapeutic end points: level of consciousness, signs of dehydration, level of $Na^+$

**Effective Communication**

- When the patient's clinical status changes, who needs to know and how will the information be disseminated?
- Where is the best place to manage the care of this patient?

**Teamwork**

- How are you going to implement the treatment strategy?
- Who is to do what and when?

Fluid, electrolyte, and endocrine-metabolic disturbances are commonly seen in hospitalized children. An individualized approach to the fluid management of these children is needed, based on the underlying diagnosis and severity of illness.

# I. FLUIDS

## A. Maintenance Fluids

The fluid intake required to maintain a euvolemic state is largely dependent on the patient's initial hydration status and underlying disease state.

The term *maintenance fluids* loosely denotes the quantity of IV fluids required to maintain hydration in an euvolemic child who is not experiencing abnormal ongoing loss of fluids as seen in gastrointestinal diseases, bleeding, and burns. The maintenance fluid calculations provide a rapid and convenient starting point for determining the amount of fluid required to maintain intravascular volume.

The Holliday-Segar method for calculating maintenance IV fluids is based on the caloric expenditure in fixed weight categories (**Table 8-1**). Calculations are based on the patient's dry/baseline weight.

Other methods are available and utilize nomograms for body surface area and caloric expenditure to determine fluid requirements. We have purposely limited ourselves to describing only one widely used methodology.

### Table 8-1. The Holliday-Segar Method for Calculating Maintenance IV Fluids

- First 10 kg: fluid requirement is 100 mL/kg/day or 4 mL/kg/h.
- 10-20 kg: for each kilogram of body weight above 10 kg, add 50 mL/kg/day or 2 mL/kg/h to the initial 40 mL/h.
- >20 kg: for each kilogram of body weight above 20 kg, add 20 mL/kg/day or 1 mL/kg/h to the 60 mL/h.

**Example:** A 26-kg child who is NPO and awaiting surgery would have a maintenance fluid requirement of 40+20+6 = 66 mL/h of IV fluid.

NPO, nothing by mouth; IV, intravenous

Maintenance fluids in children historically have been hypotonic (i.e., 0.225% normal saline [NS]). These are based on the daily electrolyte requirements in healthy children, who require approximately 2-4 mEq/kg of sodium and 1-2 mEq/kg of potassium. This translates to approximately D5 0.225% normal saline [or 0.45% NS] with 20 mEq/L of potassium chloride (KCl). This replacement fluid provides the required amount of sodium and potassium to keep these electrolytes within the normal range for patients without any significant additional losses or renal impairment. A solution with 0.45% saline or 0.9% normal saline is the preferred maintenance solution for the ill child. Evidence indicates that administration of isotonic fluids protects against acquired hyponatremia. The traditional Holliday-Segar method recommendation to use maintenance fluid therapy for sick and hospitalized children must be critically reexamined.

> *Pediatric patients have been shown to develop hyponatremia when given hypotonic fluids within the hospital setting. The use of isotonic fluids (D5NS, D5LR) in hospitalized patients is advocated to prevent the development of hyponatremia.*

Potassium in replacement IV fluids should be withheld until the patient has satisfactory urine output to avoid a risk of inducing hyperkalemia. The general practice of adding 20 mEq/L KCl to the IV fluid solution and a "one-size-fits-all" approach to KCl concentrations in IV fluids should be avoided. The amount of KCl in the IV fluid should be individualized to the patient as urine and stool output and other parameters can affect potassium requirements.

## B. Resuscitation Fluids

Resuscitation fluids in infants and children remain exclusively isotonic. Initial recommendations for treating hypovolemia include 20 mL/kg boluses of normal saline. Immediate reassessment and repeat boluses must be done quickly (up to 60 mL/kg in 30-60 minutes). Most resuscitation protocols suggest that initial fluid resuscitation should begin with crystalloid (normal saline or Ringer lactate). After 60 mL/kg of crystalloid has been administered, the use of colloid should be considered.

## C. Fluid Resuscitation in Shock

Hypovolemia remains the most common cause of shock worldwide due to gastroenteritis. Rapid restoration of intravascular volume with fluid replacement remains the key to survival. Patients with inadequate or delayed fluid resuscitation are at risk of developing organ dysfunction or progressing to irreversible shock. Regardless of the type of shock, some degree of hypovolemia is usually present and IV fluid therapy should always be considered in the initial resuscitative measures. Each bolus should be administered within 5-10 minutes or as rapidly as permitted by the vascular access. An exception to this is cardiogenic shock; these patients tend to be exquisitely sensitive to volume overload, and administration of 5-10 mL/kg of isotonic fluid must be done judiciously and ideally with central venous pressure monitoring.

Rapid IV or intraosseous access should be established to provide a means of delivering the fluid and medications required during resuscitation.

Utilizing the DIRECT algorithm (**Chapter 1**), reassessment of vital signs and clinical status must be conducted between boluses to evaluate for changes in clinical status and response to therapy.

# II. ELECTROLYTE ABNORMALITIES

Electrolyte abnormalities are common in children. Occasionally these abnormalities are due to iatrogenic causes. Severe electrolyte disturbances can present with poor feeding or irritability and can result in dehydration, shock, seizures, coma, or even death.

> *Serum osmolality can be measured in the laboratory and can also be calculated using the formula:*
> *(2 x sodium) + (glucose/18) + BUN/2.8 = serum osmolality.*
> *Normal serum osmolality range: 285-295 mOsm/L.*

## A. Sodium (Na+)

**1. Hyponatremia**

Hyponatremia is defined as a serum sodium level <135 mmol/L (<135 mEq/L). The sodium level can be decreased due to a variety of causes: increased water intake (dilute infant formula, polydipsia, infants drinking pool water), increased water retention (syndrome of inappropriate antidiuretic hormone [SIADH], renal failure), and increased sodium losses (gastroenteritis, diuretics, adrenal insufficiency).

Symptoms of hyponatremia include: irritability, poor feeding, nausea and vomiting, lethargy, seizures, and eventually coma and death. Hyponatremia may occur because of significant losses due to gastroenteritis, ostomy output, excessive sweating, cystic fibrosis, heatstroke, burns, or third spacing in pancreatitis or pleural effusions. Children on diuretics are frequently hyponatremic. Renal diseases such as renal tubular acidosis can cause loss of salt and water. In hospitalized children, excess secretion of antidiuretic hormone leads to the development of SIADH. Infants may present in the first few months of life with severe hyponatremia secondary to water intoxication from overly diluted formula or from swallowing large amounts of water in swimming or wading pools. Other causes include postobstructive uropathy and losses secondary to ventriculostomy drainage. Clinically, hyponatremia can be classified according to the patient's extracellular fluid volume status: hypovolemic, euvolemic, or hypervolemic (**Table 8-2**).

**Table 8-2  Classification of Hyponatremia According to Extracellular Fluid Volume Status**

| Euvolemia | Hypervolemia | Hypovolemia |
|---|---|---|
|  | SIADH |  |
| SIADH | Congestive Heart Failure | Diarrhea |
| Adrenal Insufficiency | Renal Failure (Acute/Chronic) | Vomiting |
| Central Nervous System Disease | Nephrotic Syndrome | Burns |
| Pulmonary Disease | Cirrhosis | Pancreatitis |

SIADH, syndrome of inappropriate antidiuretic hormone

Urgent treatment of hyponatremia should be initiated in all patients who exhibit neurological changes or seizures and if the serum sodium level is <120 mEq/L. Most frequently, 3% NaCl (513 mmol/L) is used, if available. Ideally, 3% saline should be given through a central venous line; administration through a peripheral IV or an intraosseous needle is acceptable during an emergency while awaiting placement of central venous access. The goal is to raise the serum sodium level to 120-125 mEq/L or until seizures stop. To raise the serum sodium level, administer the calculated amount of hypertonic saline over 15-20 minutes to gain rapid control of the seizures. A 1.2 mL/kg aliquot of 3% NaCl will raise the level by 1 mEq/L (0.6 mEq/kg will raise the serum sodium level by 1 mEq/L). If hypertonic saline solution is unavailable, a 20 mL/kg bolus of normal saline (0.9% NS) may be given.

Once the acute correction is completed or if the patient is not having neurological changes, correction of hyponatremia should proceed more slowly at approximately 12 mEq/L per day (0.5 to 1 mEq/L every hour). In adults, the syndrome of central pontine myelinolysis (osmotic demyelination) has been described in patients who had a rapid increase in serum sodium values.

> *It is important to correct clinically significant hyponatremia rapidly — but the total correction should be done slowly and carefully.*

The following formula is used to calculate the amount of sodium required to correct to a desired level (mEq/L):

$$0.6 \times (\text{weight in kg}) \times (\text{target Na}^+ - \text{measured Na}^+) = \text{total mEq of Na}^+ \text{ required to raise sodium level to target}$$

**Figure 8-1** illustrates how to use this formula in a clinical scenario. A good fluid to use to start replacement is either normal saline or D5NS, with or without appropriate potassium at maintenance fluid rates and with frequent electrolyte checks.

**Figure 8-1.** Sample Calculation for Determining the Amount of Sodium Required

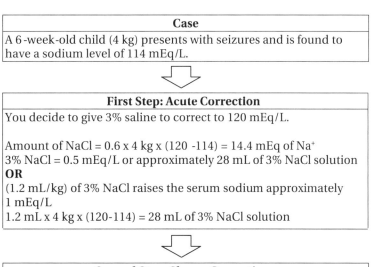

| Case |
|---|
| A 6-week-old child (4 kg) presents with seizures and is found to have a sodium level of 114 mEq/L. |

| First Step: Acute Correction |
|---|
| You decide to give 3% saline to correct to 120 mEq/L. |
| Amount of NaCl = 0.6 x 4 kg x (120 -114) = 14.4 mEq of Na$^+$ <br> 3% NaCl = 0.5 mEq/L or approximately 28 mL of 3% NaCl solution <br> **OR** <br> (1.2 mL/kg) of 3% NaCl raises the serum sodium approximately 1 mEq/L <br> 1.2 mL x 4 kg x (120-114) = 28 mL of 3% NaCl solution |

| Second Step: Slower Correction |
|---|
| You need to raise the serum sodium level an additional 12 mEq over the next 24 hours from the current 120 mEq/L. |
| 0.6 x 4 kg x (132 desired Na$^+$ − 120 actual Na$^+$) = 29 mEq/L of additional sodium needed over the next 24 hours |

### a. Syndrome of Inappropriate Antidiuretic Hormone

SIADH, by definition, is caused by an *inappropriate* release of antidiuretic hormone. When patients are hypertonic or significantly hypovolemic, there is an appropriate release of this hormone, with a resultant decrease in urine output in an effort to maximize the circulating intravascular volume. In patients with SIADH, the intravascular volume is normal or elevated and yet the urine output drops off. The diagnosis of SIADH requires three elements: low urine output, hyponatremia, and inappropriately concentrated urine (with elevated urinary sodium).

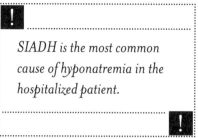

*SIADH is the most common cause of hyponatremia in the hospitalized patient.*

The causes of SIADH fall into four groups: central nervous system (CNS) abnormalities [e.g., infection, trauma, surgery, tumors, shunts, hypoxic-ischemic injury] (**Chapter 17**); pulmonary problems (e.g., pneumonia, effusions, positive pressure ventilation, asthma, tumors); drugs (e.g., carbamazepine, vinca alkaloids, narcotics, aspirin, Ecstasy, selective serotonin reuptake inhibitors); and tumors (e.g., leukemia, lymphoma, neuroblastoma).

The treatment for SIADH is water restriction. Reducing water intake to 50% of maintenance will often allow a free water diuresis and improve the serum sodium measurement. It is occasionally necessary to correct the sodium level with salt supplementation and diuretic administration.

### b. Hyponatremia Due to Water Intoxication

Water intoxication occurs when powdered infant formula is diluted with an excessive amount of water, either inadvertently (not following directions properly) or purposely (to make the formula last longer), resulting in hyponatremia. This is a common occurrence and also is seen when formula or an electrolyte solution is being diluted when an infant has gastroenteritis and diarrhea.

Infant swimming is another potential source of hyponatremia. It follows after ingestion of large amounts of water when the infant is playing in a bathtub, wading pool, or splash tub. The infant presents with irritability and poor appetite. A targeted history and check of the serum sodium level reveal the cause.

## 2. Hyponatremia and Hypovolemic States

### a. Non-renal

*Gastroenteritis.* Worldwide, gastroenteritis is the leading cause of death in children between 1 and 5 years of age. Typically the history is that of large and frequent watery stools, and the patient presents in various stages of dehydration and possibly hypovolemic shock. Depending on the severity of the hypovolemia, the patient might require aggressive and timely fluid resuscitation with isotonic fluids.

*Third Spacing.* Sepsis and peritonitis are examples of conditions where fluid can leak into the interstitial space. This can occur fairly rapidly over a matter of hours, leading to hypovolemia and hyponatremia because water and electrolytes move into the interstitial spaces. Patients present with clinical evidence of shock and hypovolemia. Serum electrolytes reveal hyponatremia, potentially hypokalemia and hypocalcemia.

*Fluid Losses.* Burns result in rapid and excessive loss of fluid due to capillary leak phenomenon. Fluid losses are both external (across the surface area involved in the burn) and internal (into the interstitial spaces). Rapid and ongoing fluid resuscitation is required in the management of burns and thermal injuries.

**b. Renal**

Diuretics can lead to hyponatremia with both short- and long-term use. Loop diuretics, such as furosemide and bumetanide, and drugs that interfere with renal tubular reabsorption, such as metolazone, can lead to significant hyponatremia. Other renal causes of hyponatremia are renal tubular acidosis, interstitial nephritis, and obstructive uropathy.

**c. Other Causes of Hyponatremia**

*Cerebral Salt Wasting (CSW).* This is a poorly understood condition in terms of exact pathophysiology. Hyponatremia occurs in the setting of normal to high urine output, and urinary sodium excretion is elevated. Patients tend to be hypovolemic and exhibit symptoms of dehydration and hyponatremia. The condition is seen in conjunction with intracranial injury, intracranial tumors, and neurosurgical procedures. It is important to distinguish CSW from SIADH, which also presents with hyponatremia but without the hypovolemia seen in CSW. Treatment of SIADH includes fluid restriction, whereas fluid and electrolyte replacement for the correction of hyponatremia is the therapeutic approach in CSW. Urinary sodium also tends to be higher in CSW (may be >100mEq/L) than in SIADH.

*Increased Total Body Sodium Associated with Serum Hyponatremia.* Congestive heart failure and nephrotic syndrome are both examples of hypervolemic conditions associated with hyponatremia despite an increase in total body sodium content. The hyponatremia is dilutional in these cases, and sodium intake restrictions are an important part of management. Treatment is directed toward the underlying condition: diuretics and inotropes for the heart failure, steroids and diuretics in nephrotic syndrome, and dialysis in renal failure.

**3. Hypernatremia**

Hypernatremia is defined as a serum sodium >145 mEq/L. At-risk groups for elevated sodium are infants, toddlers, and critically ill patients. Hypernatremia occurs when too much salt is ingested or too much free water is lost. Children who develop hypernatremia may have received concentrated formula, been breast-fed without supplementation, or been treated with salt supplements or sodium bicarbonate. Free water loss can be due to diarrhea, diabetes insipidus (central or nephrogenic), renal tubular disorders, or postobstructive diuresis.

Signs and symptoms of hypernatremia include irritability, high-pitched cry, lethargy, seizures, fever, renal failure, and rhabdomyolysis. In infants, these symptoms mimic those of infections and sepsis.

It is essential that hypernatremia be corrected gradually with frequent monitoring of electrolytes. When the sodium rises, the serum osmolality increases, and fluid moves from inside the cells to the serum in an attempt to achieve balance. This increases the osmolality inside the cell. Rapid administration of free water results in movement from low osmolality (i.e., serum) to higher osmolality (i.e., inside the cell), causing the cell to swell. This can result in cerebral edema.

It is essential to correct hypernatremia slowly. Most recommendations are to lower serum sodium values no more than 0.5 mEq/L/h or 12 mEq/L/day.

The formula for calculating the amount of free water necessary to correct the serum sodium is:

Free water deficit = (wt in kg x 0.6) x
[1 − (desired Na⁺/actual Na⁺)](1000 mL/L)

**Table 8-3** applies this formula in a clinical scenario. Frequent measurement of the serum sodium is necessary to follow the gradual fall of the sodium level and make appropriate fluid changes.

> - *1 L of 0.45% normal saline = 500 mL of free water*
> - *1 L of 0.225% normal saline = 750 mL of free water*
> - *1 L of D5 0.45% normal saline will provide 400 mL of free water and is a good starting point*

**Table 8-3.** Sample Calculation for Determining Amount of Free Water Necessary to Correct Serum Sodium

Case: A 10-month-old infant weighing 8 kg has serum sodium level of 157 mEq/L.

Free water deficit = (8 x 0.6) x [1 − (145/157)] x (1000 mL/L)
365 mL = 4.8 x 0.076(1000 mL/L)

Quick calculation: 4 mL x 8 kg x 12 mEq/L = 384 mL of free water

Maintenance fluid amounts for an 8-kg child: (100 mL/kg x 8) = 800 mL/24 h.

### a. Hypernatremia Due to Diabetes Insipidus

Diabetes insipidus (DI) is an uncommon condition that results in severe hypernatremia and excessive free water loss. It has either a CNS or nephrogenic (inherited or acquired) etiology. The diagnosis in the acute case is made by observing polyuria, a urine specific gravity <1.005, urine osmolality of <200 mOsm/L, serum hypernatremia, and hyperosmolality (serum osmolality of ≥295 mOsm/L).

> *4 mL/kg of free water will drop the sodium by 1 mEq/L*

The most common causes in the acute setting are CNS injuries, including severe head trauma and tumors (craniopharyngiomas). Elevated intracranial pressure can cause DI, and it is commonly seen in association with brain death. Nephrogenic DI is relatively rare, usually presents in a less acute setting, and is most commonly due to a hereditary defect. Treatment of DI consists of replacement of free water and administration of intranasal or IV desmopressin or vasopressin with strict monitoring of fluid balance and electrolytes.

## B. Potassium ($K^+$)

Potassium, the most abundant cation in intracellular fluid, is involved in many cellular processes, including protein synthesis. Maintenance of a transmembrane potential results in an electrical gradient across cell membranes. Changes in this resting membrane potential result in muscle excitation and nerve conduction. In particular, potassium plays a key role in myocardial contractility and function.

Potassium levels in the body are tightly regulated by renal excretion – the main mechanism being distal tubular secretion; however, patients might develop hyperkalemia due to a combination of renal dysfunction and increased potassium release from injured tissue.

### 1. Hypokalemia

Hypokalemia, defined as a potassium level <3.5 mEq/L, may occur due to inadequate intake, renal losses, and gastrointestinal losses, following insulin therapy and in association with metabolic alkalosis. Diuretics (especially furosemide and bumetanide), hyperventilation, mannitol, β-agonists (e.g., frequent use of inhaled bronchodilators), and amphotericin B can cause hypokalemia. Gastrointestinal losses via continuous nasogastric suctioning or diarrhea can also result in a significant drop in serum potassium levels.

Signs and symptoms include fatigue and paresthesias. Electrocardiogram (ECG) changes, including U waves and ventricular dysrhythmias (**Figure 8-2**), can occur when the potassium level drops below 2.5 mEq/L. Treatment of hypokalemia may include oral or IV supplementation, depending on the patient's status and the urgency of symptoms.

If the patient is receiving enteral feedings, the safest approach to correcting asymptomatic hypokalemia (no ECG changes) would be the gradual replacement of potassium by adding it to the dietary intake. Supplements of 1-3 mEq/kg/day can be administered enterally in three or four divided doses to correct hypokalemia or to prevent it in patients who are on diuretics without potassium-sparing properties. Potassium chloride can be an irritant to the gastric mucosa, might not be well tolerated, and may result in diarrhea.

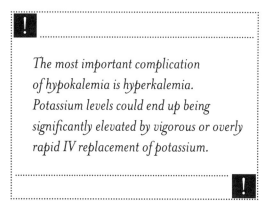

*The most important complication of hypokalemia is hyperkalemia. Potassium levels could end up being significantly elevated by vigorous or overly rapid IV replacement of potassium.*

**Figure 8-2.** Illustrated Electrocardiographic Alterations with Hypo- and Hyperkalemia

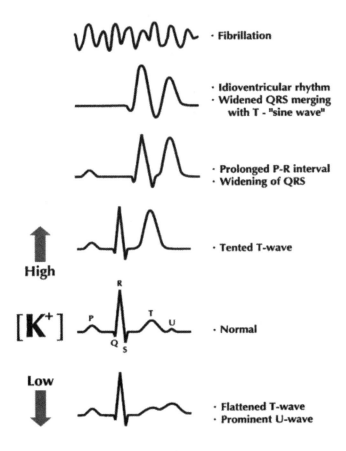

Reproduced with permission. © 2002 Elsevier. Gennari FJ. Disorders of potassium homeostasis: Hypokalemia and hyperkalemia. *Crit Care Clin.* 2002;18:273-288.

A conservative protocol for IV replacement follows:

- For K⁺ levels of 3.0-3.5 mEq/L, administer 0.25 mEq/kg IV KCl over 1 hour.

- For K⁺ levels of 2.5-3.0 mEq/L, administer 0.5 mEq/kg IV KCl over 2 hours.

- For K⁺ levels <2.5 mEq/L, administer 0.75 mEq/L IV KCl over 3 hours. A potassium level should be checked halfway through this infusion.

- A conservative and safe approach is to administer KCl in a single IV replacement dose of no more than 0.5 mEq/kg/h, with a maximum dose of 10 mEq over 1 hour. These recommendations are considerably more stringent than those employed in the care of adults.

- KCl infusion is recommended to be administered via a central venous line or a large bore IV with adequate solution dilution and ECG monitoring whenever possible.

## 2. Hyperkalemia

Hyperkalemia, or potassium levels >5.5 mEq/L, requires urgent confirmation and rapid institution of therapy to lower the levels, especially if ECG changes are present. Since renal clearance of excess potassium is fairly efficient, hyperkalemia is unusual in the setting of adequate renal function. The condition can occur as a result of renal failure (acute or chronic), hypoaldosteronism, adrenal insufficiency, metabolic acidosis, muscle and tissue necrosis (rhabdomyolysis, burns, crush injuries), tumor lysis syndrome (**Chapter 17**), and excessive intake or administration of potassium. Acidosis plays a role as well, increasing potassium levels by 0.5 mEq/L for every 0.1 decrease in the pH. Medications such as potassium-sparing diuretics (spironolactone), angiotensin-converting enzyme inhibitors, and digoxin can also lead to hyperkalemia, especially in the setting of concomitant renal dysfunction. Hemolysis from heel-stick blood sampling or tourniquet application is a common cause of false elevation of potassium levels. However, it should not be assumed that this is the cause without demonstrating normal potassium on a repeated free-flowing sample without hemolysis.

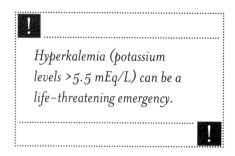

*Hyperkalemia (potassium levels >5.5 mEq/L) can be a life-threatening emergency.*

Signs and symptoms of hyperkalemia are usually related to inadequate cardiac output due to arrhythmias. ECG changes include tall, peaked T waves, widening of the QRS complex, atrioventricular block, bradycardia, and eventually ventricular tachycardia or asystole (**Figure 8-2**). Weakness and paresthesias can occur when K+ levels are >7 mEq/L.

Symptomatic hyperkalemia requires urgent intervention and therapy:

- Place the patient on a cardiorespiratory monitor with a rhythm strip and obtain a 12-lead ECG.

- Recheck the electrolytes to confirm the hyperkalemia.

- Discontinue any exogenous potassium being administered.

- Administer one or more of the following therapies:
    - Calcium gluconate: 100 mg/kg given IV over 3 minutes (1 mL/kg of 10% solution) to stabilize the myocardium and prevent arrhythmias.
    - Sodium bicarbonate: 1-2 mEq/kg given IV over 10-15 minutes. Ensure the adequacy of ventilation prior to administration. Since calcium and bicarbonate will precipitate, the line must be flushed clear between these two medications.
    - Insulin-glucose infusion to move potassium intracellularly: insulin 0.1 U/kg/h, mixed with D25% solution equivalent to 0.5 g/kg/h (2 mL/kg/h). The first hour's dose can even be administered rapidly (over 30 minutes) prior to initiating the continuous infusion. Glucose levels should be followed hourly for the duration of this infusion.
    - Albuterol by multiple-dose inhaler or nebulizer in conjunction with one or more of the above therapies. This tends to not be a very strong therapy and may not make significant changes in the potassium level, which is why it must be administered in conjunction with other therapies.

- An exchange resin, such as sodium polystyrene resin, administered 1 g/kg rectally. If the patient's hemodynamics and airway are stable, it can be administered orally or by nasogastric tube at the same dose (1g/kg) every 6 hours. The rectal route has a more rapid effect, whereas the oral/nasogastric route has a more gradual onset and a more sustained effect. This agent exchanges sodium for potassium along the gastrointestinal tract in an approximate ratio of 1 g/kg resin to 1 mEq/L decrease in $K^+$ level. Sodium levels should be monitored if more than one dose of this agent is used due to the potential for hypernatremia.

- Emergency hemodialysis should be initiated in addition to the previous steps if the hyperkalemia is life-threatening and immediate correction is desired. Because it takes time to initiate this, particularly if a large-bore indwelling line is required, all other modalities mentioned should be instituted while awaiting initiation of hemodialysis.

## C. Magnesium ($Mg^+$)

Magnesium is a cofactor for adenosine triphosphate-related functions, such as oxidative phosphorylation, protein synthesis, and DNA transcription. It is abundant in most diets and daily intake is usually adequate. Intracellular magnesium is responsible for most of the physiologic functions requiring adenosine triphosphate and magnesium. Normal plasma levels are 1.6 to 2.4 mg/dL (0.66-0.97 mmol/L).

**1. Hypomagnesemia**

Hypomagnesemia (<2 mg/dL) occurs fairly frequently (20%-50%) in intensive care unit patients, likely because of inadequate or absent dietary intake combined with increased gastrointestinal and renal losses. Pancreatitis can result in hypomagnesemia and concomitant hypocalcemia as well. Patients with renal dysfunction are less likely to develop hypomagnesemia as they have limited ability to excrete magnesium in the urine.

Hypomagnesemia is most commonly associated with hypocalcemia and may result in the clinical features of hypocalcemia, such as neuromuscular weakness, muscle wasting, ECG changes (increased PR interval, QT prolongation, and flat T waves). Hypokalemia is also associated with hypomagnesemia, and correcting the magnesium levels might help in the management of persistent hypokalemia. Laryngospasm and seizures may also be seen in severe cases.

Causes of hypomagnesemia include:

- Nothing by mouth status and lack of IV supplementation

- Malabsorption due to familial hypomagnesemia, laxative use, short bowel syndrome

- Increased renal losses secondary to diuretic use, amphotericin B, chemotherapy, aminoglycosides, intrinsic renal disease (acute tubular necrosis)

Treatment of hypomagnesemia is accomplished with slow infusions of magnesium sulfate 25-50 mg/kg over 3-4 hours. Above a serum level of 2 mg/dL (0.82 mmol/L), the kidneys will waste the rest, so no additional benefit is gained from rapid IV replacement.

## 2. Hypermagnesemia

The kidneys usually clear excess magnesium, and hence hypermagnesemia is rarely encountered except in cases of renal dysfunction. Symptomatic hypermagnesemia is seen once levels are >5 mg/dL (>2.05 mmol/L).

Signs and symptoms include nausea, vomiting, decreased tendon reflexes, and neuromuscular blockade. Cardiovascular effects include bradycardia, myocardial depression, and ECG changes, including prolonged PR interval and atrioventricular block. Neonates may present with hypotonia and apnea.

Treatment consists of administering calcium gluconate, 50-100 mg/kg IV, followed by restriction of further intake and diuresis.

# D. Calcium ($Ca^+$)

Calcium is a divalent cation, 99% of which is found in the skeleton; the remaining 1% is widely distributed throughout the body. Dietary sources of calcium include dairy products, green, leafy vegetables, and seafood with bones. Calcium is essential for teeth, bone mineralization, and muscle activity, especially myocardial excitation-contraction coupling. It also plays a pivotal role in the coagulation cascade. Recent data also suggest a role in cellular mechanisms of injury and necrosis. Excessive use of calcium during resuscitation and post-resuscitation stabilization might be detrimental to the myocardium and other tissues (**Chapter 3**).

Since almost 50% of total calcium is in the active, ionized form and most of the remaining calcium is bound to albumin and inactive, ionized calcium levels should be evaluated wherever available. Levels are closely regulated by interplay between parathyroid hormone, vitamin D, calcitonin, and renal excretion.

## 1. Hypocalcemia

Hypocalcemia is defined as total calcium <2.12 mmol/L (<8.5 mg/dL) or ionized calcium <1 mmol/L. Typically, calcium deficits occur as a result of low dietary intake and/or a lack of vitamin D or parathyroid hormone. The presentation of hypocalcemia is usually part of a more profound protein-calorie malnutrition but can occur as a stand-alone deficiency. It can occur as part of pancreatitis, but this is less common in pediatrics. The most common cause of hypocalcemia in infancy is due to congenital deficiencies of parathyroid hormone, as seen in conditions such as DiGeorge syndrome.

Hypocalcemia is a common occurrence in critically ill patients, many of whom also tend to be hypoalbuminemic. It is more relevant to measure the ionized calcium levels rather than relying solely on total calcium.

Tetany, irritability, hyper-reflexia, weakness and paresthesias, muscle fatigue, stridor, and laryngospasm are all common neuromuscular manifestations of hypocalcemia. Cardiovascular effects include hypotension, bradycardia, and arrhythmias.

### a. Neonate/Infant

Calcium levels in a term neonate drop after the first 24 hours and are then maintained by the regulatory hormones. Neonatal hypocalcemia can be encountered in association with maternal diabetes mellitus, toxemia of pregnancy, and maternal hyperparathyroidism. It can present with irritability, tetany, or seizures.

Neonates with DiGeorge syndrome (developmental anomaly of third and fourth pharyngeal pouches) can present with symptomatic hypocalcemia. These patients might exhibit lesions such as mandibular hypoplasia, hypoparathyroidism, T-lymphocyte deficiency (thymic dysfunction), and congenital heart disease (atrial septal defect, ventricular septal defect, aortic arch anomalies, pulmonic stenosis, and truncus arteriosus).

Hypocalcemia can also occur in neonates as a result of hypomagnesemia. Correction of the hypomagnesemia may also be necessary to correct the low calcium.

### b. Child

Hypocalcemia in the older child is usually a result of a disruption of one or more of the regulatory mechanisms controlling calcium levels. Hypoparathyroidism, vitamin D deficiency, inadequate dietary intake, and renal losses are common conditions resulting in hypocalcemia, but it may also be seen in any critically ill or injured child.

Aggressive calcium supplementation is reserved for symptomatic and documented hypocalcemia. It is important to evaluate renal function and check other electrolytes, particularly magnesium levels, in the evaluation and management of hypocalcemia. More detailed evaluation for the cause of hypocalcemia requires tests of parathyroid function, renal function (phosphate levels), and levels of vitamin D metabolites (25-hydroxyvitamin D and 1,25-dihydroxyvitamin D).

### c. Treatment

Therapy with IV calcium should ideally be administered through large-bore or central venous lines since calcium extravasation can result in a chemical burn with consequent tissue necrosis. Do not administer via scalp veins, intramuscularly, or subcutaneously.

Indications for IV calcium administration include hypocalcemia (low ionized calcium levels <1 mmol/L [<4 mg/dL]), hyperkalemia, calcium channel blocker overdose, hypermagnesemia, and post-arrest stabilization if there is laboratory evidence of hypocalcemia.

*Calcium Chloride.* This is the most readily bioavailable form of calcium. A 10% solution contains 1.36 mEq/mL of ionized calcium. It is administered in a dose of 10-20 mg/kg IV over 5-10 minutes through a central venous line. Rapid administration can result in bradycardia and hypotension.

*Calcium Gluconate.* This is the preferred calcium salt in neonates and may be administered orally or intravenously in the older infant and child. A 10% solution of calcium gluconate contains 0.45 mEq/mL of ionized calcium. The dosage is 50-200 mg/kg IV over 5-10 minutes for neonates and 50-125 mg/kg IV over 5-10 minutes in infants and children.

## 2. Hypercalcemia

Hypercalcemia, defined as a total calcium level >11 mg/dL (>2.75 mmol/L) or ionized calcium level >1.3 mmol/L, results from calcium release from bone. It can be seen following prolonged immobility, hyperparathyroidism, malignancies, excessive intake of vitamin A or D, and granulomatous disease.

Though relatively rare in pediatric patients, hypercalcemia can present with signs and symptoms that might lead to a wrong diagnosis. Due to the presence of hypertension and decreased level of consciousness, a patient with hypercalcemia could be mistaken for one with impending intracranial herniation. Other signs and symptoms are seen as cardiovascular and neuromuscular effects and include hypertension, shortened QT interval, irritability, lethargy, seizures, coma, nausea, vomiting, and abdominal pain.

The primary source of the hypercalcemia needs to be addressed and therapy directed specifically at lowering serum calcium levels. Acute hypercalcemia with total calcium levels >15 mg/dL requires aggressive attempts at lowering the levels.

Hydration with IV isotonic saline at 200-250 mL/kg/day in conjunction with furosemide-induced diuresis (1 mg/kg IV every 6 hours) provides a rapid response by increasing renal calcium excretion (calciuresis). Close monitoring of electrolytes, including phosphorus and magnesium, should be performed during diuresis.

Recombinant calcitonin has a rapid onset of action, acts by blocking bone resorption, and promotes calciuria. The dose of calcitonin is 10 U/kg IV, and it can be repeated every 4 to 6 hours. Mithramycin, aspirin, and indomethacin are alternative therapies that can be used to treat hypercalcemia. Glucocorticoids can reduce calcium absorption from the gastrointestinal tract. Hydrocortisone, 1 mg/kg every 6 hours, is effective in curtailing calcium absorption but is less useful in acute hypercalcemia.

# E. Phosphate ($PO_4$)

Phosphorus is present in adequate quantities in a regular diet. In the body, it is present as phosphate salts and is closely associated with calcium intake. Phosphate levels are closely regulated by renal functions of filtration and proximal renal tubular reabsorption.

The main effects of phosphate occur in membrane phospholipids, bone, adenosine triphosphate, and 2,3-diphosphoglycerate. These four systems alone make phosphate homeostasis critical to many basic functions in the body.

## 1. Hypophosphatemia

Decreased intake and excessive excretion of phosphorus occur classically in diabetic ketoacidosis. Insulin therapy further reduces phosphate levels by driving it into the cells. Renal dysfunction, such as acute tubular necrosis, renal tubular acidosis, Wilson disease, hypokalemia, and hyperparathyroidism all can lead to hypophosphatemia. Patients receiving IV fluids alone (without phosphorus supplementation), those ingesting aluminum-containing antacids, and the critically ill can become hypophosphatemic.

Signs and symptoms of hypophosphatemia in the acute setting include muscle weakness, hypoventilation, myocardial dysfunction, seizures, and coma. Treatment consists of the addition of phosphate (as sodium and potassium salts) to the IV fluids when serum phosphorus levels are below 1 mg/dL (0.323 mmol/L). Sodium phosphate contains 3 mmol (94 mg) $PO_4$ and 4 mEq/mL sodium; potassium phosphate contains 3 mmol (94 mg) $PO_4$ and 4.4 mEq/mL potassium. Replacement is given at 0.16-0.32 mmol/kg IV over 4-6 hours, and either salt can be used. If renal dysfunction coexists and potassium phosphate is used, potassium levels need to be monitored closely. Also, phosphate infusions or supplements should not be administered in the presence of hypercalcemia.

### 2. Hyperphosphatemia

Excessive intake (rare) and reduced excretion, such as in renal failure, hypoparathyroidism, and pseudohypoparathyroidism, may all result in hyperphosphatemia, as may tumor lysis syndrome and rhabdomyolysis. A hemolyzed blood sample can result in an erroneous level indicating hyperphosphatemia.

The main effect of hyperphosphatemia is the occurrence of hypocalcemia due to chelation when the total calcium measurement is multiplied by the inorganic phosphorus product >60 mg/dL. Treatment includes aluminum hydroxide antacids enterally and rehydration with isotonic fluids. Hypocalcemia should be treated aggressively as well.

# III. METABOLIC DISEASE

## A. Glucose

Glucose is essential for tissue metabolism, and its levels are maintained within a tight range by the actions of insulin. Disorders of glucose metabolism can lead to hypoglycemia and hyperglycemia with fairly significant clinical consequences.

### 1. Hypoglycemia

Hypoglycemia is defined as a serum glucose level <40 mg/dL (<2.2 mmol/L). Weakness, sweating, tachycardia, tremors, and eventually seizures might develop with hypoglycemia. The CNS symptoms are particularly evident because the brain is dependent on a steady source of glucose for neural activity. Symptoms are varied, particularly in the neonate.

Hyperinsulinism, inborn errors of metabolism, endocrine disorders (including adrenal and pituitary dysfunction), ketotic hypoglycemia, and drugs/toxins – including exogenous administration of insulin – are the broad categories of conditions leading to hypoglycemia. An extensive endocrine and metabolic workup is necessary to establish the diagnosis. Propranolol and other β-blockers might mask the symptoms (tachycardia, sweating) of hypoglycemia.

Laboratory tests, including cortisol, insulin, growth hormone, urine ketones, serum chemistry, and liver function tests, should be obtained during the hypoglycemic episode if possible.

Once hypoglycemia has been confirmed, immediate treatment with IV glucose should be initiated. Administration of 2-4 mL/kg of 25% dextrose IV will provide 0.5-1 g/kg of glucose. This solution can be diluted 1:1 so that a 12.5% solution is injected into a peripheral vein or intraosseously. Because dextrose is fairly hyperosmolar, neonates should not be given more than 12.5% dextrose. A bolus of 10 mL/kg of D5% will provide 0.5 g/kg of glucose.

### 2. Hyperglycemia

A blood glucose level >150 mg/dL is considered hyperglycemia. This condition is not unusual in the critically ill child. It is the result of a stress response and the presence of high levels of circulating epinephrine and other anti-insulin stress hormones. Glucose levels should be monitored in the post-resuscitation stabilization period.

## B. Diabetic Ketoacidosis (DKA)

Diabetic ketoacidosis (DKA), a diagnosis sometimes missed, can lead to cerebral edema with catastrophic neurologic outcomes. A newly diagnosed diabetic child (approximately 30% present in DKA) or a known insulin-dependent diabetic patient can present with this condition and require prompt attention to fluid management and correction of the acidosis.

An intercurrent illness might trigger the episode of DKA. Patients present with headaches, emesis, abdominal pain, lethargy, and clinical signs of dehydration. There may be a history of weight loss, polydipsia, and polyuria. The abdominal pain and emesis might lead to a mistaken diagnosis of an intra-abdominal process or "surgical abdomen." If the dehydration is severe, evidence of hypovolemic shock may be seen at presentation. The classic clinical signs of rapid/Kussmaul respirations have been mistaken for asthma and respiratory distress. The presence of a fruity (ketotic) odor is helpful in making the diagnosis.

### 1. Initial Stabilization

Once initial laboratory studies confirm the diagnosis, the mainstay of therapy is the administration of insulin by continuous infusion and correction of the dehydration. If the history is suggestive of an infection as the trigger, this should be investigated and appropriately treated.

An initial fluid bolus of 20 mL/kg of normal saline is administered, with an additional bolus given if the patient is hemodynamically unstable as a result of the dehydration. Only isotonic fluid should be administered during this initial fluid resuscitation phase. Lactated Ringer solution should be avoided if renal function is significantly impaired.

An insulin infusion **without a bolus** of IV insulin should be initiated at 0.05-0.1 U/kg/h. Subsequent IV fluids can be initiated using normal saline with 20 mEq/L of potassium chloride and 20 mEq/L of potassium phosphate (as long as urine output is adequate) at 1.5 to 2 times maintenance, for a total amount not to exceed 3,500 mL/m$^2$/day. Dextrose solution (D10% NS with potassium chloride and potassium phosphate) can be added once the blood glucose level is below 300 mg/dL.

Blood glucose levels should be brought down by no more than 100 mg/dL (5.5 mmol/L) every hour. A more rapid decline might require the addition of dextrose to the IV fluid sooner, even if the serum level remains elevated above 300 mg/dL. Since insulin is responsible for correction of the acidosis, the insulin infusion should be maintained while adjusting the dextrose solution as required to effect an appropriate adjustment in blood glucose level.

Hourly monitoring of blood glucose, blood gases (every 2-4 hours), and frequent monitoring of electrolytes – including sodium, potassium, calcium, magnesium, and phosphate, as well as cardiovascular ECG monitoring – should be performed.

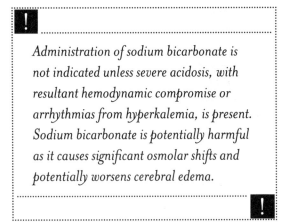

*Administration of sodium bicarbonate is not indicated unless severe acidosis, with resultant hemodynamic compromise or arrhythmias from hyperkalemia, is present. Sodium bicarbonate is potentially harmful as it causes significant osmolar shifts and potentially worsens cerebral edema.*

### 2. Cerebral Edema

Most patients in DKA might already have some degree of cerebral edema at presentation. The main risk factors for the progression are administration of large quantities of hypotonic fluids, rapid hourly declines in blood glucose levels, and hyponatremia. The latter commonly occurs in DKA and is also a result of the hyperglycemia and hypertriglyceridemia (pseudohyponatremia).

$$Na^+ \text{ corrected} = Na^+ \text{ observed} + [(\text{glucose in mg/dL} - 100/100) \times 1.6]$$

If both hyperglycemia and hypertriglyceridemia are fully corrected, the sodium level can be predicted using the following formula:

$$\{\text{Reported sodium (mEq/L)}\} \{0.021[\text{triglycerides (g/dL)} + 0.994] + 0.016 [\text{glucose (mg/dL)}]\}$$

## C. Adrenal Insufficiency

### 1. Primary Adrenal Insufficiency

Congenital adrenal hyperplasia is often seen in the first 2-3 weeks of life, presenting as shock with associated hyponatremia, hypoglycemia, and hyperkalemia. It is characterized by a group of disorders that affect mineralocorticoids and glucocorticoid production due to enzymatic deficiency in the pathways leading to the synthesis of cortisol from cholesterol. The high levels of corticotropin lead to hyperplasia of the adrenal glands. Typically, neonates with or without ambiguous genitalia will present in shock out of proportion to the duration of symptoms. They have elevated levels of steroid metabolites. Partial enzyme deficiencies may also occur and require a corticotropin stimulation test to make the diagnosis.

### 2. Tertiary Adrenal Insufficiency

This is the most common form of adrenal insufficiency presenting in the pediatric intensive care unit. Patients present with a history of weakness, emesis, abdominal pain, and fever. Tertiary adrenal insufficiency may occur because the patient is on long-term steroid therapy (such as for asthma), resulting in the suppression of the hypothalamic-pituitary-adrenal axis. An intercurrent illness might result in the patient presenting in shock out of proportion to the duration or severity of symptoms. Adrenal insufficiency should be suspected in the presence of hypoglycemia, hyponatremia, hyperkalemia, and metabolic acidosis together with azotemia. The presence of a random cortisol level of <5 μg/dL (137 mmol/L) in a stressed, critically ill patient is highly suggestive of adrenal suppression or insufficiency. Both the corticotropin and cortisol levels are low in tertiary adrenal insufficiency.

Increasingly, adrenal insufficiency is being diagnosed early in a variety of critically ill children. It should be considered in any infant or child who remains hypotensive despite adequate volume resuscitation and initiation of appropriate vasoactive agents (catecholamine-resistant shock). A random cortisol level should be obtained, and an initial dose of 2 mg/kg IV hydrocortisone may be administered and can be continued at 1 mg/kg every 6 hours if the cortisol level in a profoundly stressed patient remains below 25 µg/dL.

Alternative dosing regimens include: 0.2 mg/kg dexamethasone IV every 6 hours; or 1 mg/kg methylprednisolone IV every 6 hours. Treatment of dehydration and hypoglycemia includes adequate fluid resuscitation with normal saline boluses and the correction of hypoglycemia.

## Key Points

## Fluids, Electrolytes, and Neuroendocrine Metabolic Derangements

- Important conditions affecting sodium balance:
    - Syndrome of inappropriate antidiuretic hormone (SIADH): Low urine output, hyponatremia, and concentrated urine with high urinary $Na^+$ >30 mmol/L
    - Cerebral salt wasting: Normal to high urine output, hypovolemia, and even higher urinary $Na^+$ >100 mmol/L
    - Diabetes insipidus: High urine output, hypovolemia, hypernatremia, and dilute urine

- Acute adrenal insufficiency: Occurs in congenital adrenal hyperplasia (neonates) or as a tertiary condition in patients with long-term steroid use. Presents with hypovolemia (shock), hypoglycemia, hyponatremia, hyperkalemia, and azotemia.

- Symptomatic hyponatremia (hyponatremic seizures): Address the ABCs, then correct $Na^+$ level with IV 3% saline over 15-20 minutes. Once seizures are under control, continue to correct $Na^+$ slowly.

- In a neonate with hyponatremia, hyperkalemia, hypoglycemia, and acidosis, a diagnosis of congenital adrenal hyperplasia must be considered and immediate management started.

- Sodium should be corrected slowly (0.5-1.0 mEq/L change per hour). Too rapid of a drop can lead to cerebral edema, and too rapid of an increase can lead to central pontine myelinolysis.

- Hyperkalemia with associated electrocardiogram changes requires immediate therapy.

- Avoid hypotonic maintenance IV fluids in pediatric patients, especially those at risk of SIADH.

- Potassium in IV fluids should be adjusted to the real needs of patient urine output and potassium levels. Avoid tendency to use 20 mEq/L of potassium chloride as a "standard" additive in IV fluids in all patients.

- With significant hypovolemia, ideally give >40 mL/kg in first hour of fluid resuscitation. Rapid IV fluid resuscitation with isotonic fluid (normal saline or Ringer lactate) should be accomplished with frequent reassessment of clinical status.

- In the management of diabetic ketoacidosis (DKA), do not drop blood glucose levels by >100 mg/dL/h.

- Do not use an initial IV bolus of insulin in the treatment of DKA.

- Do not use sodium bicarbonate to correct the metabolic acidosis in DKA patients.

## Suggested Readings

1. Arora SK. Hypernatremic disorders in the intensive care unit. *J Intensive Care Med.* 2011. 2013;28:37-45.

2. Banasiak KJ, Carpenter TO. Disorders of calcium, magnesium, and phosphate. In: Nichols DG, ed. *Roger's Textbook of Pediatric Intensive Care. 4th ed.* Philadelphia, PA: Williams & Wilkins; 2008:1635-1648.

3. Brierley J, Carcillo JA, Choong K, et al. Clinical practice parameters for hemodynamic support of pediatric and neonatal septic shock: 2007 update from the American College of Critical Care Medicine. *Crit Care Med.* 2009;37:666-688.

4. Gennari FJ. Disorders of potassium homeostasis. Hypokalemia and hyperkalemia. *Crit Care Clin.* 2002;18:273-288.

5. Holliday MA, Segar WE. The maintenance need for water in parenteral fluid therapy. *Pediatrics.* 1957;19:823-832.

6. Kelly A, Moshang JR. Disorders of water, sodium, and potassium homeostasis. In: Nichols DG, ed. *Roger's Textbook of Pediatric Intensive Care. 4th ed.* Philadelphia, PA: Williams & Wilkins; 2008:1615-1634.

7. Mekitarian Filho E, Carvalho WB, Troster EJ. Hyperglycemia, morbidity and mortality in critically ill children: critical analysis based on a systematic review. *Rev Assoc Med Bras.* 2009;55:475-483.

8. Moritz ML, Ayus JC. Maintenance intravenous fluids with 0.9% sodium chloride do not produce hypernatremia in children. *Acta Paediatr.* 2012;101:222-223.

9. Neville KA, Sandeman DJ, Rubinstein A, Henry GM, McGlynn M, Walker JL. Prevention of hyponatremia during maintenance intravenous fluid administration: a prospective randomized study of fluid type versus fluid rate. *J Pediatr.* 2010;156:313-319.e1-2.

10. Reddy P. Clinical approach to adrenal insufficiency in hospitalized patients. *Int J Clin Pract.* 2011;65:1059-1066.

11. Rosenbloom AL. The management of diabetic ketoacidosis in children. *Diabetes Ther.* 2010;1:103-120.

12. Santana e Meneses JF, Leite HP, de Carvalho WB, Lopes E Jr. Hypophosphatemia in critically ill children: Prevalence and associated risk factors. *Pediatr Crit Care Med.* 2009;10:234-238.

13. Thomas CP, Fraer M. Syndrome of inappropriate antidiuretic hormone secretion. Available at: http://emedicine.medscape.com/article/924829-overview. Accessed March 15, 2013.

14. Yee AH, Burns JD, Wijdicks EF. Cerebral salt wasting: pathophysiology, diagnosis, and treatment. *Neurosurg Clin N Am.* 2010;21:339-352.

# Chapter 9

# TRAUMATIC INJURIES IN CHILDREN

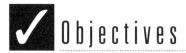 Objectives

- Rank priorities for the management of the injured child.
- Employ life-saving therapies in the injured child.
- Describe how children's patterns of injury differ from those of adults.

## I. INTRODUCTION

Trauma remains the leading cause of morbidity and mortality in children and adolescents, whose injury mechanisms and patterns can differ significantly from those of adults. Accidental and nonaccidental injuries account for a significant proportion of emergency department visits and the use of healthcare resources.

## II. THE PRIMARY SURVEY

The evaluation of an injured child begins with the primary survey, which is conducted in a systematic manner. The primary survey, recalled by the mnemonic *ABCDE*, involves evaluation and management of the airway (with spinal motion restriction), followed by assessment of breathing (with recognition and management of tension and open pneumothorax), circulation (with external hemorrhage control and intravenous fluid administration), disability (neurologic) status (with recognition of conditions requiring early neurosurgical intervention), and exposure (undressing and examining the patient while maintaining body temperature). The primary survey is designed to identify those physiologic and anatomic abnormalities that are immediately life threatening. Unless these are recognized early and corrective measures are taken, the patient may deteriorate and die in a very short time.

The paradigm of the primary survey is to assess and treat. Each life-threatening condition identified is treated before moving on to the next stage. For example, if the airway requires suctioning, this is done before assessing breathing, while if oxygen is needed, it is started before checking the circulation. Of course, with multiple providers, one provider can provide the treatment while the other continues the assessment.

It is important to restrict motion of the cervical, thoracic, and lumbar spine prior to moving a child after a traumatic event. Typically, the patient is placed in a semi-rigid extrication collar and on a long spine board at the location of the event. Prior to placement of the collar, in-line, bimanual, spinal motion restriction should be assured. If a collar is not placed at the scene, one should be applied as soon as possible. A 1-inch thick layer of padding should be placed beneath infants and young children on the long spine board from shoulders to hips, both to obtain a neutral position of the cervical spine and to minimize the development of pressure ulcers.

# A. Airway

Airway evaluation begins by assessing airway patency with the patient in the neutral position. In infants and young children, this is accomplished using the 1-inch thick layer of padding as mentioned previously. In older children, this layer should be placed beneath the entire body, including the head. This difference is due to the infant's proportionally larger head size and propensity to neck flexion when laid flat. If airway patency cannot be achieved by properly positioning the patient, several maneuvers, including a chin lift and a jaw thrust, may be used. Head tilt must be avoided to forestall potential reinjury to the cervical spinal cord.

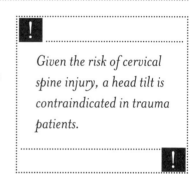

*Given the risk of cervical spine injury, a head tilt is contraindicated in trauma patients.*

*Placement of nasopharyngeal airways should be avoided in patients with midface trauma, basilar skull trauma, evidence of cerebrospinal fluid rhinorrhea, or coagulopathy.*

*Determination of correct endotracheal tube size:*
*1) Broselow Pediatric Emergency Tape*
*2) (16 + Age in years)/4*

Artificial airway adjuncts may also be helpful. These are used to displace the tongue and pharyngeal tissue from the airway. An oropharyngeal airway should be used only in an unconscious patient as it may cause significant gagging and vomiting. The length of the airway is determined by measuring the distance from the mouth to the area just cephalad to the angle of the mandible. A nasopharyngeal airway may be used in a conscious, cooperative patient. The length of the airway is determined by measuring from the tip of the nose to the tragus.

Endotracheal intubation is indicated when a patient is unable to maintain an airway because of obstruction or trauma, loss of airway tone, respiratory failure or decompensated shock, or severe neurologic dysfunction (Glasgow Coma Scale [GCS] score ≤8). It is also indicated if a patient has inhalational injury or requires airway protection from aspiration of gastric contents or blood. The correct size of endotracheal tube may be determined using either the Broselow Pediatric Emergency Tape (Armstrong Medical Industries, Inc.) or the formula shown in the box. Traditionally, uncuffed endotracheal tubes have been used for patients younger than 8 years. However, patients at risk for impaired gas exchange, such as those with acute respiratory distress syndrome, inhalation injury, or pulmonary contusions, can and should be intubated with a cuffed endotracheal tube regardless of age because they may require high ventilatory pressures to achieve adequate oxygenation and ventilation.

All trauma patients are assumed to have a full stomach. Endotracheal intubation should be performed using a rapid-sequence technique. Hypotension with administration of medications for intubation should be anticipated and measures taken to avoid this. Ketamine should be avoided where head injury is suspected because it may carry the risk of elevating intracranial pressure (ICP). Succinylcholine is contraindicated in cases of hyperkalemia, neuromuscular disease, and burns. Use etomidate cautiously, and avoid use if the patient exhibits signs and symptoms of shock.

Following neuromuscular blockade, the endotracheal tube is inserted. The tube should be advanced to a depth of 3 times the internal diameter of the tube or to a depth derived from the following formula: (age/2) + 12. Placement is checked by direct visualization of passage through the vocal cords and confirmed by bilateral chest auscultation, improvement in central color and oxygen saturation, and end-tidal carbon dioxide detection. The chest radiograph may be used to confirm proper depth of placement, but may not exclude inadvertent esophageal placement. Once the airway is secured, cricoid pressure may be removed.

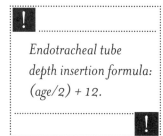

*Endotracheal tube depth insertion formula: (age/2) + 12.*

Inexperienced practitioners should not administer neuromuscular blocking agents if they are not confident that they will be able to intubate. If intubation is unsuccessful, bag-mask ventilation should be used with continued application of cricoid pressure. Advanced airway techniques may be required, such as fiberoptic intubation or use of a GlideScope (Verathon Inc.) or a gum elastic bougie. The Glidescope is a laryngoscope equipped with a camera that transmits an image to a small viewing screen accessible to multiple viewers. If endotracheal intubation is not possible or anticipated to be difficult, alternative airways such as the laryngeal mask airway or King airway may be used. A difficult airway may be anticipated in those with obvious midface trauma or cervical spine injury. When a laryngeal mask or King airway is used, it may be prudent for the patient to be taken to the operating room for conversion to an endotracheal tube and to have appropriate expertise available in the event that cricothyrotomy is necessary.

## B. Breathing

Once the airway is secured, breathing should be evaluated. The goal is normal oxygenation and ventilation. Pulse oximetry should be employed to monitor oxygen saturation with a goal of maintaining it between 94% and 99%. Oxygen may be provided by nasal cannula, face mask, nonrebreather face mask, or mechanical ventilator. Ventilation may be provided by a bag-mask device or a mechanical ventilator. Hyperventilation is not recommended in trauma patients with absent signs of cerebral herniation. In cases of suspected head injury, hyperventilation will decrease cerebral perfusion and potentially cause secondary injury. However, hyperventilation should be employed in cases of impending cerebral herniation to decrease cerebral blood flow and lower ICP. Patients with signs of tension pneumothorax require immediate needle decompression followed immediately by tube thoracostomy. Patients with signs of open pneumothorax (sucking chest wound) require an occlusive dressing followed immediately by tube thoracostomy.

## C. Circulation

The assessment of breathing is followed by the evaluation and stabilization of circulation. Hemorrhagic shock is the most frequently encountered form of shock in trauma patients.

Children may lose up to 30% of their circulating blood volume secondary to hemorrhage and still maintain normal blood pressure, so hypotension is a very late sign of pediatric shock. As such, hypoperfusion must be aggressively treated before frank hypotension develops. Applying direct pressure to actively bleeding open wounds is vital to control external hemorrhage when applicable. A commercially manufactured arterial tourniquet may be used to control hemorrhage from a bleeding extremity if direct pressure fails.

Other types of shock that may be seen in trauma victims include obstructive shock resulting from tension pneumothorax or cardiac tamponade, neurogenic shock resulting from spinal cord injury, and less commonly, cardiogenic shock resulting from trauma to the myocardium or valvular rupture.

Patients with signs of tension pneumothorax require immediate needle decompression followed by tube thoracostomy. Those with signs of hemorrhagic or neurogenic shock need volume resuscitation. Intravenous access should be obtained peripherally. After 2 unsuccessful attempts by a practitioner experienced at gaining intravenous access, an intraosseous needle should be placed, preferably in the proximal tibia. Central venous catheterization via the femoral route or venous cutdown should be considered only if a skilled practitioner is available and only if the intraosseous attempt is unsuccessful.

Once intravenous or intraosseous access is established, 20 mL/kg of isotonic crystalloid solution should be administered rapidly, and the patient should then be reassessed. If signs of shock persist, second and third boluses of 20 mL/kg should be administered. If a patient has received 40 to 60 mL/kg of fluid and is still not hemodynamically stable, 10 mL/kg of packed red blood cells should be administered. Should further transfusion be required, it should be given together with fresh frozen plasma and platelet concentrates in a ratio of 1:1:1 or 2:1:1. If 60 mL/kg is administered for neurogenic shock and the patient continues to remain hemodynamically unstable, consider vasopressor medications. A urinary catheter should be placed to monitor urine output and adequacy of resuscitation, since urine output reflects adequacy of renal perfusion. Inadequate intravascular volume and preload will be reflected by inadequate urine output. Ongoing hemodynamic instability may require operative intervention for definitive hemorrhage control.

## D. Disability

The evaluation of disability (neurologic status) follows stabilization of circulation. The level of consciousness, pupillary response, the presence of lateralizing or localizing signs, and the presence of paraplegia or paralysis should be assessed. The GCS score should be tabulated during the primary survey, again during the secondary survey, and frequently thereafter. The GCS score, used as a predictor of neurologic outcome, ranges from 3 (worst) to 15 (best). The components of the score are motor function (1-6 points), verbal response (1-5 points), and eye opening (1-4 points). Elements of the verbal score are modified to account for developmental differences in young children and infants (**Chapter 15, Table 15-1**). Any abnormality in neurologic status should prompt expeditious neurosurgical evaluation if available. Finally, hypoglycemia and hyperglycemia may each worsen neurological outcome, so a rapid blood sugar determination is essential in all critically ill or injured patients on presentation to the emergency department.

## E. Exposure

Following assessment and stabilization of neurologic status, the patients should be exposed by removing all clothing, log-rolling, and removing the backboard to allow examination of the back for life-threatening injuries. Patients should then be covered with warm blankets to prevent hypothermia. The room temperature should be warmed as should intravenous resuscitative fluids.

## F. Adjuncts to the Primary Survey

Depending on the nature of a patient's trauma, a number of additional tests, procedures, and devices may be used as adjuncts to the primary survey, including the following:

- Cardiopulmonary monitoring
- Pulse oximetry
- Blood pressure monitoring
- End-tidal carbon dioxide monitoring
- Arterial blood gas analysis
- Placement of a urinary catheter to measure output and assess renal perfusion
- Placement of a gastric tube to decompress the stomach and prevent aspiration

> *Placement of a urinary catheter should be deferred if blood is visualized at the urethral meatus.*

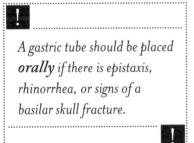

> *A gastric tube should be placed **orally** if there is epistaxis, rhinorrhea, or signs of a basilar skull fracture.*

Portable radiographs of the chest, pelvis, and (circumstances permitting) the lateral cervical spine should be obtained during the primary survey. Such radiographs may identify injuries that require immediate attention. Focused Assessment by Sonography in Trauma (FAST) may be performed by a skilled practitioner to identify pericardial, intra-abdominal, or pelvic blood or fluid.

# III. THE SECONDARY SURVEY

The secondary survey is done when the primary survey has been completed and the patient is stable. In unstable patients requiring aggressive resuscitative measures, this may be delayed. The purpose of the secondary survey is to find less obvious or physiologically disturbing injuries, or conditions that are still threatening to patient survival if not found and treated in the next few hours.

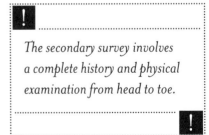

> *The secondary survey involves a complete history and physical examination from head to toe.*

## A. History

Important components of the trauma history include symptoms, allergies, medications, past medical history and pregnancy status, last meal or liquids consumed, and events and environment surrounding the injury (SAMPLE). Knowing the mechanism of injury is extremely helpful because it predicts the pattern of injuries likely to be identified. In addition, all medications and alternative preparations to which the child has been exposed should be reviewed and reconciled in the medical record.

## B. Physical Examination

The physical examination should proceed from head to toe. In an infant, the anterior fontanelle should be evaluated. The head of the patient's bed is elevated by 30 degrees (if not contraindicated) and the fontanelle is palpated. A full or bulging fontanelle is a sign of increased ICP, whereas a sunken fontanelle indicates intravascular volume loss. The head is examined for lacerations and significant irregularities indicating fractures. Raccoon eyes (periorbital ecchymosis) and the Battle sign (ecchymosis overlying the mastoid process) suggest a basilar skull fracture. The eyes are examined for pupillary response, subconjunctival hemorrhages, and extraocular movements. The nose is examined for epistaxis, rhinorrhea (suggesting leakage of cerebrospinal fluid [CSF]), and fractures. The oropharynx is evaluated for lacerations and injury to the teeth.

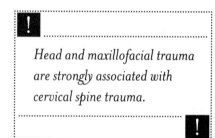

*Head and maxillofacial trauma are strongly associated with cervical spine trauma.*

In the secondary survey of the neck, the cervical collar is removed and in-line, bimanual, spinal motion restriction is temporarily applied. The neck and cervical spine are palpated for muscle spasm, step-offs and other deformities, tenderness, and crepitus. The carotid pulses should be assessed, and the position of the trachea should be evaluated. Following neck examination, the cervical collar is replaced. The chest is inspected for penetrating injuries and associated sucking chest wounds, as well as deformity or obvious fracture, and is then palpated to determine the presence of tenderness or crepitus. The lungs are auscultated for equality and clarity of breath sounds. Inequality of breath sounds may occur due to pneumothorax or hemothorax. The heart is examined with attention to the rate, rhythm, and quality of heart sounds. Distant, muffled heart sounds may represent cardiac tamponade, which may be accompanied by tachycardia with a narrow pulse pressure. The abdomen is inspected for ecchymoses, auscultated for presence and quality of bowel sounds, and palpated for tenderness, peritoneal irritation, and rigidity.

If the backboard was not removed during the primary survey, it is removed during the secondary survey. The patient is log-rolled off the backboard, and his/her back is inspected for step-offs and other deformities, as well as ecchymoses, and is palpated for tenderness. Every effort should be made to remove the backboard within 2 hours to prevent the development of pressure ulcers. Patients should be log-rolled every 2 hours thereafter to prevent pressure ulcers until the spine is cleared. The genitalia are inspected for lacerations and blood at the urethral meatus; a rectal examination is performed with assessment of tone and presence of blood in the rectal vault. The musculoskeletal system is inspected and palpated, and peripheral pulses evaluated, to identify fractures, dislocations, and physical signs suggesting compartment syndrome.

The patient's level of consciousness and pupillary response should be reassessed in the secondary survey. The GCS score should be tabulated. Reflexes should be assessed, and the presence of sensory and motor deficits should be determined. Spinal cord injury should be localized by determining the level of motor and sensory function (**Tables 9-1** and **9-2**).

**Table 9-1  Motor Levels**

| Nerve Root | Major Muscles Affected |
| --- | --- |
| C3-5 | Diaphragm |
| C5 | Elbow flexors |
| C6 | Wrist extensors |
| C7 | Elbow extensors |
| C8 | Finger flexors |
| T1 | Finger abductor (fifth finger) |
| L2 | Hip flexors |
| L3 | Knee extensors |
| L4 | Ankle dorsiflexors |
| L5 | Long toe extensors |
| S1 | Ankle plantar flexors |

**Table 9-2  Sensory Levels**

| Nerve Root | Major Sensory Area Affected |
| --- | --- |
| C4 | Clavicle |
| C6 | Thumb |
| C7 | Second and third fingers |
| C8 | Fifth finger |
| T4 | Nipples |
| T10 | Umbilicus |
| L1 | Inguinal ligament |
| L3 | Lower anterior thigh/knees |
| L5 | Big toe |
| S1 | Lateral foot |
| S3-5 | Perineum |

## C. Adjuncts to the Secondary Survey

The results of the secondary survey may point to additional studies. These may include hematologic and biochemical tests, computed tomography (CT) scans, completion of the cervical spine radiographs, additional radiographs of the thoracolumbar spine and extremities, angiography, and ultrasonography.

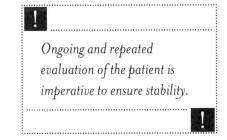

*Ongoing and repeated evaluation of the patient is imperative to ensure stability.*

Serial hematocrit measurements is important in any child with a major injury, to monitor for bleeding from a solid organ injury, such as a splenic, hepatic, or renal laceration. A rising white blood cell count, or amylase and lipase level, may be an important clue to an evolving bowel or pancreatic injury. Hepatic transaminases can provide early indication of blunt trauma injury to the liver. Urinalysis will help exclude renal contusions or lacerations. Given that anemia from blood loss and clotting dysfunction from consumptive coagulopathy commonly occur in the critically injured patient, blood samples for type and crossmatch should be sent to the laboratory together with these initial studies, so that blood products can be given as soon as they are required. Serial arterial blood gas measurements are also vitally important during the stabilization of any severely injured ventilated child, as they will guide ventilatory support. Base deficit values can guide resuscitation efforts.

# IV. MANAGEMENT OF TRAUMATIC INJURIES

## A. Traumatic Brain Injury

 Case Study

A 4-year-old boy presents to the emergency department after being struck by a taxi moving at moderate speed as he ran across the street. He sustained a brief loss of consciousness at the scene but was arousable, alternately moaning and crying, with spontaneous eye opening and the ability to follow simple motor commands when emergency medical services arrived. His vital signs remained stable, and he was immobilized with a semi-rigid collar and long spine board prior to transport. On arrival in the emergency department, he cries for his mother, opens his eyes to voice, and localizes to pain. Vital signs reveal a temperature of 96.8°F (36°C), a heart rate of 66 beats/min, a respiratory rate of 24 breaths/min, and a blood pressure of 110/67 mm Hg. $SpO_2$ is 96% on room air. Examination demonstrates a sluggishly reactive right pupil, a briskly reactive left pupil, and a large right cephalohematoma. Subsequently the boy becomes more lethargic, opening his eyes only to voice, making incomprehensible sounds, and withdrawing from pain. His right pupil is now slightly dilated. A head CT scan shows a large right biconvex extradural (epidural) mass lesion associated with midline shift and ventricular effacement, and an adjacent nondisplaced right parietal skull fracture.

**Detection**
- What are the next steps in managing this patient?
- Does this patient exhibit a classic lucid interval?

**Intervention**
- What are the most immediate treatment strategies?

**Reassessment**
- Is the current treatment strategy effective?
- Does the patient need to be intubated or receive other therapeutic interventions?

**Effective Communication**
- With this change in the patient's clinical status, who needs the information and how will it be disseminated?
- Where is the best place to manage the care of this patient?

**Teamwork**
- How are you going to implement the treatment strategy?
- Who is to do what and when?

Traumatic brain injury (TBI) contributes to a significant number of trauma deaths in children and usually occurs in motor vehicle collisions, falls, bicycle accidents, and sports injuries.

Nonaccidental trauma remains a significant cause of TBI in children younger than 2 years. TBI may be characterized as mild (GCS score 13-15), moderate (GCS score 9-12), or severe (GCS score 3-8).

Children with mild brain injury generally do well, but as many as 53% have radiographic abnormalities on head CT despite a lack of significant findings on physical examination. Up to 57% of children and 85% of infants with epidural hematomas have no apparent loss of consciousness at the time of impact, and 7% have no alteration of mental status at any time following the injury. These statistics underscore the likelihood that a life-threatening injury may exist despite a benign presentation. Children with a normal neurologic examination and a normal head CT at presentation rarely deteriorate and can be safely discharged home. Fortunately, a recently established clinical prediction rule for brain injury has shown that head CT and its attendant late cancer risks can be safely avoided in children 2 years and older who have normal mental status, no loss of consciousness, no vomiting, non-severe injury mechanism, no signs of basilar skull fracture, and no severe headache. This is also true in children younger than 2 years who have normal mental status, no scalp hematoma, no loss of consciousness or loss of consciousness for less than 5 seconds, non-severe injury mechanism, no palpable skull fracture, and who are acting normally according to the parents.

Most patients with moderate to severe TBI will not present with intracranial mass lesions but rather with diffuse cerebral swelling due to a combination of mostly vasogenic edema at the locus of injury and hyperemia elsewhere, resulting from loss of cerebral arteriolar pressure autoregulation. Such patients are managed chiefly by nonsurgical means, although drainage of CSF via ventriculostomy may be required to assist in lowering the ICP. However, intracranial mass lesions may require prompt neurosurgical evaluation, followed by neurosurgical intervention for drainage or decompression. Epidural hematomas, while uncommon in childhood, are associated with a good prognosis if promptly recognized and neurosurgically evacuated. However, as previously stated, the classic lucid interval typically observed in adults with this condition is most often absent in children. Subdural hematomas, by contrast, are both more common and far more deadly, owing to the associated cerebral tissue injury that is invariably present. Neurosurgical evacuation is indicated if a midline shift exceeds 5 mm, or if a large intracerebral hematoma is contributing to the mass effect.

The management of children with moderate to severe TBI requires careful attention to ventilatory and hemodynamic status as well as to ICP. The goal is to prevent the primary brain injury from being adversely affected by the hypoxia and hypoperfusion that may result from inadequate resuscitation, termed *secondary brain injury*. Children with moderate TBI (GCS score 9-12) may therefore require intubation and ventilation for indications other than the TBI itself. Intubation, ventilation, and ICP monitoring are indicated in those with a severe TBI (GCS score 3-8), and should be strongly considered in head-injured patients whose GCS score deteriorates rapidly by 2 or more points. When a patient with head trauma meets this criterion, the goals of mechanical ventilation are normal oxygenation ($Spo_2$ 94%-99%) and normal ventilation ($Paco_2$ 35-40 mm Hg [4.7-5.3 kPa]), since both hypercarbia and hypocarbia may worsen outcome by contributing to hyperemic or ischemic injury. Thus, hyperventilation is indicated only in cases of impending or actual cerebral herniation. Meticulous attention to respiratory and hemodynamic status is imperative, because hypoxemia and hypotension have each been shown to significantly increase morbidity and mortality in patients with TBI. Control of seizures and maintenance of normal body temperature are additionally of key importance in inhibiting the progression of brain injury to cell death and encephalomalacia. Adequate analgesia and sedation must also be provided.

The head of the patient's bed should be elevated by 30°, if not otherwise contraindicated, and the child's head should be positioned in the midline, avoiding flexion, abduction, or rotation that could impair jugular venous return.

In patients with severe TBI (GCS score 3-8), an ICP monitor may be placed in the lateral ventricle (ventriculostomy), subdural space (bolt), or brain parenchyma. Ventriculostomy catheters may be preferred because they allow both monitoring of ICP and drainage of CSF as a means of lowering ICP. Normal ICP in adults is less than 10 mm Hg, and is lower in young children and infants. Abnormal ICP exceeds 20 mm Hg at any age. Acute sustained increases (spikes) in ICP are promptly treated with bag-mask or endotracheal tube ventilation to provide mild hyperventilation. Hypertonic saline (3%) infusions or intravenous mannitol, 0.5 g/kg (range 0.25-1 g/kg), is administered to raise serum osmolality (300-310 mOsm/L) and lower ICP.

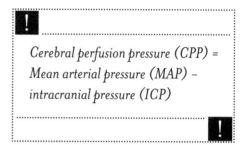

*Cerebral perfusion pressure (CPP) = Mean arterial pressure (MAP) - intracranial pressure (ICP)*

Cerebral perfusion pressure (CPP) must be monitored closely in patients with TBI. Numerically it is represented as the difference between the mean arterial pressure (MAP) and the ICP (CPP = MAP – ICP). In adults, a CPP of 60 to 70 mm Hg is usually targeted. There are no data documenting the appropriate CPP in children and infants at this time. However, given their lower MAP and ICP readings, general ranges can be extrapolated. A reasonable range is 50 to 60 mm Hg in children and 40 to 50 mm Hg in infants. Other modalities utilized for control of ICP include sedation, neuromuscular blockade, elevation of the head, maintenance of mild hypothermia (~95°F [~35°C]), strict avoidance of hyperthermia requiring active cooling modalities, use of endotracheal or intravenous lidocaine prior to suctioning, maintenance of euvolemia, and titration of serum osmolality to levels as high as 360 mOsm/L (serum sodium ~150 mEq/L) if needed.

As noted, hypertonic saline solution (3%) is preferred for control of continuous elevations of ICP, because it increases serum osmolality without causing intravascular volume depletion. In cases of intractable elevations of ICP, inotropic or vasopressor agents may also be used to optimize CPP by increasing MAP, even to the point of relative systemic hypertension. The use of mannitol to decrease cerebral edema as well as ICP has fallen out of favor except in cases of intractable intracranial hypertension, because mannitol is a potent osmotic diuretic that may cause hypotension. Moreover, ICP may rebound after its discontinuation. Corticosteroids have no role in TBI.

## B. Spinal Cord Injury

### Case Study

A 17-year-old boy presents to the emergency department after sustaining an injury during sports practice. A sharp blow resulted in severe hyperextension of his neck. He fell to the ground, unable to move his lower extremities and with significant weakness of the upper extremities. His vital signs were stable in the field, and he was immobilized with a semi-rigid collar and long spine board prior to transport. In the emergency department, the patient is awake, alert, and afebrile, with a respiratory rate of 9 breaths/min, oxygen saturation of 94% on room air, heart rate of 56 beats/min, and blood pressure of 70/40 mm Hg.

**Detection**
- What is the first step in stabilizing this patient?
- Why is this patient hypotensive?
- What is the diagnosis?

**Intervention**
- What are the most immediate treatment strategies?

**Reassessment**
- Is the current treatment strategy effective?
- Are other therapeutic interventions indicated to augment blood pressure?
- Are other therapeutic interventions indicated to augment ventilation?

**Effective Communication**
- Who needs to know about this patient's clinical status, and how will the information be communicated?

**Teamwork**
- How are you going to implement the treatment strategy?
- Who is to do what and when?

Cervical spine injury is uncommon in children. It has a mortality rate of 15% to 20%, largely due to its association with significant brain injury. Young children (<11 years) most frequently sustain cervical spine injury as the result of motor vehicle collisions, falls, and pedestrian accidents. They are at risk for high cervical injuries, cervical spine dislocations, and spinal cord injury (SCI) without radiographic abnormality (SCIWORA), the latter due to the horizontal orientation of the facet joints and the elastic nature of the intervertebral ligaments, which permits upper cervical spinal elements to shift rather than break upon application of forces, leading to angular momentum of the head and neck. Older children (>11 years) and adults are at risk for low cervical injuries and cervical spine fractures. Children ages 10 to 11 years begin to show adult patterns of injury, and their transition to those patterns is eventually completed in late adolescence. Differences in injury patterns may be attributed to anatomical differences between the young child and the older child/adult. Young children have proportionally larger heads with relatively weak neck muscles, which make them more susceptible to flexion and extension injuries. The vertebral bodies are incompletely ossified, and the intervertebral ligaments are far more elastic than those of adults. In addition, the vertebral bodies of the upper cervical spine are anteriorly wedged in children, predisposing them to forward vertebral movement and anterior dislocation, a condition termed pseudosubluxation. The fulcrum for cervical motion is at C2 to C3 in the young child compared to C5 to C6 in adolescents and adults. The young child's spinal cord may be easily stretched, torn, or sustain contusion secondary to laxity of spinal ligaments. The cord may stretch up to 5 cm without rupturing, whereas the adult cord may rupture after only 5 to 6 mm of traction.

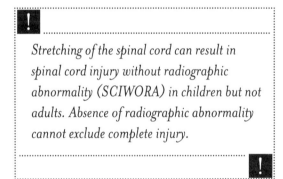

*Stretching of the spinal cord can result in spinal cord injury without radiographic abnormality (SCIWORA) in children but not adults. Absence of radiographic abnormality cannot exclude complete injury.*

Children with cervical and high thoracic SCIs are predisposed both to ventilatory compromise and neurogenic shock. The former may occur due to denervation of the intercostal muscles associated with SCIs below C4, or denervation of the diaphragm and intercostal muscles associated with SCIs above C4. The latter results from loss of sympathetic vascular tone, leading to seemingly paradoxical bradycardia despite the presence of hypotensive shock. However, even in patients with SCI, hemorrhagic shock is far more common than neurogenic shock and may coexist with neurogenic shock. As such, a careful search for sources of bleeding should be made even if SCI is present.

Respiratory failure may require intubation for diaphragmatic paralysis, pulmonary toilet, or both. Neurogenic shock is treated with aggressive volume resuscitation followed by selective use of vasopressor agents if hypotension persists despite adequate volume resuscitation. The term *spinal shock*, which refers to the truly paradoxical loss of spinal reflexes following injury, is sometimes incorrectly used to describe the hemodynamic consequences of SCI, and its use should be limited to the neurologic sequelae. Finally, great care must be taken to prevent the development of pressure ulcers, which can begin in as soon as 1 hour after SCI. There is no scientific evidence supporting the use of corticosteroids in SCI; in fact, such use is associated with increased complications, such as hyperglycemia and avascular necrosis at large joints such as the hip.

The lateral cervical spine radiograph is often used as a screening test for cervical spine injury (CSI), but it will miss 15% of all fractures. The addition of anteroposterior and odontoid views will capture most other fractures. While CT is increasingly used for definitive diagnosis of cervical spine fractures in children and adults, its use is best limited to cases in which diagnosis by standard radiograph is equivocal, due to the associated risks of late cancers. A valid clinical prediction rule for cervical spine imaging following major trauma in children has not been developed, but 8 factors are known to be associated with it: altered mental status, focal neurologic findings, neck pain, torticollis, substantial torso injury, conditions predisposing to CSI, diving, and high-risk motor vehicle crash. Absence of such factors may militate against the use of routine CT in the diagnosis of possible CSI. Regardless, cervical spine precautions, including a semi-rigid collar and thoracolumbar spinal motion restriction, must be implemented and maintained until CSI is excluded by appropriate clinical and radiological means, including spine surgery consultation and magnetic resonance imaging, when indicated.

## C. Thoracic Trauma

###  Case Study

A 4-year-old girl presents to the emergency department after falling from a second-story window. She sustained a brief loss of consciousness at the scene, but was awake, alert, and crying when emergency services arrived. Her vital signs were stable, and she was immobilized with a semi-rigid collar and long spine board prior to transport. In the emergency department, she is awake and crying for her mother. Vital signs reveal a temperature of 98.4°F (37°C), a heart rate of 120 beats/min, a respiratory rate of 50 breaths/min, and a blood pressure of 120/65 mm Hg. $Spo_2$ is 92% on room air. Her breathing pattern is paradoxical, with an asymmetric thorax.

**Detection**
- What is the source of this patient's hypoxemia?
- How will you treat her?

**Interventions**
- What are the most immediate treatment strategies?

**Reassessment**
- Is the current treatment strategy effective?
- Will she require intubation?

**Effective Communication**
- When the patient's clinical status changes, who needs to know and how will this information be disseminated?
- Where is the best place to manage the care of this patient?

**Teamwork**
- How are you going to implement the treatment strategy?
- Who is to do what and when?

Thoracic injuries, which often occur as a result of blunt trauma, are the second leading cause of death due to trauma in children (after head injuries). The overall mortality rate from thoracic trauma has been reported to be 5%, increasing to 25% when accompanied by head and abdominal trauma. In infants and toddlers, thoracic injuries occur most commonly in the contexts of motor vehicle collisions and maltreatment. School-aged children are most likely to sustain thoracic trauma due to bicycle, scooter, and skating accidents, while teenagers are most commonly injured in motor vehicle collisions.

A chest radiograph should be the initial diagnostic test in the evaluation of thoracic trauma. Due to their extremely compliant chest walls, children sustain rib fractures much less frequently than adults do and are at higher risk of pulmonary contusions. Therefore, if rib fractures are present, they signify an especially forceful impact. Pulmonary contusions are the most common thoracic injuries in children and may be associated with hypoxemia, hypoventilation, ventilation-perfusion mismatch, increased work of breathing, and decreased pulmonary compliance. There may be consolidation, edema, and alveolar hemorrhage in the area of contusion. Contusions may not be visible on early radiographs but will become apparent later. There should be high index of suspicion for thoracic trauma given an appropriate mechanism of injury. Treatment includes avoidance of fluid overload, supplemental oxygen, analgesia, incentive spirometry, and mechanical ventilation if required (**Table 9-3**).

The presence of rib fractures, particularly posterior rib fractures, should raise suspicion of physical abuse. These fractures usually occur as the result of significant compression of the chest, as happens in shaking. Other potential etiologies include birth trauma and disorders of bone ossification, such as osteogenesis imperfecta and rickets. Fractures of the first rib are associated with an especially high incidence of intrathoracic injuries, including pneumothorax and hemothorax, and should prompt CT angiography for diagnosis of significant vascular injury.

| Table 9-3 | Diagnostic Evaluation |
| --- | --- |
| **Type of Trauma** | **Diagnostic Study** |
| Any | Serial hematocrits |
| | Prothrombin time/partial prothrombin time |
| | Complete metabolic panel, including aspartate aminotransferase/alanine aminotransferase, amylase, lipase |
| | Urinalysis |
| | Radiographs of the chest, cervical spine (posteroanterior, lateral, odontoid), and pelvis |
| Head | Head CT |
| | MRI: not indicated immediately; obtain later to aid in prognostication |
| Cervical Spine | Cervical spine radiographs: posteroanterior, lateral, odontoid views |
| | Cervical spine CT: if plain radiographs are inadequate |
| | Flexion/extension radiographs: indicated when radiographs/CT scans are negative for bony injury but neck pain/tenderness is elicited; evaluates ligamentous injury |
| | MRI: indicated when radiographs/CT scans are negative for bony injury but neck pain/tenderness is elicited; evaluates ligamentous injury[a] |
| Thoracic | Chest radiograph |
| | Chest CT |
| | Chest CT angiography: indicated when serious vascular injury is suspected |
| | Electrocardiogram |
| | Echocardiogram: indicated when pericardial effusion is suspected |
| | Esophagogram: indicated when esophageal rupture is suspected |
| | Bronchoscopy/bronchography: indicated when injury to the tracheobronchial tree is suspected |
| Abdominal | Aspartate aminotransferase/alanine aminotransferase |
| | Amylase/lipase |
| | Urinalysis |
| | FAST examination |
| | Abdominal CT with oral and intravenous contrast |

CT, computed tomography; MRI, magnetic resonance imaging; FAST, focused abdominal sonography for trauma
[a]Flexion/extension films or MRI may be performed.

Multiple rib fractures have been shown to be associated with severe injury in children; mortality rates rise as the number of fractured ribs increases. Flail chest occurs when 2 or more adjacent ribs are fractured in two places each, resulting in paradoxical chest wall movement (inward movement with inspiration and outward movement with exhalation), although muscle spasm may limit the motion of small flail segments.

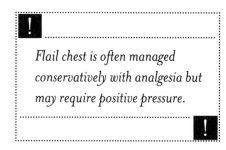

*Flail chest is often managed conservatively with analgesia but may require positive pressure.*

One-third of traumatic pneumothoraces occur in isolation, the other two-thirds in association with other injuries. Often pneumothoraces are asymptomatic and are only detected by chest radiography. Treatment is the evacuation of air with a tube thoracostomy. Accumulation of a large amount of air in the pleural space may lead to the collapse of the ipsilateral lung, with tracheal and mediastinal shift resulting in hemodynamic instability (tension pneumothorax). Signs of tension pneumothorax include tracheal shift, absence of breath sounds on the ipsilateral side, tachycardia, hypotension, dyspnea, and hypoxemia. When clinically suspected, evacuation of tension pneumothorax must not be delayed by waiting for radiographic confirmation. Prompt decompression of tension pneumothorax via needle thoracostomy, followed as soon as possible by tube thoracostomy, is imperative to prevent hemodynamic collapse. Hemothorax can develop in the context of blunt or penetrating injuries to the chest with disruption of the thoracic vessels, intercostal blood vessels, or lung parenchyma. Evacuation of significant hemothorax is important in the prevention of subsequent infection, chronic atelectasis and lung entrapment; acutely, it may compromise cardiac output due to both blood loss and obstructive shock. Ventilation-perfusion abnormalities also are possible, but evacuation should be preceded by aggressive volume resuscitation.

Cardiac contusions most frequently occur as a result of blunt trauma and may present as chest pain, dysrhythmia, or hypotension. An electrocardiogram may show ST-segment changes, atrial tachycardia, sinus tachycardia, or premature beats. Treatment is generally supportive, with cardiopulmonary monitoring required only if abnormalities appear on the electrocardiogram. Cardiac tamponade may occur if there is an accumulation of blood in the pericardial space. Patients present with tachycardia, muffled heart sounds, and a narrow pulse pressure. The diagnosis is suspected when a penetrating injury is found within an area bounded by the nipple line, midclavicular lines, and costal margins, and is confirmed by FAST or echocardiography. Treatment consists of fluid removal by pericardial window or emergency thoracotomy, although pericardiocentesis may be employed as a temporizing measure until a qualified surgeon performs evacuation, followed by definition and treatment of the bleeding source.

Diaphragmatic injuries are uncommon, but when they occur, they most frequently involve the posterolateral left hemidiaphragm. Upward coiling of a nasogastric tube and herniation of the abdominal contents into the thorax may be visualized on the chest radiograph. Up to 50% of these injuries are missed at the initial presentation, becoming apparent only on subsequent chest radiographs.

Esophageal injury is caused most frequently by penetrating injury. Blunt trauma may also induce a tear at the gastroesophageal junction due to acute movement of gastric contents into the esophagus. Gastric contents may spill into the pleural space or mediastinum. Diagnosis is made when extravasation of contrast material is seen on an esophagogram. Treatment includes antibiotics and surgical repair.

Injuries to the tracheobronchial tree are rare in children but are associated with a mortality rate of 30%. They may be caused by blunt or penetrating trauma. Patients present with subcutaneous emphysema, pneumothorax, hemoptysis, and persistent air leak following tube thoracostomy. Diagnosis may be confirmed by bronchoscopy, but bronchography may be required to visualize tears in the distal bronchial tree.

## D. Abdominal Trauma

###  Case Study

A 2-year-old girl is brought to the emergency department by her mother. The girl is lethargic and difficult to arouse. There is no history of fever, illness, ingestion, or trauma. Vital signs reveal a temperature of 96°F (36°C), a heart rate of 170 beats/min, a respiratory rate of 45 breaths/min, and a blood pressure of 64/40 mm Hg. $Sp_{O_2}$ is 95% on room air. After stabilization and removal of clothing, you find a large ecchymotic area on her abdomen.

### Detection

- What interventions would be needed to stabilize this patient?
- What is an appropriate diagnostic evaluation for this patient?

### Intervention

- What are the most immediate treatment strategies?
- Should she be intubated?

### Reassessment

- Is the current treatment strategy effective?
- Does she require additional fluid or blood products?
- Is a surgical consultation indicated?
- Are there findings suggestive of nonaccidental trauma?

### Effective Communication

- When the patient's clinical status changes, who needs to know and how will this information be disseminated?
- Where is the best place to manage the care of this child?

### Teamwork

- How are you going to implement the treatment strategy?
- Who is to do what and when?

Due to their compliant chest walls and decreased abdominal wall musculature and fat, children are at higher risk than adults of sustaining significant organ injury as a result of abdominal trauma. Multiple organs may be injured, because an impacting force will strike a relatively larger proportion of a child's body surface. Intra-abdominal injuries related to bicycle handlebars and poorly fitting car lap belts have a high likelihood of requiring surgical intervention. Physical findings include abdominal distention, abrasions, contusions, lap belt pattern ecchymoses, peritonitis, and focal or diffuse tenderness. Hemodynamically unstable patients require emergent resuscitation and laparotomy, whereas stable patients warrant further assessment.

Diagnostic assessment of abdominal trauma continues with a laboratory evaluation. Decreasing hemoglobin and hematocrit should raise suspicion of abdominal hemorrhage. Several studies have shown that elevations in the serum aspartate aminotransferase and alanine aminotransferase levels may be associated with abdominal trauma. One study found that a serum alanine aminotransferase measurement above 131 U/L with abdominal tenderness is predictive of abdominal injury with a sensitivity of 100%. Serum amylase and lipase are variable predictors of pancreatic injury. Serum amylase may be normal when obtained soon after pancreatic injury, but will be elevated 100% of the time at 3 hours or more following injury. Elevations in serum amylase may also be seen in the presence of head injury without pancreatic injury.

The FAST exam is of limited utility in the pediatric population. Most solid abdominal organ injuries in hemodynamically stable children are managed nonoperatively. The FAST examination may be useful in two specific situations in the pediatric population: (1) in multiply injured, hemodynamically unstable patients, it may be used to detect abdominal hemorrhage as the source of instability; and (2) with the laboratory evaluation and physical examination, it may serve as a screening tool to identify patients who would benefit from CT.

Indications for abdominal CT include abnormal physical examination, abnormal laboratory values, lack of a reliable physical examination due to distracting injuries or altered mental status, or a compelling need for precise information regarding specific organ injury or grade of injury. Abdominal CT is the diagnostic procedure of choice for evaluation of abdominal injury and is most useful in detecting solid organ injuries, particularly those of the liver, spleen, and kidneys. It should be performed with intravenous contrast to best delineate these injuries. Pancreatic and intestinal injuries may be missed on initial abdominal CT, particularly if it is performed soon after injury. Oral contrast may be helpful on later scans if clinical signs suggest an occult small bowel injury. Again, a recently established clinical prediction rule for intra-abdominal injury requiring acute intervention has shown that abdominal CT and its attendant late cancer risks can be safely avoided in children with no complaints of abdominal pain, no history of vomiting, no evidence of abdominal wall trauma (including seat belt sign), a GCS score ≥14, no abdominal tenderness, no evidence of thoracic wall trauma, and no decreased breath sounds.

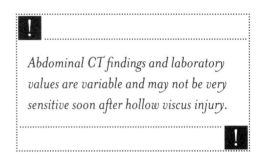

*Abdominal CT findings and laboratory values are variable and may not be very sensitive soon after hollow viscus injury.*

Splenic injury is the most common injury associated with blunt abdominal trauma. Abdominal CT with intravenous contrast is its most specific detection method. Preservation of the spleen is the standard of care in children in order to prevent immunologic compromise. Splenectomy is indicated only in cases of hemodynamic instability with irreparable splenic damage.

Liver injury, the second most common insult associated with blunt abdominal trauma, also is best diagnosed by abdominal CT with intravenous contrast. As with splenic injury, most liver injuries can be managed without surgical intervention. However, when necessary, surgical control of bleeding is typically accomplished using conservative measures rather than resection.

Kidney injuries likewise rarely require surgical intervention in childhood, except in cases of uncontrollable hemorrhage, urine leak, or renal pedicle injury. Pancreatic injury occurs much less frequently than other solid organ injuries in children, often results from impact with bicycle handlebars, and may occur as an isolated injury. Abdominal CT is the diagnostic modality of choice. Management is typically nonoperative, unless the pancreatic duct is transected.

Hollow organ injury occurs less frequently than solid organ injury and is more difficult to detect, so a high index of suspicion is required. Motor vehicle collisions in which children are restrained with poorly fitting lap belts may result in intestinal injury. Pneumoperitoneum or extravasation of oral contrast may be detected on abdominal CT. Often, free abdominal fluid is the only abnormality and remains a nonspecific finding. Similarly, motor vehicle collisions in which children are poorly restrained can also result in injury to the bladder. Disruption of the dome of the bladder, manifested by intraperitoneal extravasation of intravenous contrast, is repaired via laparotomy.

Disruption of the remainder of the bladder, detected by extraperitoneal leakage of intravenous contrast, is treated via urinary or suprapubic catheter decompression.

When physical examination or abdominal CT findings are equivocal, a high index of suspicion should be maintained and follow-up serial examinations should be performed. Diagnostic laparoscopy may be helpful in selected cases.

Abdominal compartment syndrome – defined by a sustained intra-abdominal pressure of ≥20 mm Hg in the presence of abdominal distention and oliguria or anuria, respiratory decompensation, hypotension or shock, and metabolic acidosis – is uncommon following major trauma in childhood. As in adults, timely surgical decompression is required for optimal recovery.

## E. Pelvic and Extremity Trauma

## Case Study

A 5-year-old girl is pinned against a wall when a fast moving motor vehicle jumps the curb. Vital signs were unobtainable at the scene, where she was immobilized with a semi-rigid collar and long spine board prior to transport. In the emergency department, the patient is severely agitated, moaning and crying for her mother. Vital signs reveal a temperature of 97.6°F (36°C), a heart rate of 140 beats/min, a respiratory rate of 40 breaths/min, and a blood pressure of 70/45 mm Hg. $Spo_2$ is 94% on room air. Examination demonstrates pelvic instability. The chest radiograph is normal, but the pelvic radiograph confirms multiple pelvic ring fractures.

**Detection**
- What maneuvers should be undertaken for control of bleeding?
- What additional injuries are likely to be present?

**Intervention**
- What are the most immediate treatment strategies?
- Should blood products be given?
- Should a Foley catheter be placed?

**Reassessment**
- Is the current treatment strategy effective?
- Does the patient require other therapeutic interventions for hemodynamic stability?

**Effective Communication**
- When the patient's clinical status changes, who needs to know and how will the information be disseminated?
- Where is the best place to manage the care of this patient?

**Teamwork**
- How are you going to implement this treatment strategy?
- Who is to do what and when?

Musculoskeletal trauma rarely results in life-threatening hemorrhage in children. Exceptions to this rule include unstable pelvic fractures and bilateral femur fractures. Application of a pelvic binder or sling to limit pelvic volume is the first step in controlling retroperitoneal bleeding associated with pelvic disruption, followed by aggressive volume resuscitation. Ultimately, selective embolization or external fixation may be required. Long bone fractures are immobilized as soon as possible to limit pain, lessen hemorrhage, and restore perfusion in cases where limbs are threatened by vascular compromise. Impaired limb perfusion is often associated with fractures of the elbow and knee; in-line fracture reduction may relieve external impingement upon arterial flow. Ischemic and crush injuries, most often of the distal lower extremities, may result in compartment syndrome, requiring urgent fasciotomy and aggressive hydration to preclude myoglobin deposition in the renal tubules and subsequent development of acute renal failure. Administration of sodium bicarbonate, to alkalinize the urine and further minimize tubular myoglobin precipitation, may be required in cases associated with severe myonecrosis and profound elevations in serum creatine kinase as well as myoglobin.

Fractures of the pelvis and femur that occur when pedestrians are struck by moving vehicles may be associated with head and truncal injuries, in a frequently incomplete pattern known as the Waddell triad. As previously stated, small children sustaining large force blunt trauma, such as in motor vehicle collisions, rarely sustain isolated injuries, so a careful search of the body core is warranted.

## F. Soft Tissue Trauma

All open wounds require debridement of nonviable tissue, followed by primary closure if feasible or appropriate. If this is not possible, dressing changes and local wound care should be implemented, with delayed primary closure performed once granulation tissue has formed, usually within 5-7 days. Vacuum-assisted closure of large, open, contaminated wounds, using the wound V.A.C. Therapy device (KCI) or a similar device, may facilitate healing. Fasciotomy wounds can eventually be closed using a "shoelace" technique, though skin grafting may be needed if primary closure cannot be achieved. Superficial abrasions should be cleansed and treated with topical antibiotics. Antimicrobial prophylaxis is warranted for all but clean, incisive wounds, while tetanus prophylaxis is warranted for all tetanus-prone wounds. All penetrating injuries must be considered contaminated and managed accordingly.

## G. Near Drowning

The drowning process refers to the pathological effects that occur with submersion. While less commonly used, some still characterize drowning as dry or wet. Dry drowning occurs more frequently in adults. No fluid is aspirated into the lungs. Victims develop severe laryngospasm and often have significant mucus and froth in the upper airway. Death results from cerebral anoxia. Wet drowning involves the aspiration of fluid into the lungs with resultant pathophysiologic changes.

Following submersion, a period of voluntary apnea occurs. In young children, the initial contact with the water is accompanied by the diving reflex, which shunts blood flow from the skin and splanchnic circulations to the coronary and cerebral circulations. Blood pressure is increased and heart rate is decreased. Fear and the cold water temperature amplify the diving reflex, which may partially account for the improved survival seen following long submersion in cold water. In warm water (above 59°F-68°F [15°C-20°C]), the submersion time to fatality in humans is 3 to 10 minutes. In cold water (32°F-59°F [0°C-15°C]), neurologically intact survival has been reported in submersion as long as 40 minutes. After the initial period of breath holding, a break point is reached and the victim will take a breath, resulting in aspiration of water. Initial water entry into the upper airway will lead to laryngospasm, which persists until hypoxia leads to muscle relaxation. At the same time, secondary apnea occurs, leading to involuntary gasping breaths, respiratory arrest, and eventually cardiac arrest.

Patients in the drowning process are managed much like other trauma patients. Severe electrolyte abnormalities are uncommon, and antibiotics are generally not indicated. Emerging literature in adult and neonatal populations has suggested cooling the head and therapeutic systemic hypothermia as treatments that may improve neurologic outcome in patients who have sustained a cardiac arrest.

## Key Points: Traumatic Injuries in Children

- The primary patient survey consists of an evaluation of ABCDE: airway, breathing, circulation, disability (neurologic) status, and exposure.

- Adjuncts to the primary survey include cardiopulmonary monitoring, pulse oximetry, blood pressure monitoring, end-tidal carbon dioxide monitoring, arterial blood gas analysis, urinary catheter placement, gastric catheter placement, and radiographs of the chest, pelvis, and lateral cervical spine.

- The secondary survey, history and physical examination, covers symptoms, allergies, medications, past medical history and pregnancy status, last meal, and events and environment (mechanism of injury). The physical examination proceeds from head to toe.

- Adjuncts to the secondary survey include CT scans, completion of the cervical spine radiographs, radiographs of the thoracolumbar spine and extremities, ultrasonograms, and angiograms as indicated.

- Pulmonary contusions are common in children, but rib fractures are rare due to greater chest wall compliance. Because rib fractures are usually the result of significant trauma, their existence in the absence of other significant trauma should raise a suspicion of abuse.

- The incidence of abdominal organ damage is higher in children than in adults. Splenic injury is most common, followed by liver injury. Intestinal injury is less common, and its diagnosis requires a high index of suspicion.

# Suggested Readings

1. American College of Surgeons, Committee on Trauma. *Advanced Trauma Life Support for Doctors Student Course Manual*. 9th ed. Chicago, IL: American College of Surgeons; 2012.

2. American Heart Association. *Pediatric Advanced Life Support Provider Manual*. Chicago, IL: American Heart Association; 2011.

3. Berman SS, Schilling JD, McIntyre KE, Hunter GC, Bernhard VM. Shoelace technique for delayed primary closure of fasciotomies. *Am J Surg*. 1994;167:435-436.

4. Dias MS. Traumatic brain and spinal cord injury. *Pediatr Clin North Am*. 2004; 51:271-303.

5. Holcomb JB, Wade CE, Michalek JE, et al. Increased plasma and platelet to red cell ratios improves outcome in 466 massively transfused civilian trauma patients. *Ann Surg*. 2008;248:447-458.

6. Holmes J, Lillis K, Monroe D, et al. Identifying children at very low risk of intra-abdominal injuries undergoing acute intervention [abstract]. *Acad Emerg Med*. 2011;18(5 Suppl 1):S161.

7. Holmes JF, Gladman A, Chang CH. Performance of abdominal ultrasonography in pediatric blunt trauma patients: a meta-analysis. *J Pediatr Surg*. 2007;42:1588-1594.

8. Kochanek PM, Carney N, Adelson PD, et al. Guidelines for the acute medical management of severe traumatic brain injury in infants, children and adolescents-second edition. *Pediatr Crit Care Med*. 2012;13(Suppl 1):S1-82.

9. Kochanek PM, Fink EL, Bell MJ, Bayir H, Clark RS. Therapeutic hypothermia: applications in pediatric cardiac arrest. *J Neurotrauma*. 2009;26:421-427.

10. Kragh JF, Cooper A, Aden JK, et al. Survey of trauma registry data on tourniquet use in pediatric war casualties. *Pediatr Emerg Care*. 2012;28:1361-1365.

11. Kuppermann N, Holmes JF, Dayan PS, et al, for the Pediatric Emergency Care Applied Research Network (PECARN). Identification of children at very low risk of clinically-important brain injuries after head trauma: a prospective cohort study. *Lancet*. 2009;374:1160-1170.

12. Leininger BE, Rasmussen TE, Smith DL, Jenkins TH, Coppola C. Experience with Wound VAC and delayed primary closure of contaminated soft tissue injuries in Iraq. *J Trauma*. 2006;61: 1207-1211.

13. Leonard JC, Kuppermann N, Olsen C, et al, for the Pediatric Emergency Care Applied Research Network. Factors associated with cervical spine injury in children after blunt trauma. *Ann Emerg Med*. 2011;58:145-155.

14. Levin DL, Morriss FC, Toro LO, Brink LW, Turner GR. Drowning and near-drowning. *Pediatr Clin North Am*. 1993;40:321-336.

15. Nance MD, Rotondo MF, Fildes JJ, eds. American College of Surgeons National Trauma Data Bank. Pediatric Annual Report, 2011. Available at: http://www.facs.org/trauma/ntdb/pdf/ntdbpediatricreport2011.pdf. Accessed April 21, 2012.

16. Pearn J. Pathophysiology of drowning. *Med J Aust*. 1985;142:586-588.

17. Pieretti-Vanmarcke R, Velmahos GC, Nance ML, et al. Clinical clearance of the cervical spine in blunt trauma patients younger than 3 years: a multi-center study of the American Association for the Surgery of Trauma. *J Trauma*. 2009;67:543-550.

18. Pitetti RD, Walker S. Life-threatening chest injuries in children. *Clin Pediatr Emerg Med*. 2005;6:16-22.

19. Pollack IF, Pang D. Spinal cord injury without radiographic abnormality (SCIWORA). In: Pang D, ed. New York, NY: Raven Press; 1995:509-516.

20. Potoka DA, Saladino RA. Blunt abdominal trauma in the pediatric patient. *Clin Pediatr Emerg Med.* 2005;6:23-31.

21. Rana AR, Drogonowski R, Breckner G, Ehrlich PF. Traumatic cervical spine injuries: characteristics of missed injuries. *J Pediatr Surg.* 2009;44:151-155.

22. Rice HE, Frush DP, Farmer D, Waldhausen JH, APSA Education Committee. Review of radiation risks from computed tomography: essentials for the pediatric surgeon. *J Pediatr Surg.* 2007;42:603-607.

23. Sasser SM, Hunt RC, Faul M, et al, for the Centers for Disease Control and Prevention. Guidelines for field triage of injured patients: recommendations of the National Expert Panel on Field Triage, 2011. *MMWR Recomm Rep.* 2012;61(RR-1):1-21.

24. Weed T, Ratliff C, Drake DB. Quantifying bacterial bioburden during negative pressure wound therapy: does the Wound VAC enhance bacterial clearance? *Ann Plast Surg.* 2004;52;276-279.

25. Zorrillo P, Marin A, Gomez LA, Salido JA. Shoelace technique for gradual closure of fasciotomy wounds. *J Trauma.* 2005;59:1515-1517.

# Chapter 10

# PEDIATRIC BURN INJURY

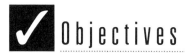 Objectives

- Explain the pathophysiology of burn injury.
- Appropriately assess and initiate management of burn injuries in children.
- Recognize inhalation injury in children and initiate appropriate airway management.
- Recognize and appropriately manage the sequelae of burn injury.

 Case Study

A 15-month-old girl is injured in a boiler explosion and partial building collapse. During initial assessment at a local emergency department, she is awake and crying, and her vital signs are remarkable for tachycardia and tachypnea. Physical exam demonstrates deep partial thickness burns involving 20% of her body surface area (BSA) and full-thickness burns involving 40% of her BSA. Approximately 40 minutes after arriving in the emergency department, the child produces black sputum and demonstrates stridor, respiratory distress, and somnolence. An arterial blood gas analysis reveals a normal $Pa_{O_2}$ of 99 mm Hg (13.2 kPa) and a $Pa_{CO_2}$ of 100 mm Hg (13.3 kPa).

**Detection**

- What are the priorities of assessment?
- What types of injury is this patient likely to have suffered? Are external burns the only possible injury?

**Intervention**

- What treatment strategies should be initiated immediately?

**Reassessment**

- Is the current treatment strategy effective?
- How much fluid is required for resuscitation? What will indicate the adequacy of resuscitation?

### Effective Communication
- When the patient's clinical status changes, who needs to know and how will the information be disseminated?
- What consultations are necessary?

### Teamwork
- How are you going to implement the treatment strategy?
- Who is to do what and when?

# I. INTRODUCTION

A burn is a traumatic skin injury that results from thermal energy or from chemical or physical agents. Annually in the United States, approximately 1.2 million people sustain burns, and one-third of burn unit admissions and deaths occur in children. Children younger than 4 years are the subset of the pediatric population at the greatest risk of burn injury, and this population also suffers the greatest risk of abuse. Overall, scald injuries represent 65% of burns suffered by children, while contact burns represent 20% of pediatric burn injuries. Despite improvements in burn care over the past 20 years, burn injury is still the fifth leading cause of unintentional injury-related death in children. Mortality is closely related to the depth and extent of injury as well as age.

# II. PATHOPHYSIOLOGY OF BURNS

The impact of a burn injury extends far beyond the involved areas of skin. The physiologic response to a burn can range from local inflammation in cases of limited injury to the systemic inflammatory response syndrome and, with more extensive injury, burn shock. Fluid loss from burned tissue is 5 to 10 times greater than that from healthy tissue and is accompanied by protein and electrolyte losses as well. Local edema is generated within 12 to 24 hours of injury and classically peaks between 24 and 48 hours. Some edema is always expected, but excessive fluid administration can contribute to pathologic edema if circumferential extremity burns are present. The systemic inflammatory response syndrome typically develops with burns of 15% to 20% BSA or greater. Temperature dysregulation, immune dysfunction with an attendant increased risk of wound infection and sepsis, and hypermetabolism are among the short- and long-term sequelae of significant burns.

## A. Approach

The approach to any emergency begins with an assessment of the airway, breathing, and circulation. The assessment of the airway and a critical appraisal of the risk of smoke inhalation and airway injury are particularly relevant to victims of a closed space fire. Supplemental humidified oxygen should be administered empirically until a thorough and definite evaluation is completed. Once the airway is assessed and stabilized, intravenous (IV) access should be established quickly, preferably with 2 large bore catheters. The volume of fluid resuscitation required is dictated by the depth and extent of injury.

# B. Initial Management

## 1. Airway Assessment

Signs of inhalation injury include respiratory distress, hypoxia, stridor, wheezing, singed nasal hairs and eyebrows, drooling, oropharyngeal blisters, tongue swelling, and production of carbonaceous sputum. If these signs are present, early intubation should be performed to protect the airway before progression to airway obstruction. Inhalation injury results from inflammation and edema generated in response to the inhalation of toxic and/or superheated products of combustion. The inflammatory reaction can lead to the formation of endobronchial casts and obstruction of the distal airways. Mucociliary clearance mechanisms are disrupted, and the accumulation of necrotic debris and products of inflammation provide an environment conducive to infection. These patients often benefit from bronchoscopy to enhance pulmonary toilet and minimize the risk of pneumonia or, when pneumonia is present, facilitate its resolution.

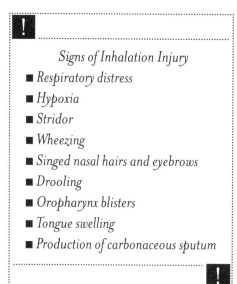

*Signs of Inhalation Injury*
- *Respiratory distress*
- *Hypoxia*
- *Stridor*
- *Wheezing*
- *Singed nasal hairs and eyebrows*
- *Drooling*
- *Oropharynx blisters*
- *Tongue swelling*
- *Production of carbonaceous sputum*

Inhalation injury may or may not be associated with carbon monoxide (CO) and cyanide (CN) poisoning. Any person exposed to fire in a confined space is at risk for CO and CN poisoning. CO poisoning may be responsible for as much as 80% of the mortality associated with inhalation injury. CO has a 250-fold higher affinity for hemoglobin than oxygen. It diminishes the oxygen-carrying capacity of hemoglobin and shifts the oxyhemoglobin dissociation curve to the left. It may also interfere with cellular oxygen metabolism at the mitochondrial level. Although measured partial pressures of oxygen are often normal in CO poisoning, there is relative tissue hypoxia. This is responsible for the delayed central nervous system sequelae of CO poisoning. This poisoning is diagnosed by measuring carboxyhemoglobin levels. Levels in excess of 5% are abnormal, and those greater than 25%, particularly when associated with headache or alteration in mental status, warrant referral to an institution where hyperbaric oxygen therapy can be delivered when feasible. In all cases, supplemental oxygen with $F_{IO_2}$ of 1.0 should be administered. The half-life of carboxyhemoglobin is 3 to 4 hours in room air, diminishes to 30 to 60 minutes at $F_{IO_2}$ of 1.0, and further decreases to 15 to 20 minutes under hyperbaric conditions at 3 atmospheres.

- *Diagnostic bronchoscopy is indicated in suspected inhalation injury to aid in definitive diagnosis.*
- *Therapeutic bronchoscopy facilitates removal of carbonaceous debris and the products of inflammation generated in response to inhalation injury.*

A high index of suspicion is necessary to diagnose CO poisoning because patients may present with nonspecific signs such as nausea, vomiting, headache, or altered sensorium. Any patient who suffers loss of consciousness at the scene of a fire should be assumed to have CO poisoning. All patients at risk for CO poisoning should receive 100% oxygen. Carboxyhemoglobin levels do not reflect the tissue burden of CO, so patients with significant neurologic abnormalities should be referred for hyperbaric oxygen therapy whenever possible.

CN poisoning results from an acute energy deficit caused by the inhibition of mitochondrial cytochrome C oxidase, rendering the cell unable to utilize oxygen. Inhalation of significant amounts of CN may therefore result in coma, seizures, apnea, and death. The historic CN antidote kit consists of inhaled amyl nitrite and IV sodium nitrite to convert hemoglobin-bound iron from the ferrous to the ferric state, thereby creating methemoglobin, to which CN preferentially binds, converting methemoglobin to cyanmethemoglobin. This is then followed by IV sodium thiosulfate, which converts cyanmethemoglobin into thiocyanate, sulfite, and hemoglobin. However, hydroxocobalamin, the hydroxyl form of vitamin $B_{12}$, combines with CN to form the nontoxic cyanocobalamin form of vitamin $B_{12}$, which is harmlessly excreted in urine. The advantage of hydroxocobalamin over the nitrites and sodium thiosulfate is that the former acts intracellularly and intravascularly, whereas the latter acts only intravascularly. Experience with hydroxocobalamin use in children remains limited, but continues to grow and is becoming the standard of care. As with the historic cyanide antidote kit, it must be administered as soon as possible following CN exposure for maximum benefit to be realized.

## 2. Fluid Resuscitation

The burn victim requires fluid resuscitation because the injury itself causes the elaboration of inflammatory mediators that produce local and systemic capillary leakage and intravascular volume loss. Superficial burns involving 10% to 15% of BSA can be managed with oral rehydration alone or with IV fluids for supplementation. Burns in excess of 15% BSA typically require IV fluid resuscitation, preferably with 2 large bore IV lines. A bladder catheter should be inserted to facilitate accurate monitoring of urine output and to assess the adequacy of the resuscitation. IV catheters can be safely placed through burned tissue, but placement distal to circumferential burns should be avoided.

The volume of fluid resuscitation that is required is dictated by the depth and extent of injury and historically was most commonly guided by use of the Parkland formula, which estimates the patient's fluid requirement to be 4 mL/kg/% BSA burn over 24 hours. Alternatives to this formula are the modified Brooke system, which recommends 2 mL/kg/% BSA burn over 24 hours, and the Brooke system as modified by O'Neill, which recommends 2 or 3 mL/kg/% BSA burn over and above maintenance IV fluids. Lactated Ringer solution is the initial resuscitation fluid, with 50% of the total volume delivered in the first 8 hours following the burn injury, and the remaining 50% over the subsequent 16 hours. Ultimately, fluid administration should be guided by repeated evaluation of the patient's intravascular volume,

---

*Fluid Resuscitation*

First 24 hours
- *Parkland formula: 4 mL/kg/% BSA burn over 24 hours*
- *Modified Brooke system: 2 mL/kg/% BSA burn over 24 hours*
- *Modified Brooke system as further modified by O'Neill: 2 to 3 mL/kg/% BSA burn over 24 hours plus maintenance IV fluids*
- *Fluids ultimately titrated to:*
  - *Heart rate*
  - *Capillary refill*
  - *Blood pressure*
  - *Urine output: 1.5 to 2 mL/kg/h (0-2 years), 1 to 1.5 mL/kg/h (2-10 years), 0.5 to 1 mL/kg/h (>10 years)*

Second 24 hours
- *Maintenance IV fluids*
- *Still may need resuscitation fluid in addition to maintenance fluid, albeit less than in first 24 hours*

which is reflected in the heart rate, blood pressure, capillary refill, and urine output, and readjusted as frequently as indicated. Adequate urine output is 1.5 to 2 mL/kg/h for children younger than 2 years, 1 to 1.5 mL/kg/h for children 2-10 years, and 0.5 to 1 mL/kg/h for children older than 10 years. Crystalloid is typically employed during the first 24 hours of resuscitation. The use of colloid in the initial resuscitation has not been shown to be beneficial. Albumin is often administered as a 5% solution at a daily dose of 0.3 to 0.4 mL/kg/% BSA, divided over 24 hours during the second 24 hours of burn resuscitation, in addition to maintenance IV fluids. As fluid resuscitation progresses, care must be taken not to overload the patient, as many burn victims receive a greater volume of fluid than that estimated by the given formulas.

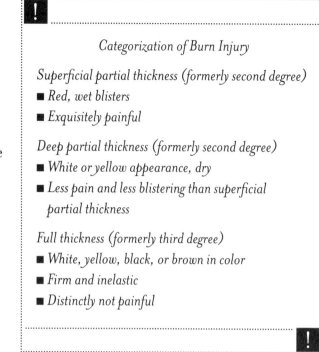

*Categorization of Burn Injury*

*Superficial partial thickness (formerly second degree)*
- *Red, wet blisters*
- *Exquisitely painful*

*Deep partial thickness (formerly second degree)*
- *White or yellow appearance, dry*
- *Less pain and less blistering than superficial partial thickness*

*Full thickness (formerly third degree)*
- *White, yellow, black, or brown in color*
- *Firm and inelastic*
- *Distinctly not painful*

### 3. Assessment of Burn Injury

The most appropriate tool to estimate the involved BSA in children younger than 15 years is the commonly published and frequently used Lund-Browder chart (**Figure 10-1**). The widely employed rule of nines is most appropriately applied to patients older than 15 years (**Figure 10-2**). Careful assessment of the depth and severity of injury is important because these factors heavily affect healing. The grading of burns as first, second, and third degree is imprecise and fails to accurately reflect the depth of injury. The current classification scheme, while more precise, is similar to the former insofar as it is also based on depth of injury relative to the anatomy of the skin. The categories are superficial, superficial partial thickness, deep partial thickness, full thickness, and deep full thickness (subdermal).

The skin is composed of 3 layers: epidermis, dermis, and subcutaneous tissue. The epidermis is the outermost layer and consists of stratified squamous epithelial cells known as *keratinocytes*. The epidermis is avascular and receives its blood supply and nutrients from the dermis. The basement membrane lies between the epidermis and dermis. The dermis is the most physiologically active layer of skin. It consists principally of fibroblasts but also contains basal epidermal cells, macrophages, and neutrophils, and is structurally supported by collagen, glycosaminoglycans, and fibronectin. The dermis contains blood vessels, lymphatic channels, sebaceous and sweat glands, and hair follicles.

The local response to burn is characterized by zones of coagulation, stasis, and hyperemia (**Figures 10-3** to **10-5**). The zone of coagulation is the most central area of injury and exhibits the necrosis that results from greatest contact with the heat source. The zone of stasis, or injury, surrounds the zone of coagulation (necrosis). The microvasculature of this tissue is disrupted, making it prone to secondary ischemic injury. Tissue within the zone of stasis has the potential for regeneration, but its circulation must be supported with fluid administration for the first 24 to 48 hours to maximize the survival of viable tissue. The zone of hyperemia, which surrounds the zone of stasis, is the minimally affected outer border of injury. Such areas heal spontaneously in 7 to 10 days.

# Pediatric Fundamental Critical Care Support

**Figure 10-1.** Lund-Browder Chart

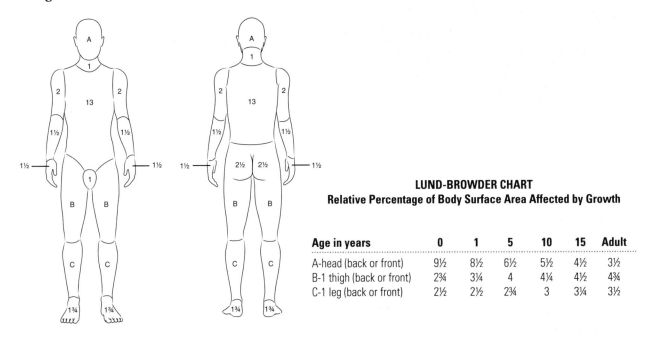

**LUND-BROWDER CHART**
**Relative Percentage of Body Surface Area Affected by Growth**

| Age in years | 0 | 1 | 5 | 10 | 15 | Adult |
|---|---|---|---|---|---|---|
| A-head (back or front) | 9½ | 8½ | 6½ | 5½ | 4½ | 3½ |
| B-1 thigh (back or front) | 2¾ | 3¼ | 4 | 4¼ | 4½ | 4¾ |
| C-1 leg (back or front) | 2½ | 2½ | 2¾ | 3 | 3¼ | 3½ |

The Lund-Browder chart is the most accurate method for estimating burn extent and must be used in the evaluation of pediatric patients under 15 years of age.

**Figure 10-2.** Rule of Nines

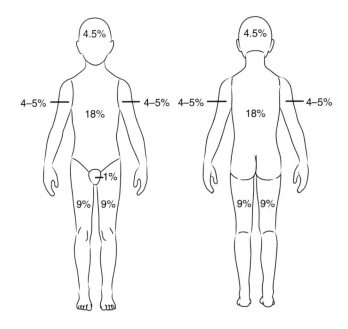

Most appropriate for children over 15 years of age.

**Figure 10-3.** Superficial Partial-Thickness Burn

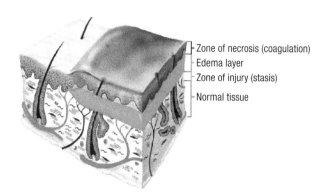

Reproduced with permission. © 2006 Elsevier. Duffy BJ, McLaughlin PM, Eichelberger MR. Assessment, triage, and early management of burns in children. *Clin Pediatr Emerg Med.* 2006;7:82-93.

**Figure 10-4.** Deep Partial-Thickness Burn

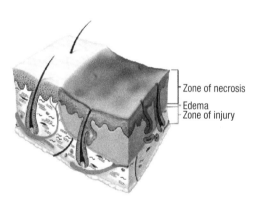

Reproduced with permission. © 2006 Elsevier. Duffy BJ, McLaughlin PM, Eichelberger MR. Assessment, triage, and early management of burns in children. *Clin Pediatr Emerg Med.* 2006;7:82-93.

**Figure 10-5.** Full-Thickness Burn

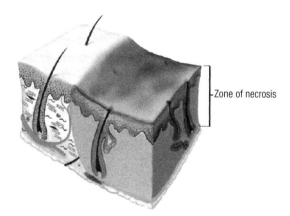

Reproduced with permission. © 2006 Elsevier. Duffy BJ, McLaughlin PM, Eichelberger MR. Assessment, triage, and early management of burns in children. *Clin Pediatr Emerg Med.* 2006;7:82-93.

Superficial burns involve only the epidermis. They are typically dry and characterized by erythema and pain without bullae. The keratinocytes slough, and epithelial cells migrate to the surface to facilitate wound closure. These injuries typically heal spontaneously within 5 to 7 days. They are managed with topical analgesics and moisturizing creams. They are not customarily included in estimating the extent of BSA burned because they heal completely without intervention.

Partial-thickness burns extend through the epidermis and into the dermis. Scalding typically produces this type of injury in children. Because partial-thickness burns are not homogeneous and can evolve over hours to days, debridement is usually necessary to accurately assess the depth of injury. Superficial partial-thickness burns, or mid-dermal burns, are erythematous and moist, and the presence of blisters is a hallmark. They are exquisitely painful because of the exposed and injured nerves. Superficial partial-thickness burns heal via re-epithelialization within 2 to 3 weeks.

Deep partial-thickness burns, characterized by a white or yellow appearance, may be less painful and demonstrate less blistering than superficial partial-thickness burns. As the depth of injury increases, the amount of pain decreases because more nerve endings are destroyed. Without intervention, deep partial-thickness burns can heal by epithelialization and contraction in 3 to 6 weeks. However, because the results are functionally and cosmetically poor, deep partial-thickness burns are typically managed with excision and grafting.

Full-thickness burns, formerly called *third-degree burns*, usually result from flame, prolonged contact, or hot oil or grease. Scalding, without prolonged exposure to hot water, rarely produces such burns. Full-thickness burns are characterized by white, yellow, brown, or black discoloration. There is severe edema without blisters, the texture of the skin is firm and inelastic, and eschar may be present. Deep full-thickness, or subdermal, burns extend to the fascia and muscle with the potential to involve tendon and bone. Usually seen in victims of house fires, deep full-thickness burns require skin grafting and may need musculocutaneous flaps.

# III. TREATMENT OF BURNS

## A. Criteria for Hospital Admission

The indications for a patient to be admitted to the hospital for burn care include superficial partial-thickness burns in excess of 10% BSA or to critical areas such as the eyes, face, ears, hands, feet, or genitals, inability to maintain adequate hydration or nutrition, caregivers who are unwilling or unable to provide burn care, burn injury in a child with a significant chronic medical condition, the need for IV analgesics or anxiolysis, and cases of suspected child abuse. The American Burn Association has established and published criteria for referring patients to burn centers (**Table 10-1**).

## B. Nonsurgical Wound Care

Among the goals of wound care are minimizing bacterial colonization and preventing infection. A variety of topical agents may be applied to superficial partial-thickness burns and deep partial- or full-thickness burns before skin grafting to prevent wound infection (**Table 10-2**). These include bacitracin, silver sulfadiazine, mafenide acetate, and silver-impregnated antimicrobial dressings.

The choice of topical agent or dressing has evolved over time based on research findings. These agents should be chosen in consultation with the burn center staff, if the patient is referred, as some agents will obscure the burn and may need to be removed for evaluation.

### Table 10-1. American Burn Association Indications for Referral to a Burn Center

- Partial thickness burns >10% total body surface area
- Burns that involve the face, hands, feet, genitalia, perineum, or major joints
- Third-degree burns in any age group
- Electrical burns, including lightning injury
- Chemical burns
- Inhalation injury
- Burn injury in patients with preexisting medical disorders that could complicate management, prolong recovery, or affect mortality
- Any patient with burns and concomitant trauma (such as fractures) in which the burn injury poses the greatest risk of morbidity or mortality. In such cases, if the trauma poses the greater immediate risk, the patient may be initially stabilized in a trauma center before being transferred to a burn unit. Physician judgment will be necessary in such situations and should be in concert with the regional medical control plan and triage protocols.
- Burned children in hospitals without qualified personnel or equipment for the care of children
- Burn injury in patients who will require special social, emotional, or rehabilitative intervention

Classified using American Burn Association/American College of Surgeons. Guidelines for the operation of burn centers. *J Burn Care Res.* 2007;28:134-141.

### Table 10-2. Topical Agents Employed in Burn Care

| Product | Application | Advantages | Disadvantages |
| --- | --- | --- | --- |
| Bacitracin | Superficial or deep partial-thickness burns, small areas | Not water soluble, good on face | Not indicated for large surface area |
| **Creams** | | | |
| Silver sulfadiazine | Deep partial- or full-thickness burns | Soothing, good for range of motion | Possible neutropenia, little eschar penetration |
| Mafenide acetate | Deep partial- or full-thickness burns | Penetrates eschar | Painful, metabolic acidosis |
| **Solutions** | | | |
| Aqueous silver nitrate (0.5%) | Deep partial- or full-thickness burns | Effective antimicrobial agent | Hyponatremia, stains wound, little penetration |
| Mafenide acetate (5%) | Graft dressing and open wound soak | Broad activity, moist dressing | |
| **Impregnated Dressings** | | | |
| Silver-containing antimicrobial barrier layer dressing (e.g., Acticoat) | Deep partial-thickness burn | Dressing change every 3 days (Acticoat 7 can be left on for 7 days) | Only deep partial-thickness burn |
| Silver-containing antimicrobial barrier containing dressing with absorptive wick-like properties (e.g., Aquacel Ag) | Deep partial-thickness burn | May be left on for 21 days | Less flexibility and ease of motion, only deep partial-thickness burns |

Bacitracin effectively protects against Gram-positive and a few Gram-negative organisms but may produce local irritation. Silver sulfadiazine is the most commonly used topical antimicrobial in burn wound management. It is bacteriocidal against Gram-positive and Gram-negative organisms and yeast. It is indicated for partial-thickness and full-thickness burns in anticipation of grafting. However, silver sulfadiazine is to be avoided in patients with sulfa allergies and glucose-6-phosphate dehydrogenase deficiency. Because it causes permanent skin staining, it is contraindicated for facial burns in children younger than 2 months. It is also contraindicated in late-term pregnant women due to the association of kernicterus and sulfonamides. Mafenide acetate is a bacteriostatic agent effective against both Gram-positive and Gram-negative organisms, including *Pseudomonas* and certain anaerobes. It is employed primarily in partial- or full-thickness burns because it can penetrate devitalized tissue. It is active in acidic (purulent) environments and is therefore particularly appropriate for eschar. Mafenide acetate can produce metabolic acidosis because it inhibits carbonic anhydrase.

A variety of relatively new, silver-impregnated, antimicrobial dressings with the ability to absorb exudate may be applied to burn wounds. The advantage of these dressings over the topical antimicrobials is that they can be left in place for several days, which eliminates the need for daily dressing changes and may in turn be associated with less pain and anxiety, thereby decreasing the need for sedation and analgesia. As yet there are no good comparative outcome data, but antimicrobial dressings appear to be equal in efficacy and cosmetic outcome compared to topical antimicrobial agents.

## C. Burn Wound Excision and Grafting

Although no controlled studies demonstrate improved outcomes with early excision and grafting of burn injuries, this practice is likely responsible for the decreased mortality from burn injuries realized over the past 20 years. The rationale for early closure of deep injuries is to reduce local infection and fluid loss and their attendant complications.

Current practice calls for grafting within 1 to 2 weeks of the injury. This should be performed by appropriately qualified surgeons, typically at a burn center.

For the young child with deep or large partial-thickness injury, it is often necessary to provide moderate to deep sedation, in addition to analgesia, to accomplish appropriate debridement and dressing changes. The depth of sedation necessary will depend on the extent of the injury, debridement required, the patient's age, and respiratory and cardiovascular status.

## D. Management of Inhalation Injury

Therapy for inhalation injury consists of aggressive pulmonary toilet, use of mucolytics, early identification and treatment of infection, and supportive care. Although no data support the routine use of mucolytics in patients with inhalation injury, many experts recommend *N*-acetyl-cysteine (3 to 5 mL of a 20% solution nebulized 3 or 4 times a day) or dornase alfa (2.5 mg nebulized once or twice daily) to help clear secretions. Routine prophylaxis with antibiotics is not used; corticosteroids are of no benefit and are potentially harmful.

The level of respiratory support that is required may range from supplemental oxygen to advanced modes of assisted ventilation and hyperbaric oxygen therapy. Supplemental humidified oxygen should be provided via nasal cannula or simple face mask. If stridor is present due to upper airway inflammation and edema, racemic epinephrine/adrenaline may be employed to transiently relieve the obstruction to airflow. Helium-oxygen admixtures (heliox) reduce resistance to turbulent airflow and, in turn, decrease the work of breathing in situations of upper airway obstruction. When the airway is compromised, however, these patients should be intubated for airway control. Based on a recent survey of pediatric burn centers, approximately 12% of pediatric burn victims require intubation, with approximately 70% of those intubated having sustained inhalation injury.

Current pediatric advanced life support guidelines support the use of cuffed tubes in all children. Ample evidence suggests that cuffed endotracheal tubes are safe and more effective in critically ill and burned pediatric patients, especially those with restrictive lung disease, in whom the presence of a leak around the endotracheal tube would impair oxygenation and ventilation. Tube size may be calculated using the formula that has been employed for uncuffed tubes: (age + 16)/4. However, children with burns and/or inhalation injury frequently experience significant airway edema; therefore, the size of the endotracheal tube should be reduced by 0.5 mm when using a cuffed tube.

The prevalence of acute respiratory distress syndrome in mechanically ventilated adults with major burns has been estimated to be as high as 54%. Although the prevalence in pediatric burn patients is likely lower, acute lung injury and acute respiratory distress syndrome represent significant clinical challenges, especially in very young patients. The level of pulmonary dysfunction should govern the mode of mechanical ventilation employed in the care of these patients. Lung-protective ventilator strategies should be used in those at risk for acute lung injury. Low tidal volume/high positive end-expiratory pressure is used initially and progresses to high-frequency oscillatory ventilation or airway pressure release ventilation in patients who require positive end-expiratory pressure in excess of 10 to 15 cm $H_2O$. Additional information on ventilator management may be found in the chapter on mechanical ventilation (**Chapter 5**).

Tracheostomy is classically utilized in patients following a prolonged course of endotracheal intubation. Although early tracheostomy (2 to 4 days after initiation of assisted ventilation) has also been used safely in a cohort of pediatric burn patients, the procedure is generally reserved for patients who have failed extubation or for those projected to require chronic mechanical ventilation, such as neurologically devastated patients.

# E. Hypermetabolism and Nutrition

The classic description of the metabolic response to injury includes an early hypometabolic "ebb," or catabolic phase, characterized by low cardiac output and a decreased metabolic rate, followed by a hypermetabolic "flow," or anabolic phase, that starts 24 to 36 hours after injury. Protein metabolism and energy expenditure increase by approximately 50% due to hypermetabolism, fluid losses, sepsis, and inflammation in children following a large burn injury, and this catabolic state can persist for 9 to 12 months. Early and aggressive nutritional therapy has been shown to reduce the elevated resting energy expenditure in burn victims. The most effective method of determining this expenditure is by indirect calorimetry; when that is not available, nutritional therapy is usually guided by a formula (**Table 10-3**).

### Table 10-3  Nutritional Therapy Formulas

| Age | Calculation |
|---|---|
| Infants (0-12 months) | 2100 kcal/m$^2$ + 1000 kcal/m$^2$ burn |
| Children (1-11 years) | 1800 kcal/m$^2$ + 1300 kcal/m$^2$ burn |
| Children (12 years and older) | 1500 kcal/m$^2$ + 1500 kcal/m$^2$ burn |

Adapted from Rose JK, Herndon DN. Advances in the treatment of burn patients. *Burns*. 1997;23(Suppl 1):S19-S26.

The enteral route is preferred for administration of nutrition. A nasogastric or nasoduodenal tube should be placed as soon as the initial evaluation and burn resuscitation are complete. In the absence of contraindications, enteral feeding should be initiated within 24 hours of injury. Feeding intolerance, as evidenced by significant gastric residual volume and diarrhea, may limit use of the gastrointestinal tract for caloric delivery. Diarrhea is a commonly encountered problem in the burn population. The etiology is likely multifactorial, usually noninfectious, and not worsened by hypoalbuminemia. Factors associated with a decreased incidence of diarrhea in burn victims include fat intake less than 20% of overall caloric intake, vitamin A intake greater than 10,000 IU per day in adults, and implementation of enteral feed within 48 hours of burn injury.

In addition to vitamin A, other vitamins, minerals, and trace elements may be required in excess of recommended daily allowances, including calcium, magnesium, vitamin D, zinc, copper, and other micronutrients. Supplementation of calcium and magnesium is recommended until serum levels are within the normal range.

In addition to early and aggressive nutritional support, attempts have been made to pharmacologically mitigate the hypermetabolic state that persists following burn injury. The hypermetabolism, which can be blunted to some extent by β-blockade, has led some to recommend the use of propranolol together with human growth hormone. However, these drugs should be used only in burn centers experienced in the care of children.

Attempts have also been made to accelerate healing through the use of anabolic agents such as oxandrolone. A recent single-center prospective trial has shown that administration of this agent improves the long-term recovery of severely burned children in terms of height, bone mineral content, cardiac work, and muscle strength, likely through decreased resting energy expenditure and increased insulin-like growth factor, benefits which appear to persist for up to 5 years post burn, without evidence of deleterious side effects. Again, use of this agent should be limited to burn centers experienced in the care of children.

## F. Hypoalbuminemia

In burn patients, hypoalbuminemia is a frequent finding. The etiology is multifactorial. Increased losses of albumin occur directly via drainage from wounds and diffusely as a consequence of profound capillary leakage, which is ignited by the cascade of inflammatory mediators triggered by the burn. Albumin production is also reduced in critical illness, likely due to an increase in production of acute phase proteins. Additionally, in the immediate post-resuscitation phase, a dilutional contribution to hypoalbuminemia may occur if intravascular volume is increased. Chronic illness and malnutrition are other potential causes of non-acute hypoalbuminemia.

Albumin contributes 80% of the normal colloid oncotic pressure; therefore, hypoalbuminemia is associated with edema, particularly of the pulmonary interstitium and bowel wall. Albumin is often administered in an effort to avoid exacerbating acute lung injury, diarrhea, feeding intolerance, impaired wound healing, and the resultant complications. However, the evidence demonstrates that mild to moderate hypoalbuminemia is well tolerated in previously healthy patients. Among burn patients with hypoalbuminemia, serum albumin gradually normalizes, especially in the context of aggressive nutritional therapy, and higher serum albumin concentration is seen in patients who receive enteral, as opposed to parenteral, nutrition. Therefore, routine albumin repletion may not be warranted. The current recommendation is to ensure appropriate caloric delivery, preferably by the enteral route, as quickly as possible. In critically ill pediatric patients; 25% albumin may be added if the serum level is below 2 mg/dL.

## G. Glycemic Control

As noted previously, protein metabolism and energy expenditure increase by approximately 50% in children following a large burn injury. The etiology of this hypermetabolic state is multifactorial but favorably affected by insulin administration. Hyperglycemia in adult burn patients is associated with increased morbidity and mortality. Although it has not been demonstrated that intensive insulin therapy can be safely and effectively implemented in the pediatric population, its use in the pediatric burn population may lower infection rates and improve survival. Careful attention must be paid to avoiding hypoglycemia. Members of the healthcare team participating in the care of pediatric burn patients should be sensitized to the importance of glucose monitoring and the recognition of hypoglycemia, especially in very young or nonverbal children. Standing insulin orders should only be written for those who demonstrate persistent hyperglycemia while they receive constant glucose delivery in the form of enteral tube feedings or parenteral nutrition; any orders must be associated with frequent bedside monitoring of serum glucose.

# IV. OUTCOME

Mortality from burns has improved over the past 20 years but may have reached a plateau in the past decade. The risk of mortality in children remains inversely proportional to age and directly proportional to extent of injury. In children older than 2 years who suffer burns to >50% BSA, mortality is approximately 20%, in younger children, mortality is approximately 50%. Early excision and closure of injured tissue is believed to be the reason for improved mortality. Smoke inhalation and thermal injury increase the risk of mortality by 20%.

Care of the pediatric burn victim has advanced in parallel with advances in burn and critical care. Early physical therapy, splinting of injured extremities, and advances in grafting techniques and skin substitutes all contribute to improvements in the quality of life following burn injury. Additional advancements in the elasticity of grafted tissues and microvascular reconstructive techniques promise to yield further improvements in cosmetic and functional outcomes.

## Pediatric Burn Injury

**Key Points**

- Initial evaluation of the pediatric burn victim begins with assessment of airway, breathing, and circulation. In addition, the extent and depth of burn injury must be assessed.

- Assess for inhalation injury, smoke inhalation, and CO and CN poisoning and treat if appropriate.

- Systemic inflammatory response syndrome, a common finding in burn victims, contributes to intravascular volume depletion and shock.

- Adequate fluid resuscitation, in the first 24 hours and beyond, is important to avoid early complications of serious burns.

- Fluid administration may be guided by the Parkland formula or modified Brooke formulas, but ultimately must be titrated to urine output and perfusion.

- Early excision and grafting are now standards of care in the management of deep partial- and full-thickness burns.

- Hypermetabolism is a significant long-term (9 to 12 months) sequela of significant burn injury, but appropriate management can significantly improve morbidity and mortality.

## Suggested Readings

1. American Heart Association. Pediatric advanced life support: 2010 American Heart Association Guidelines for Cardiopulmonary Resuscitation and Emergency Cardiovascular Care. *Circulation.* 2010;122(18 Suppl 3):S876-S908.

2. Barrow RE, Wolfe RR, Dasu MR, Barrow LN, Herndon DN. The use of beta-adrenergic blockade in preventing trauma-induced hepatomegaly. *Ann Surg.* 2006;243:115-120.

3. Duffy B, McLaughlin P, Eichelberger M. Assessment, triage, and early management of burns in children. *Clin Pediatr Emerg Med.* 2006;7:82-93.

4. Finfer S, Bellomo R, Boyce N, et al. A comparison of albumin and saline for fluid resuscitation in the intensive care unit. *N Engl J Med.* 2004;350:2247-2256.

5. Fortin JL, Giocanti JP, Ruttimann M, Kowalski JJ. Prehospital administration of hydroxocobalamin for smoke inhalation-associated cyanide poisoning: 8 years of experience in the Paris Fire Brigade. *Clin Toxicol (Phila).* 2006;44(Suppl 1):37-44.

6. Gottschlich MM, Warden GD, Michel M, et al. Diarrhea in tube-fed burn patients: incidence, etiology, nutritional impact, and prevention. *JPEN J Parenter Enteral Nutr.* 1988;12:338-345.

7. Greenhalgh DG, Housinger TA, Kagan RJ, et al. Maintenance of serum albumin levels in pediatric burn patients: a prospective, randomized trial. *J Trauma.* 1995;39:67-74.

8. Hart DW, Wolf SE, Herndon DN, et al. Energy expenditure and caloric balance after burn: increased feeding leads to fat rather than lean mass accretion. *Ann Surg.* 2002;235:152-161.

9. Jeschke MG, Finnerty CC, Kulp GA, Przkora R, Mlcak RP, Herndon DN. Combination of recombinant human growth hormone and propranolol decreases hypermetabolism and inflammation in severely burned children. *Pediatr Crit Care Med*. 2008;9:209-216.

10. Levine BA, Petroff PA, Slade CL, Pruitt BA. Prospective trials of dexamethasone and aerosolized gentamycin in the treatment of inhalation injury in the burned patient. *J Trauma*. 1978;18:188-193.

11. Mlcak RP, Jeschke MG, Barrow RE, Herndon DN. The influence of age and gender on resting energy expenditure in severely burned children. *Ann Surg*. 2006;244:121-130.

12. O'Neill JA. Fluid resuscitation in the burned child—a reappraisal. *J Pediatr Surg*. 1982;17:604-607.

13. Patterson BW, Nguyen T, Pierre E, Herndon DN, Wolfe RR. Urea and protein metabolism in burned children: effect of dietary protein intake. *Metabolism*. 1997;46:573-578.

14. Pham TN, Warren AJ, Phan HH, Molitor F, Greenhalgh DG, Palmieri TL. Impact of tight glycemic control in severely burned children. *J Trauma*. 2005;59:1148-1154.

15. Porro LJ, Herndon DN, Rodriguez NA, et al. Five-year outcomes after oxandrolone administration in severely burned children: a randomized clinical trial of safety and efficacy. *J Am Coll Surg*. 2012;214:489-504.

16. Sheridan RL, Prelack K, Cunningham JJ. Physiologic hypoalbuminemia is well tolerated by severely burned children. *J Trauma*. 1997;43:448-452.

17. Silver GM, Freiburg C, Halerz M, Tojong J, Supple K, Gamelli RL. A survey of airway and ventilator management strategies in North American pediatric burn units. *J Burn Care Rehabil*. 2004;25:435-440.

18. Suman OE, Mlcak RP, Chinkes DL, Herndon DN. Resting energy expenditure in severely burned children: analysis of agreement between indirect calorimetry and prediction equations using the Bland-Altman method. *Burns*. 2006;32:335-342.

19. Voruganti VS, Klein GL, Lu HX, Thomas S, Freeland-Graves JH, Herndon DN. Impaired zinc and copper status in children with burn injuries: need to reassess nutritional requirements. *Burns*. 2005;31:711-716.

20. Yurt RW, Howell JD, Greenwald BM. Burns, electrical injuries, and smoke inhalation. In: Rogers M, ed. *Textbook of Pediatric Intensive Care*. 4th ed. Philadelphia, PA: Lippincott Williams & Wilkins; 2008.

# Chapter 11

# NONACCIDENTAL INJURIES: DIAGNOSIS AND MANAGEMENT

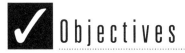 Objectives

- Identify risk factors for abuse.
- Describe injury patterns suggestive of abuse.
- Discuss the appropriate evaluation of the child with suspicious injuries.
- Describe the initial resuscitation of a child with potentially abusive injuries.
- Review the healthcare provider role as a potential/mandated reporter of suspected child abuse.

## I. INTRODUCTION

Child maltreatment is a tragically common cause of death, permanent disability, and suffering worldwide. Although many children present with histories and clinical findings that suggest abusive injuries, diagnosis and management may be complicated by atypical and delayed presentations, vague and misleading histories, and the patients' inability to communicate. Maltreatment must be considered in the differential diagnosis of any child presenting with injuries or a decreased level of consciousness.

Recognized risk factors for child maltreatment are varied, as can be seen in **Table 11-1**. Premature birth may interfere with infant-parent bonding. Babies discharged from the nursery after a prolonged hospitalization may have significant impairments, including developmental delays, feeding problems, and respiratory difficulties. They may be irritable and difficult to console, and may ultimately exhaust the ability of caregivers to cope. Toileting mishaps and irritating behaviors may result in abusive injuries to toddlers and other children in the household.

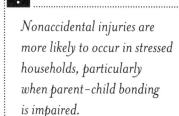

*Nonaccidental injuries are more likely to occur in stressed households, particularly when parent-child bonding is impaired.*

### Table 11-1  Risk Factors for Child Maltreatment

- Intimate partner violence
- Prior child abuse/neglect
- Substance-abusing caregivers
- Colicky/fussy child
- Prematurity or prolonged neonatal hospitalization
- Neurodevelopmental disability

# II. INJURIES THAT RAISE SUSPICION OF CHILD ABUSE

Caregivers may report mechanisms of injury that are highly unlikely at the child's developmental stage. Preverbal siblings may be blamed for injuries. Caregivers with substance abuse problems, particularly those involved in the production or sale of methamphetamine or other illegal substances may be reluctant to summon emergency medical services to the home and may opt to transport an injured child themselves despite the added risk to the child.

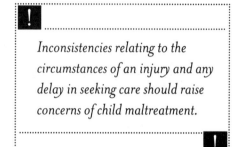

*Inconsistencies relating to the circumstances of an injury and any delay in seeking care should raise concerns of child maltreatment.*

## A. Patterns Suggestive of Abuse

Although patterns of physical injury are not absolute, among the injuries consistently found in children with witnessed, accidental injuries are epidural hematomas; simple, linear skull fractures; diaphyseal and spiral fractures in ambulatory children; and irregular, pattern-lacking, asymmetric thermal injuries that have splash marks and do not spare the popliteal or antecubital fossae. A comparison of some common accidental and nonaccidental injuries is presented in **Table 11-2**.

### Table 11-2  Accidental versus Nonaccidental Patterns of Injury[a]

| Site of Injury | Accidental Injury | Nonaccidental Injury |
|---|---|---|
| Head | Focal injuries at site of impact<br>Clear history of causative accident<br>Simple, linear skull fracture<br>Absence of other injuries | Global/widespread<br>Inconsistent description of injury<br>Diastatic, depressed skull fractures from reported short falls<br>Injuries to other body sites |
| Skeletal | Mid-shaft clavicular<br>Diaphysis of long bones in ambulatory children | Posterior ribs<br>Metaphyses of long bones in nonambulatory children<br>Vertebral body<br>Multiple sites<br>Varying ages of injury |
| Skeletal | Bruises over bony prominences in ambulatory children<br>Burns with splash appearance | Bruises to face or head in nonambulatory children<br>Bruises over padded areas, ears, neck, genitalia<br>Patterned injuries and bites<br>Burns with well-demarcated edges<br>Bruises or burns involving genitalia |

[a]No pattern of injury is diagnostic of either accident or abuse without consideration of the supporting history and developmental stage of the child.

Although accidental impact injuries to the head can result in subdural hematomas adjacent to the site of impact, such hematomas are uncommon in falls of less than 3 to 4 feet. Conversely, diffuse thin-rimmed subdural hematomas, retinal hemorrhages, posterior rib fractures, and metaphyseal fractures are more commonly found in children with inflicted injuries. Burns that are bilateral, symmetric, or of uniform depth; that have clearly defined borders, definable patterns, or evidence of healing or infection; or that include the anogenital areas should raise suspicion of maltreatment (**Figures 11-1** and **11-2**).

> *Although injury patterns may suggest either accidental or nonaccidental injury, they must be considered in the context of the description of the mishap, the child's medical and developmental history, cultural factors, and clinical findings.*

**Figure 11-1.** Burns Caused by Immersion in Hot Water

**Figure 11-2.** Small, Healed, Patterned Burns

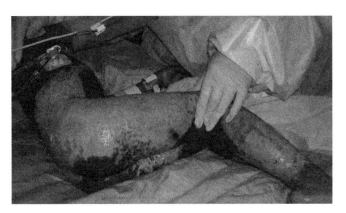

Full-thickness burns with flexure sparing due to immersion in hot water.

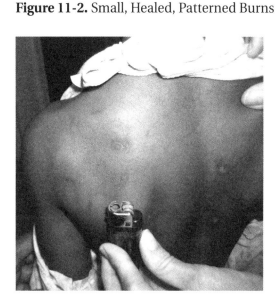

## B. Common Patterns of Maltreatment

### Case Study

A 2-month-old, previously healthy infant girl is brought to the hospital for evaluation of apnea and lethargy after having choked during a feeding. The child's mother states that the child started to have episodes of colic over the past week but was otherwise well before the mother went to work earlier that morning, leaving the baby and an older sibling in the care of her boyfriend. On initial examination, the infant is tachycardic with cool extremities, and respirations are irregular. The infant is immediately intubated and given fluid resuscitation. Although the secondary survey does not show any bruises, her anterior fontanelle is tense. Retinal hemorrhages are noted.

**Detection**

- What is the possible diagnosis?

**Intervention**

- What else needs to be done to resuscitate this infant?
- What diagnostic studies are indicated?

**Reassessment**

- What tests would be useful to evaluate the severity of the patient's condition?
- Have peripheral perfusion signs improved with resuscitation?
- Does the infant require other pharmacologic or surgical therapeutic interventions?

**Effective Communication**

- Where is the best place to manage this patient?
- Are other subspecialty consultations needed?

**Teamwork**

- How are you going to implement the treatment strategy?
- Who is to do what and when?

### 1. Abusive Head Trauma

Abusive head trauma, also known as shaken-baby or shaken-impact syndrome, is a frequently incomplete triad consisting of inflicted head injury with extra-axial hematoma, retinal hemorrhage, and skeletal injury, including metaphyseal and posterior rib fractures (**Figure 11-3**). Young infants are at the highest risk, but toddlers may display this pattern of abuse as well. A frustrated caregiver's violent shaking of a child, with or without concomitant projection onto a hard or soft surface, results in severe rotational and shearing forces capable of tearing bridging veins in the subdural and subarachnoid spaces.

Unlike children with accidental head injuries, who often present with clear histories and focal injury patterns, patients with inflicted head injuries will often present with more global cerebral findings, clinical features consistent with shock, and pallor. Caregivers commonly deny or minimize trauma. Soft-tissue swelling and bruising may or may not accompany severe inflicted head injuries, and bulging, tense fontanelles are noted. Loss of fontanelle pulsatility occurs as intracranial hypertension worsens. Cerebral edema may be fatal despite a relatively compliant infant skull (**Chapter 15**).

Inflicted skull fractures may cross suture lines, be numerous, and be widely diastatic. Inflicted primary brain injury is compounded by secondary injury resulting from hypoventilation, hypoxia, and hypoperfusion. Neurogenic fever may occur within a few hours of injury. Seizures are common in abused infants, may be subclinical, and are often very difficult to control. These secondary insults lead to profound, progressive, global cerebral edema and ischemia.

**Figure 11-3.** Radiograph From an Infant With Abusive Head Trauma

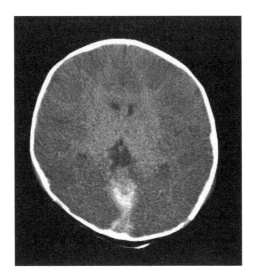

A radiograph reveals subarachnoid and subdural hemorrhages and cerebral edema consistent with abusive head trauma.

Other etiologies for intracranial pathology must be considered in the differential diagnosis of child abuse. Appropriate diagnostic testing and treatment, including antibiotics and possibly dexamethasone, should be rapidly initiated if bacterial meningitis is even a remote possibility. Acyclovir should be considered if the clinical picture suggests encephalitis. Nontraumatic causes of intracranial hemorrhage can be further investigated with neuroimaging and evaluation of coagulation or metabolic disorders.

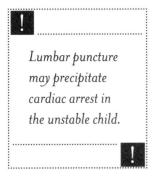

*Lumbar puncture may precipitate cardiac arrest in the unstable child.*

Lumbar puncture should be reserved for infants who do not demonstrate obvious respiratory or hemodynamic abnormalities. In general, this procedure should not be performed in the emergency department during the initial evaluation and stabilization of critically ill children. Significant risks of lumbar puncture include cardiopulmonary arrest, herniation syndromes in the presence of intracranial hypertension, and spinal epidural hematoma if the child is coagulopathic. Thus, lumbar puncture is best not performed until all such problems have been assessed or corrected.

### 2. Retinal Hemorrhages

The retinal hemorrhages that frequently, though not always, accompany extra-axial hemorrhages in inflicted head injury are the result of shear forces disrupting vulnerable tissue interfaces. The vitreous body is adherent to the retina in young children, and traction on this structure during rotational injury results in retinal hemorrhages occurring in multiple layers and extending to the periphery of the retina. This pattern is distinct

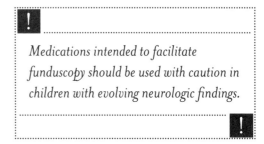

*Medications intended to facilitate funduscopy should be used with caution in children with evolving neurologic findings.*

from the focal abnormalities noted with increased intracranial pressure, sustained prolonged resuscitative efforts, and accidental traumatic brain injury. Medications that facilitate funduscopy should be used with caution in children with evolving neurologic findings because they may complicate the early diagnosis of worsening cerebral edema by precluding use of pupillary reactivity as a harbinger of evolving intracranial events.

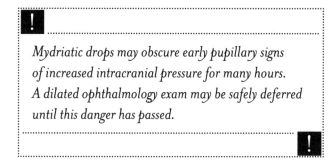

*Mydriatic drops may obscure early pupillary signs of increased intracranial pressure for many hours. A dilated ophthalmology exam may be safely deferred until this danger has passed.*

### 3. Blunt Abdominal Injury

 **Case Study**

A 3-year-old boy is found on his doorstep by his grandmother. Emergency services personnel called to the home note tachycardia and hypotension. He is resuscitated en route to the hospital. His abdomen is noted to be distended and tender to palpation.

**Detection**
- What is the possible diagnosis?

**Intervention**
- What needs to be done immediately to resuscitate this boy?
- How can the adequacy of resuscitation be determined as you proceed?

**Reassessment**
- What tests would be useful to evaluate the severity of the patient's condition?
- What radiographic studies are appropriate for evaluating the abdomen?
- What blood work should be obtained?

**Effective Communication**
- Where is the best place to manage this patient?
- Is a surgical consultation needed?

**Teamwork**
- How are you going to implement the treatment strategy?
- Who is to do what and when?

Inflicted blunt abdominal trauma is most commonly seen in mobile children, typically toddlers and children of preschool age. These injuries usually have a delayed presentation and extremely high associated morbidity. Although children in this age group may also sustain inflicted head injuries, these differ from the pattern seen in young infants in that they are usually due to direct or translational impact rather than rotational forces.

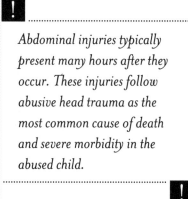

*Abdominal injuries typically present many hours after they occur. These injuries follow abusive head trauma as the most common cause of death and severe morbidity in the abused child.*

The combination of solid organ and hollow viscus injury in the absence of corroborated high-velocity impact is highly suggestive of child abuse. The following organs are the most commonly affected in inflicted abdominal injuries:

- Liver
- Spleen
- Kidney
- Pancreas
- Hollow viscus

Compressive forces may cause hematoma formation in the highly vascular duodenum. Although perforation may occur in any segment of the bowel, it is more common in the proximal jejunum due to that segment's relatively fixed position over the lumbar spine. Pancreatic contusion and transection may result in severe pancreatitis. Mesenteric disruption may compromise bowel perfusion, causing perforation. Hypovolemic shock may progress rapidly to uncompensated or even irreversible shock.

Much like inflicted severe head injuries, fatal abdominal injuries may occur without cutaneous evidence. Children may demonstrate abdominal tenderness, peritoneal signs, and distention on presentation. The diagnosis of abdominal injury may be missed in the presence of severe neurologic injury when bruising is absent. Given the life-threatening nature of abdominal injuries, they should be suspected and excluded in children presenting with other abusive injuries. Although computed tomography imaging readily demonstrates solid organ injury, hollow viscus injuries may escape detection until clinical deterioration occurs or a contrast study is performed.

### 4. Other Injury Patterns

#### a. Skeletal Trauma

Fractures involving the posterior ribs, scapulae, sternum, and spinous processes, as well as the metaphyses in nonambulatory children, are often associated with child abuse. However, any fracture that does not appear to coincide with a child's developmental stage, the related findings, and the reported mechanism of injury should raise suspicions of abuse and requires further evaluation. Posterior rib fractures in previously healthy infants indicate severe trauma to the skeletal system and, in the absence of a clear history of serious accidental trauma, are strongly linked to abuse. These fractures occur when a child is subjected to squeezing forces that cause disruption at the costovertebral junction, and they are often not visible on plain radiograph until they are in the healing phase of callus formation (**Figure 11-4**).

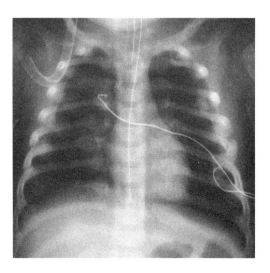

**Figure 11-4.** Numerous Healing and Acute Rib Fractures

### b. Cutaneous Injury

Bruises that occur in nonambulatory children, are clustered in a pattern, occur away from bony prominences of the body, and involve the abdomen, buttocks, back, face, ears, with or without hands should all be viewed with suspicion. Occasionally, cutaneous injuries have patterns that correlate with the object or implement used to inflict the injury (**Figure 11-5**). Bruises cannot be accurately dated by appearance, and medical professionals should be cautious in handling requests from investigative personnel to do so. Child maltreatment specialists may help determine the significance of cutaneous abnormalities in patients of specific cultural backgrounds. When the distribution of bruising does not match the history provided by family members, a past medical and family history of easy bruising and bleeding should be obtained.

### c. Sexual Abuse

Not only is sexual abuse distressingly frequent and underreported, it also often goes undiagnosed until other injuries or even pregnancy prompt evaluation. Any patient presenting with perineal trauma with or without a history of sexual abuse should be carefully evaluated; if the findings are suspicious, a report should be filed and a child abuse expert should be consulted for further examination. Of course, even in the absence of obvious perineal injury, patients presenting with clear disclosures of abuse should be reported and referred for expert evaluation.

**Figure 11-5.** Patterned Abusive Bruising

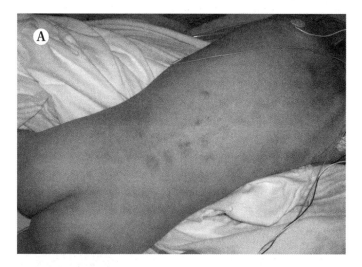

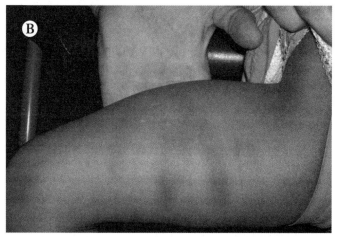

**A**, Many scratches and bruises over the back are present in this photograph. **B**, Clearly patterned bruising is visible on this child's thigh.

*Life-threatening abdominal or pelvic injury must be carefully excluded in any patient with perineal trauma.*

When a child has a history of sexual contact within the last 72 hours, an evidence collection kit must be prepared using appropriate measures to ensure that the chain of evidence is not disrupted. Anal dilatation may be an incidental finding during the initial evaluation of deeply sedated, critically ill children and may mimic sexual abuse. This and any other troubling findings are best evaluated and excluded by a pediatrician experienced in the evaluation of sexual abuse. The possibility of sexually transmitted disease must be addressed in any child presenting with suspected sexual abuse.

### d. Asphyxiation

Asphyxiation injuries may be difficult to diagnose. Smothering may share some features of near-miss sudden infant death syndrome and presents as a global hypoxic-ischemic injury with varying degrees of neurological and multiorgan dysfunction. Careful questioning after the patient's initial stabilization may elicit a history suggestive of deliberate or accidental suffocation. However, the true etiology of the infant's collapse may never be determined.

### e. Ingestions

Accidental ingestions are most common in children between 1 and 5 years of age. Ingestions in nonambulatory or preadolescent children should raise concern for abuse. All ingestions deemed to be accidental merit review of safety measures. Massive amounts of potentially lethal drugs may be forced upon children of all ages and may cause refractory hemodynamic instability with cardiac arrest. A comprehensive toxicology screen should be immediately obtained during the evaluation of any child with disturbed consciousness. Positive results for illicit drugs on screening drug tests should be confirmed to avoid reporting a potentially false-positive test. Prompt consultation with a toxicologist or a poison control center for optimal antidote and decontamination advice may be lifesaving (**Chapter 13**).

Caustic ingestions that are more severe than expected based on history or developmental stage may indicate that a child is living in a home where illegal drug use or manufacturing is occurring. This has become more common as the use of methamphetamines has increased.

### f. Medical Neglect

Medical neglect is yet another form of child maltreatment. The demands of caring for a chronically ill, technology-dependent child can become overwhelming. Substance abuse is a common comorbid factor in the negligent behavior of caregivers. Noncompliance with medical care may lead to near-fatal complications in children with diseases such as asthma, short bowel syndrome, and diabetes. Severe failure to thrive may present as a medical emergency when a child's weight is less than 70% of the predicted weight for length. Such children are at significant risk for refeeding syndrome with resultant life-threatening electrolyte disturbances and, thus, require close monitoring during the initial stages of support.

## III. ACUTE MANAGEMENT OF CHILD MALTREATMENT

Optimal care of any acutely ill or injured child begins with complete initial assessment followed by frequent, serial reassessments of the patient's **a**irway, **b**reathing, **c**irculation, and **d**isability (neurological) status, followed by **e**xposure and optimization of **e**nvironment (ABCDE). A complete set of vital signs and a Glasgow Coma Scale score must be obtained on presentation and at frequent intervals thereafter. All principles of Advanced Trauma Life Support and Pediatric Advanced Life Support should be observed when evaluating potentially injured children. Specific stabilizing measures for the initial management of pediatric trauma are described in depth in **Chapter 9**.

> *All principles of Advanced Trauma Life Support and Pediatric Advanced Life Support should be observed when evaluating potentially injured children. Specific stabilizing measures for the initial management of pediatric trauma are described in depth in* **Chapter 9**.

## IV. DIAGNOSIS OF CHILD MALTREATMENT

A thorough history must be obtained, with special emphasis on the caregiver's report of the mechanism of injury, and a complete physical examination must be performed. Caregivers and the child, if possible, must be interviewed separately as soon as possible after the incident to minimize the possibility that scripted accounts of the incident will cloud later reports. Historical details must be meticulously recorded, including but not limited to the following information: familial structure, child's previous medical condition, individuals with the child at the time of the incident, accurate description of the venue in which the reported incident has occurred, precise timeline of any and all events associated with the incident, actions taken by caregivers immediately thereafter. Physical examination must be performed with the child fully unclothed, taking care to avoid potential hypothermia. Any abnormality noted must be investigated with appropriate imaging and laboratory studies, and should be followed by serial clinical examinations as indicated.

Photographs of external findings, especially marks, bruises and superficial wounds, should routinely be obtained; such findings may change over time. Moreover, a picture will always provide a more accurate depiction than a drawing in the medical record. For photographs to have value, hospital policies must be followed and proper procedures used so that photographs identify the person depicted, date and time photo was taken, and the photographer.

Only emergent diagnostic imaging should be performed upon initial presentation. Non-emergent studies, such as a skeletal survey, should be obtained when the examination can be properly supervised by a pediatric radiologist familiar with child abuse. A poorly obtained study, even if repeated later, may present intractable problems for both investigation and prosecution. In addition, only preliminary interpretation of emergently needed imaging should be obtained initially, as all final interpretations and reports should be provided by a pediatric radiologist experienced in child abuse cases. This will minimize the risk of conflicting results or incorrect readings. Significantly, in some jurisdictions, nonemergent studies with an invasive component, such as those involving radiation, may require parental consent or court order if they are being obtained solely for forensic purposes. Finally, as with other types of traumatic injury, pediatric subspecialists, including trauma surgeons, neurosurgeons, orthopedic surgeons, anesthesiologists, intensivists, child abuse pediatricians, and child maltreatment agencies, where available, should be consulted as soon as possible, as some injuries require urgent attention in the trauma suite.

## A. Laboratory Tests

Initial laboratory studies are directed toward rapidly identifying end organ injury and its sequelae, as well as guiding critical care management (**Chapter 9**). Studies particularly relevant to the diagnosis of child abuse are delineated in **Table 11-3** and should only be ordered after consultation with a child abuse pediatrician. Calcium, phosphorus, and alkaline phosphatase levels can be obtained after stabilization to screen for systemic conditions affecting bone mineralization. Specialized studies and consultation may be indicated if a metabolic or genetic bone disease etiology for fracture is suspected.

**Table 11-3** Laboratory Studies to Consider When Child Abuse Is Suspected

| Problem | Laboratory Studies to Consider[a] |
|---|---|
| Skeletal injury | Complete blood count<br>Serum bicarbonate, creatinine phosphokinase<br>Serum calcium, phosphorus, alkaline phosphatase<br>25-OH vitamin D |
| Bruising/bleeding | Complete blood count<br>Coagulation studies<br>Von Willebrand disease panel if bruising is unexplained or if family history of bruising/easy bleeding |
| Possible blunt-force abdominal trauma | Complete blood count with serial hematocrit<br>Liver function tests<br>Amylase and lipase<br>Urine analysis |
| Altered level of consciousness | Bedside glucose and full electrolyte panel<br>Toxicology testing<br>Ammonia<br>Liver function tests |

[a]Other tests may be called for if the child's history, the family history, or the physical examination indicates other possible disease processes.

## B. Imaging

### 1. Computed Tomographic Scan

Non-contrast computed tomographic (CT) scan is the preferred study in children with suspected abusive head trauma. This study may be performed very rapidly and without sedation. Infants, toddlers, and children with decreased levels of consciousness should be immobilized for the scan in a manner that ensures airway patency, and they should be continuously observed during the study. Serial scans may be required in children found to have epidural hematomas, large evolving extra-axial collections, or a clinical picture of worsening cerebral edema.

A CT of the abdomen and pelvis will complement careful serial clinical examinations, but findings may be subtle in hollow viscus injuries. The role of ultrasonography is less clearly defined in this setting.

### 2. Magnetic Resonance Imaging

Magnetic resonance (MR) imaging is not as sensitive as CT in identifying acute hemorrhage. It is also a more lengthy study, may require additional transport of fragile patients, and often requires monitored sedation or general anesthesia with the attendant risks. In general, initial neuroimaging should be limited to a non-contrast CT of the head unless concomitant spinal cord injury is suspected. In that case, emergent MR imaging may be considered. Monitored sedation or general anesthesia is necessary to avoid added hypoxic or ischemic insult. Once past the acute phase of care, MR imaging may be helpful to child abuse investigations in determining the age of findings, such as CNS bleeds and extra-axial fluid collections. Again, it must be noted that in some jurisdictions, non-emergent studies with an invasive component, such as those involving radiation, or requiring monitored sedation or general anesthesia, may require parental consent or court order if they are being obtained solely for forensic purposes.

### 3. Skeletal Survey

A complete skeletal survey should be performed in children younger than 2 years of age when physical abuse is suspected. As discussed, this should only be done under the supervision of a pediatric radiologist experienced in child abuse, and it is not considered an emergent study. Protocols which follow the guidelines developed by the Society for Pediatric Radiology should be employed. Anteroposterior views of all extremities should be obtained, including anteroposterior feet and posteroanterior hands. Such studies should ideally be performed in the radiology suite. However, the risk of transport for an unstable patient may preclude this, and portable films may be initially obtained in the pediatric intensive care unit.

> *Initial skeletal survey must include two-view skull, two-view chest with bone technique, anteroposterior pelvis and abdomen, and lateral lumbar spine images.*

Acute fractures, particularly those involving the posterior ribs, may not be apparent on the initial skeletal survey in young children; therefore, a bone scan is recommended in conjunction with the skeletal survey once the child's condition has stabilized, because the radionucleotide tracer uptake in areas of increased bone turnover allows for identification of injuries that may go undiagnosed using standard radiographs. A repeat skeletal survey in 2 to 3 weeks to detect callus formation at fracture sites is an acceptable alternative to the bone scan in patients who cannot leave the pediatric intensive care unit. Although rib and metaphyseal fractures may not require orthopedic intervention, long bone and spinal fractures may need stabilization.

### 4. Funduscopy and Medical Photography

Funduscopy and photographic documentation by an ophthalmologist are important in establishing the extent and distribution of retinal abnormalities.

> *Photographic documentation of physical findings and retinal abnormalities is an important part of a child's evaluation but should never delay necessary interventions.*

# V. MEDICOLEGAL ASPECTS OF CHILD MALTREATMENT

Child abuse is extremely upsetting to the healthcare team. The physician and other immediate care providers must concentrate exclusively on the child's immediate medical stabilization and subsequent care. Involving social workers or child protection workers early is important. They can help gather vital information and can facilitate notification of the local child protection agency; all of these parties may act in concert with law enforcement to remove other vulnerable children from a dangerous environment.

Interactions with parents or other suspected perpetrators must remain civil. Remarks perceived as accusatory may hinder the child's medical care even if protective custody is not delayed. Unwise questioning may jeopardize the investigation.

> *The team's attention should be focused on stabilizing the child. All aspects of the investigation should be coordinated by social services and other child-advocacy professionals.*

The role of the physician and other healthcare providers includes coordination of the child's medical care as well as complete, objective, and legible documentation of all relevant findings and events. Careful, clear documentation with appropriate medical imaging and photographs obtained during the child's hospitalization will be immensely helpful if a case proceeds to criminal trial. Complete, unbiased, accurate medical information must be presented clearly and understandably to facilitate judgments that are in the child's best interest, protect the innocent, and hold offenders accountable for their actions.

Every U.S. state and territory mandates that injuries suspicious for child maltreatment must be reported by the professional caring for the child. Failure to report suspected nonaccidental injuries might enable repetitive, possibly fatal injury to the patient and endanger other children. Requirements for submitting a report – including whether such report must be personally submitted by the provider or can be done by another, such as a social worker, on the provider's behalf – often vary among jurisdictions. Thus, it is crucial to know the local statutes and regulations.

# Nonaccidental Injuries: Diagnosis and Management

- Complete initial and serial assessments of **a**irway, **b**reathing, **c**irculation, **d**isability, and **e**xposure and **e**nvironment (ABCDE) are central to the management of any seriously ill or injured child.

- All principles of Advanced Trauma Life Support and Pediatric Advanced Life Support should be observed when evaluating potentially injured children.

- Initial evaluation includes a bedside glucose measurement as well as targeted laboratory and radiologic studies.

- Multidisciplinary consultation with pediatric surgeons, anesthesiologists, and pediatric intensivists should be obtained quickly.

- Children with nonaccidental injuries typically present in a delayed fashion, complicating initial stabilization and eventual outcome.

- The team's efforts must be centered on the child's stability and comfort. Investigation of suspected abuse must be deferred to properly trained staff.

- Any negative factor, whether intrinsic to the child or to the caregiver, raises the risk of neglectful, abusive, and accidental injury.

- Patterns are suggestive, but rarely diagnostic, of abuse when compared with accidental injury.

## Suggested Readings

1. Aryan HE, Ghosheh FR, Jandial R, Levy ML. Retinal hemorrhage and pediatric brain injury: etiology and review of the literature. *J Clin Neurosci.* 2005;12:624-631.

2. Cooper A, Floyd T, Barlow B, et al. Major blunt abdominal trauma due to child abuse. *J Trauma.* 1988;28:1483-1487.

3. Dubowitz H, Bennett S. Physical abuse and neglect of children. *Lancet.* 2007;369:1891-1899.

4. Herr S, Fallat ME. Abusive abdominal and thoracic trauma. *Clin Pediatr Emerg Med.* 2006;7: 149-152.

5. Hudson M, Kaplan R. Clinical response to child abuse. *Pediatr Clin North Am.* 2006;53:27-39.

6. Lonergan G, Baker AM, Morey MK, Boos SC. Child abuse: radiologic-pathologic correlation. *Radiographics.* 2003;23:811-845.

7. McGraw EP, Pless JE, Pennington DJ, White SJ. Postmortem radiography after unexpected death in neonates, infants, and children: should imaging be routine? *AJR Am J Roentgenol.* 2002;178:1517-1521.

8. Starling SP, Patel S, Burke BL, Sirotnak AP, Stronks S, Rosquist P. Analysis of perpetrator admissions to inflicted traumatic brain injury in children. *Arch Pediatr Adolesc Med.* 2004;158:454-458.

9. Trokel M, DiScala C, Terrin NC, Sege RD. Patient and injury characteristics in abusive abdominal injuries. *Pediatr Emerg Care.* 2006;22:700-704.

# Chapter 12

# Pediatric Emergency Preparedness

## ✓ Objectives

- Discuss current issues and deficiencies in federal and state disaster plans related to the care of special populations.

- Identify the differences between caring for children and caring for adults during a disaster.

- Review select important physiological differences between children and adults.

- Describe children's unique vulnerabilities in certain disaster situations.

- Outline the importance of maintaining the family unit during a disaster.

- Summarize how to adapt current disaster plans to meet the needs of children.

## 📁 Case Study

A toxin was released near a large elementary school serving children aged 5 through 12 years. The toxin causes both shock and respiratory failure. Of the 300 children exposed, 87 will require high-end tertiary care, including mechanical ventilation. Available in the surrounding area are 30 pediatric intensive care unit beds, 20 open adult intensive care unit beds, and a total of 30 working mechanical ventilators. Eight local pediatric critical care physicians and 6 pediatric emergency medicine physicians have experience in treating shock and respiratory failure in the affected age group.

**Detection**

– What factors make children in this scenario more vulnerable to airway compromise compared to adults?

– When a minute counts, what would be the most effective way to triage a large number of pediatric victims during a disaster?

**Intervention**

– What antidotes should be used if this is a cholinergic agent and at what doses?

**Reassessment**

– Is our current local healthcare system equipped to manage a large number of pediatric patients?

– What is the next step if the number of pediatric-trained critical care, emergency medicine, or acute care personnel is insufficient?

**Effective Communication**
- Where should a first triage occur?

**Teamwork**
- Who should be directing where patients should be allocated?

# I. INTRODUCTION

In a disaster, children as a group may be at higher risk for injury than adults due in part to 2 factors: vulnerabilities related to their developmental physiology, including unique psychosocial factors such as mental health needs, school environments, and child care centers; and a disaster planning system that has historically centered on the healthcare needs of adults. Knowledge about terrorism, mass casualty incidents, and disaster response has come primarily from past military experience. For this reason, planning for disasters, including acts of terrorism, has focused almost exclusively on the adult population.

In 2010, almost one quarter of the total population of the United States was under the age of 18 years. Because the pediatric population is generally healthy compared with adults, peacetime medical systems allocate resources primarily to adults. That leaves only a few pediatric trauma centers to address critically injured children and limits the ability of community health systems to promote healthcare and disease-prevention strategies grounded in a well-child paradigm. Therefore, a disaster that affects the US population will take a higher toll among the vulnerable pediatric population and require more resources than are currently available. In previous large-scale natural disasters in the United States between 1992 and 2001, pediatric patients with an average age of 4 years represented one-third of all patients treated by disaster teams. In a recent evaluation of hospital surge capacity in New York State, area hospitals were found to have approximately one-half of the pediatric inpatient surge capacity recommended by US federal disaster-planning authorities and exceeded the recommended surge capacity for adult inpatients. Unlike the established US trauma system, nonpediatric trauma centers, and indeed all hospitals in general, will need to be prepared to receive and triage ill and injured children in a disaster. A recent study indicated that in a major pandemic, current hospital capacity to care for the expected number of critically ill or injured children would not be sufficient, even if capacity was increased by following recommendations for pediatric emergency mass critical care. Thus, hospitals that normally care for a limited number of low-acuity children will need to supplement children's hospitals that have reached maximum surge capacity, and all hospitals will require input from pediatric medical experts to provide care for pediatric patients in a disaster.

> *In a disaster, children may be at higher risk for injury than adults due in part to 2 factors: vulnerabilities related to developmental physiology and disaster planning that has historically centered on the healthcare needs of adults.*

In the current US healthcare system, because pediatric care is a specialty, only a minimal number of acute care, critical care, and emergency care providers are trained to assess, diagnose, and expeditiously treat severely injured children. Consequently, when a disaster strikes, pediatricians who may not have been trained to handle such situations will need to take leadership roles in treating pediatric patients in critical conditions. Given that pediatric emergency skills will diminish if not used or practiced, regular exercises in disaster response are critical. Equipment must be available in a range of sizes to accommodate children's differences in age, development, weight, and size. Although the majority of large medical centers may have appropriate supplies, specialty equipment may not be available at hospitals that do not routinely treat and triage children. These deficiencies in equipment and training also are reflected in disaster medical assistance teams.

In the interest of efficiency, US federal and regional medical supply stockpiles have adopted a one-size-fits-all approach. This is problematic because adult drugs may prove harmful in the younger population. Pediatric dosing requirements cannot be achieved due to how medications are stored, packaged, and prepared. The US Strategic National Stockpile of medical supplies has been modified so that a 12-hour push pack designed to supplement local supplies can be immediately dispatched after an emergency. The push pack contains medications that are approved by the Food and Drug Administration for use in children, but many of those medications arrive in adult-dose aliquots. Moreover, antidotes for chemicals used in terrorist attacks are not approved for children because significant questions remain regarding effective, nontoxic pediatric dosages. To have sufficient quantities of appropriate medicines available for children's needs in a disaster, altered standards of care would need to include dosage adjustments, changes to expiration dates, and guidelines for the use of adult-specific medications in children.

# II. UNIQUE PHYSIOLOGIC VULNERABILITIES IN CHILDREN

Because the needs of the pediatric population tend to be overlooked in disaster planning, healthcare leaders need to revisit disaster plans to ensure that they include appropriate care for children. Children are less able to escape disaster and more likely to suffer severe injury and require special care in the aftermath of disaster. Even in day-to-day situations, age-related physiological differences among children can complicate the work of providers without experience in pediatric assessment and triage (**Appendix 1**). Substantial differences based on size and physiologic and cognitive development also may increase the impact of a disaster on children.

> *Children are less able to escape disaster and are more likely to suffer severe injury and require special care in the aftermath of disaster.*

## A. Respiratory Vulnerabilities

Because children are closer to the ground than adults, they are at increased risk for severe airway injury from inhaling chemical agents that are heavier than air, such as chlorine and ammonia. A child's rapid respiratory rate and small body surface area increase the intake of agents that act on the respiratory system and the metabolic effect of those agents. Inhalational agents that cause mucosal irritation and airway edema may have more impact on children than on adults. Airway resistance increases proportionately to the fourth power of the airway's radius, so a small amount of edema or mucus can obstruct a child's airway and lead to severe respiratory compromise and death (**Chapter 2**).

In addition, children's short stature may make them more vulnerable to drowning during flooding. Over 90% of pediatric deaths during the Tōhoku earthquake and tsunami were attributed to drowning. Aspiration of water contaminated with bacteria, soil, and chemicals seen in victims of near drowning episodes will most likely predispose them to develop pneumonia and pneumonitis. This is referred to as *tsunami lung* and is well described in both the 2004 tsunami in Southeast Asia and the 2011 earthquake in Japan.

The compliant chest wall and relatively underdeveloped intercostal muscles found in infants and young children require the diaphragm to play a greater role in ventilation than it does in adults. The work of breathing may thus consume a large portion of a child's available energy and predispose them to respiratory distress and failure. A child's oxygen demand per kilogram of body weight is twice that of an adult (6-8 mL/kg as opposed to 4 mL/kg), so hypoxemia will occur more rapidly with inadequate alveolar ventilation.

Compared with adults, a child's tongue is larger in proportion to the oropharynx and may obstruct the airway in response to a minimal amount of lethargy. The trachea is flexible and narrow, which permits the airway to kink with flexion (as in inappropriate resuscitation techniques). Anatomic differences in a child's airway result in a narrow range of open airway positions, and airway occlusion with secretions or edema is common.

## B. Circulatory Vulnerabilities

A child's circulating blood volume is a larger percentage of total body weight than it is in adults (70 to 80 mL/kg versus 65 mL/kg). Due to a child's relatively small total blood volume, what may be seen as minor bleeding for an adult can be substantial blood loss in a child. Relative to body surface area, a child has a smaller fluid reserve and immature kidneys, which combine to leave the child more prone to hypovolemia and hypovolemic shock. From a global perspective, diarrhea leading to hypovolemia and shock is responsible for 17% of all deaths of children younger than 5 years. In the aftermath of a disaster, contaminated food and water supplies may contribute to severe gastrointestinal illness, causing significant morbidity and mortality in exposed children.

Children have a significant ability to compensate for volume loss by increasing heart rate. They also have a strong vascular motor response, which preserves preload. Tachycardia and vasoconstriction can mask the recognized signs of shock, like hypotension, until a child is nearly moribund. Uncompensated shock progresses more rapidly to death in children than in adults.

## C. Neurologic Vulnerabilities

Children suffer a different constellation of injuries due to trauma. A child's head is larger than an adult's, and the cranial bones and blood vessels are thinner relative to body size. This coupled with poor muscle strength in the neck predisposes children to head and neck trauma. Fractures of the C1 and C2 vertebrae account for 70% of neck fractures in the pediatric population and only 15% in the adult population. During a disaster with severe shock forces or a high-velocity explosion, children may be prone to severe, debilitating injuries that would result in their being placed in a low-priority category during triage.

Myelinization is incomplete in smaller children, which makes assessment of neurological injury and recovery potentially more difficult. Immaturity of esterase enzymes, including acetylcholinesterase, may make small children more vulnerable to pesticides and nerve agents. Children are also more prone to seizures than adults, so smaller doses of toxic agents are likely to have far greater negative consequences in terms of both morbidity and resource utilization.

## D. Musculoskeletal Vulnerabilities

A child's liver and spleen are relatively large and not as well contained within the rib cage as in adults, which causes these organs to be more vulnerable to blunt trauma. Because a child's ribs are flexible, they rarely break, and the force of an impact is transmitted to the underlying and unprotected vascular organs, which increases the risk of internal injury with hemodynamically significant hemorrhage.

A child's body surface area is largely in relation to weight, and the layers of skin are thinner than in adults. Both factors place children at increased risk for significant chemical and thermal burns and for hypothermia in response to environmental exposure. They also have consequences for treatment: large-volume, unheated adult decontamination showers will likely result in significant hypothermia in a small child.

## E. Developmental and Psychological Vulnerabilities

Children are more vulnerable during a disaster simply because they are often unable to recognize or escape danger. They may even be drawn toward dangerous situations because they are interesting. Paradoxically, they may flee rescuers due to the often frightening appearance of people in protective clothing (**Figure 12-1**). Small children are often unable to verbalize what they have experienced, which may confuse or mislead responders and result in inappropriate care.

It may be more difficult to decontaminate and evacuate children because they cannot be expected to follow group directives and require continuous psychological support. Children may have adverse reactions to caregivers, sometimes owing to fear of strangers or pain. Certain procedures, such as open wound management, will be more time-consuming in frightened children. With their larger body surface areas, children will also lose heat more rapidly than adults, which may lead to hypothermia. Members of the care team with experience in calming and reassuring children should be placed in charge of such situations. Because they are unable to care for themselves, large numbers of children who are not injured may wander around and require shelter.

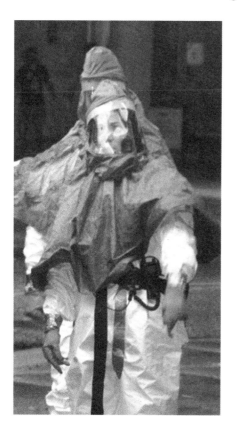

**Figure 12-1.** Rescuer in Protective Clothing

# III. TREATING CHILDREN'S DISASTER-RELATED INJURIES AND ILLNESSES

Despite their greater vulnerabilities, children with acute injuries or illnesses are more likely than adults to respond to rapid and efficient medical care and so will significantly benefit from appropriate preparation. In a disaster, most care will be supportive. Simple interventions such as supplemental oxygen and appropriately delivered intravenous fluids will save many injured children. We will address children's specific needs in a variety of disaster situations.

## A. Exposure to Chemical Agents

Children are vulnerable to injury from chemical agents in gaseous form due to their rapid respiratory rates. Gases that are heavier than air, like chlorine and ammonia, may accumulate in the small child's breathing space more rapidly than in an adult's. Nerve agent intoxication may manifest differently in children than in adults. During acetylcholine overload caused by nerve agents, children may be more prone to dehydration and shock from fluid loss due to gastrointestinal secretions. Children are also more likely than adults to have seizures during cholinergic crisis.

Antidotes to nerve agents and pesticides are often available in auto-injectors, but both the dose and the needle length may be inappropriate for children. Neither pralidoxime nor atropine has been extensively tested in children, and newer antidotes have not been tested in children at all. In cases of severe exposure, if adult-size Mark 1 auto-injectors are the only source of antidote, they should be used in even the smallest children. Dosing recommendations for atropine and pralidoxime in children are given in **Table 12-1**.

With their thin skin, children may be more vulnerable to the effects of vesicants, which place them at increased risk for systemic absorption. Given their higher ratio of body surface area to weight, children may lose a larger percentage of their skin than adults when exposed to the same volume of chemical agent. Children with large chemical burns are thus at higher risk for dehydration, hypovolemic shock, and hypothermia.

They may inhale vesicants, such as mustard agents, that are delivered in explosive blasts; these agents may more readily cause occlusion of children's small airways. Decontamination may be more difficult because children cannot follow directions and may need to be held throughout the procedure. High-pressure washing may injure small children, and cold-water washing may cause hypothermia and shock. Children are best decontaminated by attendants using warm water, but such a labor-intensive approach may not be practical during a disaster without meticulous advance planning and dedicated teams of responders at the scene.

### Table 12-1  Antidote Dosing for Anticholinesterase Exposure in Children

| Agent | Dose and Management | Mark 1 Auto-Injector Dosing for Severe Symptoms | | |
|---|---|---|---|---|
| | | 3-7 years or 13-25 kg | 8-14 years or 26-50 kg | >14 years or >50 kg |
| Atropine | 0.05 mg/kg IV or IM for moderately severe symptoms, up to 0.1 mg/kg IV or IM in clear cholinergic crisis every 2-5 min as needed for marked secretions, bronchospasms, hypoxia, respiratory compromise | 1 injector delivers 0.08-0.13 mg/kg | 2 injectors deliver 0.08-0.13 mg/kg | 3 injectors deliver <0.11 mg/kg |
| Pralidoxime chloride | 20-50 mg/kg IV or IM to a maximum 1 g IV or 2 g IM; may repeat every 30-60 min for weakness or high atropine requirement up to 2000 mg/h | 1 injector delivers 24-46 mg/kg | 2 injectors deliver 24-46 mg/kg | 3 injectors deliver <35 mg/kg |
| Diazepam | 0.05-0.3 mg/kg IV | | | |
| Lorazepam | 0.1 mg/kg IV or IM | | | |
| Midazolam | 0.1-0.2 mg/kg IV or IM | | | |

IV, intravenous; IM, intramuscular; N/A, not available
Classified using data from *America's Children in Brief: Key national indicators of well-being*. Federal Interagency Forum on Child and Family Statistics; 2012. http://www.childstats.gov/americaschildren/demo.asp. Accessed November 14, 2012. Rotenberg JS, Newmark J. Nerve agent attacks on children: diagnosis and management. *Pediatrics*. 2003;112:648-658.

## B. Radiation Exposure

The same factors that increase a child's risk of inhaling chemical agents also increase the risk of inhaling radioactive gases. Radiation-induced cancers occur more often in children than in adults exposed to the same dose. In utero exposure to radiation can cause intellectual disability and other congenital anomalies. Human breast milk is quickly contaminated with radiation, so infants of exposed mothers may not be able to breastfeed. Treatment with potassium iodide is recommended for children younger than 17 years and for pregnant and lactating women at lower exposure levels than those for other adults. To protect the thyroid from radioactive iodine, treatment with potassium iodide is indicated if the exposure projected by government sources is >0.05 Gy (>5 rad). Neonates treated with potassium iodide should have their thyroid function checked between 2 and 4 weeks after a single dose.

## C. Exposure to Biological Agents

The signs and symptoms of exposure to biological agents in children will be similar to those seen in adults. Fluoroquinolones and tetracycline (both used for anthrax and plague exposure) are contraindicated in growing children. See **Table 12-2** for acceptable alternative treatments.

### Table 12-2  Treatment for Exposure to Biological Agents

| Infectious Agent | Pediatric Prophylaxis | Pediatric Therapy | Notes |
|---|---|---|---|
| Inhalational anthrax | Ciprofloxacin 10-15 mg/kg PO every 12 h (maximum 500 mg/dose) for 60 days or doxycycline 2.2 mg/kg PO every 12 h (maximum 100 mg/day) for 60 days | Ciprofloxacin 10-15 mg/kg IV every 12 h (maximum 400 mg/dose) or doxycycline 2.2 mg/kg IV every 12 h (maximum 100 mg/day) and clindamycin 10-15 mg/kg IV every 8 h and penicillin G 250-600 U/kg/day divided every 4 h | Patients who are clinically stable can be switched to a single oral agent (ciprofloxacin or doxycycline) to complete a 60-day course of therapy |
| Cutaneous anthrax due to terrorism | | Penicillin V 25-50 mg/kg/day PO divided every 6 h or amoxicillin 40-80 mg/kg/day PO divided every 8 h or ciprofloxacin 10-15 mg/kg PO (maximum 1 g/day) every 12 h or doxycycline 2.2 mg/kg PO every 12 h (maximum 100 mg/day) | |
| Gastrointestinal anthrax | Same as inhalational anthrax | | |
| Plague | Gentamicin 2.5 mg/kg IV every 8 h or doxycycline 2.2 mg/kg IV (maximum 200 mg/day) or ciprofloxacin 15 mg/kg IV | Gentamicin 2.5 mg/kg IV every 8 h or streptomycin 15 mg/kg IM every 12 h or ciprofloxacin 15 mg/kg IV every 12 h (maximum 400 mg/dose) or doxycycline 2.2 mg/kg IV every 12 h (maximum 200 mg/day) or chloramphenicol 25 mg/kg every 6 h (maximum 4 g/day) | Chloramphenicol may be preferable in plague meningitis; use in young children may be associated with serious side effects |
| Tularemia | | Same as for plague | |
| Botulism | | Supportive care; antitoxin from CDC | |
| Brucellosis | | TMP/SMX 30 mg/kg PO every 12 h for 6-week course and rifampin 15 mg/kg every 24 h or gentamicin 7.5 mg/kg IM every day for 5 days | |

IV, intravenous; PO, by mouth; IM, intramuscular; CDC, Centers for Disease Control and Prevention; TMP/SMX, trimethoprim and sulfamethoxazole
Classified using data from *America's Children in Brief: Key national indicators of well-being.* Federal Interagency Forum on Child and Family Statistics; 2012. http://www.childstats.gov/americaschildren/demo.asp. Accessed November 14, 2012.

Children may be at increased risk for infection with smallpox because they have no immunity to the virus, whereas adults who were vaccinated as children may be protected. Children are efficient vectors for infectious agents spread by droplets and may be affected in numbers out of proportion to the global population. Due to their increased susceptibility to respiratory failure, in an epidemic of respiratory illness, children may have an increased need for mechanical ventilation and be at increased risk for fatal outcomes. Oseltamivir phosphate, which may be effective against influenza when used within the first 48 hours of symptom onset, is not approved for use in children younger than 2 weeks of age. Moreover, there is very little research to support the use of oseltamivir before, during, or after a pandemic. Zanamivir, another neuraminidase inhibitor approved for pediatric use in those as young as 7 years, has a more promising profile than oseltamivir for seasonal as well as pandemic flu. Those strains have not shown any resistance to zanamivir.

## D. Triage

During a disaster when resources are limited, hospitals must have rapid and reliable triage systems to prioritize the care of patients by severity and resource availability. Without an effective triage system, any emergency room can be quickly overwhelmed during a mass casualty incident. Here, we discuss a few popular triage systems that may be applied during a disaster when the main goal becomes allocating limited resources quickly to salvageable patients.

**Figure 12-2.** JumpSTART Pediatric Mass Casualty Triage

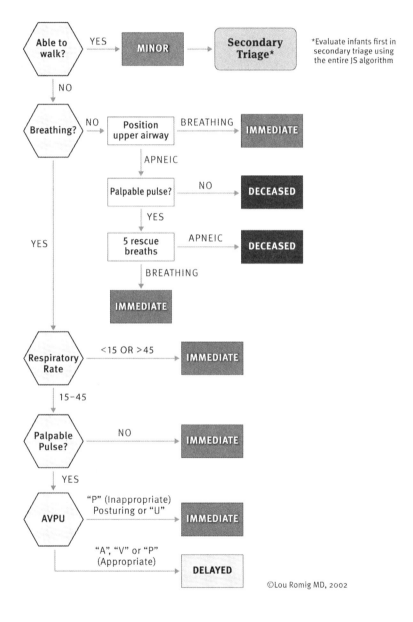

The Simple Triage and Rapid Transport (START) triage algorithm, developed in 1983, has an inherent advantage during a time of resource scarcity because it is quick and requires only vital signs and observational data. Later, Romig developed JumpSTART, a modified version of START for pediatric patients between infancy and young adulthood (early puberty) (**Figure 12-2**). Differences between the START and JumpSTART algorithms reflect physiological differences between adults and children. For example, a child with apnea is more likely to have a primary respiratory problem than an adult with apnea. Nevertheless, a child is more likely to be salvageable with restoration of ventilation and oxygenation. It is important to remember that no prehospital mass-casualty incident triage system has been validated for use for patients of any age during a disaster.

AVPU, alert, verbal, painful (stimuli), unresponsive
Reproduced with permission from Lou E. Romig, MD, FAAP, FACEP and Team Life Support, Inc. The JumpSTART Pediatric MCI Triage Tool Web site. http://www.jumpstarttriage.com/JumpSTART_and_MCI_Triage.php. Updated May 29, 2012. Accessed November 20, 2012.

While START and JumpSTART are examples of primary triage systems, the purpose of tertiary triage is to determine where the patients will be ultimately placed in the hospital (i.e., emergency room, inpatient ward, operating room, or critical care unit) or to determine if the patient must be stabilized and transferred to another facility with greater capacity or capabilities. Thus, tertiary triage helps to utilize limited resources in the most effective way during a disaster. The Sequential Organ Failure Assessment (SOFA) score is a relatively new organ failure score system developed to measure outcomes of intensive care unit patients. The mean and highest SOFA scores during an intensive care unit stay have been shown to be particularly reliable predictors of mortality, whereas an initial SOFA score higher than 11 can predict a mortality rate >90% (**Table 12-3**). A SOFA score and keen clinical judgment may help intensivists to determine which patients will most likely survive and which will not. The original SOFA score has not been validated in a pediatric population. No such score exists for children, and the difficult issue of predicting mortality in this population is made more difficult due to both this and to the special emotional bonds adults share with children. Both under- and over-triage, however, will cause significant additional mortality and morbidity during a disaster.

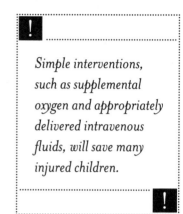

*Simple interventions, such as supplemental oxygen and appropriately delivered intravenous fluids, will save many injured children.*

### Table 12-3  Sequential Organ Failure Assessment Score

| Organ System | Score | | | | |
| --- | --- | --- | --- | --- | --- |
| | 0 | 1 | 2 | 3 | 4 |
| Respiratory: $Pao_2/Fio_2$ | >400 | ≤400 | ≤300 | ≤200 | ≤100 |
| Renal: creatinine (μmol/L) | ≤110 | 110-170 | 171-299 | 300-440; urine output ≤500 mL/day | >440; urine output <200 mL/day |
| Hepatic: bilirubin (μmol/L) | ≤20 | 20-32 | 33-101 | 102-204 | >204 |
| Cardiovascular: hypotension | No hypotension | MAP <70 mm Hg | Dopamine ≤5[a], dobutamine (any dose) | Dopamine >5[a] or epinephrine ≤0.1[a] or norepinephrine ≤0.1[a] | Dopamine >15[a] or epinephrine >0.1[a] or norepinephrine >0.1[a] |
| Hematologic: platelet count | >150 | ≤150 | ≤100 | ≤50 | ≤20 |
| Neurologic: Glasgow Coma Scale score | 15 | 13-14 | 10-12 | 6-9 | <6 |

[a]Adrenergic agents administered for at least 1 hour (doses given are in μg/kg/min).
MAP, mean arterial pressure
Reproduced under the terms and conditions of the Creative Commons Attribution License. Zygun D, Berthiaume L, Laupland K, et al. SOFA is superior to MOD score for the determination of non-neurologic organ dysfunction in patients with severe traumatic brain injury: A cohort study. *Crit Care.* 2006;10:R115.

# IV. PRESERVING THE FAMILY UNIT

Children are not self-sufficient and depend on family and caregivers. Adult patients will often place the needs of children above their own, and it may be difficult or inadvisable to separate children from adults in a disaster situation. If children must be separated from parents and families, specific measures must be taken to reunite them, particularly if the children are young and preverbal. It may be more efficient to leave family units together so that even injured adults can participate in the care of small children. When family members are separated, children are at greater risk for intentional injury, exposure, and accidents in the post-disaster period. If family members must be separated, emergency workers must get complete identification, and personnel must be assigned to the task of caring for the child until the family can be reunited.

Attention must be given to caring for the entire family unit. After Hurricane Katrina, children who were separated from their parents during the evacuation remained separated afterward and suffered psychological trauma. When children are evacuated with adults, the relationship between the children and their adult caregivers must be identified, and guardianship status must be determined.

In a disaster that occurs without warning, children may be at school or day care. Disaster plans should not assume that children will be in the custody of their parents when disaster strikes. Planning must take into account children who are not injured but need sheltering and evacuation. Although that may not be the job of hospital-based disaster healthcare providers, pediatricians need to ensure that local and regional planning accounts for the requirements of those who are not injured but cannot take care of themselves.

*If children must be separated from parents and families, specific measures must be taken to reunite them, particularly if the children are young and preverbal. It may be more efficient to leave family units together so that even injured adults can still participate in the care of small children.*

# V. ADAPTING DISASTER PLANS TO ADDRESS THE NEEDS OF CHILDREN

The needs of children are consistently overlooked in planning for disaster in part because there are already so many other shortcomings in the planning process. Many preparations made for adults may apply to children when disaster plans are tailored to include the pediatric population.

## A. Emergency and Prehospital Planning for Children

Pediatric-specific triage protocols should be taught to and practiced by first responders at the local, state, and national levels, and support for their development must come from the federal level. The specific educational needs of physicians, nurses, and respiratory care providers who will likely care for children in a disaster should be assessed. Emergency medical services personnel and response vehicles should be furnished with pediatric-specific equipment and medications. Pathways for communication, referral, and transport should be assessed and bolstered as necessary.

## B. Hospital Planning for Children

Disaster planning that considers the needs of children must prepare for situations in which the number of children who require medical care is out of proportion to normal numbers. When children are affected in proportion to their share of the total population, the hospital census will show a higher than normal percentage of pediatric patients. If a disaster occurs at a school, at a day care center, or on a school bus, the number affected could be even greater. In many cases, children may need to be cared for in nonpediatric units.

In general, hospitals that do not routinely care for large numbers of children need to include pediatricians on their disaster management planning teams. If pediatricians lack specific training in disaster management, appropriate education should be provided. The pediatricians, in turn, can identify and enhance areas of planning where the needs of children differ from those of adults. Plans to manage the surge of pediatric patients during a disaster may include organizing teams in which care providers with pediatric-specific skills supervise those without such skills.

Communication and modes of transport between community hospitals and children's hospitals should be detailed, including written transfer agreements that specify triage criteria. Equipment and pharmaceutical supplies should be evaluated for appropriateness for children. In institutions that do not regularly care for children, supplies may need to be augmented with pediatric-specific equipment, pharmaceuticals, and supplies (e.g., decontamination units and Mark 1 kits). Drills that include pediatric patients should be conducted.

In some cases, when large numbers of families are affected, units that normally do not care for entire families may need to be adapted. Such changes need to be planned and drilled in advance.

> *Disaster planning that includes the needs of children must prepare for situations in which the number of children who require medical care is out of proportion to usual numbers.*
>
> *Children's hospitals must serve as referral centers that take the majority of pediatric casualties when feasible and set the standard for pediatric disaster management.*

## Key Points

# Pediatric Emergency Preparedness

- The unique physiology of the developing child requires that disaster responders be familiar with the differences between children and adults with respect to disaster planning and response.

- A child's position within a family unit requires disaster planners and responders to plan for caregiving and family reunification.

- It is incumbent on caregivers and medical professionals to help families develop plans for disaster response well in advance of any incident.

- Disaster drills must be conducted with the child's unique physiology and position within the family unit in mind.

- The child's need may disrupt other elements of a disaster plan, as key personnel may not be available because they are taking care of their own children. Mechanisms to care for children of key personnel should be considered when developing site-specific disaster plans.

## Suggested Readings

1. American Academy of Pediatrics Committee on Environmental Health. Radiation disasters and children. *Pediatrics*. 2003;111:1455-1466.

2. Black RE, Morris SS, Bryce J. Where and why are 10 million children dying every year? *Lancet*. 2003;361:2226-2234.

3. Dolan MA, Krug SE. Pediatric disaster preparedness in the wake of Katrina: lessons to be learned. *Clin Pediatr Emerg Med*. 2006;7:59-66.

4. Eichelberger MR. *Pediatric Trauma: Prevention, Acute Care, Rehabilitation*. St. Louis, MO: Mosby; 1993.

5. Ferreira FL, Bota DP, Bross A, Melot C, Vincent JL. Serial evaluation of the SOFA score to predict outcome in critically ill patients. *JAMA*. 2001;286:1754-1758.

6. Furhman B, Zimmerman J, eds. *Pediatric Critical Care*. 3rd ed. St. Louis, MO: Mosby; 2005.

7. Hagan JF; American Academy of Pediatrics Committee on Psychosocial Aspects of Child and Family Health; Task Force on Terrorism. Psychosocial implications of disaster or terrorism on children: a guide for the pediatrician. *Pediatrics*. 2005:116;787-795.

8. Jenkins JL, McCarthy ML, Sauer LM, et al. Mass-casualty triage: time for an evidence based approach. *Prehosp Disaster Med*. 2008;23:3-8.

9. Kanter RK. Strategies to improve pediatric disaster surge response: potential mortality reduction and tradeoffs. *Crit Care Med*. 2007;35:2837-2842.

10. Kanter RK, Moran JR. Pediatric hospital and intensive care unit capacity in regional disasters: expanding capacity by altering standards of care. *Pediatrics*. 2007:119;94-100.

11. Lynch EL, Thomas TL. Pediatric considerations in chemical exposures: are we prepared? *Pediatr Emerg Care*. 2004;20:198-208.

12. Mace SE, Bern AI. Needs assessment: are disaster medical assistance teams up for the challenge of a pediatric disaster? *Am J Emerg Med.* 2007;25:762-769.

13. Middleton KR, Burt CW. Availability of pediatric services and equipment in emergency departments: United States, 2002-2003. *Adv Data.* 2006;367:1-16.

14. National Commission on Children and Disasters. 2010 Report to the President and Congress. AHRQ Publication No. 10-M037, October 2010. Rockville, MD: Agency for Healthcare Research and Quality; 2010. http://archive.ahrq.gov/prep/nccdreport. Accessed April 23, 2013.

15. Romig LE. The JumpSTART pediatric MCI triage tool and other pediatric disaster and emergency medical resources. http://www.jumpstarttriage.com. Accessed April 23, 2013.

16. Rotenberg JS, Newmark J. Nerve agent attacks on children: diagnosis and management. *Pediatrics.* 2003;112:648-658.

17. Waisman Y, Amir L, Mor M, et al. Prehospital response and field triage in pediatric mass casualty incidents: the Israeli experience. *Clin Pediatr Emerg Med.* 2006;7:52-58.

# 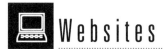 Websites

1. Chemical Hazards Emergency Medical Management. U.S. Department of Health & Human Service. http://chemm.nlm.nih.gov/.

2. Chemical Terrorism. New York State Department of Health. http://www.health.ny.gov/environmental/emergency/chemical_terrorism/poster.htm.

3. Children and Disasters. American Academy of Pediatrics. http://www2.aap.org/disasters/.

4. FEMA for Kids. US Department of Homeland Security Federal Emergency Management Agency. http://www.fema.gov/kids/.

5. Helping Kids Cope with Disaster. US Department of Homeland Security Federal Emergency Management Agency. http://www.fema.gov/coping-disaster#4.

# Chapter 13

# Management of the Poisoned Child and Adolescent

## ✓ Objectives

- Discuss the strategies to resuscitate, evaluate, and stabilize the poisoned patient.
- Compare indications and contraindications of decontamination and elimination techniques.
- Review common toxidromes, their presentations, and therapies.
- Explore two specific poisonings and therapy.

## Case Study

A 2-year-old girl is brought to the emergency department with minimal response to painful stimuli. Her heart rate is 80 beats/min, blood pressure is 70/40 mm Hg, and respiratory rate is 12 breaths/min. She has normal pupillary size and response.

**Detection**
- What is this child's physiologic status?
- What should be included in the differential diagnoses?

**Intervention**
- What are the immediate treatment priorities?
- Does the airway need to be secured?
- Any fluid boluses required?

**Reassessment**
- Is the treatment strategy effective?
- What is the etiology of the patient's altered mental status?
- Is any history available from the family?
- Is this child at risk for ongoing toxin exposure or absorption?
- Is any decontamination required?

**Effective Communication**

- Does the poison center need to be consulted?
- When the patient's clinical status changes, who needs the information and how will it be disseminated?
- Where is the best place to manage the care of this patient?

**Teamwork**

- How are you going to implement the treatment strategy?
- Who is to do what and when?

# I. INTRODUCTION

There are two major groups of poisoned children: those younger than 6 years in whom 99% of poisoning is unintentional, and adolescents in whom one must consider intentional causes. Children younger than 6 years tend to ingest a single agent in a small amount, which is usually nontoxic, and they present for medical attention shortly following the ingestion. Adolescent poisoning tends to result in more fatalities. These deaths are due to suicide, mixed ingestions, experimentation, intentional abuse, and delay in seeking medical attention. In all age groups, the most common class of substances resulting in fatalities in developed countries is analgesics, including acetaminophen (paracetamol) and salicylate. Other classes that result in fatalities include antidepressants, stimulants, and street drugs. In developing areas, pesticides, antimalarials, metals (including iron and lead), plants, and envenomation remain major sources of poisoning. In general, the mortality rate is low at a rate of 0.008 for all children <19 years old, and even lower at a rate of 0.003 for US children younger than 6 years in 2011.

In developing countries, most acute poisoning cases are unintentional and due to industrial toxins, such as organophosphates and envenomation from snake, arachnid, and insect bites. Acute and chronic poisoning can also follow the ingestion of fake, tainted, and "traditional" medications and foodstuffs, and the consumption of toxic plants by curious or hungry children. Chronic poisoning by water and food contaminated with heavy metals is also relatively common. Pediatric substance abuse is comparably rare in most developing countries with certain exceptions (i.e., street children and child soldiers).

## A. Resuscitation and Stabilization

As with all acutely ill children, the first step is prompt recognition and intervention in life-threatening conditions. A primary survey or rapid cardiopulmonary assessment focuses on the A (*airway*), B (*breathing*), C (*circulation*), D (*depressed level of consciousness, disability, drugs, decontamination*) approach. Vital signs should be obtained immediately and age-related norms considered. Isotonic fluids such as normal saline should be the

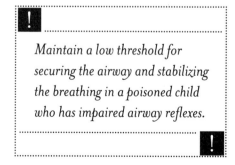

*Maintain a low threshold for securing the airway and stabilizing the breathing in a poisoned child who has impaired airway reflexes.*

first-line therapy for hypotension before the institution of vasopressors. Considerations during initial management of the patient with a depressed level of consciousness should include administration of dextrose, naloxone, and flumazenil.

Following stabilization, a secondary survey is conducted, which includes a more focused history to determine substance, quantity, and time of ingestion. In addition to vital signs and general physical examination, mental status, whether agitated or depressed, pupillary size, presence of nystagmus, and seizure often suggest a specific toxicologic syndrome, or *toxidrome*. Hypothermia, hypotension, or bradycardia suggests toxic ingestion of narcotics, sedative/hypnotics, or antihypertensives. Hyperthermia, hypertension, or tachycardia suggests anticholinergics, sympathomimetics, cocaine, or amphetamines. Dilated pupils are consistent with amphetamines, cocaine, anticholinergics, antihistamines, and sympathomimetics, while constricted pupils suggest narcotics, cholinergics, organophosphates, and phencyclidine. Nystagmus can be present with toxic ingestions of alcohols, carbamazepine, carbon monoxide, phencyclidine, ketamine, phenytoin, or sedative/hypnotics, while seizures can be caused by a number of agents (**Table 13-1**).

### Table 13-1  Signs and Symptoms Associated With Pediatric Ingestions

| Symptom | Toxic Causes | Clinical Tip |
| --- | --- | --- |
| Hypoxic Child | Carbon monoxide, methemoglobinemia, cyanide | |
| Hypoxia and Pulmonary Edema | Cocaine, amphetamines, metal fumes, nitrogen dioxide, opioids, salicylates and smoke inhalation | |
| Wheezing Child | Beta-blockers, irritant gases (chlorine), hydrocarbons, isocyanates, organophosphates, carbamates, smoke inhalation, and food-borne sulfites | |
| Increased Osmolar Gap[a] | Acetone, ethanol, ethyl ether, ethylene glycol, isopropyl alcohol, mannitol, methanol, propylene glycol, renal failure, and ketoacidosis (diabetic and alcoholic) | Calculated osmolality = 2 x Na$^+$ (mEq/L) + glucose (mg/dL)/18 + blood urea nitrogen (mg/dL)/2.8. Normal osmolar gap (between measured and calculated) = 3-10 mOsm/kg |
| Increased Anion Gap[a] | Methanol, uremia, diabetic ketoacidosis, paraldehyde, iron, inhalants (carbon monoxide, cyanide, toluene), isoniazid, ibuprofen, lactic acidosis, ethylene glycol, ethanol ketoacidosis, salicylates | Normal anion gap = [Na$^+$] - ([Cl$^-$] + [HCO$_3^-$]) Normal = 8-12 mEq/L |
| Methemoglobinemia | Benzocaine, dapsone, inhaled nitric oxide, lidocaine, naphthalene, nitrates, nitrites, nitroprusside, phenazopyridine, prilocaine, sulfonamides | |
| Tachyarrhythmia | Amphetamines, cocaine, caffeine, chloral hydrate, aromatic hydrocarbons, anticholinergics, and theophylline | |
| QT Prolongation | Amiodarone, arsenic, chloroquine, quinine, quinidine, organophosphates, tricyclic antidepressants | More agents have been shown to prolong QT; check current references. If the cause of QT prolongation is sodium channel blockade, administration of 1-2 mEq/kg sodium bicarbonate or administration of 3% saline may be helpful. |
| Sleepy Child | Antihistamines, any sedative hypnotic, alcohols, gamma-hydroxybutyrate, tricyclic antidepressants, opioids, carbon monoxide, cyanide, and hypoglycemic agents | Naloxone, glucose, or flumazenil may be diagnostic for reversing opioids, hypoglycemia, or benzodiazepines, respectively. |

| Table 13-1 | Signs and Symptoms Associated With Pediatric Ingestions (continued) | |
|---|---|---|
| **Symptom** | **Toxic Causes** | **Clinical Tip** |
| Seizures | Amphetamines, anticholinergics, antihistamines, butyrophenones, caffeine, camphor, carbamates, carbon monoxide, cocaine, cyanide, ethylene glycol, hypoglycemic agents, methanol, methylene dioxy-methamphetamine (MDMA), meperidine, isoniazid, lithium, nicotine, organophosphates, phencyclidine, phenothiazines, phenylpropanolamine, tricyclic antidepressants, salicylates, strychnine, theophylline, venlafaxine, *Gyromitra* (mushroom species) | Pyridoxine for isoniazid-induced seizures<br>Avoid phenytoin or fosphenytoin |
| Tachycardia | Amphetamines, caffeine, cocaine, theophylline, carbon monoxide, cyanide, hydrogen sulfide, anticholinergics (antihistamines, phenothiazines, tricyclic antidepressants, and atropine), ethanol, withdrawal from any psychoactive drug | |
| Bradycardia | Digoxin, organophosphates, carbamates, physostigmine, beta-blockers, clonidine, opioids, calcium channel blockers, and lithium | |

ᵃPlease see **Chapter 8** for an expanded discussion regarding osmolar and anion gap.
Classified using Pulsus Group, Inc. Koren G. A primer of paediatric toxic syndromes or 'toxidromes.' *Paediatr Child Health*. 2007;12:457-459.

With the possible exception of a blood glucose or arterial blood gas measurement, laboratory tests in poisoned patients are often not necessary for the initial resuscitation and stabilization. At the start of treatment, the determination of the anion and osmolar gaps, electrolytes, renal function, and specific serum quantitative tests can provide valuable information in mixed or unknown ingestions, and can help assess the need for antidotes or elimination therapies. Quantitative tests in pediatric toxicology (**Table 13-2**) should always include acetaminophen/paracetamol and salicylate levels as they represent common, treatable, and potentially lethal ingestions. Qualitative tests, such as those obtained using a urine toxicology screen, provide confirmation, assist in evaluation of altered mental status, and help determine the need for counseling. Other supportive tests include an electrocardiogram, co-oximetry, venom detection kits, and pregnancy testing in older girls.

| Table 13-2 | Useful Quantitative Tests in Pediatric Toxicology | |
|---|---|---|
| | • Acetaminophen (paracetamol)<br>• Anticonvulsants (e.g., carbamazepine, phenytoin, valproic acid)<br>• Barbiturates<br>• Carboxyhemoglobin<br>• Digoxin<br>• Ethanol<br>• Ethylene glycol | • Iron<br>• Lead<br>• Lithium<br>• Methanol<br>• Methemoglobin<br>• Salicylate<br>• Theophylline |

Adapted with permission. © 2005 McGraw-Hill. Hoffman RJ. Laboratory testing. In: Erickson TB, Ahrens WR, Aks SE, et al, eds. *Pediatric Toxicology*. 1st ed. New York, NY: McGraw-Hill; 2005:151-159.

## B. Gastrointestinal Decontamination

Gastrointestinal (GI) decontamination refers to measures to minimize absorption of the ingested toxin from the GI tract.

### 1. Syrup of Ipecac

> *Syrup of ipecac is no longer recommended for routine use in the home or hospital.*

Syrup of ipecac has not been shown to demonstrate any benefit, may interfere with charcoal administration, and may lead to complications like aspiration pneumonitis. As such, the American Academy of Pediatrics and the American Academy of Clinical Toxicology have recommended that ipecac no longer be used to treat ingestions.

### 2. Gastric Lavage

Gastric lavage, using a large orogastric tube and either saline or water, has no definite indications, with studies demonstrating lack of improvement in outcome. Thus, routine use is not recommended by the American Academy of Clinical Toxicology. Lavage may be considered under the following conditions: within 1 hour of ingestion; when a rapid deterioration in mental status is expected, such as with tricyclic antidepressants; or when even a minimal decrease in toxic exposure might be critical, such as may occur with ingestion of calcium channel blockers or lithium. The contraindications to gastric lavage include: ingestions of caustic agents, large foreign bodies, and sharp objects; the inability to protect the airway; and when the agent is not expected to be in the stomach. Complications include aspiration, esophageal or gastric perforation, decreased oxygenation during the procedure, hyponatremia, and water intoxication. The presence of a cuffed endotracheal tube may decrease, but may not eliminate, the risk of aspiration.

> *The contraindications to gastric lavage include:*
> - *Ingestion of caustic agents, large foreign bodies, or sharp objects*
> - *Inability to protect the airway*
> - *When the agent is not expected to be in the stomach*

### 3. Activated Charcoal

Activated charcoal (AC) has increased particle surface area to adsorb the toxins and is most likely to be of benefit if administered within 1 hour of ingestion. However, patients with salicylate ingestions may benefit from delayed administration due to delayed absorption and gastric emptying. The recommended dose is 1 g/kg, with a maximum recommended dose of 100 g. AC is effective for most tablet ingestions, though not for agents such as iron, lithium, alcohols, strong acids and alkalis, cyanide, and hydrocarbons. Multiple doses of AC have been shown to decrease serum levels of theophylline, dapsone, phenobarbital, carbamazepine, and quinine; however, the use of multiple doses has not been demonstrated to improve patient outcomes. Aspiration is a potential complication so AC should not be administered unless the patient is able to protect the airway or the trachea has been intubated. AC is contraindicated in patients with suspected bowel obstruction or perforation.

## C. Whole Bowel Irrigation

Whole bowel irrigation (WBI) using a polyethylene glycol solution (given orally or by nasogastric tube) produces a rapid catharsis with expulsion of the GI contents. Small children should receive 0.5 L/h, whereas older children and adolescents should receive 1.5-2 L/h. Infusion for 4 to 6 hours is usually required to achieve a clear effluent. No indications for use of WBI have been established due to a lack of demonstrated outcome benefit. WBI may be considered in potentially toxic ingestions of sustained-release or enteric-coated medications and drugs that are not well adsorbed by charcoal, such as iron, lithium, and lead. WBI may also facilitate removal of ingested packets of illicit drugs. The irrigation solutions can liberate toxins from AC and potentially interfere with its efficacy; therefore, activated charcoal should be administered before WBI. Contraindications to the use of WBI include the presence of ileus, bowel obstruction, bowel perforation, hemodynamic instability, and unprotected airway.

## D. Cathartics

Cathartic agents alone have not been shown to be beneficial, and their routine use in children is not recommended. However, because salicylate levels may increase due to its release from charcoal, administration of AC mixed in sorbitol is reasonable. Sorbitol has shorter transit times than any magnesium preparation.

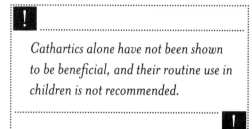

*Cathartics alone have not been shown to be beneficial, and their routine use in children is not recommended.*

## E. Enhanced Elimination

Forced diuresis, urinary alkalinization, hemodialysis, continuous renal replacement therapies, and charcoal hemoperfusion are attempts at enhanced toxin elimination with varying efficacies. Forced diuresis has been shown to be ineffective and is not recommended. Alkaline diuresis can increase the elimination of weak acids, such as salicylates and phenobarbital, and is indicated with ingestion of these agents. A general goal of urinary alkalinization is to maintain a urine pH >7.5.

Hemodialysis uses a semipermeable membrane to remove specific toxins from the blood against a concentration gradient. It should be used for substances that have a small molecular weight, are water soluble, have a small volume of distribution, and are not highly protein bound. Patients poisoned with substances resulting in renal failure, coma, or progressive instability and who meet the appropriate pharmacokinetic criteria should be considered as candidates for hemodialysis. These substances include ethylene glycol, methanol, phenobarbital, procainamide, lithium, valproic acid, carbamazepine, and salicylate.

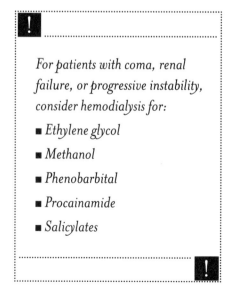

*For patients with coma, renal failure, or progressive instability, consider hemodialysis for:*

- *Ethylene glycol*
- *Methanol*
- *Phenobarbital*
- *Procainamide*
- *Salicylates*

Charcoal hemoperfusion uses a cartridge of AC to remove toxins from the blood and can be used for overdoses involving carbamazepine, phenobarbital, procainamide, and theophylline.

## F. External Decontamination

In the case of dermal exposure to toxins, any residual agent must be removed as soon as possible, with care taken to prevent others from becoming exposed. Running large volumes of lukewarm soapy water over the naked child is safe for most toxins, but not certain powder-based chemical weapons. Attention must be paid to the child's core temperature to avoid hypothermia. Contaminated clothing and runoff can be a source of secondary intoxication. Some volatile agents are toxic when exhaled, as are certain poisons in the vomitus and feces.

# II. TOXIDROMES

The most common toxidromes seen in children are summarized in **Table 13-3**. Recreational drugs causing hospital admissions are listed in **Table 13-4**.

## A. Sympathomimetic

Sympathomimetic poisoning syndrome presents with hypertension, tachycardia, seizures, central nervous system excitation, and mydriasis. Cocaine and amphetamines are the typical ingestants. Additional findings on physical examination include tremor, warm skin, diaphoresis, hypoactive bowel sounds, restlessness, paranoia, hallucinations, mania, and insomnia. Treatment is mainly supportive with benzodiazepines and short-acting antihypertensive agents for easy titration when necessary. Patients should be monitored for myocardial ischemia, stroke, and rhabdomyolysis.

## B. Narcotic

Overdose with a narcotic agent presents with a triad of miosis, respiratory depression, and depressed level of consciousness. Ingestion of heroin, morphine, or codeine can present with these findings, as well as hypotension, bradycardia, hypothermia, hypoactive bowel sounds, hyporeflexia, and confusion. Treatment for opioid toxicity is supportive, with naloxone as a specific antidote. The half-life of naloxone may be much shorter than that of the opioid, and repeat doses – or rarely, an infusion – of naloxone might be required. Also, the administration of naloxone might result in unmasking of pain, tachycardia, and systemic and pulmonary hypertension; thus it should be used with caution in patients at risk of pulmonary hypertension. Administration of naloxone for a patient with chronic exposure to narcotics may precipitate severe withdrawal crisis.

### Table 13-3  Common Toxidromes

| Toxidromes | BP | Pulse | RR | Temp | Mental Status | Pupil size | Peristalsis | Diaphoresis | Reflexes | Other | Common Causative Agents |
|---|---|---|---|---|---|---|---|---|---|---|---|
| Anticholinergic | N↑ | ↑ | ± | ↑ | Delirium | ↑ | ↓ | ↓ | N | Dry mucous membranes, flush, urinary retention, mumbling speech, picking movements; mnemonic: "blind as a bat, mad as a hatter, red as a beet, hot as a hare, and dry as a bone" | Antihistamines, atropine, antipsychotic drugs, scopolamine, tricyclic antidepressants |
| Cholinergic (muscarinic) | ± | ↓ | N↑ | N↓ | Normal to depressed | N↓ | ↑ | ↑ | N | Mnemonic SLUDGE: salivation, lacrimation, urination, diarrhea, GI upset and emesis; bronchorrhea | Organophosphates, physostigmine, pilocarpine, pyridostigmine |
| Cholinergic (nicotinic) | ↑ | ↑ | ± | N | Depressed | ↑ | ± | N↑ | ↓ | Fasciculations, paresis, abdominal pain, headache | Nicotine |
| Opioid | N↓ | N↓ | ↓↓ | N↓ | Depressed | ↓ | ↓ | N | N↓ | Some opioids (meperidine, tramadol) may not cause miosis | Opioids |
| Sedative/Hypnotic | N↓ | N↓ | N↓ | N↓ | Depressed | N↓ | | ↑ | N↓ | Ataxia | Barbiturates, benzodiazepines (clonazepam, alprazolam) |
| Sympathomimetic | ↑ | ↑ | ↑ | ↑ | Agitated | ↑ | N↑ | ↑ | ↑ | Tremor, seizures | Amphetamines, cocaine, caffeine, theophylline |
| Serotonin Syndrome | ↑ | ↑ | N↑ | N↑ | Variable | ↑ | N↑ | ↑ | ↑ | Clonus and rigidity greater in lower extremities | Citalopram, fluoxetine, paroxetine, sertraline |
| Withdrawal (ethanol/sedative hypnotic) | ↑ | ↑↑ | ↑ | ↑ | Agitated, disoriented | ↑ | ↑ | ↑ | ↑ | Tremors, seizures | Ethanol, barbiturates, benzodiazepines |
| Withdrawal (opioids) | ↑ | ↑ | N | N | Normal, anxious | ↑ | ↑ | ↑ | N | Vomiting, rhinorrhea, piloerection, diarrhea, yawning | Opioids |

BP, blood pressure; RR, respiratory rate, Temp, temperature; ↑, increased; ↑↑, very increased; N↑, no change or increased; ±, variable; N, change unlikely; ↓, decreased; N↓, no change or decreased

## C. Sedative/Hypnotic

Sedative or hypnotic poisoning presents with a depressed level of consciousness, respiratory depression, and hyporeflexia. Typical agents include benzodiazepines and, less commonly, barbiturates. Additional findings could include confusion, delirium, ataxia, blurry vision due either to miosis or mydriasis, and nystagmus. The mainstay of therapy is observation and supportive care, with cautious consideration of flumazenil as it may induce seizures. Once again, the half-life of flumazenil is relatively short and repeated doses might be needed if apnea recurs. Flumazenil is not recommended in the patient who received benzodiazepines to control seizures with resultant apnea/respiratory depression, and it is contraindicated in comatose patients if the diagnosis has not yet been made. Its use in tricyclic antidepressant overdose and in those regularly taking benzodiazepines may precipitate intractable seizures.

## Table 13-4  Common Causes of Recreational Poisoning

| Agent/Club Drug[a] | Mechanism of Toxicity | Clinical Features | Management |
|---|---|---|---|
| **Amphetamine (e.g., methamphetamine, paramethoxyam-phetamine)** *Speed, meth, ice, uppers, death* | Sympathomimetic: adrenergic receptor stimulation | **Cardiovascular:** tachycardia, hypertension, palpitations, arrhythmias, coronary ischemia **Metabolic:** hyperthermia, rhabdomyolysis, diaphoresis **Nervous system:** seizures, intracranial hemorrhage | • Supportive care and monitoring • Fluid and electrolyte balance • Benzodiazepines for seizures, hypertension, and sedation • Active cooling measures – ice packs; may need sedation and paralysis • Sodium bicarbonate for wide complex tachyarrhythmias |
| **Ecstasy (3,4-methylene-dioxmethamphetamine [MDMA])** *XTC, E, eccies, adam* | Sympathomimetic, serotonergic, SIADH | See amphetamines + hyponatremia, seizures, bruxism | • Avoid beta-blockers and phenytoin |
| **Cocaine** *Snow, crack, coke, rock* | Sympathomimetic, local anesthetic action, cardiac Na channel blockade | See amphetamines | • Antihypertensive agents • Nitrates and opiate analgesia for coronary ischemia • Sodium bicarbonate for wide complex tachyarrhythmias |
| **Ketamine (PCP is similar)** *Special K, Vitamin K, ket, cat valium* | Sympathomimetic | See amphetamines + altered sensory perception, injuries and trauma, emergence phenomena | • Consider multisubstance abuse |
| **Dextromethorphan** *DM, Dex* | Pro-serotonergic | Dissociative "high," dysphoria; if taken with MAOI or SSRI, will present with serotonin syndrome | • Patients may have anticholinergic appearance if the combination product contains antihistamine. • Check acetaminophen levels. |
| **Nitrates (amyl nitrate, butyl nitrate)** *Blue bottles, poppers, liquid incense* | Vasodilation, heme moiety oxidation | Hypotension, syncope, methemoglobinemia | • Supportive care, methylene blue for methemoglobinemia |
| **γ-Hydroxybutyrate (and precursors, GBL, BD)** *GHB, GBH-grievous bodily harm, easy lay, liquid G* | GABA receptor activation | Sedation, coma, myoclonus, seizures | • Supportive care |
| **Benzodiazepines** *Valium, Xanax, Ativan* | GABA receptor activation | Sedation, coma, hypotension | • Supportive care, flumazenil |
| **Anticholinergic agents** *Angel's trumpet, Datura sp* | Muscarinic receptor blockade | Delirium, dry skin and mucous membrane (inability to sweat), flushing of the skin, hyperthermia, visual impairment (mydriasis, loss of lens accommodation), urinary retention ("blind as a bat, red as a beet, hot as a hare, dry as a bone, mad as a hatter") | • Low stimulus, benzodiazepine sedation, physostigmine |
| **Methylene-dioxypyrovalerone (MDPV), mephedrone** *Bath salts, Ivory Wave, Vanilla Sky* | Sympathetic stimulation | See amphetamines + profoundly alerted mental status, sweating, mydriasis, muscle tremors and spasms, stroke, cerebral edema, respiratory distress, myocardial infarction, severe panic attacks, agitation, paranoia, hallucinations, and violent behavior | • Supportive care • Benzodiazepines (for sedation, to control seizures, or both) • Intravenous fluids, especially if suspicion of rhabdomyolysis |
| **Dihydrodesoxy-morphine-D, desomorphine** *Crocodile* | 8-15 times more potent than morphine, typically has impurities | Similar to morphine + skin in places of injection becomes grey and green, scabrous, flakes off so it resembles the skin of a crocodile; may cause peripheral limb ischemia with necrosis and possible secondary infection; may smell of iodine | • Supportive care • Naloxone |

[a]Street names are given in italics.
SIADH, syndrome of inappropriate antidiuretic hormone secretion; MAOI, monoamine oxidase inhibitor; SSRI, selective serotonin reuptake inhibitor; GBL, gamma butyrolactone; BD, 1-2-butanediol; GABA, gamma-aminobutyric acid

## D. Anticholinergic

The anticholinergic toxidrome includes thirst, hyperthermia, mydriasis, delirium, tachycardia, and dry skin, the latter of which differentiates anticholinergic and sympathomimetic toxidromes. Causative agents include atropine, diphenhydramine, antihistamines, tricyclic antidepressants, and antipsychotics. Many hallucinogenic plants (i.e., *Datura*, angel's trumpet, jimson weed) are anticholinergics. Other presentations could include hypertension, psychosis, chorea, seizures, coma, depression, confusion, hallucination, and urinary retention. Treatment is supportive with a focus on cooling and antihypertensive therapy. Benzodiazepines can be helpful in the agitated patient.

## E. Cholinergic

The cholinergic syndrome is classically described by the mnemonic *SLUDGE*: salivation, lacrimation, urination, defecation, GI upset, emesis; and the "killer B's": bronchorrhea, bronchospasm, and bradycardia. Organophosphates, found in some insecticides and in nerve gases like sarin, are agents that inhibit cholinesterase so that acetylcholine accumulates in the affected tissues. SLUDGE represents the muscarinic receptor toxicity, in addition to bradycardia, tachypnea, hypothermia, miosis, and bronchorrhea, while nicotinic receptor stimulation produces tachycardia, hypertension, fasciculations, confusion, weakness, paralysis, drowsiness, coma, and mydriasis. Children may present only with the central symptoms and with tachycardia instead of bradycardia, as nicotinic effects predominate over the muscarinic effects; however, miosis is usually present, as well as a garlic odor, which may suggest the diagnosis. Atropine, a competitive inhibitor of only the muscarinic acetylcholine receptor, and pralidoxime, an enzyme that reverses cholinesterase inhibition at both muscarinic and nicotinic receptors, are effective antidotes.

# III. SPECIFIC AGENTS AND ANTIDOTES

Common toxins and their antidotes are listed in **Table 13-5**; however, a more detailed discussion of acetaminophen/paracetamol and salicylate poisonings is warranted as they represent frequent, potentially fatal but treatable ingestions.

## A. Acetaminophen/Paracetamol

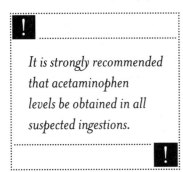

*It is strongly recommended that acetaminophen levels be obtained in all suspected ingestions.*

Acetaminophen is the most commonly reported potentially toxic pharmaceutical agent and the cause of the greatest absolute number of fatalities from poisoning in developed countries, given that it is a prevalent co-ingestant and has an increased incidence of therapeutic overuse. With the recognition of its role as a frequent cause of hepatotoxicity, liver failure, and death, and the availability of an effective antidote, it is strongly recommended that acetaminophen levels be obtained in all suspected ingestions.

### Table 13-5  Toxic Ingestions and Specific Therapies

| Agent | Therapy |
|---|---|
| Acetaminophen | N-acetylcysteine |
| Amphetamine | Benzodiazepine |
| Anticholinesterase | Atropine, pralidoxime |
| Benzodiazepine | Flumazenil |
| β-adrenergic blocker | Glucagon |
| Calcium channel blocker | Calcium, glucagon, insulin |
| Carbamate | Atropine, pralidoxime |
| Carbon monoxide | Oxygen, hyperbaric oxygen |
| Cocaine | Benzodiazepine |
| Cyanide | Amyl and sodium nitrite, thiosulfate, hydroxocobalamin |
| Tricyclic antidepressant | Sodium bicarbonate |
| Digoxin | Digoxin-specific Fab fragments |
| Ethylene glycol | Fomepizole, ethanol |
| Heavy metal | British antilewisite, ethylenediaminetetraacetic acid (EDTA), penicillamine, 2,3-dimercaptosuccinic acid (DMSA) |
| Heparin | Protamine |
| Hypoglycemic agent | Glucose, octreotide, glucagon |
| Iron | Deferoxamine |
| Isoniazid | Pyridoxine |
| Lead | British antilewisite, 2,3-dimercaptosuccinic acid (DMSA) |
| Lithium | Hemodialysis |
| Methanol | Fomepizole, ethanol |
| Methemoglobin | Methylene blue |
| Nitrites | Methylene blue |
| Opioids | Naloxone, nalmefene |
| Organophosphate | Atropine, pralidoxime |
| Phenothiazine | Diphenhydramine |
| Salicylate | Sodium bicarbonate, hemodialysis |
| Theophylline | Charcoal, hemoperfusion |
| Warfarin derivative | Vitamin $K_1$, fresh frozen plasma |

Metabolism in the liver is predominantly by glucuronidation and sulfonation; when these systems are overwhelmed by toxic ingestions, the cytochrome P450 system produces a highly reactive and toxic metabolite, N-acetyl-para-benzoquinone imine (NAPQI). This is usually reduced by glutathione into a nontoxic metabolite, but when glutathione stores are depleted, NAPQI increases and causes hepatocellular damage. Less lethal toxicity is seen in children as they have more glutathione than adults.

An acetaminophen dose of 150 mg/kg is potentially toxic, although much lower doses can be fatal in those children with glutathione depletion (i.e., malnourished) and chronic liver disease. Drug levels should be obtained 4 hours after ingestion, or as soon as possible thereafter, to assess the risk of toxicity using the Rumack-Matthew nomogram. The nomogram is not useful earlier than 4 hours post-ingestion as distribution following a single acute ingestion will not have occurred. A second level should be obtained 4 hours after the first when extended release formulations are suspected. The nomogram is only useful for acute exposure and does not apply to patients on long-term acetaminophen therapy. The antidote for acetaminophen poisoning is N-acetylcysteine (NAC), which acts as a precursor for glutathione and increases

> **Acetaminophen poisoning:**
> - *150 mg/kg may be lethal, lower doses in the malnourished and those with liver disease*
> - *Obtain serum level >4 hours post-ingestion*
>
> *RX:*
> - *Administer charcoal within 1 hour*
> - *Give NAC IV or PO when IV not available within first 8 hours*

non-toxic sulfation metabolism, among other mechanisms. NAC, available in both oral and intravenous forms, is most effective if administered within 8 hours of ingestion, but it should be given whenever acetaminophen toxicity is suspected. Activated charcoal binds to NAC, but losses due to charcoal binding are not clinically significant; therefore, charcoal should not be withheld in isolated acetaminophen ingestion presenting within 4 hours or with a potential co-ingestant.

## B. Salicylates

Although the overall incidence of salicylate poisoning has declined and there have been no fatalities in US children in 2011, these agents still have the potential to be a problem as they can be found in a number of over-the-counter oral and topical preparations, such as bismuth subsalicylate and oil of wintergreen. Physiologically salicylate poisoning initially causes a respiratory alkalosis by direct stimulation of the medulla, followed by an increased anion gap metabolic acidosis through a number of mechanisms. Thus, the initial blood gas measurement may be misleading to the uninitiated. Patients present with nausea, vomiting, tinnitus, cerebral edema, central nervous system disturbances, fever, coagulopathy, pulmonary edema, hepatotoxicity, rhabdomyolysis, hypoglycemia, hypokalemia, and dehydration. Infants and children may not manifest the initial respiratory alkalosis.

Ingestion of more than 150 mg/kg of salicylate should be considered toxic. A ferric chloride test, where 1 to 2 drops of $FeCl^3$ in 1 mL of urine produces a purple color change in the presence of any salicylate, or the Phenistix test (Miles Laboratories), which produces a brown color change, may be performed as a screen, when salicylate levels are not readily available. A quantitative test will be necessary to determine therapy. In acute ingestions, symptoms are typically present with levels >30 mg/dL (2.15 mmol/L); patients with levels >100 mg/dL (7.14 mmol/L) should undergo dialysis. In long-term ingestions, serum levels are unreliable in predicting severity of illness; however, a level >60 mg/dL (4.3 mmol/L) may be a relative indication for dialysis, as are seizures, altered mental status, refractory acidosis, or deterioration despite adequate supportive care.

> **Salicylate poisoning:**
> - *>150 mg/kg is toxic*
> - *Symptoms with blood levels >30 mg/dL*
>
> *RX:*
> - *Use GI emptying and activated charcoal*
> - *Alkalinize urine for serum level >40 mg/dL*
> - *Consider dialysis for serum levels >100 mg/dL*

The treatment plan should include GI decontamination with gastric emptying in an acute overdose and AC for large ingestions. Aggressive fluid resuscitation is an important first step. Urine alkalinization to trap ions and thereby prevent tubular absorption in the kidney should be instituted for serum levels >40 mg/dL (2.2 mmol/L) or in the presence of signs and symptoms of salicylism. Acetazolamide is not recommended; although it alkalinizes the urine, it acidifies the serum.

## C. Antivenom

Antivenoms are available for certain reptile and arthropod venoms. Most are purified polyvalent immunoglobulins produced by injection of small amounts of venom into dedicated horses or sheep. As foreign proteins, they have a risk of inducing hypersensitivity reactions, both type I and type III. In view of this and their cost, they are indicated only for cases of envenomation, not after all bites. High-quality antivenoms exist for all major venomous Australian, European, and North American snakes, and many Asian, African, and South American snakes, various arthropods, and the Australian box jellyfish (*Chironex fleckeri*) and stonefish. It is important to ensure that the product used is appropriate for the likely species, has been appropriately stored, and is a genuine product from a reputable supplier. Low-quality and fake antivenoms are a major problem in several countries, particularly in Asia and Africa.

# Management of the Poisoned Child and Adolescent

**Key Points**

- After addressing the *ABCD* of resuscitation, administration of dextrose, naloxone, or flumazenil should be considered in patients who present with a depressed level of consciousness.

- Neither flumazenil or naloxone should be administered in any patient with a history of chronic benzodiazepine or narcotic administration, respectively, as administration may precipitate drug withdrawal.

- Initial blood tests should always include acetaminophen/paracetamol and salicylate levels as they represent common treatable and potentially lethal ingestions.

- Syrup of ipecac is no longer recommended for routine use in the home or hospital.

- For the majority of ingestions, administration of activated charcoal or gastric lavage is only indicated if the patient presents within 1 hour of ingestion.

- Knowledge of the symptoms of common toxidromes will allow rapid identification of the most likely cause and timely initiation of appropriate treatment of the poisoned patient.

# Suggested Readings

1. Abbruzzi G, Stork CM. Pediatric toxicologic concerns. *Emerg Med Clin North Am.* 2002;20: 223-247.

2. Bronstein AC, Spyler DA, Cantilena LR, et al. 2011 annual report of the American Association of Poison Control Centers' National Poison Data System (NPDS): 29th Annual Report. *Clin Toxicol.* 2012;50:911-1164.

3. Hoffman RJ. Laboratory testing. In: Erickson TB, Ahrens WR, Aks SE, Baum C, Ling LJ, eds. *Pediatric Toxicology.* 1st ed. New York, NY: McGraw Hill; 2005:151-159.

4. Larson AM, Polson J, Fontana RJ, et al. Acetaminophen-induced acute liver failure: results of a United States multicenter, prospective study. *Hepatology.* 2005;42:1364-1372.

5. Mazor S, Aks SE. Antidotes. In: Erickson TB, Ahrens WR, Aks SE, Baum C, Ling LJ, eds. *Pediatric Toxicology.* 1st ed. New York, NY: McGraw Hill; 2005:121-131.

6. Osterhoudt KC, Ewald MB, Shannon M, Henretig F. Toxicologic emergencies. In: Fleisher G, Ludwig S, Henretig F, eds. *Textbook of Pediatric Emergency Medicine.* 5th ed. Philadelphia, PA: Lippincott Williams and Wilkins; 2006:951-1007.

7. Position paper: cathartics. American Academy of Clinical Toxicology; European Association of Poisons Centers and Clinical Toxicologists. *J Toxicol Clin Toxicol.* 2004;42:243-253.

8. Position paper: whole bowel irrigation. American Academy of Clinical Toxicology; European Association of Poisons Centers and Clinical Toxicologists. *J Toxicol Clin Toxicol.* 2004;42:843-854.

9. Tenenbein M. Recent advances in pediatric toxicology. *Pediatr Clin North Am.* 1999;46:1179-1188.

10. Vale JA, Kulig K, American Academy of Clinical Toxicology, European Association of Poisons Centers and Clinical Toxicologists. Position paper: gastric lavage. *J Toxicol Clin Toxicol.* 2004;42:933-943.

# Chapter 14

# Transport of the Critically Ill Child

## ✓ Objectives

- Describe the communication process for the safe transport of the critically ill child.
- Specify the information the referring institution should provide to the transport team and accepting facility to facilitate stabilization, appropriate referral, and timely transfer.
- Outline methods for stabilization of the critically ill child prior to transfer.
- Identify the factors that influence transport team composition and the mode of transport.
- Recognize problems and complications related to ground and aeromedical transport.
- Describe pretransport communication and coordination.
- Itemize and identify the equipment and monitoring necessary for safe transport and optimal outcomes.

## Case Study

A 2-year-old girl who is intubated secondary to smoke inhalation injury is being transported to a regional children's hospital. During transport, the ventilator alarm sounds for high pressure and the child's oxygen saturation drops below 90% despite the increase of $F_{IO_2}$ to 1.0. The high-pressure alarms persist even after suctioning, and oxygenation continues to deteriorate. The child is now becoming bradycardic and hypotensive, and she develops poor perfusion.

**Detection**

- What is this child's physiologic status or Pediatric Early Warning Score? (Refer to **Chapter 1**, **Table 1-1**.)
- What are the most likely diagnosis and the worst possible diagnoses?

**Intervention**

- What are the priorities to stabilize the patient?

**Reassessment**

- Is the current treatment strategy effective?
- Does the patient need other therapeutic interventions?

**Effective Communication**
- What information should be communicated to the medical control person?
- What type of equipment should be accompanying this patient on transport?

**Teamwork**
- How are you going to implement the treatment strategy?
- Who is to do what and when?

# I. INTRODUCTION

Critically ill pediatric patients are at increased risk of morbidity and mortality during transport to access care that is not available at the existing location, such as care in a diagnostic department, operating room, specialized unit within the hospital, or another medical facility. The decision to transport these patients is based on an assessment of the potential benefits versus the potential risks associated with the transport itself. Risk is not isolated to the patient but may extend to some degree to the accompanying personnel. The risks of transport can be minimized by careful planning, the use of appropriately qualified personnel, and the availability of appropriate equipment.

# II. GENERAL CONSIDERATIONS

Many critically ill pediatric patients may require lengthy transport to an appropriate regional pediatric tertiary care facility. Initially most critically ill or injured children are taken to the closest medical facility for primary stabilization. Once stabilized, these children will require transport to a facility with an appropriate level of care and expertise. Interhospital transport services are a vital link in the system of emergency and critical care for children, bridging the patient's initial stabilization with definitive care in the tertiary care center. This transport from one hospital to another should be from a lower level of care to a higher one.

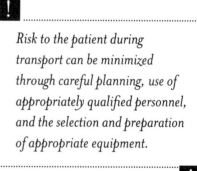

*Risk to the patient during transport can be minimized through careful planning, use of appropriately qualified personnel, and the selection and preparation of appropriate equipment.*

During transport, a patient is potentially at risk for instability and deterioration. Therefore, transport for a diagnostic test or a procedure that is unlikely to alter the management or outcome must be questioned. Whenever possible, diagnostic testing or simple procedures should be attempted at the bedside to avoid subjecting a patient to the risks associated with transport.

The transport team is selected according to training and skills, and the available equipment and supplies are assembled to provide for any ongoing or anticipated needs for acute care. There should be minimal disturbance in the monitoring or maintenance of the patient's vital functions during transport. Ideally, all transports of critically ill pediatric patients, both intrahospital and interhospital, would be performed by specially trained individuals, but that is not always possible.

Given that not all transferring facilities have access to a dedicated pediatric critical care transport team, contingency plans for using locally available resources should be developed. The standards for organized transport services as set forth by the American Academy of Pediatrics (AAP) and the Society of Critical Care Medicine (SCCM) are rigorous. A comprehensive and effective interhospital transfer plan for facilities that do not have access to an organized pediatric critical care transport team can be developed in 4 steps:

1. A multidisciplinary team of physicians, nurses, respiratory therapists, hospital administrators, and local emergency medical services personnel is formed to plan and coordinate the process.

2. The team conducts a needs assessment that focuses on patient demographics, transfer volume, transfer patterns, available resources (personnel, equipment, emergency medical services, communication), and receiving facilities.

3. A standardized transfer plan is written.

4. The transfer plan is regularly evaluated and refined after use and at periodic intervals using a standard quality improvement process.

Transport to a tertiary care setting should be coordinated with the receiving providers to ensure that the patient travels safely and arrives in stable or improved condition. Ideally, the transport is supervised in person or in communication with a physician who has experience and training in pediatric emergency medicine or pediatric critical care.

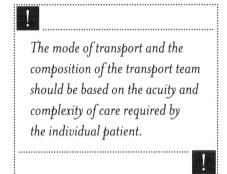

*The mode of transport and the composition of the transport team should be based on the acuity and complexity of care required by the individual patient.*

The mode of transportation for a critically ill patient is an important aspect of comprehensive care. Ground ambulances, helicopters, and fixed-wing aircraft are the principal vehicles available for interfacility transport. Depending upon geographic location and resources, other vehicles may be needed, including, but not limited to, boats, private vehicles, carts, and bicycles. The composition of the accompanying team will also depend upon the resources available but should include individuals with the skills and experience that best meet the needs of the patient during transport.

Pediatric transport medicine is a relatively new field of clinical interest that has developed rapidly over the past 3 decades. The AAP has stated that the goal of pediatric interfacility transport is to improve outcomes of critically ill or injured pediatric patients who are not in proximity to a hospital that provides the required level of care. Advances in technology and transportation have allowed dedicated pediatric critical care transport teams to offer many therapies that were previously restricted to use within the intensive care unit (ICU). This can minimize transport-associated risks and improve outcomes.

Every pediatric tertiary care facility should have an organized pediatric transport system. Ideally, the system is regional, with central medical control under the direction of a physician trained in pediatric emergency medicine or pediatric critical care medicine.

# III. INTRAFACILITY TRANSPORT

The basic reason for moving a critically ill pediatric patient within the facility is the need for additional care that utilizes technology and/or specialists not available in the child's current location. This may require moving a patient within the hospital to a diagnostic testing area, operating room, or pediatric intensive care unit (PICU). The transport process must be organized and efficient due to the potential risks it entails for the patient. Intrahospital transport is not benign and physiological adverse events can occur during transfer. Safe transport of the critically ill pediatric patient requires coordination, communication, and appropriate equipment and monitoring to ensure stability and prevent clinical deterioration in the patient's clinical condition.

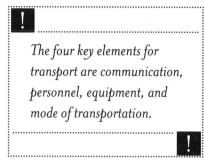

*The four key elements for transport are communication, personnel, equipment, and mode of transportation.*

## A. Pre-transport Communication and Coordination for Intrafacility Transport

Physician-to-physician and nurse-to-nurse communication regarding the patient's condition and treatment should occur both prior to and at the completion of any transport (**Appendix 14**). Detailed handoff communication should occur whenever a patient's management will be assumed by a different team, whether related to transfer from unit to unit or to testing or interventions performed outside the PICU.

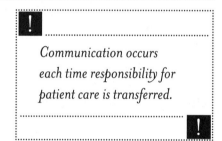

*Communication occurs each time responsibility for patient care is transferred.*

Pre-transport confirmation should indicate that the area to which the patient is being transported (e.g., radiology, operating room, nuclear medicine) is ready to receive and immediately begin the specified procedure or test. Ancillary services and other members of the healthcare team (e.g., security, respiratory therapy, escort) should be notified of the timing of the transport and the equipment and monitoring that will be required. The responsible physician should either accompany the patient or be notified that the patient is out of the PICU and at risk of an acute adverse event in another area of the hospital. Monitoring and resuscitation equipment must be equivalent to that of the PICU and, if necessary, additional monitoring should be provided during transport to ensure safe transport. The medical record should document the indications for transport and the patient's status and interventions performed during the transport process.

## B. Personnel During Intrafacility Transport

It is strongly recommended that a minimum of 2 people accompany a critically ill pediatric patient. One should be a nurse who has completed a competency-based orientation and has met the prescribed standards for pediatric critical care nurses. Additional personnel may include a respiratory therapist, registered nurse, or critical care technician as needed. It is strongly advised that a healthcare professional (physician, nurse practitioner, physician assistant) with training in airway management, advanced pediatric life support, critical care, or the equivalent accompany intubated or unstable critically ill patients.

When a procedure is anticipated to be lengthy and the receiving location is staffed by appropriately trained personnel, patient care may be transferred to those individuals if this action is acceptable to both groups. This allows for maximum utilization of staff and resources. If care responsibility is not transferred, the transport personnel should remain with the patient until return to the PICU.

## C. Equipment and Monitoring During Intrafacility Transport

Minimum equipment and monitoring are recommended to accompany all patients during the transport process. All critically ill patients require a blood pressure monitor, a pulse oximeter, and a cardiac monitor/defibrillator. It is recommended that transport monitoring be equivalent to the level delivered in the ICU. At the very minimum, it should include continuous electrocardiography monitoring, continuous pulse oximetry, and periodic measurement of blood pressure, pulse rate, and respiratory rate. Selected patients may also benefit from end-tidal capnography, continuous intra-arterial blood pressure monitoring, and central venous pressure and intracranial pressure monitoring.

When available, monitors with the capacity for storing and reproducing patient bedside data should be utilized to allow for review of data collected during the procedure and transport. The minimum requirements are shown in **Table 14-1**.

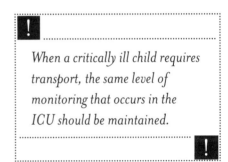

*When a critically ill child requires transport, the same level of monitoring that occurs in the ICU should be maintained.*

Airway management equipment, including a resuscitation bag and face mask of proper size and fit for the patient's age and size, should accompany the patient. It is also important to have an oxygen source of ample supply to provide for the patient's projected needs during transport plus an additional 30 minutes of oxygen in reserve.

### Table 14-1  Minimum Monitoring Equipment Required for Transport

- Electrocardiographic monitor
- Pulse oximeter
- Defibrillator with battery backup and transcutaneous pacing capability
- Oxygen analyzer and oxygen tank
- Ventilator appropriate for infants, children, and adults
- Infusion pumps
- Noninvasive blood pressure monitor
- Portable suction unit

Standard resuscitation drugs, such as epinephrine (adrenaline) and antiarrhythmic agents, should be transported with each patient in the event of sudden cardiac arrhythmia or arrest. A more complete array of pharmacologic agents should either accompany the patient or be available from supplies in the emergency resuscitation carts or crash carts located along the transport route and at the transport destination. In many hospitals, pediatric patients share diagnostic and procedural facilities with adult patients, so a complete set of pediatric resuscitation equipment and medications must accompany infants and children and also be available at their destination. Supplemental medications, such as narcotics and sedative agents, are to be considered on a case-by-case basis.

An appropriate supply of intravenous fluids and continuous drip medications, administered and regulated on battery-operated infusion pumps, should be ensured. All battery-operated equipment must be fully charged and capable of functioning for the duration of the transport. Backup batteries and electric cords for the equipment should be included. If a healthcare professional capable of medical decision making will not be accompanying the patient during transport, protocols or communication mechanisms must be in place to permit the administration of medications and fluids by appropriately trained personnel under emergency circumstances.

Bag-mask ventilation is the most commonly employed ventilation method during intrahospital transports. However, portable mechanical ventilators are gaining in popularity and use because they are capable of more reliably administering prescribed minute ventilation and desired oxygen concentrations. In children, a default oxygen concentration of 100% is frequently used. However, oxygen concentration must be precisely regulated for neonates and patients with congenital heart disease who have single ventricle physiology or who are dependent on a right-to-left shunt to maintain systemic blood flow. For patients receiving mechanical ventilatory support, equipment similar to that used in the PICU is preferred at the receiving location; otherwise, the equipment used in the PICU is transported to meet the patient at the destination.

The position of a patient's endotracheal tube must be noted and confirmed radiologically before transport. The adequacy of oxygenation and ventilation is confirmed with either bag-mask ventilation or trial on transport ventilator. Occasionally, patients may require modes of ventilation or ventilator settings that are not replicable during transport or at the receiving location. In such cases, alternative modes of mechanical ventilation must be tested before transport to ensure appropriateness of therapy and patient stability. If a patient cannot be maintained safely with alternative therapy, the risks and benefits of the transport must be reexamined.

Transport ventilators must have alarms for both disconnection and excessively high airway pressures. Pediatric patients with tracheostomy tubes must be transported with great caution because most home or transport ventilators are not capable of sensing disconnection and alarms will be delayed. Any ventilator must have a backup battery power supply, and electrical cords must accompany the patient during transport.

## IV. INTERFACILITY TRANSPORT

The two general indications that a critically ill child requires interfacility transport are that the referring hospital lacks the resources to care for the patient beyond initial stabilization and that the patient has a diagnosis or severity of illness that requires comprehensive subspecialty care best accomplished at a regional pediatric tertiary care center. Transport should be arranged promptly

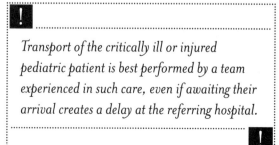

*Transport of the critically ill or injured pediatric patient is best performed by a team experienced in such care, even if awaiting their arrival creates a delay at the referring hospital.*

when the referring facility has assessed the child and determined that its resources are not adequate or that subspecialty support is required.

Timely recognition of a child in need of transport is critical. Favorable patient outcomes depend on the expertise and availability of nursing and medical personnel and the technologic support in the referral facility.

Delays are inherent in arranging an interfacility transport, particularly when a specialized team from the receiving hospital is necessary. Therefore, the child's clinical deterioration must be anticipated and expected, and an appropriate team must be mobilized as soon as possible during the initial stabilization.

Rapid transport seldom is the sole concern in interfacility transport and rarely supersedes stabilization. The level of care that can be provided during transport is an equally important consideration in recognizing and preventing clinical deterioration and providing continued stabilization. The transport team should be capable of providing an equal or higher level of care than the referring hospital and have the means to maintain that level of care during transport. The vehicle type, mode of transport, and team composition should be selected to best meet the needs of the patient during transport (**Appendix 15**).

> *Difficulty in achieving and ensuring adequate stabilization in a patient may be considered a relative contraindication to transport. However, the problem may be that true stabilization is possible only at the receiving facility.*

Healthcare practitioners must be aware of their local, regional, and national laws regarding interfacility patient transfers. In the United States, federal regulations define the legal responsibilities of the hospitals involved. Financially motivated transfers are illegal and put both the institution and the individual practitioner at risk for serious penalty. Current U.S. regulations and best practices require that a competent patient, or the legally authorized representative of a minor child or incompetent patient, give informed consent prior to interfacility transport. This must include the disclosure of risks versus benefits of transport, documentation in the medical record, and a signed consent form. If circumstances do not allow for informed consent, both the indications for transport and the reason for not obtaining consent must be documented. Transfer and transport agreements must be completed in advance to prevent needless delays. A transfer algorithm showing the sequence of events involved in an interfacility patient transport is presented in **Figure 14-1**.

## A. The Transport Process

Once the transport decision has been made, the patient must be prepared. The goal is optimal stabilization. The patient's condition and the trajectory of illness or injury must be considered. Whenever possible, medical interventions aimed at stabilizing the patient should be discussed with the receiving physician and the transport team. Airway patency must be assured.

> *If there is any concern about maintaining airway patency for the duration of the transport process, the patient must be intubated.*

**Figure 14-1.** Transport Algorithm

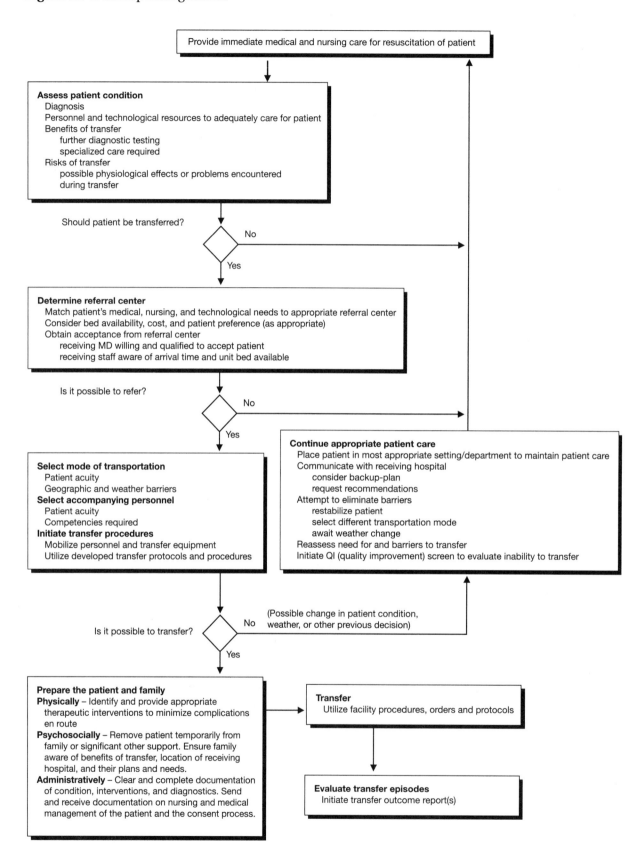

If necessary, intubation should be performed by the most experienced individual available, whether it is someone at the referring facility or a member of the transport team. Once the airway is stabilized and secured, adequate ventilation and oxygenation are ensured. Circulation must be assessed and stabilized. Maintaining adequate intravenous access is important. In most circumstances, two functional intravenous lines are preferred during transport. Appropriate temperature control is also essential, especially between buildings and within vehicles.

While the patient is being stabilized, the medical record, laboratory reports, radiographs, and any additional imaging studies are copied to accompany the patient. At least one parent or legal guardian should remain with the child during preparations, ensuring that necessary information and consent are obtained prior to the actual transport. Often, at least one parent or legal guardian may accompany the child throughout the transport process.

## B. Mode of Transport

To ensure a successful interfacility transport, the most appropriate vehicle type and the best team composition should be requested. Interfacility transport is typically accomplished through the use of a ground ambulance, critical care mobile ICU ambulance, helicopter, or fixed-wing aircraft, but other modes of transport may be dictated by regional or local resources. The following factors must be considered when selecting the optimal mode of interfacility transport for a critically ill pediatric patient:

- Diagnosis and severity of illness
- Risk of deterioration during transport
- Team capabilities
- Urgency to arrive at the tertiary care facility and team response time
- Distance between the two facilities
- Local geography, weather, and traffic conditions
- Availability of vehicles or aircraft

After these factors have been weighed, the relative cost and availability of resources, both personnel and equipment, must be considered for each practical option.

The transport team must review the constraints of the transport environment (**Table 14-2**), which is small and confined, with finite resources. Consequently, team members' sensory perception, communication, and range of motion are limited.

### Table 14-2  Comparison of Modes of Transport

| | Ground Ambulance | Fixed-Wing Aircraft | Helicopter |
|---|---|---|---|
| Availability[a] | Excellent | Fair | Good |
| Safety | Good | Good | Good |
| Cabin environment (space, noise, vibration) | Fair-Good | Good | Poor |
| Transport time | Fair | Good | Excellent |
| Range | <100 miles (160 km) (typically) | 200-2000 miles (322-3218 km) | 100-150 miles (160-241 km) |
| Special issues | Road and weather conditions | Need for multiple transfers | Weather conditions |

[a]Depends upon local geographic characteristics and regional resources.
Adapted with permission. © 1997 Wolters Kluwer Health. Durbin DR. Preparing the child for interhospital transport. In: Henretig FM, King C, eds. *Textbook of Pediatric Emergency Procedures.* Baltimore, MD: William & Wilkins; 1997.

Compared to other modes of transport, ground ambulances are readily available, relatively inexpensive, and spacious. On average, they are the most common mode of interfacility transport. They are operable in most weather conditions and can be brought to a halt if interventions or procedures are required. In some cases, weather may necessitate that a ground ambulance be used, even if the distance between facilities is significant. Ambulances are generally considered safer than either helicopters or fixed-wing aircraft. Disadvantages associated with ground transportation include increased transport time over long distances and the risk of traffic and weather-associated delays.

The distinct advantages of a helicopter versus a ground ambulance are faster transport to the receiving facility over a wider distance and avoidance of traffic congestion. Helicopters are best utilized when speed of transport is the most critical factor in the management of a patient. Monitoring and evaluating the pediatric patient are extremely difficult during helicopter transport. The small space inside the cabin and the constant noise and vibration from the rotors limit the ability to perform procedures during flight. In addition, helicopter transport is more costly than ground transport. Weather conditions preclude flying up to 15% of the time, limiting this mode of travel.

Fixed-wing aircraft are typically used for transports of more than 150 miles (~240 km). Depending upon the type of aircraft, the cabin environment may permit excellent patient monitoring and assessment. Many of these aircraft are pressurized and land at controlled sites. Interventions can be performed more easily than in rotor-wing aircraft. The disadvantages of fixed-wing transport are long start-up times (though this may be offset by the speed of the flight) and the need to move the patient multiple times, typically using a ground ambulance between the hospital and the aircraft.

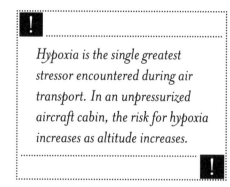

*Hypoxia is the single greatest stressor encountered during air transport. In an unpressurized aircraft cabin, the risk for hypoxia increases as altitude increases.*

Multiple transfers increase the risk of such difficulties as airway deterioration, intravenous catheter malfunction, and equipment failure. Altitude may also increase the risk of adverse effects: hypoxia, gas expansion, and reactions to temperature, humidity, and gravitational forces that are unique to air transport.

A patient's initial compensatory response to hypoxia is an increase in respiratory rate and effort. Supplemental oxygen should be provided, especially when a child's pulmonary status may be compromised. Additionally, as altitude increases, gas volume increases proportionally. Physiologically, a patient with a small pneumothorax may develop a clinically significant tension pneumothorax with increases in altitude due to decreases in barometric pressure. Similarly, pneumocephalus may expand to further complicate a closed head injury. Nasogastric tubes must be connected to a functioning suction unit to decompress the stomach. Pressurized equipment may need adjustment at high altitudes to maintain the appropriate negative pressure. The high-volume, low-pressure cuff on an endotracheal tube should be slightly deflated before flight, and periodically checked and adjusted during flight, to the minimal volume needed to maintain an adequate seal. Nonetheless, despite the many added considerations, the time saved by flying may overset the potential risks.

## C. Configuration of the Transport Team

The primary responsibility for a patient typically stays with the referring institution until arrival at the accepting facility, unless the transport team is sent from the accepting facility. During transport, a patient should not be put at increased risk by any decrease in the level of care. Careful attention must be paid to the qualifications and experience of the transport personnel.

Variations in team composition are possible, as shown in **Table 14-3**. The composition will be dictated by the patient's needs and the hospital's available resources. The team may include physicians, nurses, respiratory therapists, paramedics, and emergency medical technicians. No single team composition is preferred over all others.

### Table 14-3 Comparison of Transport Team Configurations

| Transport | Advantages | Disadvantages |
|---|---|---|
| Private vehicle | Cost, speed, accessibility | No care en route, unreliable |
| Emergency medical services/ambulance | Cost, speed, some monitoring | Limited skills/interventions |
| Emergency medical services team and skills + nurse and/or physician | Improved skills/monitoring | Scarce resources depleted |
| Broad-based critical care team | Cost, speed, improved monitoring, and intervention | Limited pediatric critical care skills/knowledge |
| Specialized pediatric critical care transport team | Highest level of care, monitoring, and skills | Limited availability |

Adapted with permission. © 1997 Wolters Kluwer Health. Durbin DR. Preparing the child for interhospital transport. In: Henretig FM, King C, eds. *Textbook of Pediatric Emergency Procedures.* Baltimore, MD: William & Wilkins; 1997.

Team members may be drawn from local emergency medical services personnel, medical personnel from the referring hospital, hospital-based critical care teams that typically transport adult and trauma patients, and dedicated pediatric and neonatal transport teams. Patient safety and the availability of needed medical care are factors to consider when creating a team for a specific transport. Although local emergency medical systems tend to offer rapid response times, their personnel usually do not have the training, experience, or equipment to transport a critically ill or injured child. Healthcare professionals from the referring hospital may be rapidly mobilized, but their absence may place their facility at a disadvantage. Personnel with limited experience in pediatric prehospital or critical care will find patient management difficult in the mobile transport environment. Adult-based critical care transport services offer both ground and flight resources but often have limited expertise and equipment for the care of critically ill children.

Specialized pediatric and neonatal transport systems offer personnel (nurses, respiratory therapists, nurse practitioners, physicians, and emergency medical technicians) who are skilled in the care of critically ill pediatric patients. These specialized teams offer the optimal level of care during transport and often provide continuity of care from transport to the PICU. They are usually based at the regional tertiary care center, making them somewhat slower to arrive at the referring facility, and they may be costly in comparison to other ground transport methods. Unfortunately, such teams are not available in all areas, and they may not have access to all types of transport vehicles. When available, these teams should be used to transport the most unstable patients, even if they require more time to arrive or to stabilize a patient.

# V. PREPARING A PATIENT FOR INTERFACILITY TRANSPORT

## A. Pre-transport Coordination and Communication for Interfacility Transport

Every facility should establish a plan with protocols that outline the process for obtaining appropriate transport once it is determined to be needed. A list of names and telephone numbers of facilities equipped to manage critically ill children should be compiled and be readily available in the emergency department. There should also be a list of contact numbers for transport systems capable of accommodating these patients, if transport will not be provided by the receiving tertiary care facility.

One of the most important steps in the interfacility transport of a critically ill pediatric patient is the initial referral call. Based on the information exchanged, the receiving hospital must determine the most appropriate bed assignment (PICU or general pediatric floor) and anticipate the patient's need for specialized diagnostic or therapeutic modalities. If a specialized pediatric transport team from the receiving hospital is mobilized, the optimal team composition must be determined. The key patient information for the initial referral call should include:

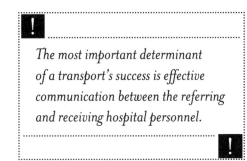

*The most important determinant of a transport's success is effective communication between the referring and receiving hospital personnel.*

- Patient's identifying information
- Referring physician's name
- Facility name, location, and contact telephone number
- Brief summary of the patient's condition

- Vital signs and weight
- Pertinent findings of physical exam
- Relevant laboratory and radiographic results
- Significant interventions performed and patient response

The receiving physician may provide advice about further evaluation or interventions. Before transport can be initiated, that physician must accept the patient and confirm the availability of appropriate resources at the receiving hospital. The mode of transport will be determined by the transferring physician in consultation with the receiving physician and based on patient acuity, time, weather, any medical interventions required for continued stabilization, and available personnel and resources.

If the transport team is not associated with the referring or receiving facility, the staff at the referring hospital must assist in the arrangements for efficient patient transfer. The transport provider should be contacted to confirm availability, capabilities, and details of the patient's status and anticipated needs during transport. An estimate of preparation and transport time should also be shared (**Table 14-4**).

### Table 14-4 Information Required by the Transport Team

- Patient's name, weight, age, sex, date of birth
- Patient's location (unit and hospital facility) at both transferring and receiving hospitals, including addresses and telephone numbers
- Names and contact telephone numbers for both transferring and receiving attending physicians
- Basic diagnosis
- Method of transport (ground, fixed-wing aircraft, helicopter)
- Nature of transport (incubator, pediatric stretcher, adult stretcher)
- Team composition (number of team members)
- Reason for mode of transport (patient acuity, traffic or weather conditions, etc.)
- Equipment required or anticipated for transport
- Patient status, including interventions already instituted

Classified using Freedman SH, King BR. Aeromedical transport procedures. In: Henretig FM, King C, eds. *Textbook of Pediatric Emergency Procedures*. Baltimore, MD: William & Wilkins; 1997.

A nurse-to-nurse report should be provided to the unit at the accepting facility. If that receiving facility is not involved in the transport process, the referring physician should telephone the receiving physician immediately before the patient's departure and report the most recent vital signs, current clinical status, and estimated time of arrival.

While awaiting the arrival or coordination of the transport team, staff at the referring hospital should ensure that the patient is optimally prepared for transport. The medical record and laboratory and radiographic studies should be copied, monitoring and assessment should be continued, and necessary procedures should be performed by the most experienced personnel. If airway patency or ventilatory status is questionable, the airway should be secured with an endotracheal tube. All intravascular lines should be checked for patency and taped securely in place. The cervical spine and any fractured bones should be stabilized and/or immobilized before transport. The patient should be given nothing by mouth throughout the transport process. Nasogastric tubes should be connected to a functioning suction unit. If clinically significant pneumothorax or hemothorax is present, a chest tube must be inserted and fluid or air collections evacuated prior to transport. In addition, the patient's family members should be informed of the nature of the child's illness or injury and why transport is being arranged so that they can provide informed consent. The responsibilities of the referring hospital are summarized in **Table 14-5**.

| Table 14-5 | Responsibilities of the Referring Hospital |
|---|---|

- Stabilize patient.
- Communicate with accepting facility early in the process.
- Notify the family and obtain consent for transfer/transport.
- Secure vascular access and tracheal tube.
- Stabilize the cervical spine and any fractures (as indicated).
- Copy all patient records and radiographic studies, including transfer summary, medication list, and laboratory results.
- Provide transport team with telephone number to call for results of pending laboratory studies.
- Prepare blood products, if indicated.

## B. Personnel for Interfacility Transport

In addition to the vehicle operators, a minimum of two people should accompany the patient. At least one person must be a nurse, physician, or advanced emergency medical technician capable of providing advanced airway management, including endotracheal intubation, intravenous therapy, interpretation and treatment of dysrhythmia, and basic and advanced cardiac and trauma life support. When a physician does not accompany the patient, the transport team must be available to communicate with a healthcare clinician who is capable of providing advice and medical orders if the patient's clinical condition changes. If this is not technically possible, the team should have standing orders to perform acute lifesaving interventions.

## C. Minimum Required Equipment During Interfacility Transport

A list of the minimum necessary equipment should be reviewed and discussed regardless of who transports the patient. Ideally, transport packs containing correctly sized equipment and medications for pediatric patients should be prepared in advance and be readily available for emergency situations. **Tables 14-6** through **14-8** list recommended respiratory equipment, transport equipment, and transport medications for pediatric patients. These items should accompany the patient during interfacility transport. A range of equipment and medications may be necessary to cover the pediatric age spectrum. The supplies may be adapted to meet a given patient's clinical needs or mode of transport.

### Table 14-6  Minimum Recommended Respiratory Equipment

- 500-mL resuscitation bag
- 1-liter resuscitation bag with oxygen reservoir
- Oxygen supply tubing: #2
- Manometer with tubing and adapter
- Nasal cannulas: neonatal, pediatric, adult
- Non-rebreather masks: pediatric, adult
- Resuscitation face masks, 1 each: neonate, infant, toddler, pediatric, small adult, large adult
- End-tidal carbon dioxide monitors (disposable): pediatric, adult
- End-tidal carbon dioxide supplies, 1 each: endotracheal tube adapter, supply tubing, pediatric and adult cannulas
- Positive end-expiratory pressure valve (adjustable)
- Flexible adapters to connect bag-valve system to endotracheal/tracheostomy tube
- Oral airways, 1 each: 5, 6, 7, 8, 9 (pediatric sizing); 0, 1, 2, 3, 4 (adult sizing)
- Nasal trumpets, 1 each: 14F, 16F, 18F, 20F, 22F, 24F, 26F, 30F
- Nebulizer setup with mask and endotracheal tube adapter
- MacIntosh laryngoscope blades: #1, #2, #3, #4
- Miller laryngoscope blades: #0, #1, #2
- Endotracheal tube stylets, 1 each: small, medium, large
- Magill forceps, 1 each: pediatric, adult
- Laryngoscope handles: pediatric, adult
- Extra laryngoscope batteries and light bulbs
- Adhesive tape: 1-inch roll
- Booted hemostat
- 10 mL syringes: 2
- Endotracheal tubes, 2 each: uncuffed 2.0 ,2.5, 3.0, 3.5, 4.0, 4.5 (mm); cuffed 3.0, 3.5, 4.0, 4.5, 5.0, 5.5, 6.0, 6.5, 7.0, 8.0 (mm)
- Water-soluble lubricant
- Suction catheters, 2 each: 6F, 8F, 10F, 12F, 14F
- Tonsil tip suction
- Swivel adapter
- Stethoscope
- Continuous positive airway pressure prong setup with tubing: extra small, small, large
- Scalpel with blade for cricothyrotomy
- Needle cricothyrotomy kit

### Table 14-7  Minimum Recommended Transport Equipment

- Adhesive tape
- Alcohol swabs
- Arm boards: pediatric, adult
- Arterial line tubing
- Intraosseous needles
- Blood pressure cuffs: neonatal, infant, child, small adult, large adult
- Butterfly needles: 23-gauge, 25-gauge
- Communications backup (e.g., cellular telephone)
- Defibrillator electrolyte pads (pediatric and adult) or jelly
- Point-of-care testing capability for glucose
- Electrocardiography electrodes: infant, pediatric, adult
- Flashlights with extra batteries
- Heimlich valve (chest evacuation valve)
- Infusion pumps
- Intravenous fluid tubing: pediatric, adult
- Y tubing for blood administration
- Extension tubing
- Microbore tubing for syringe pumps
- 3-way stopcocks
- Intravenous catheters: 14- to 24-gauge
- Intravenous solutions (plastic bags)
- 1000 mL, 500 mL of normal saline
- 1000 mL of Ringer lactate
- 250 mL of 5% dextrose
- Irrigating syringe (60 mL), catheter tip
- Kelly clamp
- Hypodermic needles, assorted sizes
- Hypodermic syringes, assorted sizes
- Normal saline for irrigation
- Pressure bags for fluid administration
- Pulse oximeter with multiple-site adhesive or reusable sensors: neonatal, pediatric, adult sensors
- Salem sump nasogastric tubes: assorted sizes
- Soft restraints for upper and lower extremities
- Stethoscope
- Suction apparatus
- Suction catheters
- Surgical dressings (sponges, conforming gauze, woven gauze)
- Tourniquets for venipuncture/intravenous access
- Scissors
- Spinal and cervical spine immobilization devices
- Thermometer
- Sterile and nonsterile gloves
- Chest tubes: 12F, 16F, 20F, 26F
- Chest tube insertion kits
- Nasogastric tubes: 8F, 10F, 12F, 14F
- Urinary Foley catheters and urinary collection bags
- Clear dressings for intravenous catheter sites

### Table 14-8  Minimum Recommended Transport Medications

- Pediatric emergency medication reference guide
- Adenosine
- Albuterol
- Amiodarone
- Atropine
- Calcium chloride
- Topical anesthetic spray: oral, dermal mucous membrane
- Dextrose 25%
- Dextrose 50%
- Digoxin
- Diltiazem
- Diphenhydramine
- Dopamine
- Epinephrine/adrenaline, 1 mg/10 mL (1:10,000)
- Epinephrine/adrenaline, 1 mg/1 mL (1:1000) multiple-dose vial
- Fosphenytoin (must be refrigerated)
- Furosemide
- Glucagon
- Heparin, 1000 units/1 mL
- Isoproterenol
- Labetalol
- Lidocaine, 100 mg/10 mL
- Lidocaine, 2 g/10 mL
- Magnesium sulfate
- Mannitol
- Methylprednisolone
- Metoprolol
- Naloxone
- Narcotic analgesics (e.g., morphine, fentanyl)
- Neuromuscular blocking agents (e.g., vecuronium, pancuronium, rocuronium)
- Nitroglycerin injection
- Nitroglycerin tablets
- Nitroprusside
- Normal saline, for injection
- Phenobarbital
- Potassium chloride
- Procainamide
- Prostaglandin $E_1$ (must be refrigerated)
- Pulmonary surfactant
- Sedatives/hypnotics (e.g., lorazepam, midazolam, ketamine)
- Sodium bicarbonate
- Sterile water, for injection
- Terbutaline
- Verapamil

## D. Monitoring During Interfacility Transport

At a minimum, interfacility transport must provide the same level of monitoring as in the intrafacility process (**Table 14-1**). Some patients may benefit from arterial blood pressure, central venous pressure, intracranial pressure, and/or end-tidal carbon dioxide monitoring. For those who require mechanical ventilatory support, the position of their endotracheal tubes should be noted and secured prior to transport. The adequacy of oxygenation and ventilation must be reconfirmed frequently. The mode of mechanical ventilation must be evaluated before transport to ensure acceptability and stability during travel. The child's status, interventions, and management during transport must be documented in the patient medical record. The receiving facility should be given copies of all transport documentation along with the information from the referring institution.

# Transport of the Critically Ill Child

## Key Points

- Staff at the referring hospital should carry out all interventions to stabilize a pediatric patient, including performing or assisting the transport team in any procedures necessary to prevent clinical deterioration during transport.

- To allow safe transport, patients should be transported only when sufficiently stabilized.

- Adequate information is required to determine a patient's optimal mode of transport and the composition of the transport team.

- Early contact must be established with the receiving physician and facility to ensure the most expedient transfer of a patient.

- Whenever possible, all appropriate materials (medical record, laboratory results, radiographic studies, and contact phone numbers) should be prepared prior to transport.

- The transport team and receiving physician/facility should be informed about any changes in the clinical condition of the patient.

- The appropriate equipment must accompany a patient during all inter- and intrafacility transports.

- The referring transport team should provide all necessary equipment and medications, including sufficient materials to sustain the patient for a minimum of 30 minutes beyond the expected transport time.

## Suggested Readings

1. American Heart Association. *PALS Provider Manual*. Dallas, TX; 2011.

2. Henretig FM, King C, eds. *Textbook of Pediatric Emergency Procedures*. Baltimore, MD: Lippincott Williams & Wilkins; 1997.

3. Kanter RK, Tompkins JM. Adverse events during interhospital transport: physiologic deterioration associated with pretransport severity of illness. *Pediatrics*. 1989;84:43-48.

4. McCloskey K, Orr R, eds. *Pediatric Transport Medicine*. St. Louis, MO: Mosby; 1995.

5. Wallen E, Venkataraman ST, Grosso MJ, Kiene K, Orr RA. Intrahospital transport of critically ill pediatric patients. *Crit Care Med*. 1995;23:1588-1595.

6. Warren J, Fromm RE, Orr RA, Rotello RC, Horst HM. SCCM guideline for the inter- and intrahospital transport of critically ill patients. *Crit Care Med*. 2004;32:256-262.

7. Woodward GA, ed. *Guidelines for Air and Ground Transport of Neonatal and Pediatric Patients*. 3rd ed. Elk Grove Village, IL: American Academy of Pediatrics; 2007.

# Chapter 15

# Neurologic Emergencies

## ✓ Objectives

- Describe the normal physiology of the intracranial vault and cerebral blood flow.
- Review the emergent neurological assessment of the pediatric patient.
- Summarize the acute management of seizures and status epilepticus.
- Describe the approach to the patient with altered mental status or coma.
- Review the current management of intracranial hypertension.

## 📁 Case Study

A 3-year-old girl presents to the emergency department after being found febrile, unresponsive, and exhibiting rhythmic, jerking movements on her right side. History reveals that she was found unresponsive by her parents in their living room, with an open, empty bottle of tablets by her side. The emergency medical personnel were called and found her apneic and bradycardic. Bag-mask ventilation was started, and the girl was transferred to the hospital. You are called to assist in her evaluation and management.

**Detection**

— What is the most likely diagnosis?

**Intervention**

— Does the patient need to be immediately intubated?

— What airway maneuvers and/or adjuncts should be considered?

— Should dextrose be administered?

**Reassessment**

— Should reversal agents such as naloxone be given?

**Effective Communication**

— Who should be contacted about this patient?

**Teamwork**

— Who is to do what and when?

# I. INTRODUCTION

An increasing understanding of neuron physiology and pathophysiology has led to a commensurate increase in targeted neuroprotective therapies.

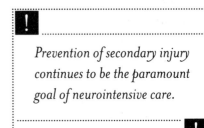

*Prevention of secondary injury continues to be the paramount goal of neurointensive care.*

Because the homeostatic reflexes all serve to preserve cerebral function and neuronal survival under pathophysiologic conditions, altered or depressed neurologic function in a child should be considered an emergent situation. Functional recovery requires prompt resolution of the insult and minimization of secondary injury. Thus, maintenance of normal oxygen delivery to the central nervous system (CNS) while minimizing cerebral oxygen utilization remains the primary goal in patients with neurologic injury.

Establishing a patent airway and effective breathing and circulation (ABC) takes priority in neurologic emergencies as in any other emergent situation. However, in neurologic emergencies, any known or suspected trauma requires cervical spine stabilization during airway manipulation (**Chapters 2** and **9**).

Patients with neurologic disease may suffer respiratory insufficiency for a variety of reasons, including hypoventilation and airway obstruction. Deteriorating neurologic status raises the possibility of impending respiratory failure, and establishment of an artificial airway should be promptly considered. Generally, elective intubation prevents hypoxemia and hypercarbia and is safer than emergent intubation. Finally, isotonic or hypertonic fluids should be used for resuscitation to minimize the risk of cerebral edema.

1. *Maintenance of adequate airway, breathing, and circulation (ABC) takes priority in neurologic emergencies.*
2. *Early intubation protects against hypoxemia and hypercarbia.*
3. *The cervical spine must always be immobilized during neurologic emergencies if any known or suspected trauma.*
4. *Isotonic or hypertonic fluids should be used for resuscitation.*

# II. BASIC PHYSIOLOGY OF THE INTRACRANIAL VAULT

Many neurologic emergencies share common pathophysiologic processes that affect the pressure within the cranial vault and/or impair cerebral blood flow (CBF). The human body has a number of regulatory mechanisms that help to reduce these changes and their impact on neurologic function. A basic understanding of these mechanisms, their derangements, and the methods of improvement are imperative for persons treating children with neurologic conditions.

# A. Intracranial Pressure

The Monro-Kellie doctrine states that the cranial vault contains a fixed volume consisting of 3 basic components—brain (80%), blood (10%), and cerebrospinal fluid (CSF) (10%)—encased by the thick, inelastic dura mater and the semirigid cranium. These components exist in a state of volume-pressure equilibrium, and expansion of one induces a reduction in the volume of one or both of the others. **Figure 15-1** illustrates intracranial compliance. The interaction of these 3 components (brain, blood, CSF) and the physiologic mechanisms controlling each of them provides the framework for neurointensive care.

Infants with open fontanelles may be prone to intracranial hypertension because the inelastic dura mater, which encases the brain, limits expansion of the intracranial compartment. Furthermore, infants have a shorter craniospinal axis (measured from the cranial dura down the length of the spinal canal to the lumbosacral area) than the adult; this provides less space to allow for the displacement of CSF or cerebral blood volume (CBV). **Figure 15-2** demonstrates how the intracranial compartment can compensate for a change in the volume of a component.

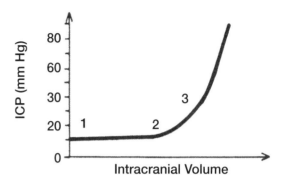

**Figure 15-1.** Intracranial Compliance

Between points 1 and 2, although intracranial volume is increased (i.e., by tumor, edema, or hemorrhage), the intracranial contents remain at a constant pressure. Displacement of cerebrospinal fluid and intracerebral blood into the spinal space accommodates this increased volume. At point 2, although the intracranial pressure (ICP) is normal, any further increases in volume (e.g., tumor, edema, obstructive hydrocephalus, or intracranial hemorrhage) will produce an exponential rise in ICP, which may be life-threatening. Point 3 represents a decompensated state and a neurosurgical emergency with dangerously high ICP.

**Figure 15-2.** Interactions Among Intracranial Compartments

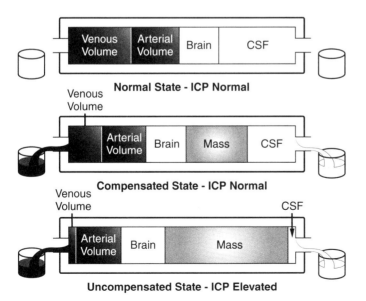

The top diagram illustrates the 3 components of the intracranial vault in equilibrium with normal intracranial pressure (ICP). The middle diagram represents an increasing mass lesion (e.g., hemorrhage); the compensatory mechanisms include the extrusion of cerebrospinal fluid (CSF) and venous blood volume. This corresponds to a move from point 1 to point 2 in **Figure 15-1**, and the ICP remains normal. The bottom diagram illustrates the uncompensated state, which occurs following maximal compensatory fluid displacement from the intracranial space, producing an elevated ICP. This corresponds to a move from point 2 to point 3 in **Figure 15-1**. The interaction of these 3 components and the physiologic mechanisms controlling each provide the framework for neurointensive care.

### 1. The Brain

The brain constitutes the largest volume (80%) of the intracranial vault. The brain parenchyma is composed of neurons (50%) and glial and vascular elements. Neurons require a significant amount of energy to produce neurotransmitters and are electrically active cells. However, because the brain contains only minimal energy stores, increases in CBF must occur in response to increased metabolic needs, such as during seizures and hyperthermia.

The brain's volume is dynamic and may respond to cellular edema or an increase in the extracellular fluid (ECF) space. Cellular injury produces edema (cytotoxic edema) due to a failure of the mechanisms that maintain cellular homeostasis. Cytotoxic edema responds particularly poorly to osmotic therapy and often portends a poor prognosis. The ECF volume increases with any process that increases the blood-brain barrier permeability (vasogenic edema). Both forms of edema contribute to increased brain volume, and thus increased intracranial pressure (ICP), in many pathologic processes.

### 2. Cerebral Blood Volume

Blood in arteries, veins, and capillaries occupies approximately 10% of the intracranial space. CBF changes in response to alterations in brain metabolism, blood pressure, and arterial $Pa_{CO_2}$ and $Pa_{O_2}$. Arteriolar tone regulates these changes, so CBF must be altered to effect changes in CBV. Although increased arteriolar tone (e.g., by decreasing $Pa_{CO_2}$ via hyperventilation) produces a rapid decrease in CBV (and consequently ICP), this places the brain at risk for ischemic injury. Therefore, recommendations support only brief manipulation of $Pa_{CO_2}$ to reduce CBV and ICP.

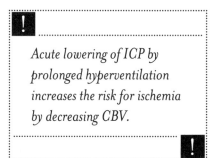

*Acute lowering of ICP by prolonged hyperventilation increases the risk for ischemia by decreasing CBV.*

### 3. Cerebrospinal Fluid

CSF accounts for approximately 10% of the intracranial volume. The brain essentially floats in the CSF, which provides a protective cushion and prevents traction on nerve roots, blood vessels, and delicate membranes. The actual intraventricular volumes are approximately 40 to 60 mL in infants, 60 to 100 mL in young children, 80 to 120 mL in older children, and 100 to 160 mL in adults. The choroid plexus produces approximately 70% of the CSF, and the remainder is formed in the extrachoroidal sites, including the ventricular ependyma, sylvian aqueduct, subarachnoid pial surface, and brain and spinal cord parenchyma. The rate of formation is approximately 0.35 to 0.40 mL/min, or 500 to 600 mL/day, independent of age. The turnover time for CSF is 5 to 7 hours.

*CSF is produced at a steady rate, independent of age. Obstruction to flow, increased production, or impaired resorption of CSF can increase ICP.*

**Figure 15-3** shows the normal pathway of CSF flow, which is generated by pressure gradients as well as cilia on the ependymal surfaces. The arachnoid villi on the superior surface of the brain resorb the CSF and drain into the superior sagittal sinus.

**Figure 15-3.** Flow of Cerebrospinal Fluid

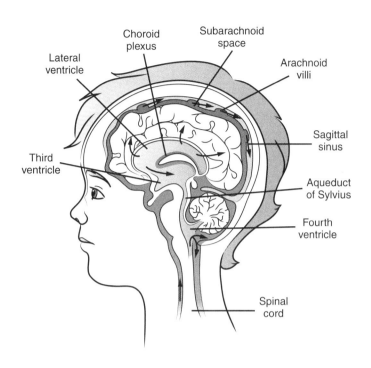

Increased production, impaired resorption, or obstructed flow can all increase CSF volume and ultimately ICP. CSF provides a chemically appropriate environment for neurotransmission and the removal of metabolic by-products. As an ultrafiltrate of plasma, CSF contains the same electrolyte concentrations as serum and the rest of the ECF. Glucose and other larger molecules are transported into the CSF across the impermeable blood-brain barrier, so alterations in the barrier can disrupt neurologic function. The use of osmotically active substances to reduce brain water in the treatment of intracranial hypertension requires an intact blood-brain barrier.

## B. Cerebral Blood Flow

The brain depends entirely upon exogenous glucose for its metabolic needs, and CBF is tightly matched to metabolic demands. Not surprisingly, CBF to gray matter (active neurons) exceeds that to white matter, which is less metabolically active. Other factors affecting CBF include mean arterial pressure, $Pa_{CO_2}$, $Pa_{O_2}$, and age; in adults the normal CBF is 50 mL/100 g/min, whereas it is 40 mL/100 g/min in neonates and 100 mL/100 g/min in children. The critical threshold below which ischemia develops, producing electroencephalographic (EEG) changes, is 20 mL/100 g/min in the adult and 5 to 10 mL/100 g/min in the infant.

As with all organs, the perfusion pressure is determined by the difference between the upstream and downstream pressures. In the brain, either the central venous pressure (CVP) or the ICP may provide the greater downstream pressure. Therefore, cerebral perfusion pressure (CPP) = mean arterial pressure (MAP) − (ICP or CVP), whichever is higher.

The body maintains a stable CBF over a wide range of arterial pressures through autoregulation, producing dilation or constriction of the precapillary arterioles, as necessary. **Figure 15-4** depicts autoregulation in a normal adult. At extremely low CPP, CBF decreases and ischemia ensues. At CPP above the autoregulatory range, high CBF produces cerebral edema. With time, the range over which autoregulation occurs adjusts to the patient's normal blood pressure. Generally, the lower limit for autoregulation is 25% below the patient's baseline MAP, and this should be the maximal induced reduction in blood pressure used to decrease the risk of cerebral ischemia. Due to the lower prevailing MAP in young children and infants, the acceptable CPP is slightly lower than the value targeted in adults (60 to 70 mm Hg), but the optimal value has not been scientifically determined.

**Figure 15-4.** Autoregulation of Cerebral Blood Flow

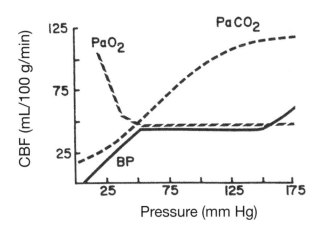

CBF, cerebral blood flow

> !
> 1. *Chronic hypertension shifts the autoregulatory curve rightward, so an acute drop in MAP >25% from the baseline may place the patient at risk of ischemia.*
> 2. *Hypercarbia and hypoxia both dilate cerebral blood vessels.*
> 3. *Increased brain activity (including seizures) increases CBF, possibly ICP.*

CBF correlates linearly with $Pa_{CO_2}$, ranging from 20 to 80 mm Hg (2.7-10.7 kPa). The changes in CBF with altered $Pa_{CO_2}$ occur independently of a change in arterial pH. Hyperventilation to lower $Pa_{CO_2}$ provides an effective means of rapid reduction in CBV and, consequently, ICP. However, as mentioned previously, this may place the patient at risk of cerebral ischemia. Hypoxemia below 40 to 50 mm Hg (5.3-6.7 kPa) also dilates the cerebral blood vessels, resulting in increased CBF and maintenance of cerebral oxygen delivery to areas of very low levels of oxygen content. However, this occurs at the expense of increased CBV and possibly increased ICP. Finally, anything that increases the metabolic demands of the brain, including hyperthermia and seizures, increases CBF.

# III. EMERGENT NEUROLOGIC ASSESSMENT OF THE PEDIATRIC PATIENT

## A. Level of Consciousness

The neurologic examination in emergencies is geared at assessing the level of consciousness and signs of intracranial hypertension or focal pathology. Certain aspects of the exam cannot be assessed in young children due to their inability to follow commands or communicate verbally. Careful serial assessment of the level of consciousness is the most important component of this exam. Combative behavior may be a sign of impaired neurologic function. A quiet child with eyes closed may be asleep or may have depressed consciousness. The response to noxious stimuli in such patients often provides clues to the degree of altered consciousness. The Glasgow Coma Scale (GCS) score is widely used in adult patients, and a modified pediatric scale exists for infants and children (**Table 15-1**).

### Table 15-1 Glasgow Coma Scale Modified for Infants and Children

| Clinical Parameter | Infants (Ages 0-12 Months) | Children (Ages 1-5 Years) | Points[a] |
|---|---|---|---|
| Eye opening | Spontaneous | Spontaneous | 4 |
| | Response to speech | Response to speech | 3 |
| | Response to pain | Response to pain | 2 |
| | No response | No response | 1 |
| Verbal response | Coos/babbles | Appropriate words | 5 |
| | Irritable cries | Inappropriate words | 4 |
| | Cries | Persistent cry | 3 |
| | Moans | Grunts | 2 |
| | No response | No response | 1 |
| Best motor response | Normal | Spontaneous | 6 |
| | Withdraws to touch | Localized pain | 5 |
| | Withdraws from pain | Withdraws from pain | 4 |
| | Flexor response | Flexor response | 3 |
| | Extensor response | Extensor response | 2 |
| | No response | No response | 1 |

[a]Total Glasgow Coma Scale score = eye + verbal + motor points; best possible score = 15; worst possible score = 3.

## B. Movement

Careful observation for asymmetric movements of the extremities and facial/ocular muscles may also provide diagnostic clues. Abnormal movements may indicate seizures (clonic, stereotyped), toxins or metabolic disease (tremors, asterixis, myoclonus), or basal ganglia injury (chorea, dystonia). Abnormal postures in response to stimulation, including that from suctioning and other procedures, consist of flexor posturing, extensor posturing, and flaccidity. All 4 extremities should be checked for response by applying pressure with a pen or similar object across the nail bed. Appropriate responses indicate intact sensory and effectors pathways. The terms *decorticate posture* and *decerebrate posture* are oversimplifications, but progression along this spectrum generally indicates more severe or more caudal lesions. Care should be taken to ensure responses are not stereotypical, such as the triple flexion response in the lower extremities.

> 1. Motor and sensory function must be evaluated in all 4 extremities.
> 2. Pressure on the nail beds using a pen or similar object produces a strong stimulus without injury.
> 3. Evidence of a motor or sensory level deficit strongly suggests a spinal cord lesion.

In cooperative patients, careful assessment for a motor or sensory level response may pinpoint the location of any spinal cord lesion.

## C. Motor and Sensory Evaluation

Brainstem reflexes (cranial nerve exam) allow for localization of the lesion, provide diagnostic clues, and indicate whether the airway reflexes and respiratory drive remain intact. Pupillary, corneal, oculocephalic (doll's eye), vestibular (cold-water calorics), and gag reflexes should be assessed in patients with depressed consciousness to help determine the location and severity of the lesion. In patients with possible cervical spine injury, oculocephalic reflexes should not be tested.

In patients treated with neuromuscular blockade, pupillary reactions may constitute the entire neurologic exam. Pupillary reactivity can persist in deep coma caused by metabolic disease, but its absence indicates a lesion of the third cranial nerve or midbrain, including possible herniation syndromes. An absent or diminished gag reflex places the patient at increased risk of airway obstruction.

## D. Respiratory Patterns

Respiratory patterns may indicate specific lesions (**Table 15-2**) or the need to secure an artificial airway. In Cheyne-Stokes respiration, a gradually increasing period of hyperventilation then diminishes to hypoventilation and apnea in a regularly alternating pattern. Sustained hyperventilation (with large tidal volumes) indicates rostral brainstem injury. This must be distinguished from the hyperventilation induced by pulmonary edema, which may also be caused by neurologic disease (neurogenic pulmonary edema). Patients with true central hyperventilation have elevated (or at least normal) arterial $Pao_2$ and increased arterial pH. On the other hand, patients may have Kussmaul respirations (large, rapid breaths) as compensation for a metabolic acidosis (such as with diabetic ketoacidosis). Caudal lesions produce apneustic breathing, which consists of inspiratory pauses, typically lasting 2 to 3 seconds. Ataxic breathing, the irregular alteration between deep and shallow breathing, occurs with lesions of the medulla. The lower the lesion, the more likely the patient will require mechanical ventilation, and patients with apneustic or ataxic breathing have a high likelihood of requiring complete mechanical respiratory support.

**Table 15-2** Respiratory Patterns in Diseases of the Central Nervous System

| Respiratory Pattern | Description | Lesion Localization |
|---|---|---|
| Cheyne-Stokes | Crescendo-decrescendo | Deep cortical or diencephalon |
| Central hyperventilation | Elevated $Pao_2$ | Rostral brainstem |
| Apneustic | Inspiratory pause | Mid-caudal pons |
| Ataxic | Random deep/shallow | Central medulla |

## E. Herniation Syndromes

With herniation of CNS components into another compartment, several discrete syndromes may be seen, any of which portends a poor prognosis and requires immediate intervention for recovery. Central herniation occurs when the hemispheres and basal nuclei are displaced downward through the tentorial notch. Initially, patients have depressed or altered consciousness, Cheyne-Stokes respirations, and small, reactive pupils. The eyes usually remain conjugate at this stage. With progression, patients may develop flexor posturing of the upper extremities. Further progression produces central hyperventilation, fixed mid-position pupils, and extensor posturing often confused with seizures. At this stage, patients may also have disconjugate eye movements in response to oculocephalic testing or cold-water calorics.

Uncal herniation occurs when a lateral lesion pushes the medial uncus and hippocampal gyrus over the lateral edge of the tentorium. The most consistent early sign is the unilaterally dilated pupil. Patients with uncal herniation may progress in an extremely rapid fashion to depressed consciousness with extensor then flexor posturing, typically of the contralateral extremities. They also develop disconjugate gaze.

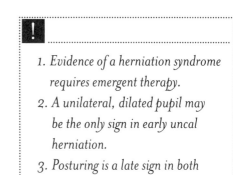

1. *Evidence of a herniation syndrome requires emergent therapy.*
2. *A unilateral, dilated pupil may be the only sign in early uncal herniation.*
3. *Posturing is a late sign in both uncal and central herniation.*

# IV. STATUS EPILEPTICUS

 Case Study

While visiting with her grandparents, an 18-month-old child was noted to feel warm to the touch. She was not eating well and was put to bed for a nap. The grandparents heard a loud noise and found the child having generalized tonic-clonic movements. Emergency medical services responded and transported the child. With a non-rebreather face mask in place, oxygenation saturation was 92% on $F_{IO_2}$ 1.0. Upon arrival, the child had a temperature of 104°F (40°C) and was lethargic.

**Detection**
– What is the likely diagnosis of this patient?

**Intervention**
– Which, if any, antiepileptic medication(s) should be considered?

**Reassessment**
– When, if at all, would you consider a second antiepileptic medication?
– What are the indications for an imaging study?
– What are the indications for performing a lumbar puncture?

**Effective Communication**
– Where is the best place to manage the care of this patient?

**Teamwork**
– How are you going to implement the treatment strategy?

Status epilepticus (SE) is a common pediatric neurologic emergency. It is estimated to affect between 25,000 and 50,000 children annually, with 40% occurring in children younger than 2 years of age. Etiologies of SE are summarized in **Table 15-3**.

### Table 15-3. Etiology of Status Epilepticus in Pediatric Patients

| | |
|---|---|
| Antiepileptic noncompliance | Drug toxicity (penicillin, ciprofloxacin, theophylline, cyclosporine, amitriptyline, phenothiazines, lidocaine, imipenem, tacrolimus, cocaine, sympathomimetics, isoniazid, ethanol) |
| Cerebrovascular accidents (stroke, AVM) | Fever |
| CNS infections (meningitis, encephalitis) | Drug withdrawal |
| CNS tumors | Malignant hypertension |
| Head trauma (accidental, nonaccidental) | Underlying CNS disorders |
| Hypoxic-ischemic injury | Neurocutaneous syndromes (Sturge-Weber, tuberous sclerosis, NF1) |
| Electrolyte disorders (glucose, sodium, calcium) | |

AVM, arteriovenous malformations; CNS, central nervous system; NF1, neurofibromatosis type 1

The current operational definition of generalized convulsive SE in adults and older children (>5 years) refers to ≥5 minutes of continuous seizure or ≥2 discrete seizures between which there is incomplete recovery of consciousness. The authors of this definition cite a paucity of pediatric data to allow recommendations in children younger than 5 years. Although there is general agreement that seizures continuing for longer than 5 minutes should usually be treated, overaggressive treatment may lead to avoidable morbidity.

## A. Pathophysiology and Organ Dysfunction

Seizures result from abnormal synchronous electrical discharges (depolarization) of a group of neurons in the CNS. Depolarization stems from the influx of sodium into the neuron, whereas repolarization results from the egress of potassium from the cell, which restores the resting negative electrical potential. This potential is regulated by a sodium-potassium pump that is driven by adenosine triphosphate.

Prolonged seizures may cause selective neuronal loss in the hippocampus, cortex, and thalamus, areas rich in glutamate receptors. This calcium-mediated neuronal cell death is referred to as the excitotoxic theory, which is similar to that proposed to occur in CNS ischemia. Although prolonged seizures may be sufficient to cause neuronal damage, the superimposition of hypoxia, hypotension, acidosis, and hyperpyrexia exacerbate the degree of damage.

SE may be divided into 2 stages. The first 30 minutes are characterized by increased autonomic activity: hypertension, tachycardia, hyperglycemia, diaphoresis, and hyperpyrexia. This is followed by a second stage, characterized by multiorgan involvement, and includes respiratory failure (hypoxemia, hypercarbia), decreased CBF, increased ICP, and a dropping arterial blood pressure. Severe acidosis ensues, and the patients may develop leukocytosis, hyperkalemia, and an elevated creatine kinase (secondary to increased muscle activity). The characteristics of early versus late SE are compared in **Table 15-4**.

A relative decrease in CBF occurs at a time when demands for cerebral energy substrates (oxygen, glucose) are markedly increased and cerebral autoregulation is depressed. This signals the failure of adaptive mechanisms.

| Table 15-4 | Physiologic Derangements in Early Versus Late Status Epilepticus |

|  | Early (<30 Minutes) | Late (>30 Minutes) | Complication |
| --- | --- | --- | --- |
| Blood pressure | ↑ | ↓ | Hypotension |
| $Pao_2$ | ↓ | ↓ | Hypoxia |
| $Paco_2$ | ↑ | Variable | ↑ ICP |
| Serum pH | ↓ | ↓ | Acidosis |
| Autonomic | ↑ | ↔ | Arrhythmias |
| CK | Normal | ↑ | Renal failure |
| $K^+$ | Normal | ↑ | Arrhythmias |
| CBF | ↑ 900% | ↑ 200% | CNS bleed |
| $CMRo_2$ | ↑ 300% | ↑ 300% | Ischemia |

CK, creatine kinase; CBF, cerebral blood flow; $CMRo_2$, cerebral metabolic rate of oxygen consumption; ICP, intracranial pressure
Adapted with permission. © 1987 Wolters Kluwer Health. Dean JM, Singer HS. Status epilepticus. In: Rogers MC, ed. *Textbook of Pediatric Intensive Care Medicine*. Baltimore, MD: Williams & Wilkins; 1987:618.

Respiratory failure associated with SE may be due to an increase in $CO_2$ production from the hypermetabolic state, a decrease in respiratory drive (due to muscle fatigue or medications used to suppress the seizure), and increased mechanical load on the respiratory muscles. There may also be concomitant aspiration or neurogenic pulmonary edema, which can contribute to both hypoxemia and respiratory acidosis.

The cardiovascular changes and initial hyperadrenergic state are due to the release of endogenous catecholamines. Patients have an initial increase in systemic vascular resistance that will decrease over time. As the seizure continues, hyperpyrexia must be prevented because it contributes to neuronal cell death. Studies in adult patients have shown that a CSF pleocytosis is possible; however, any elevation in the CSF count in a pediatric patient is suggestive of possible infection. Appropriate cultures should be obtained and therapy instituted. The prolonged muscle activity may lead to an elevation in creatine kinase and production of myoglobin with subsequent myoglobinuria; therefore, careful attention to the patient's hydration status and renal function is essential. The massive catabolic stress of SE may also lead to hyperkalemia, so attention to electrolyte status is required. Acidemia may be worsened by impaired ventilation, hypoxemia, and anaerobic metabolism.

## B. Evaluation and Management of Status Epilepticus

The therapeutic goals for SE include: (1) general supportive care, (2) termination of SE, (3) prevention of seizure recurrence, (4) correction of the precipitating causes, and (5) prevention and treatment of potential complications. Immediate attention to the airway, breathing, and circulation are essential. Status epilepticus requires management and evaluation to be performed simultaneously. A suggested clinical approach to SE is outlined in **Table 15-5**.

# Pediatric Fundamental Critical Care Support

### Table 15-5  Treatment Algorithm for Status Epilepticus

1. **Out-of-hospital treatment:** Consider lorazepam 2-4 mg PR or 5-10 mg diazepam PR
2. **Arrival to ED.** Assess ABCs. Apply oxygen, establish airway and ventilation. Reassess throughout management. Consider airway adjuncts: nasopharyngeal tube and $F_{IO_2}$ 1.0 via non-rebreather.
3. Establish IV or IO access. Labs for initial studies. Administer dextrose if hypoglycemic. Isotonic fluid boluses for inadequate perfusion and/or hypotension.
4. Pharmacotherapy
    a. Administer lorazepam, 0.1 mg/kg IV (maximum 4 mg); may repeat one time.
       **Alternatives:** diazepam, 0.5 mg/kg PR; midazolam, 0.2 mg/kg IM.
    b. Administer fosphenytoin, 20 mg/kg IV, no faster than 150 mg PE/min immediately after initial dose of benzodiazepine. May give an additional 5-10 mg/kg of fosphenytoin prior to start of barbiturates if seizures continue. Assess and monitor airway and hemodynamics.
       **Alternative:** phenytoin, 20 mg/kg, no faster than 1 mg/kg/min with a maximum rate of 50 mg/min.
       **Anticipate need for endotracheal intubation.**
       **Continuous cardiopulmonary monitoring.**
    c. If seizures persist after initial benzodiazepine and fosphenytoin, consult neurology and administer **PHENobarbital**, 20 mg/kg IV, no faster than 1 mg/kg/min up to a maximum rate of infusion 50 mg/min. Monitor blood pressure and consider elective endotracheal intubation.
       **Anticipate need for endotracheal intubation.**
       **Continuous cardiopulmonary monitoring.**
    d. If seizures persist, initiate refractory SE treatment: midazolam bolus of 0.2 mg/kg and midazolam infusion beginning with 0.1 mg/kg/h, increased every 15 min until seizure activity stops. Monitor ECG, blood pressure, and EEG.
       **Anticipate need for endotracheal intubation.**
       **Continuous cardiopulmonary monitoring.**
    e. If seizures persist, administer **PENTobarbital**, 5 mg/kg IV, up to a maximum rate of 50 mg/min. Begin infusion at 1 mg/kg/h. Additional boluses of 5 mg/kg may be given to achieve either burst suppression pattern on EEG or cessation of seizure activity.
       **Anticipate need for endotracheal intubation.**
       **Continuous cardiopulmonary monitoring.**
       Other pharmacologic agents used for refractory SE include valproic acid (20 mg/kg IV) or levetiracetam (20-30 mg/kg IV load)
    f. Clinical seizure activity may cease, but non-convulsive SE may persist. EEG evaluation is warranted in patients who do not return to baseline neurological status.
5. Diagnostic evaluation. Treat underlying causes and systemic complications.

PR, per rectum; ED, emergency department; ABC, airway, breathing, and circulation; IV, intravenous; IO, intraosseous; IM, intramuscular; PE, phenytoin sodium equivalents; SE, status epilepticus; ECG, electrocardiogram; EEG, electroencephalogram

Although most seizures are self-limited and stop in ≤5 minutes, most children who arrive to the emergency department or pediatric intensive care unit have been seizing for a significant length of time. This may include time seizing prior to discovery, time waiting for emergency personnel, and time spent en route to the hospital. Many patients may have already received medications from family members or emergency medical services (EMS) personnel, which may contribute to any respiratory depression seen on arrival.

*Management of SE includes:*
1. *General supportive care*
2. *Termination of SE*
3. *Prevention of seizure recurrence*
4. *Correction of precipitating causes*
5. *Prevention and treatment of potential complications*

### 1. Airway Management

The immediate assessment of the airway begins with a check for patency and reflexes. The airway may be secured by simple maneuvers, such as suctioning, positioning, and the use of airway adjuncts (nasal trumpets). High-flow oxygen should be administered and pulse oximetry instituted to evaluate oxygenation status. The presence of nasal flaring, poor chest rise, retractions, cyanosis, abdominal paradoxical breathing, diminished breath sounds, or apnea suggests that the patient should be endotracheally intubated and mechanically ventilated. If the patient requires the administration of a neuromuscular blocking agent for intubation, one with a short half-life should be used. This will stop the motor component of the seizure but will do nothing to stop the underlying electrical activity. Patients who are under continued paralysis should be monitored with continuous EEG.

### 2. Cardiovascular Management

Tachycardia, cool extremities, delayed capillary refill, diminished pulses, and poor urine output suggest hypovolemia. This and the resulting poor perfusion may be exacerbated by the addition of medications and positive pressure ventilation. The Pediatric Advanced Life Support (PALS) guidelines should be followed to obtain vascular access, through which the patient may receive isotonic fluid boluses (20 mL/kg). Antipyretics should be administered early in the management of the patient in SE.

### 3. Investigations

Specific studies should be tailored to match the patient history; however, serum glucose should be checked immediately, particularly in young infants. Other blood work may include testing serum electrolytes (sodium, calcium, and magnesium) and liver function, measuring arterial blood gas and antiepileptic drug levels, and ordering urine toxicology screening. In patients with altered mental status and signs of focality, an imaging study (non-contrast computed tomography [CT] scan) should be considered prior to a lumbar puncture for CSF examination. Antibiotics and antivirals (if indicated) should be promptly administered and the lumbar puncture delayed in the event that there are severe respiratory, cardiovascular, or other contraindications, such as a coagulopathy or elevated ICP.

Non-convulsive SE is possible in patients who do not quickly return to the baseline. Electrographic seizure activity has been reported in up to 15% of patients whose overt clinical seizures are pharmacologically controlled. This form of SE presents with altered mentation and absent or subtle motor findings (i.e., finger twitch), so is defined by EEG criteria. The incidence of non-convulsive SE in pediatrics is currently unknown, but adult studies have shown a mortality rate between 30% and 50%.

## C. Pharmacotherapy

The goal of administering an antiepileptic drug is to achieve rapid and safe termination of the event and to prevent recurrence. Common first-line medications are the benzodiazepines (diazepam, lorazepam, and midazolam), and second-line agents include phenytoin, fosphenytoin, and phenobarbital. The pharmacology and routes of administration of these agents are presented in **Table 15-6**. Common errors in the management of SE include insufficient drug dosages, delay in advancing to a second-line drug, and inadequate supportive care.

### Table 15-6  Pharmacologic Agents to Treat Status Epilepticus

| Drug | Dosage | Onset | Duration |
|---|---|---|---|
| Lorazepam | 0.1 mg/kg/dose IV/IO; may repeat once<br>Maximum: 4 mg/dose | 2-3 min | >6 h |
| Midazolam | 0.05-0.2 mg/kg/dose IV/IO/IM<br>Maximum: 5 mg/dose<br>Infusion: 1 μg/kg/min (range, 1-18 μg/kg/min)<br>PR: 0.5-1 mg/kg/dose | 2-5 min | 30-60 min |
| Diazepam | 0.1-0.3 mg/kg/dose<br>Maximum: 10 mg/dose<br>PR: 0.3-0.5 mg/kg/dose | 2-5 min | 60-90 min |
| Fosphenytoin | 20 mg/kg load IV/IM PE<br>3 mg/kg/min up to 150 mg/min | IV: 10-30 min<br>IM: >30 min | >10 h |
| Phenytoin | 20 mg/kg load IV<br>1 mg/kg/min up to 50 mg/min | 15-30 min | >10 h |
| PHENobarbital | 20 mg/kg load IV/IM<br>1 mg/kg/min up to 100 mg/min | 20-30 min | >50 h |
| PENTobarbital | 5-15 mg/kg load IV<br>Maximum rate of 50 mg/min<br>Infusion 1 mg/kg/h | 20-30 min | >72 h |
| Valproic acid | 20 mg/kg load IV<br>Infusion 3-6 mg/kg/h | 5-15 min | >10 h |
| Levetiracetam | 20-30 mg/kg load IV, then infusion<br>5 mg/kg/min (maximum 3 g) | 60 min | >24 h |

IV, intravenous; IO, intraosseous; IM, intramuscular; PR, per rectum; PE, phenytoin sodium equivalents

## D. Refractory Status Epilepticus

Refractory SE is defined as a continuing episode despite the administration of multiple agents, including benzodiazepines, fosphenytoin or phenytoin, and phenobarbital. Other drugs that are used for refractory SE include: valproic acid, pentobarbital, levetiracetam, and propofol. Often these patients have had continuous (clinical and/or electrographic) seizure activity for several hours. Their care should be a collaborative effort between intensive care specialists and neurologists, and requires standard invasive intensive care monitoring as well as 24-hour availability of an EEG.

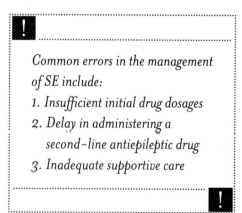

*Common errors in the management of SE include:*
1. *Insufficient initial drug dosages*
2. *Delay in administering a second-line antiepileptic drug*
3. *Inadequate supportive care*

# V. ALTERED MENTAL STATUS AND COMA

## Case Study

A 15-year-old boy arrives at the emergency department after becoming combative and disoriented at school after he was involved in an altercation. His mental status has continued to deteriorate, and the staff called you to assist in his intubation and further management.

**Detection**
- What is the most likely diagnosis?

**Intervention**
- What are the indications and techniques to consider in the airway management of a head-injured patient?
- What medications should be considered for the intubation of a head-injured patient?

**Reassessment**
- What is the differential diagnosis for a patient with an altered level of consciousness?

**Effective Communication**
- Who needs to be contacted about this patient?

**Teamwork**
- How are you going to implement the treatment strategy?

The differential diagnosis of coma and altered mental status includes neurologic and non-neurologic diseases and constitutes a true emergency. A systematic approach to these patients increases the likelihood of making the specific diagnosis. Maximal functional recovery depends upon resolution of the primary insult, if possible, and prevention of any secondary injury.

## A. Etiologies

Depressed consciousness results from either involvement of both cerebral cortices or the brainstem reticular activating system (RAS). This represents an emergency because a prolonged episode potentially limits the likelihood of full recovery. A wide variety of conditions produce alteration of consciousness in children. **Table 15-7** lists the etiologies that produce altered mental status and coma. Trauma, including head trauma, both accidental and nonaccidental, is a common cause of coma in the pediatric patient and is discussed in **Chapters 9** and **11**.

### Table 15-7  Etiologies of Altered Mental Status and Coma in Children

| Ischemic | Infection | Toxins |
|---|---|---|
| Cardiac arrest, cerebrovascular accident, near drowning, shock | Meningitis, encephalitis, brain abscess | Organophosphates, hypoglycemics, drugs of abuse, accidental ingestion |
| **Metabolic** | **Trauma** | **Neoplastic** |
| Diabetic ketoacidosis, hypoglycemia, sodium or osmolar abnormalities, hypoxia, hypercarbia, hyperammonemia | Accidental, nonaccidental | Mass lesions, obstructive hydrocephalus, overproduction of cerebrospinal fluid (choroid plexus) |
| **Inflammatory** | | |
| Systemic lupus erythematosus cerebritis | | |

Cerebral hypoxia and hypoxia-ischemia cause a significant proportion of comas in pediatric patients. (See **Chapter 3** for a discussion of global ischemia.) Cerebrovascular accidents (CVAs) producing focal ischemia occur much less commonly in pediatric patients than in adults, but those predisposed to thromboembolic disease may present with focal ischemic CVA. Congenital heart disease places patients at risk for paradoxical emboli and increases their risk for thrombosis formation. Thromboembolic CVA may also occur in patients with hemoglobinopathies and hypercoagulable states, including nephrotic syndrome, and protein C and protein S deficiencies. To result in coma, embolic CVAs must involve both cerebral hemispheres (uncommon) and the vertebrobasilar system, which supplies the RAS. Dural sinus thrombosis occurs in severely dehydrated neonates and following infections of the orbit or paranasal sinuses (particularly the sphenoid sinus). This may produce venous infarction of the brainstem and result in coma.

Intoxication may result from either exogenous or endogenous toxins. Hypoglycemia, hyper- or hypocalcemia, hyper- or hypomagnesemia, and hyper- or hypo-osmolality may all produce altered mental status. Any cause of severe acidosis (lactate, inborn error of metabolism) or hyperammonemia (liver failure, inborn error) may also produce altered mental status. Toddlers may accidentally ingest any substance in the home, whereas teenagers may intentionally consume a wide variety of substances. Sedatives (benzodiazepines, barbiturates, and alcohols), tricyclic antidepressants, stimulants (phencyclidine, amphetamines, cocaine), opiates, salicylates, organophosphates, and many other drugs may cause altered mental status (**Chapter 13**).

Seizures from any cause may depress consciousness both during (ictal) and following (postictal) the actual seizure. Historic evidence for the seizure may be subtle. Prolonged postictal states may occur due to persistence of the cause of the seizure (hypoglycemia, CVA, hyponatremia) or as a consequence of the seizure itself. Neuronal energy demands increase markedly with seizures, and inadequate augmentation of supply may produce an ischemic injury.

Meningitis, encephalitis, brain abscess, and subdural empyema may all cause altered mental status. This may result from elevation of ICP, direct inflammation of the RAS, vasculitis, and subsequent infarctions and seizures. Collagen vascular diseases (systemic lupus erythematosus) may similarly affect the level of consciousness, as may tumors, particularly with acute enlargement (hemorrhage into the tumor) or acute obstructive hydrocephalus.

# B. Evaluation

Serial examinations of the level of consciousness are the most important aspect of the neurologic exam. As in all cases, assurance of adequate airway control, respiratory effort, and hemodynamic status is of paramount importance. Because hypoglycemia occurs more commonly in critically ill young children and infants than in adults, the ABCs should be expanded to include D for checking a dextrose (glucose) level and for disability—signs or symptoms of CNS emergencies, such as dilated pupils or the Cushing triad (hypertension, bradycardia, and abnormal respirations). A significant alteration in any of these vital functions may produce altered mental status in a patient. During the resuscitation of comatose patients, 2 key points must be considered. First, if trauma is known or suspected, cervical spine immobilization must be maintained at all times, including during establishment of an artificial airway (**Chapter 2**). Second, fluids for resuscitation should be isotonic or hypertonic to minimize the possibility of cerebral edema and increased ICP.

> *Altered mental status constitutes a medical emergency. ABCs still receive top priority, but now include D for disability (signs of herniation, cervical spine, or other trauma) and dextrose.*

Once initial stability has been established and supported, specific evaluation for the cause of the altered/depressed mental status should begin. Many possibilities must be considered in the differential diagnosis of coma or altered mental status in children (**Table 15-7**). Life-threatening causes should be ruled out quickly with a careful history and physical exam, looking for signs of trauma, meningismus, elevated ICP (papilledema), or a toxidrome (**Chapter 13**). Historical information may be limited or difficult to obtain. Specific considerations include the following: Is the patient's mental status worsening/improving? How/where was the patient found, and what was nearby? Were any medications given by family or emergency medical services personnel?

Emergent imaging using a CT scan identifies significant intracranial hemorrhage, mass lesions, midline shift, skull fractures, or signs of intracranial hypertension, such as effacement of the sulci or basilar cisterns. The most important consideration prior to a CT scan is whether the patient is stable enough for the procedure. Patients must be adequately resuscitated, and those with compromised airway protective reflexes or respiratory effort should have an airway secured before imaging.

A lumbar puncture (LP) permits determination of the opening pressure, cell counts, protein and glucose levels, and culture with Gram stain. As with CT, cardiorespiratory function must be adequate before performing LP, particularly in infants and small children whose respiratory function can be severely impaired by positioning for the procedure. There is controversy over whether a CT scan must be performed in all patients prior to LP because it might precipitate herniation in patients with mass lesions or elevated ICP.

> 1. *If cervical spine injury is known or suspected, intubation requires 2 people to provide immobilization. Fiberoptic techniques may be required.*
> 2. *Resuscitation should proceed with isotonic or hypertonic fluids.*
> 3. *Rule out life-threatening causes first and treat while the workup proceeds.*

However, negative CT scans do not rule out all situations where subsequent herniation may occur after LP (e.g., meningitis). Patients with suspected CNS infection and contraindication to LP should be treated with empiric antibiotics (and antiviral agents when appropriate), obtaining CSF when deemed safe and with neurosurgical assistance if required.

In addition to checking whole-blood glucose, serum electrolytes (including calcium, magnesium, and phosphorus), liver and renal function, arterial blood gas, lactate, and ammonia should all be measured in the patient with altered mental status. A complete blood count may provide evidence of an infectious process or anemia consistent with chronic disease. Urine and serum toxicology screens should be obtained, ideally prior to the administration of sedatives or analgesics.

## C. Therapy

Therapy for coma is directed at the underlying cause, while maintenance of normoxia, normocarbia, and normal perfusion is of paramount importance. Treatment of hypoglycemia with 25% dextrose (2 mL/kg) or 10% dextrose (5 mL/kg) rapidly restores serum glucose levels. Further monitoring and maintenance of normoglycemia (80-150 mg/dL or 4.4-8.3 mmol/L) appears prudent. Symptomatic hyponatremia requires an initial, rapid increase in serum sodium to levels that do not produce symptoms; an increase of 5 mEq/L usually will suffice, and 6 mL/kg of 3% hypertonic saline will provide this increase.

> 1. *When elevated ICP is suspected, an adequate airway and circulatory support should precede diagnostic procedures (CT scan, magnetic resonance imaging, lumbar puncture).*
> 2. *Presumptive therapy for intracranial hypertension or CNS infection should be instituted expectantly if diagnostic procedures are delayed.*
> 3. *Negative findings on a head CT do not rule out possible herniation after LP if clinical signs of intracranial hypertension are present.*

# VI. INTRACRANIAL HYPERTENSION

## Case Study

A 2-year-old boy has been brought to the emergency department after falling down a flight of stairs. Combative on arrival, he had a room-air pulse oximetry value of 82%, and he has been intubated with cervical spine precautions. You have been called to assist in his management. During your exam, he becomes stiff, his blood pressure increases to 150/90 mm Hg, and his heart rate decreases to 55 beats/min.

**Detection**
- What are the clinical signs and symptoms associated with an ICP elevation?
- What is the Cushing triad?

**Intervention**

– What are the indications for administration of mannitol and/or hypertonic saline?

**Reassessment**

– What other therapies could be considered for ICP elevation?

**Effective Communication**

– Who needs to know about this patient?

**Teamwork**

– How are you going to monitor this patient?

Although intracranial hypertension (increased ICP) has a number of etiologies, specific management is imperative to promote adequate cerebral perfusion pressure and CBF.

# A. Manifestations

The Monro-Kellie doctrine states that intracranial hypertension results from any process that increases the volume of the brain, CSF, or CBV, without a compensatory decrease in the other components. **Table 15-8** lists some common entities that may increase ICP. At least initially, such increase must be inferred from clinical manifestations. Increased ICP itself produces minimal findings (except papilledema and headache) unless mass effect produces local ischemia or herniation of intracranial components. Chronic, slowly progressive increases in ICP are particularly well tolerated. Evidence of increased symptoms at night (increased $Paco_2$), upon awakening (with position changes), or with coughing (increased CBV) may all indicate an elevated ICP. Acute increases produce mental status changes and cranial nerve findings much more rapidly. Once intracranial hypertension is suspected, therapy should be instituted immediately and consideration given to monitoring the ICP.

### Table 15-8 Entities That Produce Increased Intracranial Pressure

| | |
|---|---|
| A | Alcohol |
| E | Electrolytes, Encephalitis |
| I | Ingestion, Infection, Insulin |
| O | Opiates |
| U | Uremia |
| T | Trauma |
| H | Hyper/Hypoglycemia, Temperature, Blood Pressure |
| I | Intussusception |
| P | Psychiatric |
| S | Seizures, Structural |

## B. Monitoring Intracranial Pressure

ICP can be monitored in a number of locations (intraventricular, intraparenchymal, subarachnoid/subdural, and epidural) and by different techniques. The "gold standard" is placement of an intraventricular catheter because it allows drainage of CSF, which provides a therapeutic option for increased ICP. The main disadvantages are the difficulty of placement, particularly in patients with compressed ventricles; the increased risk and consequences of infection; and the possibility of malfunction as the ventricles become progressively smaller. The ultimate goal is to recognize elevated ICP. Although ICP >20 mm Hg often triggers interventions, CPP <65 mm Hg (and perhaps between 40 and 50 mm Hg in infants) warrants therapy to raise MAP and/or lower ICP.

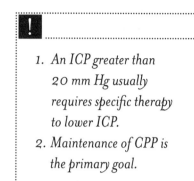

1. *An ICP greater than 20 mm Hg usually requires specific therapy to lower ICP.*
2. *Maintenance of CPP is the primary goal.*

## C. Therapy

Assurance of adequate respiratory and circulatory function should receive top priority in all patients, including those with intracranial hypertension. During endotracheal intubation, special attention should be paid to use drugs that do not increase ICP and to provide adequate anesthesia to blunt ICP spikes with laryngoscopy. Fever should be aggressively treated to prevent increased cerebral metabolism and CBF. Similarly, seizures should be aggressively treated. Adequate analgesia and sedation during painful procedures also reduce ICP.

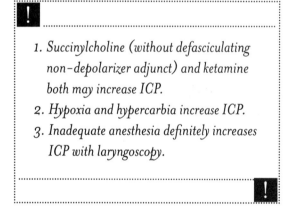

1. *Succinylcholine (without defasciculating non-depolarizer adjunct) and ketamine both may increase ICP.*
2. *Hypoxia and hypercarbia increase ICP.*
3. *Inadequate anesthesia definitely increases ICP with laryngoscopy.*

Therapy for elevated ICP begins with brief induced hyperventilation and sedation, as well as midline neck positioning and elevation of the head of the bed to 30° (when not contraindicated) to maximize venous drainage. Other therapies aim to reduce the volume of the intracranial contents and/or to minimize cerebral metabolic demands.

When intracranial hypertension is suspected, one of the most difficult decisions is determining when to electively sedate and intubate the patient who is otherwise maintaining adequate gas exchange. Although sedation will obscure the clinical neurologic exam, elective intubation is much safer than emergent intubation when apnea or hypoventilation occurs. Once a patient is intubated, however, the need for ICP monitoring increases due to the lack of exam criteria. If a ventricular drain is present, CSF drainage is the next line of therapy. Placement of an extraventricular drain is particularly useful in the initial management of patients with ventricular shunt malfunction, infection, or obstructive hydrocephalus due to neoplasm. Neuromuscular blockade may further lower ICP, even in patients who appear adequately sedated, and has the added benefit of lowering systemic oxygen consumption.

Osmolar therapy constitutes the next line in medical therapy of intracranial hypertension. Either mannitol (0.5 g/kg [range 0.25-1 g/kg] intravenously as needed) or hypertonic saline (HTS) may be used to raise serum osmolarity. Controlled hypovolemia is not appropriate because it places the patient at risk for hypotension and decreased CPP. The diuretic effect of mannitol must be considered in this regard. However, diuretics do have a role in the euvolemic or volume-expanded patient with inadequate response to mannitol. Some evidence suggests that higher serum osmolality can be achieved with HTS (up to 360 mOsm) than with mannitol (320 mOsm) without increased risk of side effects, but the choice of agent generally depends on rapid availability and the patient's volume status. The HTS dose depends on the concentration of the solution. Because sodium distributes in the extracellular fluid space, 0.6 mEq/kg will raise the serum sodium by 1 mEq/L (**Chapter 8**). Infusions of 3% HTS (between 0.1 and 1 mL/kg/h) may be used to maintain the serum sodium (and osmolality) at a level that reduces ICP. Importantly, this circumstance differs dramatically from correction of hypotonicity in that increases in osmolality must often occur at rates >0.5 mEq/L/h. Normalization of ICP (and CPP) predominates over a specific target for the rate of increase in serum osmolality, so the frequency of HTS boluses and rate of infusions will depend on the patient's response as long as serum osmolality remains below 360 mOsm.

> *Hypertonic saline bolus dosing: 3 mEq/kg of 3% HTS will raise the serum sodium by 5 mEq/L, which corresponds to a dose of 6 mL/kg of 3% HTS.*

Other medical therapies have beneficial effects in certain situations. Corticosteroids (dexamethasone) reduce peritumor edema but have no beneficial effects in non-neoplastic causes of intracranial hypertension. Careful consideration should be given to gastrointestinal prophylaxis with antacid medications when using corticosteroids because these patients have an increased risk of intestinal ulceration and hemorrhage (Cushing ulcer). High-dose barbiturates inducing pharmacologic coma have proven benefits in reducing ICP, though their effect on outcome remains less clear. In addition, they reduce cerebral oxygen consumption, providing another possible benefit. Barbiturate coma may also be necessary in patients with refractory seizures, which increase ICP.

Two medical therapies deserve special mention. First, aggressive hyperventilation ($Paco_2$ <35 mm Hg [<4.7 kPa]), which may be required for an acute increase in ICP, has no place in the long-term management of intracranial hypertension. As mentioned earlier, the reduction in CBF places the brain at risk of ischemia. Also, since the response depends on pH change in the CSF, accommodation occurs with sustained hypocapnia. Note that this also means that a patient with metabolic acidosis (i.e., diabetic ketoacidosis) may require a lower $Paco_2$ to maintain a pH of 7.35 to 7.4 and normal CBF until the acidosis is corrected. Secondly, hypothermia theoretically promotes a number of conditions that reduce ICP. Several studies of traumatic brain injury in animal models and children have documented decreased cerebral oxygen consumption, decreased CBF, reduced inflammation, and altered intracellular signaling with hypothermia. Initiation of moderate hypothermia (90-92°F [32-33°C]) for 48 hours after severe traumatic brain injury may be considered.

> *Hyperventilation ($Paco_2$ <35 mm Hg [4.7 kPa]) has no place in the long-term management of increased ICP.*

Surgical therapies for elevated ICP include removal of mass lesions (tumor, hematoma) or cranial bones (craniectomy) to increase the compliance of the cranial space. Limited comparative data support the use of decompressive craniectomy in particular clinical conditions, but it can reduce ICP in patients with medically refractory intracranial hypertension. Another second-line surgical option is the placement of a lumbar drain in patients with slit-like ventricles and increased ICP but with open basilar cisterns. Limited data suggest that this lowers ICP and does not promote herniation.

# VII. CEREBROVASCULAR ACCIDENTS

 ## Case Study

Early in the day, a 5-year-old girl with sickle cell disease complained of headache; later, her mother found her less responsive, with slurred speech and decreased movement of her left arm. She brought the girl to the emergency department, where you were consulted to assist in her care. She is dysarthric, hemiparetic on the left, with mildly decreased level of alertness. Her vital signs are significant for mild tachycardia but otherwise normal.

**Detection**

– What are the common presenting signs and symptoms of a CVA in a pediatric patient?

**Intervention**

– What laboratory studies should be obtained in a patient with a suspected CVA?

– What neuroimaging studies are required in a patient with a suspected CVA?

**Reassessment**

– What is the differential diagnosis of suspected CVA?

**Effective Communication**

– Who should be contacted and where should this patient be managed?

**Teamwork**

– What should the treatment strategy be for a pediatric patient with a CVA?

Although CVAs occur much less commonly in children than in adults, the reported incidence (about 2 cases per 100,000 children each year) closely approximates that of childhood brain tumors. This incidence increases further in specific at-risk populations. Furthermore, CVAs rank among the top 10 causes of death in pediatric patients. Therefore, anyone providing emergency care for children must have the skills to recognize and manage CVAs. As in adults, therapies must be instituted rapidly to promote maximal functional recovery.

## A. Manifestations of Cerebrovascular Accidents

The manifestations of a CVA depend in part on the type of event (hemorrhagic versus thromboembolic) and on the location of the injury. The majority of pediatric CVAs involve the intracranial branches of the carotid artery, specifically the middle cerebral artery. Lesions in this distribution produce hemiparesis, hemianesthesia, hemianopia, and, when affecting the dominant hemisphere, aphasia. Because the sensorimotor function for the lower extremities resides on the medial aspect of the cortex, lesions of the anterior cerebral artery affect those functions, as well as emotional control and intellectual function. Lesions of the posterior cerebral artery affect vision or the deep structures of the brainstem, producing motor and sensory defects, pupillary abnormalities, and depressed consciousness. Finally, the vertebrobasilar system (posterior circulation) supplies the lower brainstem and cranial nerves; therefore, deep coma, cranial nerve abnormalities, and cerebellar signs occur with CVAs in that distribution.

## B. Hemorrhagic Cerebrovascular Accident

Hemorrhagic stroke, which has a higher mortality rate than ischemic stroke, has both aneurysms and arteriovenous malformations (AVMs) as primary etiologies, although conversion of initially ischemic events may occur (particularly for venous infarctions). Aneurysms occur either with congenital defects in the muscular layer of arteries or in association with neurocutaneous syndromes and inherited defects of connective-tissue components (i.e., Ehlers-Danlos syndrome). Nearly half of aneurysms occur in the posterior circulation, and many occur distally and deep within the brain substance.

Both the requisite increase in ICP and vasospasm contribute to the decreased CBF following aneurysmal bleeding. Blood in the basilar cisterns compromises blood flow to the hypothalamus, resulting in abnormalities of adrenergic tone. This likely contributes to the dysrhythmia and electrocardiogram changes seen with subarachnoid hemorrhage (SAH). Increased sympathetic tone probably produces the neurogenic pulmonary edema seen in these patients.

SAH in adults is different than in children. First, the role of vasospasm in children remains less clear than that in adults. Although some studies have suggested similar rates of vasospasm and others less in children, children suffer fewer symptoms when it occurs. Generally, the therapy for vasospasm parallels that for CVAs, with maintenance of adequate CBF being the primary goal. However, in patients with untreated aneurysms, induced hypertension carries a significant risk of rebleeding and should be avoided. Also, calcium channel blockade probably has a limited role in the treatment of pediatric SAH. Finally, children have a much lower incidence of rebleeding than adults, reducing the need for emergent surgical intervention in the absence of significant mass lesion or intracranial hypertension.

Arteriovenous malformations present most frequently in the second decade of life. Again, most are supratentorial, involving some component of the middle cerebral artery distribution. More than half of patients have intraparenchymal involvement in the hemorrhage, but while SAH may result from extension to the ventricular system or cerebral convexities, blood typically does not involve the basilar cisterns. Therefore, vasospasm is not a concern, although other aspects of therapy for arteriovenous malformations are similar to those for aneurysmal bleeding. Definitive treatment by surgical excision or, in some cases, embolization eradicates the 2% to 3% risk of rebleeding per year.

## C. Thromboembolic Cerebrovascular Accidents

Thromboembolic disease, which produces ischemic strokes, affects the middle cerebral artery distribution in most cases. Various diseases predispose patients to thromboembolic disease. Cardiac disease, either acquired or congenital, is the most common predisposing factor. Sickle cell disease represents a well-studied predisposition and the only one for which controlled clinical trials have been performed. Infections, including meningitis and paranasal sinus infections, form another large category. Finally, many metabolic and inherited hematologic disorders predispose children to stroke.

Unfortunately, the majority of pediatric patients with ischemic CVAs present late. Intravenous thrombolytic therapy is contraindicated after 3 hours of symptoms. Intra-arterial therapy may be performed up to 8 hours from onset depending on the arterial territory. Abbreviated diffuse weighted magnetic resonance imaging will help differentiate those patients that may be candidates for thrombolytic therapies. However, thrombolysis in pediatric CVAs remains an infrequent therapy. Most treatment aims to prevent secondary injury by promoting adequate oxygen supply to marginal regions. As mentioned, decreased blood volume, hypotension, and hypocarbia all exacerbate cerebral ischemia. In fact, some authors recommend volume expansion with colloid to induce hemodilution and improve the microvascular rheology. Although this approach may remain controversial, prevention of hyperviscosity by limiting hematocrit to the normal range seems appropriate.

Generally speaking, thromboembolic CVAs should remain clinically static after presentation because the embolic event has already occurred. Therefore, deterioration of the neurologic exam should raise suspicion of a secondary insult. Possibilities include hyponatremia, hyper- or hypoglycemia, worsened perfusion, or hemorrhagic conversion. Another possibility is recurrent embolism or extension of clot. Also, edema surrounding the infarcted area typically increases over the first 24 to 48 hours before reaching its zenith. Prompt evaluation of each possibility is required. Peak cerebral edema occurs later in patients suffering secondary insults, such as recurrent emboli, cerebral ischemia secondary to hypotension, or ECF hypotonicity. If other investigations fail to determine the etiology of the deterioration, consideration should be given to systemic anticoagulation with heparin. Heparinization also may be indicated in patients with documented thrombus and acute thromboembolic CVA if the initial head CT does not detect hemorrhage.

# VIII. CEREBROSPINAL FLUID SHUNTS

## Case Study

A 14-year-old boy, who received a ventriculoperitoneal shunt at birth for aqueductal stenosis and underwent a shunt revision 3 months ago, presents with a headache and complaints of not feeling right. He has not gone to school in several days, and he vomited 3 times before arriving in the emergency department. His mother reports that he has a flu-like illness. While being interviewed, the patient has a 1-minute right-sided seizure and seems a bit dazed as you try to continue your history and physical exam. He has a respiratory rate of 20 breaths/min, heart rate of 70 beats/min, blood pressure of 150/90 mm Hg, and temperature of 100.8°F (38.2°C). His mother asks what you think is going on.

### Detection

- What are the common signs and symptoms of ventriculoperitoneal shunt malfunction?
- What are the major complications in patients with shunted hydrocephalus?

### Intervention

- What laboratory and neuroimaging studies should be performed?

### Reassessment

- What interventions are indicated?

### Effective Communication

- Who needs to be contacted about this patient?

### Teamwork

- How are you going to implement the treatment strategy?

Patients who present with shunt obstruction may show signs of increased ICP that include headache, nausea, vomiting, lethargy, and papilledema. It is crucial to involve the neurosurgeon early in the evaluation and management of these patients. Evaluation begins with a thorough history and physical exam. Following the ABCs, imaging studies are performed and include a head CT and a shunt series (lateral radiograph of the skull and an anteroposterior view to include the neck, chest, and abdomen to check the shunt position and connections). After these images are reviewed with the neurosurgeon, an attempt to obtain CSF from the shunt is made in a sterile fashion. If this fails or an elevated opening pressure suggests a shunt obstruction, a surgical revision may be necessary. If CSF is obtained, testing includes cell count, culture, Gram stain, and a glucose and protein determination.

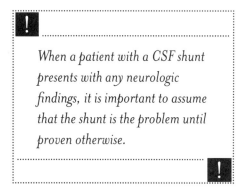

*When a patient with a CSF shunt presents with any neurologic findings, it is important to assume that the shunt is the problem until proven otherwise.*

Serious complications that may occur in patients with CSF shunts include mechanical failure (proximal or distal obstruction) and infection. The risk of shunt failure is greatest in the first months following placement. Many, if not all, of these children are admitted to the pediatric intensive care unit for observation preceding the surgical repair. Common signs and symptoms include headache, vomiting, nausea, altered mental status, lethargy, and a general feeling of malaise.

Obstruction is the most frequent cause of shunt malfunction, with proximal obstruction occurring more frequently than distal. The proximal end of the catheter may become occluded with choroid plexus, ependymal cells, glial tissue, brain debris, fibrin, or blood, or the tip of the catheter may migrate into the brain parenchyma. Distal obstruction may result from kinking or disconnection of the tubing, migration of the catheter outside the peritoneum, intra-abdominal infection, or pseudocyst formation. Regardless of the etiology of the obstruction, occlusion will prevent the egress of CSF from the ventricular system, which will ultimately lead to a buildup of CSF in the ventricular system and a rise in ICP.

The incidence of CSF shunt infections is between 5% and 8%. Infection may involve the shunt equipment, the wound, the CSF, or the distal site where the shunt drains. Approximately 70% of shunt infections occur within the first 2 months following surgery, and almost 90% will occur in the first 6 months. The organisms most frequently isolated include *Staphylococcus epidermidis* (40%) and *S. aureus* (20%), with the remainder caused by enterococci, streptococci, Gram-negative rods, and yeast. Clinical signs depend on the site of the infection (**Table 15-9**). Wound infections manifest with fever and reddening of the incision or shunt tract, with a discharge of pus along the incision as the infection progresses. Patients with ventriculitis and meningitis have fever, headache, irritability, and neck stiffness or nuchal rigidity. The treatment of choice is removal of the shunt hardware with placement of an external ventricular drain and administration of parenteral antibiotics. Infections of temporarily placed external ventricular drains are managed in the same manner.

**Table 15-9** Symptoms of Shunt Malfunction

| Infants | Toddlers | Adolescents |
|---|---|---|
| Fever, vomiting | Fever, vomiting | Fever, vomiting |
| Head enlargement | Headache | Headache |
| Tense fontanelle | Irritability and tiredness | Vision problems |
| Prominent scalp veins | Swelling along shunt track | Irritability and/or tiredness |
| Swelling along shunt track | Loss of prior abilities (sensory or motor) | Personality change or decline in school performance |
| Irritability and tiredness | Seizures | Loss of coordination |
| Downward eye deviation | | Difficulty in waking or staying awake |

## Neurologic Emergencies

**Key Points**

- In the young child, irritability is an early sign of change in mental status.

- Acute changes in neurologic function, including altered mental status and weakness, require emergent evaluation and treatment to promote maximal recovery.

- Preservation of cerebral blood flow is of paramount importance in any neurologic emergency.

- Hypoxemia, hypercarbia, and hyperthermia should be aggressively prevented in a patient with any neurologic abnormality.

- Intracranial hemorrhage in the young infant can cause hemodynamically significant blood loss.

- Hypoglycemia is common in stressed infants and must be corrected promptly.

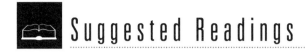

# Suggested Readings

1. Avner JR. Altered states of consciousness. *Pediatr Rev.* 2006;27:331-338.

2. Bratton S, Bullock R, Carney N. Guidelines for the management of severe traumatic brain injury. *J Neurotrauma.* 2007;24(Suppl 1):S1-S105.

3. Emeriaud G, Pettersen G, Ozanne B. Pediatric traumatic brain injury: an update. *Curr Opin Anaesthesiol.* 2011;24:307-313.

4. Forsyth LL, Liu-DeRyke X, Parker D, Rhoney DH. Role of hypertonic saline for the management of intracranial hypertension after stroke and traumatic brain injury. *Pharmacotherapy.* 2008;28:469-484.

5. Fuhrman BP, Zimmerman JJ, eds. *Pediatric Critical Care.* 4th ed. Philadelphia, PA: Mosby; 2011:805-870, 893-906.

6. Issacman DJ, Trainor JL, Rothrock SG. Central nervous system. In: Gausche-Hill M, Fuchs S, Yamamoto L, eds. *The Pediatric Emergency Medicine Resource.* 4th ed. Sudbury, MA: Jones and Bartlett Publishers; 2004:146-185.

7. Kligman RM, Stanton BF, St. Geme JW, eds. *Nelson Textbook of Pediatrics.* 19th ed. Philadelphia, PA: Saunders; 2011:1998-2108.

8. Kochanek PM, Carney N, Adelson PD, et al. Guidelines for the acute medical management of severe traumatic brain injury in infants, children, and adolescents-second edition. *Pediatr Crit Care Med.* 2012;13(Suppl 1):S1-S82.

9. Posner JB, Saper CB, Schiff N, Plum F. *The Diagnosis of Stupor and Coma.* 4th ed. Cambridge, MA: Oxford University Press; 2007.

10. Shearer P, Riviello J. Generalized convulsive status epilepticus in adults and children: treatment guidelines and protocols. *Emerg Med Clin North Am.* 2011;29:51-64.

11. Shu S. Section VI. Neurologic. In: Perkin RM, Swift JD, Newton DA, eds. *Pediatric Hospitalist Medicine: Textbook of Inpatient Management.* 2nd ed. Philadelphia, PA: Lippincott Williams & Wilkins; 2008:259-276.

12. Wheeler DS, Wong HR, Shanley TP. *Pediatric Critical Care Medicine: Basic Science and Clinical Evidence.* London, UK: Springer-Verlag; 2007:865-1012.

# Chapter 16

# MANAGEMENT OF THE CHILD WITH CONGENITAL HEART DISEASE

## 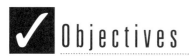 Objectives

- Identify congenital cardiac defects in neonates who present with low cardiac output.
- Discuss initial management and diagnostic testing of a cyanotic infant.
- Review the evaluation and treatment of children with acyanotic congenital heart disease.
- Understand the most common causes of low cardiac output syndrome in the postoperative pediatric cardiac surgical patient.
- Outline the evaluation and management of low cardiac output syndrome.
- Summarize the most common postoperative arrhythmias.

##  Case Study

A 6-day-old male newborn presents to the pediatric unit with a 2-day history of decreased feeding, increasing tachypnea, and lethargy. His vital signs are heart rate 195 beats/min, respiratory rate 90 breaths/min, and room air saturations 87% via pulse oximetry when measured in both the right arm (preductal) and right leg (postductal). There are no intercostal or suprasternal retractions noted. Rales, but not wheezing or stridor, are heard on auscultation. Pulses in all four extremities are difficult to palpate.

**Detection**

- What are the most important initial steps in evaluating this newborn?
- What should be included in the differential diagnosis?
- What is the most likely diagnosis?

**Intervention**

- Which studies and treatment strategies take priority?

**Reassessment**

- Is the current treatment strategy effective?
- Does the patient need other therapeutic interventions?

#### Effective Communication
- Who needs to be aware of this patient?
- Where is the best place to manage the care of this patient?

#### Teamwork
- How are you going to implement the treatment strategy?
- Who is to do what and when?

# I. INTRODUCTION

The purpose of this chapter is to consider the principal issues involved in the care of the pediatric cardiac patient. Although many facets of care are common to all cardiac patients, pediatric cardiac intensive care requires a clear understanding of a patient's native cardiac anatomy and physiology, as well as the changes to the circulation that occur following surgical intervention.

# II. NEONATES WITH LOW CARDIAC OUTPUT

## A. Hypoplastic Left Heart Syndrome

Hypoplastic left heart syndrome (HLHS) describes a spectrum of congenital heart diseases characterized by varying degrees of hypoplasia of the left-sided heart structures. The incidence in the United States is 2.4 cases per 10,000 live births. HLHS is characterized by a tiny left ventricle, incapable of supporting the systemic circulation, and underdevelopment of the mitral and aortic valves. The central anatomic feature in the most common form is aortic valve atresia with hypoplasia of the ascending aorta and aortic arch. In the case of aortic atresia and mitral atresia, the ascending aorta is typically very small and is perfused through retrograde aortic arch flow via the ductus arteriosus. Survival beyond birth depends on persistent patency of the ductus arteriosus to maintain the systemic circulation. Without intervention, HLHS is fatal within the first few days after birth. Neonates typically present with mild cyanosis, tachypnea, and signs of shock after the ductus arteriosus, upon which the systemic circulation depends, begins to close.

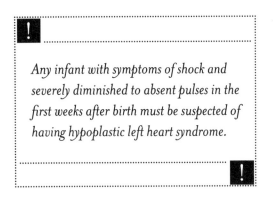

*Any infant with symptoms of shock and severely diminished to absent pulses in the first weeks after birth must be suspected of having hypoplastic left heart syndrome.*

An arterial blood gas will show a lactic acidosis and hypoxemia, typically with a $Pa_{O_2}$ <100 mm Hg (<13.3 kPa). The physical findings of a mild cyanosis, respiratory distress, and impending cardiovascular collapse are nonspecific and do not help to distinguish this ductal-dependent cardiac lesion from others that present in the neonatal period. The electrocardiogram will show right ventricular forces predominantly, as in normal neonates. Cardiomegaly and pulmonary edema will be present on the chest radiograph. Echocardiogram confirms the diagnosis and should be performed urgently.

Timely and appropriate initial medical management is lifesaving. A prostaglandin $E_1$ ($PGE_1$) infusion should be initiated rapidly to reopen the ductus arteriosus and restore perfusion to the descending aorta and, through retrograde flow, to the ascending aorta and coronary circulation. The usual starting dose of $PGE_1$ is 0.05 µg/kg/min (range 0.025-0.1 µg/kg/min). The major side effects of $PGE_1$ include apnea and peripheral vasodilatation, so the clinician must be prepared to provide mechanical ventilatory support and administer additional fluids and/or inotropic agents if needed. Infants who are diagnosed prenatally or who present with stable hemodynamics may benefit from spontaneous breathing. However, the infant who presents in cardiogenic shock with critically low oxygen delivery requires control of the airway and hemodynamic support with intubation and mechanical ventilation.

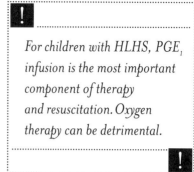

*For children with HLHS, $PGE_1$ infusion is the most important component of therapy and resuscitation. Oxygen therapy can be detrimental.*

Once the ductus arteriosus has reopened and distal perfusion is restored, maintaining a favorable balance between the systemic and pulmonary circulations is critical for preserving distal organ perfusion while maintaining adequate pulmonary blood flow. Hyperventilation and hyperoxia will both lead to preferential pulmonary blood flow through the ductus at the expense of systemic blood flow. Judicious fluid administration (with 10-20 mL/kg of 0.9% saline or 5% albumin) and inotropic support (with 3-10 µg/kg/min dopamine or 0.01-0.1 µg/kg/min epinephrine) may be necessary in certain cases to support low cardiac output.

The specifics of surgical palliation for HLHS may vary, but in most centers, a staged surgical approach is undertaken during the first week after birth to create a neo-aorta and provide adequate pulmonary circulation (**Table 16-1**). The three goals of stage I reconstruction for HLHS are: 1) to provide systemic perfusion independent of the ductus arteriosus, 2) to preserve

### Table 16-1 Staged Surgical Repair of Hypoplastic Left Heart Syndrome

| Procedure | Age of Patient | Actions Performed |
| --- | --- | --- |
| Norwood procedure | First weeks after birth | Patent ductus arteriosus is ligated. |
| | | Main PA is separated from branch PAs and used in the creation of a neo-aorta using the main PA, diminutive ascending aorta, and vascular allograft. |
| | | Pulmonary blood flow is reestablished via modified Blalock-Taussig shunt (innominate or subclavian artery to ipsilateral PA) or Sano shunt (right ventricle to PA conduit). |
| | | Atrial septectomy is performed. |
| | | Regulation of pulmonary blood flow with a shunt of fixed diameter and length, coupled with nonrestrictive interatrial communication via the atrial septectomy, enables normal development of the pulmonary vasculature while avoiding excessive ventricular volume overload. |
| Modified bidirectional Glenn anastomosis | 3-6 months | Take down of modified Blalock-Taussig shunt or right ventricle to PA conduit (Sano shunt). |
| | | Distal superior vena cava is sewn into the top of the right PA (end-to-side anastomosis). |
| Modified Fontan | 2-4 years | Inferior vena cava is connected to the branch PA via an extracardiac procedure conduit or intracardiac tunnel. |

PA, pulmonary artery

ventricular function, preventing volume and pressure overload, and 3) to allow normal maturation of the pulmonary vasculature. The procedure consists of: 1) anastomosing the main pulmonary trunk to the underside of the diminutive aortic arch with arch reconstruction and coarctectomy; 2) creation of a systemic to pulmonary artery shunt, either with an innominate to pulmonary artery graft or via a right ventricle to pulmonary artery conduit to provide a source of pulmonary blood flow; and 3) atrial septectomy to avoid pulmonary venous hypertension. A cavo-pulmonary anastomosis, connecting the superior vena cava to the right pulmonary artery (bidirectional Glenn), is performed at ~6 months. The third stage (Fontan operation) incorporates the inferior vena cava into the pulmonary circulation and is performed at approximately 2 years of age. Successful completion of the third stage allows the entire systemic venous return to completely bypass the right side of the heart and flow directly into the pulmonary arteries. Long-term survival with good neurologic outcome is dependent upon high surgical volumes, so families who opt for surgery for HLHS should be referred to regional centers that specialize in complex congenital cardiac surgery.

## B. Aortic Stenosis

In the United States, aortic stenosis occurs in 3% of children with congenital heart disease (CHD). The commissures of the aortic valve are fused, resulting in a thickened, domed valve with a stenotic orifice. The presenting symptoms and findings on physical examination are variable and relate to the degree of valve narrowing. Patients will have a systolic ejection murmur loudest at the upper right sternal border with radiation into the neck. Often a click will be audible. Patients with critical aortic stenosis have decreased systemic perfusion resulting in cardiogenic shock. They will have poor oral intake with decreased urine output. On examination, these infants will be tachypneic and lethargic, with diminished peripheral pulses throughout. Children with mild or moderate stenosis are normally asymptomatic and present with a loud systolic murmur.

Neonates with critical aortic stenosis present with cardiovascular collapse and require emergent treatment with $PGE_1$ infusion to reestablish ductal-dependent systemic flow. Intubation, mechanical ventilation, and inotropic support are needed in these critically ill neonates.

Balloon valvuloplasty is often successful at treating this lesion, though severe aortic regurgitation at the time of the procedure and restenosis afterward are known significant risks. Surgical valve replacement with a prosthetic mechanical valve or the patient's native pulmonary valve (Ross procedure) is recommended for patients in whom the valve annulus is very small or after failed valvuloplasty. Enlargement of the left ventricular outflow tract with a patch (Konno procedure) may be required at the time of the valve replacement to make additional room for the valve in the left ventricular outflow tract.

## C. Coarctation of the Aorta

Coarctation of the aorta (CoA), which occurs in 5% of children with CHD, is a narrowing of the descending aorta that usually occurs opposite to the ductus arteriosus. The symptoms in these patients will vary depending on the degree of obstruction. Infants with critical CoA will present in the neonatal period with cardiogenic shock, while children with mild disease will often present later with hypertension or an asymptomatic murmur.

Infants with critical CoA are fussy, have difficulty feeding, and become lethargic over time. On exam, femoral pulses are decreased while pulses in the right upper extremity may be normal or bounding. If the diagnosis is missed, these patients progress to cardiogenic shock with respiratory failure and/or congestive heart failure.

> *Infants with critical coarctation present with shock in the first week after birth, after spontaneous closure of the ductus arteriosus. Left ventricular ejection fraction decreases acutely in response to the increased afterload, leading to elevated ventricular wall tension, decreased myocardial perfusion pressure, and the risk of myocardial ischemia.*

Most children with CoA undergo surgical repair, although balloon angioplasty or stent implantation can be performed in selected older patients. Many older children with CoA have postoperative hypertension that is usually responsive to β-receptor blockade agents or angiotensin-converting enzyme inhibitors. In the immediate postoperative period, esmolol (50-250 μg/kg/min) has the advantage of a very short half-life, which allows for easy titration. Patients normally transition to oral therapy with either atenolol (0.5-2 mg/kg/day) or enalapril (0.05-0.25 mg/kg given twice daily), titrating the dose as necessary (maximum dose 5 mg) to maintain a normal blood pressure.

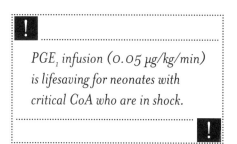

> *$PGE_1$ infusion (0.05 μg/kg/min) is lifesaving for neonates with critical CoA who are in shock.*

## D. Myocarditis and Cardiomyopathies

Myocarditis and cardiomyopathies may present in the neonatal period but are much more common at older ages. Both lesions are characterized by ventricular dysfunction. Patients typically present with signs and symptoms of congestive heart failure (**Tables 16-2** and **16-3**) but may also present in cardiogenic shock.

### Table 16-2  Common Symptoms of Heart Failure

| Infants | Children |
| --- | --- |
| Tachypnea | Failure to thrive |
| Diaphoresis | Decreased energy |
| Feeding intolerance | Exercise intolerance |
| Decreased urine output | Frequent respiratory infections |
| Failure to thrive | Chest pain |

### Table 16-3  Common Physical Findings of Congestive Heart Failure

| | |
| --- | --- |
| Tachycardia | Tachypnea |
| Displaced and dampened apical impulse | Failure to thrive |
| Gallop rhythm (S3 and S4) | Pulmonary rales |
| Hepatomegaly | Peripheral edema |

Myocarditis is most often associated with a viral illness, whereas the cardiomyopathies have an extensive list of etiologies (such as inborn errors of metabolism) that extends beyond the scope of this chapter. Patients with either entity may show significant improvement with appropriate medical therapy (afterload reduction, diuretics) or their condition may not improve, necessitating heart transplantation.

The causes of low cardiac output in newborns are listed in **Table 16-4**, and a summary of the initial evaluation and treatment of low cardiac output is presented in **Table 16-5**.

### Table 16-4  Causes of Low Cardiac Output in Newborns

| | |
|---|---|
| Coarctation of the aorta | Myocarditis |
| Hypoplastic left heart syndrome | Pericardial tamponade |
| Critical aortic stenosis | Pneumothorax |
| Interrupted aortic arch | Hydrops fetalis |
| Arrhythmia (tachycardic or bradycardic) | Sepsis (decompensated, late-stage) |
| Cardiomyopathy (hypertrophic from maternal diabetes) | |

### Table 16-5  Initial Evaluation and Treatment of Newborns with Low Cardiac Output

| Initial Evaluation | Initial Treatment |
|---|---|
| Blood culture | Intravenous fluid resuscitation: 10 mL/kg bolus of normal saline or 5% albumin or packed red blood cells (if anemic). Repeat if clinically indicated. |
| Arterial blood gas | |
| Central venous oxygen saturation | Inotropic agents (**Table 16-9**) |
| Lactate | Prostaglandin $E_1$ (for ductal-dependent lesions): 0.05 µg/kg/min intravenously |
| Chest radiograph | Treatment of underlying arrhythmia |
| Electrocardiogram | Intravenous immune globulin for myocarditis |
| Echocardiogram | Antibiotics |

NOTE: Oxygen can be detrimental in hypoplastic left heart syndrome.

# III. CYANOTIC CONGENITAL HEART DISEASE

 Case Study

A 12-hour-old female neonate is noted to be cyanotic with preductal (right arm) and postductal (right leg) pulse oximetry readings of 70%. She is mildly tachypneic but is alert, awake, and appears to be in no distress.

**Detection**

– What are the most important initial steps in evaluating this newborn?

- What should be included in the differential diagnosis?
- What is the most likely diagnosis?

**Intervention**
- Which studies and treatment strategies take priority?

**Reassessment**
- Is the current treatment strategy effective?
- Does the patient need other therapeutic interventions?

**Effective Communication**
- Who needs to be aware of this patient?
- Where is the best place to manage the care of this patient?

**Teamwork**
- How are you going to implement the treatment strategy?
- Who is to do what and when?

Both central cyanosis and acrocyanosis may be seen in newborns. Acrocyanosis involves the hands and the feet and does not represent true arterial hypoxemia. Central cyanosis is present throughout the body, but it is more evident in the mucous membranes, lips, and tongue and represents true hypoxemia. For central cyanosis to be recognized clinically, more than 5 g/dL of hemoglobin must be deoxygenated.

# A. Cyanotic Congenital Heart Disease with Decreased Pulmonary Blood Flow

Patients with cyanotic CHD and decreased pulmonary blood flow have obstructed pulmonary blood flow and right-to-left shunting of blood at either the atrial or the ventricular level. In the neonatal period, patients with these defects are usually cyanotic in proportion to the degree of pulmonary stenosis, but they are rarely dyspneic as there is an absence of congestive heart failure.

### 1. Tetralogy of Fallot

Tetralogy of Fallot (TOF) is the most common form of cyanotic CHD, occurring in 7% of children in the United States with congenital heart disease. The tetralogy consists of:

- Pulmonary stenosis (subvalvular, valvular, and/or supravalvular)
- Ventricular septal defect (VSD)
- Aorta overriding the ventricular septum
- Right ventricular hypertrophy

From a pathophysiologic standpoint, the dominant features of TOF are the VSD and the degree of right ventricular outflow tract obstruction (RVOTO). Patients with mild RVOTO will have signs of overcirculation due to a left-to-right shunt through the VSD. These patients have normal saturations ("pink TOF") and signs of congestive heart failure. However, in patients with severe

RVOTO, significant right-to-left shunt occurs at the VSD level. In these patients, a patent ductus arteriosus (PDA) maintains normal pulmonary blood flow in the immediate postnatal period. The degree of cyanosis will depend on the severity of the pulmonary stenosis and will worsen as the PDA closes. A hypercyanotic spell, or tetralogy spell ("tet spell"), is a characteristic sequence of clinical events in older infants and children that begins with irritability and hyperpnea and is followed by a prolonged period of profound cyanosis leading to syncope.

> !
>
> *Characteristic sequence of hypercyanotic spell:*
> - Irritability and hyperpnea
> - Intense cyanosis
> - Syncope
>
> *Treatment:*
> - Place the child in knee–chest position.
> - Provide maximal supplemental oxygen.
> - If necessary, give morphine 0.1 mg/kg intramuscularly.
>
> !

Medical treatment is lifesaving in children with hypercyanotic spells. Initially, attempts should be made to calm the child, who then should be placed in a knee-to-chest position. Maximal supplemental oxygen by face mask should be provided. If the spell continues, morphine (0.1 mg/kg) may be given intramuscularly; if it persists, more aggressive therapy is initiated, including rapid placement of an intravenous catheter followed by administration of isotonic intravenous fluid (20 mL/kg of 0.9% saline) and sodium bicarbonate (1-2 mEq/kg). Sometimes, administration of a β-blocker may be needed to relax the RVOTO and increase pulmonary blood flow. In severe cases that do not respond to these measures, intubation and administration of an α-adrenergic agonist (phenylephrine) may be needed to increase systemic vascular resistance and decrease right-to-left shunting at the VSD. Anemia (hemoglobin <10 g/dL), when present, often precipitates a hypercyanotic spell, and blood transfusion may be required.

Surgical repair of TOF is indicated for any child with hypercyanotic spells or increasing cyanosis (oxygen saturation <75%). Until recently, patients with symptomatic TOF were repaired utilizing a staged approach, with placement of a modified Blalock-Taussig shunt (a polytetrafluoroethylene tube connection between the innominate artery and the pulmonary artery) in early infancy as a palliative measure. Definitive repair, with pulmonary valvotomy, resection of right ventricular infundibular muscle bundles, and VSD closure, was then performed at 3 or 4 years of age.

With advances in medical and surgical management of younger infants with CHD, definitive repair is now optimally performed as a single surgical procedure at about 6 months of age.

### 2. Tricuspid Atresia

Tricuspid atresia with normally related great arteries is a rare form of CHD in which the tricuspid valve orifice is not patent. A patent foramen ovale or atrial septal defect must be present to allow systemic venous blood to shunt from right to left. The right ventricle and pulmonary outflow tract are typically hypoplastic unless a large VSD is present. Patients with tricuspid atresia and normally related great arteries present in the immediate neonatal period with cyanosis (oxygen saturations of ~70%). Initial medical therapy includes the initiation of $PGE_1$ infusion (0.05 µg/kg/min) to maintain the patency of the ductus arteriosus. Palliative surgery is performed in the first week after birth and consists of placement of a modified Blalock-Taussig shunt. A bidirectional Glenn (cavo-pulmonary anastomosis connecting the superior vena cava to the right pulmonary artery) insert is performed at approximately 6 months as a staged approach, followed by the modified Fontan procedure at approximately 2 years of age. The modified Fontan procedure allows systemic venous blood to completely bypass the right side of the heart by directing the inferior vena cava through an extracardiac conduit into the pulmonary arteries. This staged surgical repair is summarized in **Table 16-1**.

### 3. Pulmonary Stenosis

Pulmonary stenosis occurs in 9% of children with heart disease, most of whom will present with a harsh systolic ejection murmur at the upper-left sternal border with radiation to the back. Infants with critical pulmonary stenosis will be cyanotic and have ductal-dependent pulmonary blood flow. This critical form of stenosis may also be included in the category of cyanotic CHD with decreased pulmonary blood flow due to a large obligatory right-to-left atrial shunt. Newborns with critical pulmonary stenosis need to be treated with $PGE_1$ infusion. Balloon valvuloplasty of the pulmonic valve is usually successful in the immediate newborn period. Surgery is considered only in children with severely dysplastic and hypoplastic valves or those with additional obstruction at the subvalvular or supravalvular levels.

## B. Cyanotic Congenital Heart Disease with Increased Pulmonary Blood Flow

Cardiac lesions with cyanosis and increased pulmonary blood flow can be classified further into those with increased pulmonary arterial vascularity in which there is hilar prominence on the chest radiograph (transposition of the great arteries and truncus arteriosus) and those with increased pulmonary venous vascularity in which the chest radiograph typically shows a ground-glass or white-out appearance (total anomalous pulmonary venous connection with pulmonary venous obstruction and hypoplastic left heart syndrome). In clinical practice these two groups often cannot be accurately distinguished from one another based on signs, symptoms, or radiographic findings, and echocardiography is needed to make the diagnosis.

### 1. Transposition of the Great Arteries

In dextrotransposition of the great arteries (d-TGA), the aorta arises from the right ventricle while the pulmonary artery arises from the left ventricle. The pulmonary and systemic circulations are configured in parallel rather than in series, resulting in cyanotic blood circulating back to the systemic circulation. Cyanosis usually appears in the delivery room while cardiac examination may otherwise be normal. The chest radiograph may be normal, although the cardiac silhouette may occasionally resemble an "egg on a string" as a result of the right ventricular predominance and a narrow superior mediastinum. Pulmonary markings are normal or slightly increased. In newborns with d-TGA, initiation of $PGE_1$ infusion (0.05 μg/kg/min) can help increase oxygen saturations while awaiting balloon septostomy as a more definitive palliation. Balloon atrial septostomy (BAS) is often necessary to alleviate profound cyanosis because mixing occurs most optimally between the low-pressure atria rather than at the ductus level. Furthermore, BAS is effective in decompressing the left atrium, which is often distended as pulmonary blood flow increases in the first few days after birth. However, neonates who undergo BAS are at increased risk of adverse neurologic outcomes, and some centers are performing the procedure only in unstable patients.

Many neonates undergo surgical repair of the defect in the first week after birth, although palliation with BAS allows for stabilization and some flexibility in timing. Infants with d-TGA and a moderate to large VSD may not be diagnosed this early since interventricular mixing leads to minimal cyanosis. However, as pulmonary vascular resistance decreases during the first weeks after birth, findings of a large left-to-right shunt with signs of congestive heart failure (e.g., poor feeding, tachypnea) will develop. The arterial switch operation, in which the pulmonary artery is re-anastomosed to the right ventricle and the aorta to the left ventricle, with transfer of the coronary arteries, is now the surgical procedure of choice for the correction of d-TGA.

> *Transposition of the great arteries is the most common form of cyanotic heart disease to present on the first day after birth. It should be suspected in any cyanotic infant, especially if poor response to supplemental oxygen is seen.*

### 2. Truncus Arteriosus

Truncus arteriosus is a rare form of CHD in which a large single (truncal) valve provides a common outlet for the right and left ventricles. A large VSD allows for mixing of blood from both ventricles. This common vessel, the truncus arteriosus, gives rise to the aorta, coronary arteries, and pulmonary arteries. The classification of truncus depends on the location of the pulmonary artery or its branches as they arise from the trunk. The mixing of saturated and unsaturated blood at the ventricular level and the ejection through the single truncal valve leads to mild cyanosis. Increased pulmonary blood flow with onset of congestive heart failure quickly develops as pulmonary vascular resistance drops. The chest radiograph shows a normal or increased heart size, with increased pulmonary markings and, in some cases, a right aortic arch. A significant percentage of these patients have a 22q11 microdeletion resulting in DiGeorge syndrome. Therefore, patients with truncus should be evaluated immediately for hypocalcemia (secondary to hypoparathyroidism) and T-cell immunodeficiency. Irradiated blood cells should be used for transfusions to prevent the development of graft-versus-host disease in patients in whom DiGeorge syndrome is suspected. Definitive surgical repair can usually be performed in the first week after birth. A valved homograft conduit is placed between the right ventricle and the main pulmonary artery, after separating the branch pulmonary arteries from the truncus arteriosus, and the VSD is closed in such a way as to direct the left ventricular blood through the truncal valve into the aorta. Subsequent surgical procedures are necessary to increase the size of the conduit as the child grows.

> *Blood from both ventricles is ejected into the truncal artery. Systemic and pulmonary circulation mixes and the arterial oxygen saturation depends on the amount of pulmonary blood flow. As pulmonary vascular resistance decreases, pulmonary blood flow will increase, leading to left ventricle overload, pulmonary edema, and decreased systemic oxygen delivery.*

### 3. Total Anomalous Pulmonary Venous Connection

Patients with total anomalous pulmonary venous connection, a rare form of CHD, have their entire supply of oxygenated pulmonary venous blood returning to the systemic venous circulation. This admixture of oxygenated and desaturated systemic venous blood produces cyanosis. The four subtypes of total anomalous pulmonary venous connection are based on the location of pulmonary venous return:

> *Neonates with obstructed total anomalous pulmonary venous connection present with severe cyanosis.*

supracardiac (to the innominate vein or superior vena cava), intracardiac (to the coronary sinus or right atrium), infracardiac (below the diaphragm to the hepatic, portal, or umbilical venous system), and mixed (a combination of subtypes). The degree of obstruction to the pulmonary venous blood return determines the timing of presentation and the severity of cyanosis. Neonates with total anomalous pulmonary venous connection and significant obstruction frequently present in extremis with profound cyanosis. Neonates without obstruction are only mildly cyanotic and have a pulmonary flow murmur, so the diagnosis may be missed initially. Surgical repair is done immediately upon presentation with good long-term results.

**Table 16-6** lists the causes of cyanosis in newborns, and **Table 16-7** outlines the initial evaluation and treatment of cyanotic newborns.

### Table 16-6  Causes of Cyanosis in Newborns

**Cyanotic heart disease**

With decreased pulmonary vascularity

- Tetralogy of Fallot
- Tricuspid atresia

Critical pulmonary stenosis

With increased pulmonary blood flow

- Transposition of the great arteries
- Truncus arteriosus
- Total anomalous pulmonary venous connection

**Respiratory diseases**

**Hematologic disorders (methemoglobinemia)**

**Neuromuscular disorders (hypoventilation)**

### Table 16-7  Initial Evaluation and Treatment of Cyanotic Newborns

**Initial Evaluation**

Chest radiograph

Electrocardiogram

Hyperoxia test:
- Obtain $Pa_{O_2}$ on room air and after 10 minutes on 100% $F_{IO_2}$
- If preductal $Pa_{O_2}$ >150 mm Hg (>19.9 kPa), then no cyanotic congenital heart disease

Consult cardiology for echocardiography as appropriate for definitive diagnosis of suspected congenital heart disease.

**Initial Treatment**

Airway, circulation, breathing

Prostaglandin $E_1$ infusion at 0.05 μg/kg/min

Once diagnosis of cyanotic congenital heart disease is confirmed, titrate $F_{IO_2}$ to achieve oxygen saturations appropriate for the specific lesion.

# IV. ACYANOTIC CONGENITAL HEART DISEASE

## Case Study

A 2-month-old male infant presents to the emergency department after several days of tachypnea, diaphoresis, poor feeding, and decreasing activity. His vital signs include a pulse of 180 beats/min and respiratory rate of 75 breaths/min. A harsh systolic regurgitant murmur is detected. His liver is palpable 6 cm below the right costal margin.

**Detection**
- What are the most important initial steps in evaluating this infant?
- What should be included in the differential diagnosis?
- What is the most likely diagnosis?

**Intervention**
- Which studies and treatment strategies take priority?

**Reassessment**
- Is the current treatment strategy effective?
- Does the patient need other therapeutic interventions?

**Effective Communication**
- Who needs to be aware of this patient?
- Where is the best place to manage the care of this patient?

**Teamwork**
- How are you going to implement the treatment strategy?
- Who is to do what and when?

## A. Acyanotic Congenital Heart Disease with Increased Pulmonary Blood Flow

### 1. Ventricular Septal Defect

VSD is the most common form of CHD. Its signs and symptoms are the result of the amount of left-to-right ventricular shunting. The size and direction of the shunt depend on the relative pressures and/or resistances of both the systemic and pulmonary circulations. Neonates with VSD are often asymptomatic until the pulmonary vascular resistance drops at approximately 2 to 6 weeks of age, resulting in an increased shunt and the appearance of clinical symptoms.

An infant with a small to moderate VSD will present with a holosystolic (regurgitant) murmur and remain asymptomatic. The intensity of the murmur is inversely proportional to the size of the defect. Children with larger VSDs will have less impressive murmurs and typically develop signs and symptoms of heart failure (**Tables 16-2** and **16-3**). With these large defects, right ventricle and pulmonary artery pressure will increase to systemic levels. Smaller defects create a pressure difference between the left and right ventricles.

With advances in the medical and surgical care of children with CHD, cardiothoracic surgery can now be performed safely, even in small infants. Percutaneous transcatheter closure is used in muscular and residual postoperative VSDs. Although the technique is safe and effective, patient size is a limitation. Indications for surgical closure include the following:

- Uncontrolled congestive heart failure
- Increased pulmonary vascular resistance with a risk for pulmonary vascular obstructive disease
- Failure to thrive despite maximum medical therapy
- Recurrent pulmonary infections
- Endocarditis
- Paradoxical emboli

Eisenmenger syndrome develops if a significant left-to-right shunt lesion remains unrepaired and long-standing pulmonary hypertension progresses to irreversible pulmonary vascular obstructive disease with resultant right-to-left ventricular shunting and cyanosis. Death follows as a result of pulmonary hemorrhage, infection, and/or paradoxical emboli.

## 2. Atrial Septal Defect

Atrial septal defect (ASD) is present in 10% of children with congenital heart disease. It is found more frequently in females than males (at a ratio of 2:1). ASDs occur in 3 separate locations in the atrial septum:

- *Ostium primum* defects are located in the lower third of the atrial septum, near the atrioventricular valves.
- *Ostium secundum* defects are found in the middle portion of the septum and are the most common.
- *Sinus venosus* defects occur in the posterior portion of the septum, adjacent to the venae cavae.

The direction and amount of atrial level shunting is determined by the relative compliances of the right and left ventricles and the size of the defect. Typically, the right ventricle is more compliant, so left-to-right shunting occurs more frequently.

With rare exception, patients with an ASD are asymptomatic and classically have a fixed split $S_2$ with a systolic ejection murmur at the upper-left sternal border due to relative pulmonary stenosis. If symptoms are present, they develop later in childhood and are frequently related to arrhythmias. Indications for closure of an ASD are right ventricular volume overload, arrhythmias, paradoxical emboli, and elevated pulmonary vascular resistance. Closure may be performed by placing a device during cardiac catheterization or by suturing the defect primarily or with a patch. Both approaches are associated with low morbidity and mortality rates.

### 3. Patent Ductus Arteriosus

As an isolated anomaly, PDA occurs in approximately 1 in 2000 to 2500 live births. Its incidence increases in premature infants and is inversely proportional to their gestational age. The ductus arteriosus, an embryologic structure connecting the main pulmonary artery to the descending aorta, normally closes within the first few days after birth. Patients with PDA have left-to-right shunting dependent on the same issues of anatomic shunt size and relative resistance that govern VSD flow. In the presence of increased pulmonary vascular resistance, shunting through the PDA may be bidirectional. Infants with a large PDA, especially premature infants, will have symptoms of heart failure. Those with a small to moderate PDA will present with an asymptomatic continuous murmur over the upper-left sternal border.

Indomethacin is successful in closing many PDAs in premature infants. In older patients, catheter-based closure or surgical ligation is extremely effective, with essentially no morbidity or mortality.

### 4. Atrioventricular Septal Defect

Atrioventricular septal defect occurs in 7% of children with congenital heart disease. It is commonly found in children with trisomy 21 defect (Down syndrome). The lesion consists of a large defect in the atrial and ventricular septum with a common atrioventricular valve that is the inlet to both ventricles. Children with this defect are usually diagnosed in the first weeks after birth due to a systolic regurgitant murmur. If undiagnosed, patients will usually develop typical signs and symptoms of heart failure in their first months, as pulmonary vascular resistance decreases, and the degree of left-to-right shunting increases. To avoid acute and long-term consequences of pulmonary hypertension, surgical repair is required in infancy, ideally at 3 to 6 months of age.

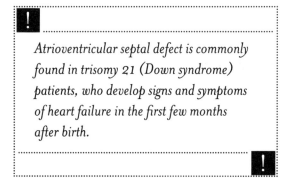

*Atrioventricular septal defect is commonly found in trisomy 21 (Down syndrome) patients, who develop signs and symptoms of heart failure in the first few months after birth.*

To review the causes of acyanotic heart disease, see **Table 16-8**. An overview of the evaluation and treatment of acyanotic heart disease can be found in **Table 16-9**.

## Table 16-8  Causes of Acyanotic Congenital Heart Disease

Acyanotic congenital heart disease with increased pulmonary blood flow (shunt lesions)
- Ventricular septal defect
- Atrial septal defect
- Patent ductus arteriosus
- Atrioventricular septal defect

Acyanotic congenital heart disease with obstruction
- Pulmonary stenosis (valvular, supravalvular, subvalvular)
- Aortic stenosis (valvular, supravalvular, subvalvular)
- Coarctation of the aorta

Other causes of heart failure
- Arrhythmia
- Cardiomyopathy
- Myocarditis
- Coronary artery anomalies

## Table 16-9  Initial Evaluation and Treatment of Acyanotic Heart Disease

**Initial Evaluation**

Chest radiograph
Electrocardiogram with rhythm strip
Echocardiography

**Initial Treatment**

Diuretics
- Loop diuretic (furosemide 1-2 mg/kg/dose orally or IV every 6-12 h)
- Thiazides (chlorothiazide 2-5 mg/kg/dose IV every 12 h)
- Potassium-sparing (spironolactone 0.5-3 mg/kg/day divided, every 6-24 h)

Afterload-reducing agents
- ACE inhibitors: enalaprilat 5-10 µg/kg/dose IV every 8-12 h; enalapril 0.05-0.25 mg/kg/day divided every 12-24 h PO
- Milrinone 0.25-0.75 µg/kg/min IV
- Nitroprusside 0.5-10 µg/kg/min IV
- Nitroglycerine 0.5- 5 µg/kg/min IV

Inotropic agents
- Digoxin 8-10 µg/kg/day divided every 12 h (dose is age dependent)
- Dopamine 5-10 µg/kg/min (adrenergic agonist)
- Dobutamine 5-15 µg/kg/min (adrenergic agonist)
- Epinephrine/adrenaline 0.05-0.1 µg/kg/min (adrenergic agonist)
- Milrinone 0.25-0.75 µg/kg/min (phosphodiesterase inhibitor)

*NOTE:* Optimal use of oxygen; hyperoxia can increase left-to-right shunting.

IV, intravenous; PO, by mouth; ACE, angiotensin-converting enzyme

# V. LOW CARDIAC OUTPUT SYNDROME

 **Case Study**

A 4-year-old boy presents to the emergency department with lethargy 2 weeks after an uncomplicated surgical repair of an atrial septal defect. He is found to be tachycardic and tachypneic. An arterial blood gas measurement shows a marked lactic acidosis.

**Detection**

- What are the most important initial steps in evaluating this child?
- What should be included in the differential diagnosis?
- What is the most likely diagnosis?

**Intervention**

- What studies and treatment strategies take priority?

**Reassessment**

- Is the current treatment strategy effective?
- Does the patient need other therapeutic interventions?

**Effective Communication**

- Who needs to be aware of this patient?
- Where is the best place to manage the care of this patient?

**Teamwork**

- How are you going to implement the treatment strategy?
- Who is to do what and when?

Low cardiac output syndrome (LCOS) describes a clinical and biochemical state of inadequate systemic oxygen delivery to meet the patient's metabolic demands. The syndrome is frequently seen in patients with severe sepsis, myocarditis, and cardiomyopathies and after pediatric cardiac surgery. Postoperative physiologic changes in response to cardiopulmonary bypass, residual lesions, cardioplegia, ventriculotomy, changes in the loading conditions of the myocardium, or myocardial ischemia during aortic cross-clamping all may contribute to the development of LCOS.

When unrecognized or inadequately treated, LCOS can lead to irreversible end-organ failure, cardiac arrest, and death. Although precise and accurate assessment of oxygen delivery in critically ill children is challenging, hemodynamic and biochemical parameters can guide the clinician at the bedside. Arterial lactate and central venous oxygen saturation are two important biochemical markers in patients with LCOS. Severe LCOS is a form of cardiogenic shock, although it may have etiologies other than poor myocardial contractility.

Common causes of low cardiac output are presented in **Tables 16-10** and **16-11**. The findings associated with LCOS are listed in **Table 16-12**, but a patient need not have all findings to be diagnosed. The goal is to make the diagnosis early in order to identify treatable causes and institute timely therapy to prevent irreversible end-organ injury.

### Table 16-10 Causes of Postoperative Low Cardiac Output

- Arrhythmias
- Hypovolemia
- Anemia
- Myocardial dysfunction
- Residual cardiac lesions
- Pulmonary hypertension
- Cardiac tamponade

### Table 16-11 Possible Residual Lesions after Surgery

- Valvular stenosis
- Valvular insufficiency
- Arterial stenosis
- Residual shunts
- Outflow tract obstruction

### Table 16-12 Signs and Symptoms of Low Cardiac Output Syndrome

- Tachycardia
- Poor peripheral effusion
- Decreased urine output
- Lactic acidosis
- Elevated or rapidly rising lactate levels (>0.75 mmol/L/h [>6.76 mg/dL])
- Widened arterial-mixed venous oxygen saturation difference (>30-40%)
- Altered mental status
- Late findings
    - Increased creatinine
    - Increased liver enzymes
    - Seizures
    - Hypotension

## A. Arrhythmias

The cardiac rhythm must be determined when assessing an unstable postoperative patient. A 12-lead electrocardiogram with a long rhythm strip should be performed as soon as possible. Descriptions of the most common arrhythmias following congenital heart surgery and their usual modes of treatment are presented in **Table 16-13**. Electrocardiographic images are shown in **Figures 16-1** through **16-4**. These rhythms can also occur without any underlying structural heart disease, as in myocarditis or Kawasaki disease.

> *The development of LCOS after surgery should prompt a reevaluation for the presence of residual hemodynamic lesions, tamponade, or arrhythmia.*
>
> *An unstable patient with a wide complex tachycardia should be presumed to have ventricular tachycardia and be treated immediately with direct-current cardioversion at 2-4 J/kg.*

### Table 16-13 Common Arrhythmias Following Congenital Heart Surgery and Usual Treatments

| Arrhythmia | Signs/Symptoms | Circumstances | Treatment |
| --- | --- | --- | --- |
| Junctional ectopic tachycardia | Narrow (normal) complex tachycardia<br>Rate ≥180 beats/min<br>VA relationship is 1:1 (with retrograde P wave or greater) | Most common after surgeries involving the ventricular septum:<br>  Tetralogy of Fallot<br>  VSD<br>  Atrioventricular septal defect | Pace the atrium to restore AV synchrony<br>Treat hyperthermia, agitation<br>Minimize β-adrenergic dosing<br>Amiodarone (5 mg/kg/dose IV given over 20-60 min)<br>Procainamide (3-6 mg/kg/dose IV) |
| Heart block | *First degree:* prolonged PR interval<br>*Second degree:*<br>Type I/Wenckebach: progressive prolongation of the PR interval until AV conduction is lost<br>Type II: AV conduction that occurs in a fixed ratio other than 1:1<br>*Third degree:* complete loss of AV conduction | Most common after surgeries around the AV node:<br>  VSD repairs<br>  Mitral valve replacement<br>  Enlargement of left ventricular outflow tract (Konno procedure)<br>  L-looped heart (ventricular inversion) is additional risk factor | None (first degree and Wenckebach often asymptomatic)<br>Temporary or permanent pacing<br>First degree and Wenckebach: in setting of tachycardia and very prolonged AV interval (can be similar to junctional ectopic tachycardia)<br>Second degree, type II, and third degree block: always require dual chamber pacing<br>If dual chamber pacing is not possible, ventricular pacing will prevent ventricular asystole. |
| Orthodromic reciprocating tachycardia | Reentrant tachycardia (normal conduction from atria to ventricles across AV node with atrial reentry via an accessory pathway) with P in T wave<br>VA relationship always 1:1<br>Sudden onset and cessation of tachycardia | Wolff-Parkinson White syndrome<br>Hidden accessory pathway | Adenosine (100-300 µg/kg IV rapid push)<br>Synchronized direct current cardioversion (0.5-2 J/kg)<br>Amiodarone or β-blocker (atenolol) for recurrent episodes<br>Atrial overdrive pacing |
| Atrial flutter | Reentrant tachycardia within the atrium<br>Narrow QRS complex, usually with 2:1 or 3:1 AV conduction | Most common with severe right atrial enlargement or extensive atrial surgery:<br>  Fontan procedure (atriopulmonary connection or lateral tunnel) years after surgery<br>  Ebstein anomaly<br>  Mustard procedure (for transposition of the great arteries)<br>  Senning procedure (for transposition of the great arteries) | Adenosine (does not alter atrial rate, but can help in diagnosis)<br>Synchronized cardioversion (0.5-2 J/kg)<br>Rapid atrial pacing (at rate greater than the atrial rate)<br>Amiodarone or other antiarrhythmics (for recurrent episodes) |
| Ventricular tachycardia | Wide complex tachycardia<br>Rare in pediatrics | Most common in:<br>  Sick ventricles with poor hemodynamics<br>  Severely hypertrophied ventricle | Direct current cardioversion (2-4 J/kg)<br>Amiodarone (5 mg/kg IV)<br>Lidocaine (0.5-1.5 mg/kg IV) |

VA, ventricular to atrial; AV, atrioventricular; VSD, ventricular septal defect; IV, intravenous

**Figure 16-1.** Third Degree Atrioventricular Block

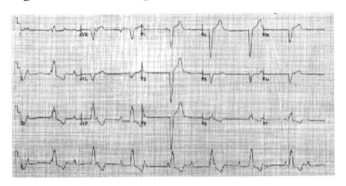

Complete atrioventricular block (third degree), either congenital or acquired, is the most common bradyarrhythmia in children. Lack of conduction between the atria and the ventricles is seen as a slow QRS rate and a regular atrial rhythm with an irregular PR interval.
Courtesy of Ana Lia Graciano, MD, FAAP.

**Figure 16-2.** Supraventricular Tachycardia

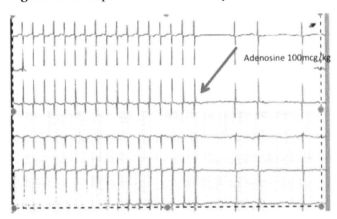

In paroxysmal supraventricular tachycardia (SVT), the electrocardiogram demonstrates regular RR interval and narrow QRS. SVT is usually caused by a re-entry circuit involving the atrioventricular node; adenosine causes a temporary block in the node, interrupting the re-entry circuit.
Courtesy of Ana Lia Graciano, MD, FAAP.

**Figure 16-3.** Wolff-Parkinson-White Syndrome

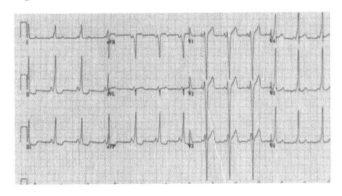

In Wolff-Parkinson-White syndrome, the impulse is carried in antegrade manner through the atrioventricular node (orthodromic conduction), resulting in a normal QRS complex, and in retrograde manner via the accessory pathway to the atrium, perpetuating the tachycardia. The typical electrocardiogram pattern with an upstroke of the QRS (delta wave) is recognized after cessation of the tachycardia.
Courtesy of Ana Lia Graciano, MD, FAAP.

**Figure 16-4.** Atrial Flutter

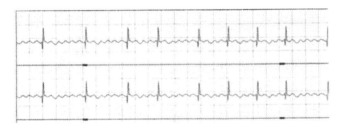

Atrial flutter is characterized by rapid, regular sawtooth flutter waves at rates between 250 to 500 per minute. Atrioventricular conduction is blocked to some degree, resulting in the ventricle responding irregularly every 2 to 4 atrial beats.
Courtesy of Ana Lia Graciano, MD, FAAP.

## B. Cardiac Tamponade

One important cause of LCOS that requires immediate recognition and management is cardiac tamponade, a clinical syndrome caused by the accumulation of fluid in the pericardial space and leading to impaired ventricular filling and subsequent hemodynamic compromise. Echocardiography can confirm the diagnosis by demonstrating a collection of pericardial fluid with associated atrial compression or collapse during ventricular systole. The diagnosis of tamponade must be considered in any postoperative patient with LCOS – even in the absence of high filling pressures, or radiographic or echocardiographic changes – because even a small fluid collection can cause tamponade if it results in impaired myocardial filling. Cardiac tamponade is treated by clearing occluded chest tubes, by pericardiocentesis, or by mediastinal re-exploration. Rapid fluid resuscitation may be necessary to support the circulation until adequate pericardial drainage is achieved.

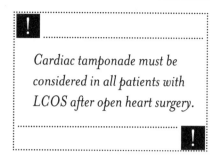

*Cardiac tamponade must be considered in all patients with LCOS after open heart surgery.*

## C. Myocardial Dysfunction

Myocardial contractility can be enhanced by using β-adrenergic agonists or phosphodiesterase inhibitors (**Table 16-9**). Cardiomyocyte contractility and relaxation occur due to rapid calcium cycling within the cells. β-adrenergic agonists work by increasing intracellular cyclic adenosine monophosphate (cAMP), which subsequently increases calcium cycling in both systole and diastole. Given that cAMP is degraded by phosphodiesterases, phosphodiesterase inhibitors also serve to increase cAMP.

Milrinone, a selective phosphodiesterase III inhibitor, potentiates cAMP effect, leading to an increase in intracellular calcium and contractile force in cardiac muscle. At infusion rates of 0.75 µg/kg/min, milrinone has been shown to prevent LCOS following surgical repair of CHD. Phosphodiesterase inhibition is not receptor dependent and therefore is not altered by receptor down-regulation that occurs during chronic adrenergic stimulation. Another advantage of these drugs is that they promote afterload reduction for the systemic (and pulmonary) ventricle, hence the name inodilators.

Blood pressure is determined by both the cardiac output and the systemic vascular resistance, and systemic vascular resistance and cardiac contractility have an inverse relationship. Therefore, use of vasodilators for afterload reduction results in an increase in cardiac contractility, cardiac output, and oxygen delivery, albeit often at a lower blood pressure. When vascular tone is high, either intrinsically or secondary to the use of higher doses of adrenergic agonists, and cardiac output is low, pure vasodilating agents can be used to improve oxygen delivery. Nitroprusside (0.5-10 µg/kg/min) and nitroglycerine (0.5-5 µg/kg/min) are commonly used for this purpose, particularly in combination with low dose epinephrine/adrenaline (0.01-0.05 µg/kg/min), to improve cardiac contractility. Caution should be used with nitroprusside as cyanide toxicity can occur when infused at high doses for several days.

When blood pressure is too low to maintain adequate organ perfusion, it is preferable to maximize preload and contractility before resorting to increasing systemic vascular resistance. Such an approach is preferred due to the inverse relationship between afterload and cardiac function and the likelihood that the increase in blood pressure will come at the cost of a decrease in cardiac output and oxygen delivery. An exception to this relationship occurs when coronary perfusion is critically low. Under these conditions, increasing systemic vascular resistance will increase oxygen delivery to the myocardium and thus improve myocardial function. Despite the inverse relationship between ventricular function and afterload, it is sometimes necessary to increase systemic vascular resistance to achieve an acceptable blood pressure. Commonly used vasopressors include epinephrine/adrenaline and norepinephrine/noradrenaline (both of which also have significant α-adrenergic agonist effects) and, more recently, vasopressin (0.0003-0.002 U/kg/min), which does not bind to adrenergic receptors and therefore may be effective in catecholamine-resistant states. Persistent hypotension refractory to fluids and catecholamines may indicate adrenal insufficiency, and supplementation with corticosteroids like hydrocortisone may stabilize blood pressure in patients with refractory hypotension.

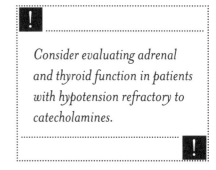

*Consider evaluating adrenal and thyroid function in patients with hypotension refractory to catecholamines.*

The neonatal heart has an immature calcium-handling system and is more dependent on extracellular calcium for contractility. Laboratory and anecdotal evidence suggest that maintenance of ionized calcium levels 20% to 30% above the normal physiologic range is associated with improved hemodynamics during the early period following neonatal cardiac surgery. Hypocalcemia, either secondary to genetic issues (such as chromosome 22 deletions) or as a result of citrate in packed red blood cells, should be aggressively treated.

Optimal management of the pediatric patient with cardiac disease requires a comprehensive understanding of the basic principles of oxygen delivery, cardiovascular physiology, and the anatomy and physiology of CHD. Signs and symptoms of LCOS should be treated aggressively, and diagnostic and therapeutic strategies should address both common and lesion-specific problems.

The tests used to evaluate patients with low cardiac output are summarized in **Table 16-14**.

**Table 16-14 Evaluation of Patients with Low Cardiac Output**

Chest radiograph
Electrocardiogram
Arterial blood gas
Complete blood counts
Serum electrolytes
Echocardiogram
Central venous and arterial blood pressure monitoring

# Management of the Child With Congenital Heart Disease

## Key Points

- Infants who present with low cardiac output or shock in the first weeks of life must be evaluated for congenital heart disease.

- Most forms of congenital heart disease can be categorized into 2 groups—acyanotic and cyanotic—and a presumptive diagnosis can be made by integrating information obtained from the history, physical examination, chest radiograph, and pulse oximetry. Definitive diagnosis can often be confirmed with an echocardiogram.

- Initiation of prostaglandin $E_1$ infusion can be lifesaving in children with congenital heart disease and ductal-dependent blood flow, and should be considered in any neonate who presents with shock or cyanosis.

- Prompt recognition and appropriate treatment of low cardiac output syndrome is essential for preserving organ function in pediatric patients with congenital heart disease.

## Suggested Readings

1. Fuhrman BP, Zimmerman JJ, eds. *Pediatric Critical Care*. 4th ed. Philadelphia, PA: Saunders Elsevier; 2011:319-321, 340-343.

2. Garson A Jr, Bricker JT, Fisher DJ, Neish SR, eds. *The Science and Practice of Pediatric Cardiology*. 3rd ed. Baltimore, MD: Williams and Wilkins; 2005.

3. Hoffman TM, Wernovsky G, Atz AM, et al. Efficacy and safety of milrinone in preventing low cardiac output syndrome in infants and children after corrective surgery for congenital heart disease. *Circulation*. 2003;107:996-1002.

4. Keane JF, Lock JE, Fyler DC, eds. *Nada's Pediatric Cardiology*. 2nd ed. Philadelphia, PA: Saunders Elsevier; 2006.

5. Kolovos NS, Bratton SL, Moler FW, et al. Outcome of pediatric patients treated with extracorporeal life support after cardiac surgery. *Ann Thorac Surg*. 2003;76:1435-1441.

6. Mackie AS, Gauvreau K, Booth KL, Newburger JW, Laussen PC, Roth SJ. Hemodynamic correlates of serum cortisol in neonates after cardiopulmonary bypass. *Pediatr Crit Care Med*. 2011;12: 297-303.

7. McQuillen PS, Hamrick SE, Perez MJ, et al. Balloon atrial septostomy is associated with preoperative stroke in neonates with transposition of the great arteries. *Circulation*. 2006;113: 280-285.

8. Nichols D, Greeley WJ, Lappe DG, Wetzel RC, eds. *Critical Heart Disease in Infants and Children*. 2nd ed. Philadelphia, PA: Mosby Elsevier; 2006.

9. Wheeler D, Wong H, Shanley T, eds. *Pediatric Critical Care Medicine: Basic Science and Clinical Evidence*. New York, NY: Springer-Verlag; 2007:672-706.

Chapter 17

# ONCOLOGIC AND HEMATOLOGIC EMERGENCIES AND COMPLICATIONS

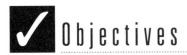 Objectives

- Describe risk factors unique to the immunosuppressed pediatric patient.
- Recognize and treat causes of shock in the pediatric cancer patient.
- Recognize and treat causes of respiratory failure in the pediatric cancer patient.
- Review metabolic abnormalities associated with tumor lysis syndrome and list treatment priorities.
- Describe risk factors associated with hyperleukocytosis.
- Identify and treat spinal cord compression.

 Case Study

A 12-year-old girl with acute lymphocytic leukemia, who was recently released from the hospital after induction chemotherapy, presented to a referring hospital with a 2-hour history of fever, shaking, and chills after having her central line flushed with heparin. On admission, her temperature is 102.6°F (39.2°C), heart rate is 156 beats/min, blood pressure is 82/35 mm Hg, and respiratory rate is 28 breaths/min. Laboratory data obtained on admission show a white blood cell (WBC) count of $0.1 \times 10^9$ cells/L, hemoglobin 7.2 g/dL (72 g/L), and platelet count of $45,000 \times 10^9$ cells/L. Her electrolytes are normal except for a $K^+$ of 2.8 mEq/L (2.8 mmol/L). Blood culture 12 hours after admission is growing Gram-positive cocci. You have been asked to evaluate the patient.

**Detection**
 – What is this patient's physiologic status?
 – What is the most likely diagnosis?

**Intervention**
 – Which treatment strategies take priority?

**Reassessment**
 – Is the current treatment strategy effective?
 – Does the patient need more fluids? Is a blood transfusion indicated?

**Effective Communication**

- When the patient's clinical status changes, who needs this information and how will it be disseminated?
- Where is the best place to manage the care of this patient?

**Teamwork**

- How are you going to implement the treatment strategy?
- Who is to do what and when?

# I. INTRODUCTION

This chapter is designed to provide essential information on aspects of care that may be critical in the management of medical complications in the pediatric oncology/hematology patient.

Recent evidence supports the use of aggressive therapies early in the course of the patient's acute illness. These may include broad-spectrum antimicrobial coverage, fluid resuscitation, and early respiratory and inotropic support. The therapeutic goals should be discussed with the primary attending, the patient's guardian, the patient (if appropriate), and the intensive care unit team. Decisions concerning continuation or limitations of care should be frequently explored based on the patient's primary diagnosis, oncologic prognosis, and clinical course.

# II. FEVER AND NEUTROPENIA

## A. Definitions

Neutropenic fever, a common complication seen during the treatment of pediatric malignancies, is defined as a single oral temperature over 100.9°F (38.3°C) or a sustained temperature over 100.4°F (38°C) for ≥1 hour. Rectal temperature measurements are contraindicated in neutropenic patients due to the potential disruption of the rectal mucosal barrier, which creates a route for infection. Febrile neutropenia is an absolute neutrophil count of either <500 x $10^9$ cells/L or <1000 x $10^9$ cells/L with an expected persistent decrease over the next 2 or 3 days.

## B. Risk Factors

The risk of infection increases with the degree and duration of neutropenia. Patients in whom a neutropenic period is anticipated to last <7 days have a low risk; this applies to most patients with solid tumors who are undergoing standard chemotherapy regimens. Neutropenic episodes lasting between 7 and 10 days have an intermediate risk, and this is seen in patients with lymphoma, chronic leukemia, and autologous stem cell transplant. Episodes lasting >10 days have a high risk of infection, and this is associated with acute leukemia and allogeneic stem cell transplant. Certain clinical and laboratory risk factors are also associated with serious infections. The clinical risk factors include: hemodynamic instability (shock), pneumonia, neutropenic enterocolitis, severe oral mucositis, diarrhea, perianal lesions, catheter-related infections, and persistent and rising temperature >102.2°F (39°C) despite single-agent broad-spectrum intravenous (IV) antibiotic use. Laboratory risk factors include: elevated C-reactive protein >10 mg/L (>95.2 nmol/L), absolute monocyte count <100 x $10^9$ cells/L, and the presence of Gram-negative bacteremia.

## C. Treatment

The standard of care for patients with fever and neutropenia requires immediate empiric inpatient IV antibiotic therapy with close observation for at least 3 days. The patient requires a thorough history and physical examination and a full laboratory workup with complete blood cell count, full chemistry studies, specimen culture of all indwelling catheters (blood culture, urine culture, peritoneal catheter culture), *Clostridium difficile* toxin and other stool studies in patients with diarrhea, a chest radiograph, and lumbar puncture when clinically indicated. Early drainage of any fluid collection (abscess, effusion, and empyema) for culture and symptom relief is highly recommended.

The organisms associated with serious infections in children and the suggested antimicrobials and dosages are summarized in **Table 17-1**. Febrile neutropenic patients without a focus of infection may be treated with a single broad-spectrum antibiotic with antipseudomonal coverage, such as cefepime, meropenem, or piperacillin/tazobactam. A dual coverage of aminoglycosides and antipseudomonal β-lactams has to be considered in patients who present with Gram-negative bacteremia or sepsis. Empiric coverage should be continued even on afebrile patients until the absolute neutrophil count is >500 x $10^9$ cells/L. The antimicrobial spectrum should be broadened to include coverage for anaerobes, drug-resistant Gram-negative agents, Gram-positive organisms, and fungus in persistently febrile neutropenic patients. The addition of vancomycin is recommended in those with positive cultures for Gram-positive bacteria or when a catheter-related infection is suspected. Following a diagnosis of a catheter-related infection, catheter removal is warranted in hemodynamically unstable patients, those with persistent bacteremia despite treatment with an appropriate agent, and patients whose infections are caused by fungi, mycobacteria, *Staphylococcus aureus*, *Acinetobacter baumannii*, *Pseudomonas aeruginosa*, *Stenotrophomonas maltophilia*, and vancomycin-resistant *Enterococcus*.

Colony-stimulating factors may be used in high-risk patients to shorten the duration of neutropenia. These agents have been utilized with increasing frequency for patients with neutropenia and multiple-organ-system failure, sepsis or septic shock, and/or invasive fungal disease. Granulocyte colony-stimulating factor given IV or subcutaneously in a dose of 5 to 10 μg/kg/day stimulates the release of neutrophils. Granulocyte-macrophage colony-stimulating factor in a dose of 5 μg/kg/day IV or subcutaneously enhances the release of neutrophils and macrophages and may be considered for patients in whom fungal disease is confirmed or strongly suspected. Either medication

> *Fever and Neutropenia*
> - *Blood culture, urine culture, and chest radiograph*
> - *Immediate empiric intravenous antibiotic therapy:*
>   *Cefepime: 150 mg/kg/24 h ÷ every 8 h IV/IM ±*
>   *Vancomycin: 60 mg/kg/24 h ÷ every 6 h IV*
>   *(verify local resistance patterns)*
> - *Consider granulocyte colony–stimulating factor:*
>   *5–10 μg/kg/day IV or SC in high–risk patients with bacteremia and septic shock*
> - *Close monitoring in an inpatient setting*

should be continued until the absolute neutrophil count exceeds 1000 x 10$^9$ cells/L for 3 consecutive days. A study showed a reduction in the duration of neutropenia, length of antibiotic treatment, and number of hospital days with the use of colony-stimulating factors.

### Table 17-1 Treatment Recommendations for Serious Infections in Immunosuppressed Children[a]

| Organism | Treatment |
| --- | --- |
| **Gram-positive organisms** Coagulase-negative *Staphylococcus*, α-hemolytic *Streptococcus*, *Enterococcus*, *Corynebacterium* | Vancomycin[b]: 15 mg/kg every 6 h IV <br> Linezolid: 10 mg/kg every 8 h IV; maximum dose, 1200 mg/24 h <br> Daptomycin[b]: 4-6 mg/kg every 24 h IV (not approved for children <18 years) |
| **Gram-negative organisms** *Klebsiella, Bacillus, Pseudomonas, Escherichia coli* | Cephalosporins[b]: <br> – Cefepime: 50 mg/kg every 8 h IV/IM; maximum dose, 6 g/24 h <br> – Ceftazidime: 50 mg/kg every 8 h IV/IM; maximum dose, 6 g/24 h <br> Aminoglycosides[b]: <br> – Gentamicin: 2.5 mg/kg every 8 h IV <br> – Tobramycin: 2.5 mg/kg every 8 h IV <br> Carbapenems[b]: <br> – Imipenem-cilastatin: 25 mg/kg every 6 h IV; maximum dose, 4 g/24 h <br> – Meropenem: 40 mg/kg every 8 h IV; maximum dose, 6 g/24 h |
| **Fungi** *Candida, Aspergillus* | Fluconazole[b]: loading dose, 12 mg/kg IV; maintenance, 6 mg/kg IV every 24 h after loading dose; maximum loading dose, 400 mg <br> Liposomal amphotericin B: 3-5 mg/kg every 24 h IV <br> Caspofungin: loading dose, 70 mg/m$^2$ IV; maintenance, 50 mg/m$^2$ IV every 24 h after loading dose; maximum loading dose, 70 mg <br> Voriconazole: loading dose, 6 mg/kg every 12 h IV x 2 doses; 4 mg/kg every 12 h IV |
| **Anaerobes** | Clindamycin: 10 mg/kg every 6-8 h IV/IM; maximum dose, 2800 mg/24 h <br> Metronidazole: 7.5 mg/kg every 6 h IV/PO; maximum dose, 4 g/24 h |
| **Antivirals** <br> – Respiratory syncytial virus | Ribavirin: 6 g by aerosol (small-particle aerosol generator) over 12-18 h daily for 3-7 days (6 g in 300 mL preservative-free sterile water)[c] |
| – Influenza type A | Amantadine: <br> – 1-9 years: 5 mg/kg PO once daily; maximum dose, 150 mg/24 h <br> – >9 years (<40 kg): 5 mg/kg PO once daily; maximum dose, 200 mg/24 h <br> – >40 kg: 200 mg once daily <br> Rimantadine: <br> – 1-9 years: 5 mg/kg PO once daily; maximum dose, 150 mg/24 h <br> – >10 years (<40 kg): 5 mg/kg PO once daily; maximum dose, 150 mg/24 h <br> – >40 kg: 100 mg PO twice daily |
| – Influenza types A and B | Zanamivir: >7 years <br> – Day 1: 2 doses (5 mg via inhalation) at least 2-12 h apart <br> – Days 2-5: 2 doses (5 mg via inhalation) every 12 h for 4 days; initiate within 2 days of symptom onset <br> Oseltamivir[b]: <br> – <15 kg: 30 mg PO twice daily <br> – >15-23 kg: 45 mg PO twice daily <br> – >23-40 kg: 60 mg PO twice daily <br> – >40 kg: 75 mg PO twice daily <br> – >12 years: 75 mg PO twice daily for 5 days |

### Table 17-1  Treatment Recommendations for Serious Infections in Immunosuppressed Children[a] (continued)

| Organism | Treatment |
| --- | --- |
| **Antivirals** (continued) | |
| - Parainfluenza | Ribavirin may be beneficial if used early (see respiratory syncytial virus treatment for dose) |
| - CMV pneumonia | Ganciclovir[b]: 5 mg/kg every 12 h IV |
| | OR |
| | Foscarnet[b]: 90 mg/kg every 12 h IV |
| | AND |
| | Immunoglobulin: 0.5 g/kg daily IV |
| *Pneumocystis jiroveci* | Trimethoprim-sulfamethoxazole[b]: 5 mg/kg trimethoprim component every 6-8 h IV. |
| | Methylprednisolone: 1 mg/kg every 12 h; should be started within 72 h in patient presenting with hypoxia ($Pa_{O_2}$ <70 mm Hg [9.3 kPa] on room air) |

IV, intravenous; IM, intramuscular; PO, orally; CMV, cytomegalovirus
[a]These recommendations are general guidelines only. Specific antibiotic choices should be individualized, taking into consideration clinical circumstances (renal function, liver function), patient age, immunization status, and local microbial virulence, sensitivities, and patterns of resistance. The antibiotic dosing, interval, and frequency should be discussed with a pediatric intensivist or pediatric infectious disease expert.
[b]Adjust for renal failure.
[c]Reserved for severe cases.

## D. Complications of the Febrile Neutropenic State

### 1. Bacteremia

Up to 40% of febrile neutropenic patients will have documented bacteremia, with catheter-related infections being the most frequent cause. In the United States, the most common infective agents are coagulase-negative staphylococci, *S aureus*, and enterococci. Patients with acute myelogenous leukemia have a high risk for *Streptococcus viridans* infections. The rate of infections caused by Gram-negative organisms appears to be increasing.

### 2. Lower Respiratory Tract Infections

 Case Study

An 11-year-old boy who underwent peripheral blood stem cell transplant 12 days ago is admitted to the intensive care unit from the bone marrow transplant ward because of respiratory distress and hypoxia, $Sp_{O_2}$ of 89% on an $F_{IO_2}$ of 0.5. A chest computed tomographic (CT) scan shows a diffuse ground-glass pattern. His WBC is $0.2 \times 10^9$ cells/L.

**Detection**

- What is this child's physiologic status?
- What is the most likely diagnosis?

### Intervention

- Which treatment strategies take priority?

### Reassessment

- Is the current treatment strategy effective?
- Is the patient a candidate for noninvasive mechanical ventilation? Would you intubate now?

### Effective Communication

- When the patient's clinical status changes, who needs to know and how will the information be disseminated?
- Where is the best place to manage the care of this patient?

### Teamwork

- How are you going to implement the treatment strategy?
- Who is to do what and when?

The immune deficiency of the primary disease and/or the toxicity of the therapy make pediatric cancer patients susceptible to a wide range of infectious and noninfectious problems that may progress rapidly to respiratory failure. Initiation of broad-spectrum antibacterial, antifungal, and antiviral therapy is often indicated in patients with rapid clinical or radiologic deterioration. High-resolution CT to identify pulmonary pathology should be utilized in all patients with respiratory symptomatology, irrespective of the plain radiograph findings. Bronchoscopy with bronchoalveolar lavage or open lung biopsy should be considered early in the course of the patient's illness. This may help differentiate infectious from noninfectious etiologies (diffuse alveolar hemorrhage), particularly in patients who have undergone bone marrow and stem cell transplantation.

Community-acquired viral infections, such as influenza, respiratory syncytial virus (RSV), and parainfluenza, can have devastating effects in pediatric oncology patients, and transplant patients in particular. Patients with RSV infections may benefit from ribavirin, palivizumab, and RSV immunoglobulin. Patients with influenza infections will benefit from the early use of antiviral medications (amantadine, rimantadine, zanamivir, or oseltamivir). No effective therapy exists for parainfluenza pneumonia. Mortality from cytomegalovirus (CMV) pneumonitis in bone marrow transplant patients is high. The recommended initial treatment for CMV pneumonia is a combination of IV ganciclovir and immune globulin. *Pneumocystis jiroveci* (formerly *Pneumocystis carinii*) and CMV pneumonia should be included in the differential of any immunocompromised patient who presents with respiratory symptoms, hypoxemia, and diffuse patchy infiltrates on the chest radiograph. The treatment of choice for *P jiroveci* pneumonia is IV trimethoprim-sulfamethoxazole (pentamidine in allergic patients). Corticosteroids (methylprednisolone 1-2 mg/kg/day IV divided, then given every 6 hours) should be initiated in patients with moderate or severe *P jiroveci* pneumonia ($Pa_{O_2}$ <70 mm Hg [9.3 kPa] on room air) within 72 hours of initiating antibiotic therapy.

Pediatric oncology patients presenting with respiratory failure should promptly receive noninvasive positive-pressure ventilation or be intubated and mechanically ventilated as indicated. Recent data support placing pediatric stem cell recipients with acute respiratory failure on high-frequency oscillatory ventilation within 6 hours of initiating mechanical ventilation. These data demonstrated the potential for improved outcome with early application of lung-protective strategies in the acute lung injury process.

### 3. Neutropenic Enterocolitis (Typhlitis)

Neutropenic enterocolitis is a necrotizing inflammatory process that affects the mucosal wall of the cecum and colon. The pathogenesis is not clear, but may be related to a combination of factors, including neutropenia, mucositis, direct cytotoxic effect of chemotherapy and, in some cases, neoplastic infiltration on the intestinal wall that creates a dysfunctional mucosa prone to microbial invasion, overgrowth, hemorrhage, and necrosis. The typical presentation of neutropenic enterocolitis mimics acute appendicitis. Most patients present with fever, abdominal pain, watery or bloody diarrhea, nausea, and vomiting. The diagnostic modality of choice is CT scan, which demonstrates the increase in bowel wall thickness. Ultrasonography may also be useful as a bedside diagnostic tool, particularly in critically ill patients, and as a follow-up tool to assess the evolution of changes to the bowel wall. Sepsis and perforation are the most common associated complications. Early diagnosis is essential for a good outcome. The treatment of choice is conservative medical management and includes bowel rest with nasogastric decompression, platelet and red cell infusions, parenteral nutrition, and broad-spectrum antimicrobial therapy including anaerobic, Gram-negative, and antifungal coverage. Surgical interventions are indicated for patients showing clinical deterioration despite adequate medical management, abscess formation, persistent abdominal bleeding, or bowel perforation.

### 4. Invasive Fungal Infections

Approximately 15% to 45% of patients with persistent neutropenic fever may have invasive fungal infections. Recurrent episodes of prolonged neutropenia, exposure to immunosuppressive agents, and chronic steroid use place pediatric oncology patients at high risk for developing these types of infections. The most common fungal infections are caused by *Candida albicans*, non-*albicans Candida* species, and *Aspergillus fumigatus*. The increase in non-*albicans Candida* ssp. is attributed to fluconazole resistance. Neutropenic patients with persistent fever lasting longer than 3 to 5 days should receive empiric antifungal coverage. Amphotericin B is the drug of choice for empiric antifungal coverage. Combination antifungal therapy with caspofungin and liposomal amphotericin B, followed by voriconazole maintenance, has proven to be a safe regimen for immunosuppressed children with invasive pulmonary aspergillosis.

The management of infectious complications in the febrile neutropenic pediatric patient requires an aggressive multidisciplinary approach. The emergency department physician, nursing staff, respiratory therapist, hospitalist, and intensivist should work in conjunction with the pediatric oncology and infectious disease teams to develop the best management strategy for these patients.

# III. SHOCK IN THE PEDIATRIC ONCOLOGY PATIENT

 Case Study

A 5-year-old boy with a history of acute lymphocytic leukemia is brought into the pediatric intensive care unit (PICU) from a referring hospital, where he presented 24 hours ago with fever, neutropenia, and thrombocytopenia. He was treated with ceftriaxone and acetaminophen (paracetamol). He became oliguric, tachycardic, and hypothermic. He received 500 mL of normal saline prior to transfer. On arrival to the PICU, he is found to be lethargic, with a temperature of 95.9°F (35.5°C), blood pressure of 70/30 mm Hg, and heart rate of 175 beats/min.

**Detection**
- What is this child's physiologic status?
- What is the most likely diagnosis?

**Intervention**
- Which treatment strategies take priority?

**Reassessment**
- Is the current treatment strategy effective?
- Does this patient need additional fluids?
- Would you consider vasopressors?
- Is endotracheal intubation indicated?

**Effective Communication**
- When the patient's clinical status changes, who needs the information and how will it be disseminated?

**Teamwork**
- How are you going to implement the treatment strategy?
- Who is to do what and when?

## A. Risk Factors

Shock and respiratory failure are the most common reasons for any child to be admitted into a PICU. Even though the clinical presentation of septic shock in oncology patients may be similar to that of noncancer patients (**Chapter 6**), the critically ill oncology patient presents additional challenges to the healthcare provider. These patients typically present with neutropenic fever, septic shock, and preexisting end-organ dysfunction.

## B. Treatment

The general principles for the management and diagnosis of septic shock are covered in **Chapter 6**. The ultimate therapeutic goal in septic shock is to restore and maintain optimal organ perfusion within 1 hour. Strategies for maximizing the potential for a positive outcome include: aggressive fluid management (possibly more than 60 mL/kg in the first hour); broad-spectrum antimicrobial coverage that includes Gram-positive, Gram-negative, antifungal, and antiviral medications (depending on the clinical presentation); early use of inotropic and vasopressor support; and positive-pressure ventilation. Early implementation of renal replacement therapy is indicated in the fluid-overloaded patient with renal insufficiency. The practitioner should be attentive to oncology patients presenting in shock but not responding to conventional resuscitative measures. Dilated cardiomyopathy secondary to medications (anthracyclines, high-dose cyclophosphamide, 5-fluorouracil) or radiation may be a contributing factor to the shock state in these patients.

Corticosteroid use is indicated in patients with fluid-refractory vasopressor-resistant shock, purpura fulminans, or suspected or proven adrenocortical insufficiency. The recommended initial hydrocortisone dose is 1 to 2 mg/kg/day for *stress* coverage, to 50 mg/kg/day titrated to reversal of *shock*. Early transfer to a PICU for inotropic and vasopressor support and invasive cardiopulmonary monitoring is indicated in patients who do not respond to fluid resuscitation.

The care of these patients should be carefully directed to avoid end-organ failure, as they have substantially greater risk of mortality than do noncancer patients, due to the complex nature of their disease process and immunocompromised state.

> *Inotropic/Vasopressor Support in Sepsis*
> - *Norepinephrine (noradrenaline) 0.05-2 µg/kg/min for warm shock*
> - *Epinephrine (adrenaline) 0.05-2 µg/kg/min for cold shock*
> - *Hydrocortisone 2 mg/kg x 1 or 50 mg/m²/day for **stress** dosing*

## C. Prognosis

Although the survival rates for pediatric cancer patients with septic shock are lower than the survival rates for non-cancer pediatric patients, recent data support an aggressive approach in the care of these patients.

# IV. FLUID AND ELECTROLYTE DISORDERS

Water and electrolyte disorders (**Chapter 8**) are common in the pediatric oncology patient. These disorders are usually the result of the primary tumor's impact on the kidney and/or the urinary tract, or secondary to the toxic renal effects of chemotherapy.

## Case Study

A 12-year-old, previously healthy girl presents to the emergency department with fever, tachypnea, oliguria, petechiae, and generalized edema. Her initial complete blood count shows: WBC count, 250,000 x $10^9$ cells/L; platelets, 32,000 x $10^9$ cells/L; hemoglobin, 7.2 g/dL; lactate dehydrogenase, 3000 IU/L; uric acid, 12 mg/dL; potassium, 6.2 mEq/L (6.2 mmol/L); phosphorus, 9 mg/dL (2.9 mmol/L); and calcium, 6 mg/dL (1.5 mmol/L).

**Detection**
- What is this child's diagnosis?
- What is she at risk for?

**Intervention**
- Which treatment strategies take priority?
- Would you consider an exchange transfusion?
- Should you treat her hypocalcemia?

**Reassessment**
- Is the current treatment strategy effective?
- Does she need more fluids?
- What types of fluids are indicated?
- Is a blood transfusion needed?
- Is a platelet infusion indicated?

**Effective Communication**
- Do you need to contact the nephrologist now?
- Where is the best place to manage the care of this patient?

**Teamwork**
- Who is to do what and when?

## A. Tumor Lysis Syndrome

Tumor lysis syndrome (TLS) is a life-threatening complication resulting from massive cellular lysis and release of intracellular metabolites, including nucleic acids, proteins, phosphorus, and potassium. It most often develops approximately 12 to 72 hours after the initiation of chemotherapy but may also occur spontaneously or after administration of steroids, hormones, or radiation therapy.

### 1. Diagnosis

Tumor lysis most frequently occurs in patients with large tumor burden (Burkitt lymphoma, lymphoblastic lymphoma, and leukemia) or in instances where a tumor is widely disseminated, rapidly proliferating, or highly sensitive to chemotherapy. The 2004 Cairo and Bishop Classification system defines 2 TLS categories:

#### a. Laboratory Tumor Lysis Syndrome (most common)

Occurrence of >2 of the following values within 3 days before to 7 days after initiation of cancer treatment:

- Uric acid: increase of 25% from baseline or value ≥8 mg/dL (>475.8 µmol/L)
- Potassium: increase of 25% from baseline or value ≥6 mEq/L (>6 mmol/L)
- Phosphorus: increase of 25% from baseline or value ≥6.5 mg/dL (>2.10 mmol/L)
- Calcium: decrease of 25% from baseline or value ≤7 mg/dL (<1.75 mmol/L)

### b. Clinical Tumor Lysis Syndrome

Presence of the above laboratory values and at least 1 of the following clinical manifestations:

- Renal failure (estimated glomerular filtration rate of ≤60 mL/min)
- Cardiac arrhythmia
- Seizures

## 2. Symptoms

The symptoms most commonly found in patients with TLS include: anorexia, malaise, weakness, vomiting, hiccups, paresthesia, tetany, carpopedal spasm, oliguria, anuria, lethargy, encephalopathy, seizures, electrocardiogram changes with high peaked T waves to life-threatening arrhythmias, syncope, shock, and death if uncorrected.

## 3. Pathophysiology

The high cell turnover with the release from cellular breakdown, accentuated by chemotherapy, leads to a dramatic rise in plasma levels of uric acid, urea nitrogen, phosphorus, and potassium that rapidly saturates renal homeostatic mechanisms. The glomerular filtration rate declines and progresses to renal failure, as a result of the precipitation of calcium phosphate in the microvasculature and uric acid crystals in the renal tubules.

## 4. Treatment

The key to the management of TLS is early diagnosis of the primary condition, rapid recognition of the risk factors, and prompt initiation of preventive treatment. A summary of TLS treatment is presented in **Table 17-2**. Essential treatment measures are as follows.

---

**Table 17-2  Treatment of Tumor Lysis Syndrome**

- Hydrate with 5% dextrose in normal saline at least 2 times maintenance. Monitor urine output continuously.
- Control uric acid:
  - Rasburicase: 0.2 mg/kg once daily in a 30-min intravenous infusion, may repeat for 3-5 days. Contraindicated in patients with glucose-6-phosphate dehydrogenase deficiency and methemoglobinemia.
  OR
  - Allopurinol: 100 mg/m$^2$ orally 24-48 h prior to initiation of chemotherapy
- Maintain specific gravity ~1.010 and urinary output at least 3 mL/kg/h.
- Restrict potassium and phosphorus; monitor hyperkalemic patients with a cardiopulmonary monitor.
- Replace calcium only in symptomatic patients.
- Consider early renal replacement therapy in patients with refractory hyperkalemia or with rapid decline in renal function.

---

### a. Monitoring

Patients with TLS, or at risk to develop TLS, should be monitored for electrocardiographic changes associated with hyperkalemia (prolonged PR, flattened P, widened QRS, and peaked T wave) and/or hypocalcemia (prolonged QT interval). Patient levels of sodium, potassium, phosphorus, calcium, magnesium, creatinine and urea nitrogen, lactate dehydrogenase, and uric acid, should be monitored every 6 hours for the first 24 hours, then every 12 hours for the next 3 days, and once daily subsequently.

#### b. Hydration

IV hydration should begin at least 48 hours before specific tumor therapy is initiated. The infusion rate should be at least twice the maintenance requirement. Urine output should be continuously monitored and kept at least at 3 mL/kg/h. Furosemide or mannitol may be required to maintain this urinary output, but such use is discouraged in the volume-depleted patient.

#### c. Urine Alkalinization

Urine alkalinization is no longer recommended. It may improve uric acid solubility, but it does not increase the solubility of xanthine and hypoxanthine metabolites after or during allopurinol treatment, resulting in a possible xanthine-obstructive uropathy. Urine alkalinization may also contribute to calcium-phosphate precipitation that may worsen TLS.

#### d. Hyperkalemia and Hyperphosphatemia

Potassium and phosphorus replacements should be restricted.

#### e. Uric Acid Control

Uric acid control may be obtained with allopurinol in the low-risk patient and rasburicase (recombinant urate oxidase) in the high-risk patient. Allopurinol should be administered orally at a dose of 100 mg/m² twice daily at the same time that hydration is started. A single dose of rasburicase should be administered at a dose of 0.2 mg/kg IV given over 30 minutes, once daily. The first dose should be administered at least 4 hours before tumor-specific therapy and can be continued daily for 3 to 5 days if needed. Concomitant use of both is not recommended. Rasburicase is contraindicated in patients with glucose-6-phosphate dehydrogenase deficiency and methemoglobinemia. Rasburicase is the drug of choice for clinical TLS therapy and for TLS prevention in high-risk patients.

#### f. Management of Severe Electrolyte Disturbances

Patients with hyperkalemia (>6 mEq/L [>6 mmol/L]) or with electrocardiographic signs of hyperkalemia should receive insulin, glucose, bicarbonate, and calcium (**Chapter 8**). Diuretics should be used with caution in dehydrated patients. Sodium polystyrene sulfonate, taken orally at 1 g/kg, may be helpful in preventing potassium rebound after the transient effect of acute hyperkalemia treatment. Patients with hyperphosphatemia should receive oral phosphate binders, such as sevelamer hydrochloride, calcium carbonate, calcium acetate, or aluminum hydroxide.

Calcium replacement with a single dose of calcium gluconate, 50 mg/kg, is indicated during TLS only in patients with neuromuscular irritability secondary to hypocalcemia, including seizures, arrhythmias, or positive Chvostek or Trousseau sign. Renal replacement therapy (hemodialysis, continuous venovenous hemofiltration) should be initiated in patients with refractory hyperkalemia, severe metabolic acidosis, volume overload unresponsive to diuretics, and uremic symptoms including pericarditis and encephalopathy or in patients with rapidly declining renal function.

# V. NEUROLOGIC EMERGENCIES

## A. Hyperleukocytosis

### 1. Definition

Hyperleukocytosis is defined as a WBC count of ≥100,000 x $10^9$ cells/L in the peripheral blood.

### 2. Risk Factors

Hyperleukocytosis occurs in children with acute myelocytic leukemia (AML), acute lymphocytic leukemia, chronic myelogenous leukemia, and myeloproliferative disorders. Children with hyperleukocytosis are at increased risk for pulmonary and central nervous system (CNS) complications due to leukostasis (sludging of leukemic cells in capillary vessels). Children with AML are at the greatest risk because monocytic blasts are more adherent to vessel walls. Patients with hyperleukocytosis are at risk for TLS, cerebral stroke, and pulmonary stasis.

### 3. Clinical Findings

Clinically significant hyperleukocytosis occurs with a WBC count of ≥200,000 x $10^9$ cells/L in patients with AML and in excess of 300,000 x $10^9$ cells/L in patients with acute lymphocytic leukemia and chronic myelogenous leukemia. Most patients are asymptomatic at presentation, but some may present with subtle CNS signs, such as headaches, tinnitus, dizziness, and blurred vision. The presentation sometimes is more dramatic and includes full-blown symptoms of cerebral stroke (changes in mental status, focalization, seizures, and increased intracranial pressure). Pulmonary manifestations include tachypnea, dyspnea, hypoxia, and acidosis.

Children with hyperleukocytosis often develop a consumptive coagulopathy, likely through activation of the extrinsic pathway. The platelet count, prothrombin time (PT), partial thromboplastin time (PTT), and fibrinogen level should be monitored frequently. CT and/or magnetic resonance imaging (MRI), with and without contrast, is useful in evaluating the nature and extent of a stroke.

### 4. Treatment

The treatment of hyperleukocytosis aims at the prevention of TLS, reduction of tumor burden through hydration, tumor-specific management through leukapheresis or exchange transfusion. The management of stroke and pulmonary leukostasis is supportive. Treating the underlying malignancy may prevent additional strokes and help decrease further pulmonary involvement. The platelet count should be maintained at >50,000 x $10^9$ cells/L. Coagulation disorders should be corrected promptly. Packed red blood cell (PRBC) transfusions are discouraged in patients with asymptomatic anemia because of the risk of worsening hyperviscosity.

## B. Spinal Cord Compression

###  Case Study

A 15-year-old high school basketball player presents to the emergency department with a 1-month history of progressive back pain radiating to the right lower extremity, which was initially relieved by ibuprofen. The patient now complains of right lower-extremity weakness and paresthesias. Physical examination reveals tenderness to percussion on the back, decreased strength and hyporeflexia of the right lower extremity, and poor sphincter tone on rectal examination.

**Detection**
- What is the possible diagnosis?

**Intervention**
- What diagnostic modality is indicated?
- Which pharmacologic treatment should be initiated?
- Should you contact neurosurgery?

**Reassessment**
- Is the current treatment strategy effective?

**Effective Communication**
- Who needs to know if the patient continues to have neurologic deterioration?
- Where is the best place to manage this patient?

**Teamwork**
- How are you going to implement the treatment strategy?
- Who is to do what and when?

### 1. Pathophysiology

Spinal cord compression in children with cancer most frequently results from metastatic spread (85%) of the tumor rather than primary disease. The most common metastatic tumors involving the spinal cord are sarcomas (Ewing sarcoma, osteosarcoma), neuroblastomas, lymphomas, germ cell tumors, and metastatic CNS neoplasms. Tumors typically infiltrate by local extension into the epidural space through the intervertebral foramina from nearby structures or by hematogenous spread. Most tumors are primarily located in the lumbosacral region and surround the spinal cord. The spinal cord and the vertebral venous plexus become progressively compressed by the encircling tumor, resulting in vasogenic cord edema, hemorrhage, and ischemia.

### 2. Symptoms

Pain, either local or radicular, is the most frequently encountered presenting sign of spinal cord compression in children (80%). The onset of pain is often insidious and follows a gradually progressive course (weeks to months). Pain associated with epidural compression of the spinal cord is exacerbated when the patient is recumbent and improves when the patient is in upright position. Once motor weakness and sensory deficits appear, progression of the disease may be rapid. Autonomic dysfunction (bladder or bowel incontinence) is a late and ominous sign of epidural compression. Lesions above T10 produce hyperreflexia, a positive Babinski reflex, whereas lesions below T10 that compress the conus or cauda equine produce hyporeflexia.

### 3. Diagnosis

For children with suspected spinal cord involvement, MRI with gadolinium enhancement of the entire spine is the recommended diagnostic modality. Craniospinal T1-weighted and T2-weighted MRI allows demonstration of epidural involvement, intraparenchymal spread, and compression of nerve roots. Conventional radiographs may reveal bone destruction but do not provide information about the spinal cord structure. Lumbar puncture is relatively contraindicated in spinal cord tumors except in leptomeningeal disease.

### 4. Treatment

Early diagnosis and treatment is vital for a child with cancer with confirmed spinal cord compression. High-dose steroids (dexamethasone 1-2 mg/kg) should be administered immediately, followed by lower doses (0.25-0.5 mg/kg IV every 6 h) once the diagnosis is confirmed. Emergent laminectomy with posterior decompression, radiation therapy, and chemotherapy should be initiated as indicated. Non-oncologic diagnoses must be excluded (tuberculosis, osteomyelitis). Prompt referral to a pediatric hospital for pediatric neurosurgery and a pediatric oncology evaluation is warranted. The prognosis for recovery in those with neurologic dysfunction is related to the severity and duration of symptoms at the time of diagnosis. About 66% of children treated regain some motor and sensory function.

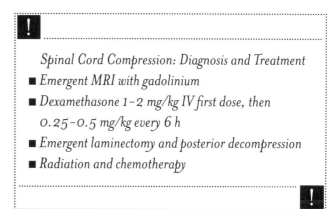

*Spinal Cord Compression: Diagnosis and Treatment*
- *Emergent MRI with gadolinium*
- *Dexamethasone 1-2 mg/kg IV first dose, then 0.25-0.5 mg/kg every 6 h*
- *Emergent laminectomy and posterior decompression*
- *Radiation and chemotherapy*

# VI. HEMATOLOGY: COAGULATION AND TRANSFUSIONS

 Case Study

An 8-year-old, African-American girl undergoing chemotherapy for acute lymphoblastic leukemia is in the clinic to receive her regular red blood cell transfusion (every 3-4 weeks). After 30 minutes of the transfusion, she develops chills, fever, hypotension, gross hematuria, and extensive bleeding from her mucosal membranes. Her initial laboratory results show: WBC count, $32,000 \times 10^9$ cells/L (68% neutrophils, 20% bands, 12% lymphocytes); hemoglobin, 4.5 g/dL; platelet count, $54,000 \times 10^9$ cells/L; PT, 38 sec; activated partial thromboplastin time, 58 sec; fibrinogen, 50 mg/dL (1.47 μmol/L); and D-dimer >10,000 ng/mL (normal, 0-230 ng/mL).

**Detection**

- What is the most likely diagnosis?

**Intervention**

- Which treatment strategies take priority?
- What diagnostic modality is indicated?
- Is a blood transfusion indicated?

**Reassessment**

- Is the current treatment strategy effective?

**Effective Communication**

- When the patient's clinical status changes, who needs this information and how will it be disseminated?
- Should the patient be transferred to the PICU?

**Teamwork**

- How are you going to implement the treatment strategy?
- Who is to do what and when?

For this particular case, the transfusion needs to be stopped immediately, critical care support given, and depleted coagulation factors and red blood cells should be replaced with fresh frozen plasma (FFP), cryoprecipitate, and PRBCs. Empiric antibiotics should be given to treat possible transfusion-associated bacterial infection.

Hemostasis is maintained through a delicate balance between procoagulant and antithrombotic factors. Severe deficiency of coagulation proteins can lead to bleeding or clotting. Clinically significant decreases in red blood cells, platelets, or coagulation factors require therapeutic intervention. Transfusion of blood products can assist in oxygen-carrying capacity, expanding the vascular volume, and improving coagulation and hemostasis. PRBCs are the most common blood component used, followed by platelets and FFP.

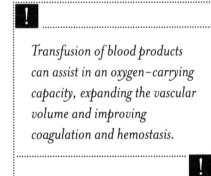

*Transfusion of blood products can assist in an oxygen-carrying capacity, expanding the vascular volume and improving coagulation and hemostasis.*

# A. Coagulopathies

Disseminated intravascular coagulation (DIC) due to malignancy, infection, or intravascular hemolysis can cause microangiopathy with hemolytic anemia and consumption of platelets and coagulation factors. DIC can result in life-threatening bleeding, large vessel thrombosis, or gangrenous limbs or digits. The main causes of DIC in children are infection (e.g., meningococcemia), malignancy, massive tissue damage, and immunologic reaction.
The focus should be on treating the underlying condition and replacing deficient coagulation factors and cellular elements with transfusions of FFP, cryoprecipitate, PRBCs, or platelets for bleeding symptoms.

DIC is a thrombotic disorder, but may lead to thrombosis or hemorrhage. Thrombin formation and hemorrhage are the 2 primary manifestations in DIC. Patients often present with signs and symptoms of end-organ dysfunction secondary to microvascular fibrin formation or abnormal bleeding. The type of manifestation is dependent on the underlying problem.

Microthrombi can result in purpura fulminans or skin necrosis, organ failure, or gangrene. Thrombosis in the microvasculature results in a significant decrease in platelets and coagulation factors. The consumption of factors presents as purpura fulminans, mucosal bleeding, petechial hemorrhages, bleeding from central and peripheral lines, and possibly intracranial bleeding.

The diagnosis of DIC is not made based on a specific test, but rather is made when the proper laboratory evidence and clinical findings are present. Common laboratory findings in DIC consists of an elevated PT and activated partial thromboplastin time, decreased fibrinogen, elevated D-dimer, decreased platelet count, decreased concentration of factors V and VIII, and fragmented red blood cells on the peripheral smear. These abnormalities are a reflection of the excessive thrombosis, resulting in the consumption of platelets, coagulation factors, and fibrinolysis.

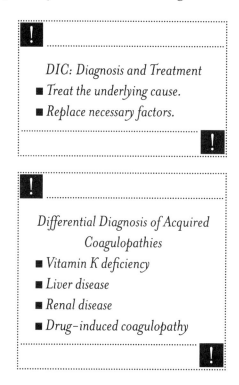

*DIC: Diagnosis and Treatment*
- *Treat the underlying cause.*
- *Replace necessary factors.*

*Differential Diagnosis of Acquired Coagulopathies*
- *Vitamin K deficiency*
- *Liver disease*
- *Renal disease*
- *Drug-induced coagulopathy*

The most effective therapy begins with the treatment of the underlying illness, thus eliminating the catalysts of intravascular coagulation. Replacement therapy prior to the treatment of the underlying illness is important. In most critical care settings, treatment of the catalyst and replacement of factors is performed simultaneously. The replacement should begin with platelets and FFP. Transfusion of cryoprecipitate is required for the replacement of fibrinogen. Follow-up laboratory studies are necessary to monitor the correction of deficiencies.

## B. Blood Products

The transfusion of blood products in patients newly diagnosed with a malignancy is frequently a necessary treatment in the critical care setting, but it is not without risk or complication. These complications arise from both infectious and noninfectious origins. Over the past 20 years, significant advances in the screening of blood products has led to a decrease in the incidence of infections. Still, the possibility continues and must be carefully weighed. The decision to transfuse a patient should only be made when it is clinically indicated. Informed consent should always be obtained before the administration of blood products.

To decrease the chance of clerical error, all blood products drawn for typing and crossmatching must be clearly labeled with the patient's identification information. Before initiating the transfusion, the patient's identification band must be checked and blood type verified. Administration of incompatible blood products can result in serious consequences, including death.

Nucleic acid screening for human immunodeficiency virus types 1 and 2, hepatitis B and C viruses, and human T-lymphotropic virus types I and II has virtually eliminated these infections from the blood supply, though a statistically calculable risk remains. Bacterial infections still occur in 1 in 2000 platelet transfusions and a smaller proportion of PRBC transfusions. Despite the improvements in screening, the risks have not been completely eradicated. Some of the pathogens transmitted by transfusions include: CMV, *Bartonella* species, *Borrelia* species, *Brucella* species, *Leishmania* species, *Parvovirus*, plasmodia, rickettsiae, *Toxoplasma* species, prions, and certain *Trypanosoma* species.

**1. Red Blood Cells**

Anemia is frequently encountered in the critical care setting. Red blood cells should only be administered with the consideration of clinical signs and symptoms (**Table 17-3**). A sudden loss of blood can compromise the cardiovascular system. Healthy, young individuals can tolerate a loss of approximately 30% of their blood volume. Unless there is rapid intervention, patients who lose 50% of their blood volume proceed to heart failure and death.

---

**Table 17-3   Clinical Signs and Symptoms of Anemia**

**General:** Patients with sudden loss of blood can present with confusion and decreased responsiveness, as seen in patients with hypovolemic shock. Patients with a gradual onset of anemia have decreased stamina, headache, irritability, and anorexia.

**Skin color:** Check for pallor in the normally pink mucosa and nail beds, mottling, cool clammy skin, and delayed capillary refill. Prolonged iron deficiency can lead to softening and spooning of the fingernails.

**Tachypnea:** Rapid breathing and air hunger are important signs of anemia in infants and young children. Healthy adolescents tolerate moderately severe anemia with only dyspnea associated with exercise.

**Tachycardia:** Patients with hypovolemic shock will have a rapid and thready pulse; those with prolonged anemia have an audible flow murmur on auscultation.

---

Patients with slow blood loss or chronic anemia are usually well-compensated. Subsequently, these patients may lack symptoms and not seek medical attention immediately, but they may quickly decompensate if otherwise stressed. These patients often present with clinical signs and symptoms of anemia that include headache, fatigue, dyspnea, irritability, anorexia, and tachycardia.

The underlying reason for anemia should be determined and, when possible, corrected to avoid additional transfusions. Anemia can be caused by a number of factors, such as active bleeding, chronic inflammation, tumor infiltration of the bone marrow, bone marrow failure, nutritional deficiency, chemotherapy, and radiation therapy. The transfusion of PRBCs should be considered when the hemoglobin level falls below 7 g/dL. However, the decision to transfuse should be based on clinical parameters and context, not solely on a laboratory value. The volume of PRBCs transfused in small pediatric patients who require less than 1 U should be based on body weight. As a general rule, 10 mL/kg of PRBCs will increase the recipient's hemoglobin by approximately 1.5 g/dL.

Severely anemic patients scheduled to undergo a surgical procedure or radiation therapy should be transfused prophylactically. Care should be taken not to rapidly transfuse these patients, because it may induce congestive heart failure; it is preferable to transfuse the severely anemic patient in smaller aliquots. Consider transfusion in patients with a hemoglobin <5 g/dL at the rate of 1 mL x hemoglobin (g)/kg if there is evidence of cardiovascular instability. One unit of PRBCs may contain 225 to 350 mL and, depending on the blood bank, may have a hematocrit of

55% to 80%. PRBCs are the product of choice to restore oxygen carrying-capacity and red cell mass. PRBCs must be ABO and Rh(D) compatible to prevent a massive transfusion reaction. Crossmatching is required to prevent transfusion of incompatible minor blood-group antigens. Only in a life-threatening emergency should O-negative products be utilized.

> *Anemia can be caused by a number of factors, such as active bleeding, chronic inflammation, tumor infiltration of the bone marrow, bone marrow failure, nutritional deficiency, chemotherapy, and radiation therapy.*

The use of leukocyte filters has become standard practice in many institutions. Leukocyte-depleted red blood cells reduce the incidence of febrile reactions and other cytokine-induced adverse events. The filters remove 99.9% of the leukocytes, which cause fever. Additionally, washed PRBCs effectively remove the unwanted cells, while maintaining approximately 85% of the red cell mass. The use of irradiated blood is standard practice in cancer centers but is normally reserved for patients likely to undergo a bone marrow transplant. Indications for red blood cell transfusion are listed in **Table 17-4**.

### Table 17-4 Indications for Red Blood Cell Transfusion

1. Infants <4 months old
    a. Hgb level <13 g/dL in neonates <24 h old
    b. Hgb level <13 g/dL and presence of severe pulmonary disease, cyanotic heart disease or heart failure
    c. Acute blood loss of at least 10% of total blood volume
    d. Phlebotomy losses of at least 10% of the total blood volume
    e. Hgb level <9 g/dL in infants with clinical manifestations of anemia
2. Children >4 months of age
    a. Symptomatic anemia
    b. Hgb level <7 g/dL
    c. Hgb level <8 g/dL in patients undergoing surgery or invasive procedures
    d. Intraoperative blood loss of 10% to 15% or more of total blood volume, postoperative Hgb level <8 g/dL, and signs or symptoms of anemia
    e. Hgb level <9 g/dL in patients with symptomatic anemia
    f. Hgb level <10 g/dL in patients receiving radiation therapy
    g. Acute blood loss with hypovolemia unresponsive to crystalloid or colloid

Hgb, hemoglobin

There is a high incidence of inherited defects in the globin structure in patients of African, Indian, Asian, and Mediterranean populations. The homozygous form of sickle cell anemia is a debilitating disease. Early in life, these patients present with severe hemolytic anemia and vaso-occlusive disease. Patients with sickle cell anemia are at an increased risk of death secondary to sepsis or CNS thrombosis. Patients with hemoglobinopathies, such as sickle cell disease, are at increased risk for vaso-occlusive infarction of marrow, the spleen, and renal medullary tissue. They often have recurrent painful crises.

Hypertransfusion therapy of PRBCs and maintaining the hemoglobin levels above 10 g/dL decreases production of sickle red blood cells. This significantly decreases morbidity, the risk of other life-threatening events, and the frequency of painful crises. Patients with sickle cell disease have an increased risk of stroke and hyperviscosity, and, therefore, should not be transfused to a hemoglobin level above 12 g/dL.

Hypertransfusion is also effective in minimizing the production of hemoglobin S. Because of the inherent risks, prophylactic transfusions are reserved for patients who are severely ill, and recommended for patients with a history of CNS thrombosis or transcranial Doppler blood flow velocities >200 cm/sec in the middle cerebral or internal carotid arteries.

The use of exchange transfusion in sickle cell patients is also effective in reducing the sickle cells. This modality is beneficial to patients with recurrent stroke, because there is no increase in hematocrit or blood viscosity. Exchange transfusions are also indicated in patients with hyperleukocytosis or hyperbilirubinemia.

Pediatric oncology patients commonly are anemic at diagnosis. In addition, patients may be significantly anemic while undergoing chemotherapy and are routinely transfused with PRBCs. They are usually transfused if the hemoglobin level is <7 g/dL and to maintain a level above 10 g/dL when receiving radiation therapy. All hematology-oncology patients should receive irradiated blood products to prevent transfusion-associated graft-versus-host disease.

*Dosage*. The dose of PRBCs is dependent on the desired hemoglobin or hematocrit level, the rate of red cell destruction, and the presence of blood loss. Patients with severe anemia, but no ongoing blood loss, who receive 10-15 mL/kg should increase hemoglobin by 2.5 to 3 g/dL and the hematocrit by 10%.

2. Platelets

Platelets have an important role in hemostasis and coagulation. An adequate number of functional platelets are required for hemostasis. After vascular injury, the formation of the primary hemostatic plug prevents the flow of blood from small- and medium-sized blood vessels. In addition, platelets release thromboxane $A_2$, which mediates the change in vascular tone and platelet activation.

A healthy individual with functional platelets can withstand a platelet count as low as 10,000 x $10^9$ cells/L. Individuals with fever or infection or who are acutely ill have a much higher risk of bleeding, even with platelet counts as high as 30,000 x $10^9$ cells/L.

Clinical signs and symptoms of a reduced platelet count, known as *thrombocytopenia*, are nonspecific but primarily consist of gingival bleeding, epistaxis, hematuria, and petechial rash. The rash is most commonly seen on the upper and lower extremities. Diagnosis of thrombocytopenia is based upon the platelet count.

Platelet transfusion is used to prevent bleeding and to treat bleeding secondary to thrombocytopenia or platelet dysfunction. It is not indicated for patients with rapid destruction problems, such as immune thrombocytopenic purpura (ITP). In this circumstance, a transfusion is only indicated with life-threatening hemorrhage. Platelet transfusions are useful in the bleeding patient with a consumptive coagulopathy, such as DIC. Platelets are frequently administered to patients receiving chemotherapy or who have bone marrow infiltration. Indications for platelet transfusions are listed in **Table 17-5**.

| Table 17-5 | Indications for Platelet Transfusions |

**Premature or sick infants**

- Platelet count <50,000 x $10^9$ cells/L
- Platelet count <100,000 x $10^9$ cells/L for hemodynamically unstable infants

**Children**

- Platelet count <10,000 x $10^9$ cells/L with evidence of failure of platelet production
- Active bleeding with a qualitative platelet defect
- Platelet count <30,000 x $10^9$ cells/L with active bleeding
- Platelet count <50,000 x $10^9$ cells/L with an anticipated minor invasive procedure and less than 100,000 x $10^9$ cells/L with an anticipated major surgery

**Oncology**

- Platelet count <10,000 x $10^9$ cells/L without active bleeding and failure of platelet production
- Platelet count <10,000 x $10^9$ cells/L when undergoing induction chemotherapy for acute lymphocytic leukemia
- Platelet count <20,000 x $10^9$ cells/L when undergoing induction chemotherapy for acute myelogenous leukemia
- Platelet count <30,000 x $10^9$ cells/L for patients with tumors in the central nervous system
- Platelet count <20,000 x $10^9$ cells/L prior to lumbar puncture
- Platelet count >100,000 x $10^9$ cells/L in patients with a high risk of traumatic taps
- Platelet count <50,000 x $10^9$ cells/L in a bleeding patient with normal coagulation studies
- Platelet count <20,000 x $10^9$ cells/L prior to an intramuscular injection

*Dosage.* Random platelets, 1 U/10 kg, will increase the platelet count by approximately 50,000 x $10^9$ cells/L if there is no active consumptive process (fever, ITP, sepsis, alloimmunization, DIC) or sequestration. The platelet count should be checked 1 to 2 hours posttransfusion to identify refractory patients.

If the platelet count does not increase as expected following two separate transfusions, the patient may have immune-mediated platelet refractoriness secondary to alloantibodies. Nonimmune causes of this condition are common and include splenomegaly, fever, infection, DIC, and the use of amphotericin.

For refractory patients, a trial of crossmatched platelets should be given. Should this fail, other possibilities for treatment include leukocyte-depleted human lymphocyte antigen-matched platelets or massive transfusion with random donor platelets, the latter of which will saturate the antibody concentration.

Pheresis platelets are harvested from a single donor and generally contain >30,000 x $10^9$ cells/L platelets, which is equal to 6 to 8 units of random donor platelets. The volume is usually 250 to 300 mL. The use of platelets from single-donor apheresis is indicated for patients who are frequently transfused or need multiple units to decrease donor exposure and the inherent risks.

## 3. Plasma Derivatives

### a. Fresh Frozen Plasma

Patients with severe clotting deficiencies or with a consumptive coagulopathy may require derivatives of plasma. FFP is a rich source of clotting factors, containing a high concentration of fibrinogen, factor VIII, von Willebrand factor, and factor XIII. It is frequently used in patients unable to synthesize clotting factors due to liver disease or in those with a consumptive coagulopathy secondary to trauma.

FFP is plasma that has been harvested from whole blood. The whole blood is centrifuged, and the excess plasma is then frozen within 8 hours of collection. FFP can be stored for 1 year at -4°F (-20°C). It is thawed at 98.6°F (37°C) for 30 to 60 minutes prior to transfusion. To increase the likelihood of the product remaining sterile and containing adequate levels of coagulation factors, FFP must be administered within 8 hours of thawing. Additionally, the product must be ABO compatible with the patient's blood type.

Patients with a significantly prolonged PT and PTT have approximately 15% to 25% of their normal factor levels. Large amounts of FFP are required to increase the coagulation factor levels above 30%. Each unit contains about 250 mL of plasma and yields only a 3% increase in coagulation factor levels. Indications for transfusion of FFP are listed in **Table 17-6**.

### Table 17-6. Indications for Transfusion of FFP

- Emergency reversal of warfarin anticoagulation
- Disseminated intravascular coagulation
- Thrombotic thrombocytopenic purpura
- Prolonged partial thromboplastin time >60 s
- Prolonged prothrombin time >18 s despite administration of vitamin K
- Liver disease
- Massive blood loss

*Dosage.* FFP is administered at 10 to 20 mL/kg and should be infused at a maximum rate of 0.5 mL/kg/min.

The use of FFP should be reserved for situations in which a concentrate of coagulation factors is not necessary and/or not available. Generally FFP is no longer used for administration of factor VIII or IX.

### b. Cryoprecipitate

The preparation of cryoprecipitate consists of flash freezing fresh plasma. It is then thawed at 39.2°F (4°C). The residual precipitate contains 150 to 200 mg of fibrinogen per 15 mL. Cryoprecipitate also contains factor VIII, factor XIII, von Willebrand factor, and fibronectin at much higher concentrations than in FFP. The use of cryoprecipitate is indicated when fibrinogen levels are <100 mg/dL. It should be transfused within 4 hours of thawing.

*Dosage.* Cryoprecipitate dosing is 1 unit per 5 to 10 kg. One unit contains 10 to 15 mL of volume and will raise the fibrinogen level by 5 to 10 mg/dL per unit. With proper dosing, the expected rise should be 60 to 100 mg/dL. The therapeutic goal is a fibrinogen level >100 mg/dL.

## C. Adverse Reactions

The main cause of acute hemolytic reactions is ABO incompatibility. Treatment seeks to eliminate the precipitating agent and provide general supportive care.

The incidence of adverse reactions associated with the transfusion of blood products is about 5%. Most are mild urticarial reactions that can be treated by stopping the transfusion for 30 minutes, followed by the administration of antihistamines. If the symptoms subside, the transfusion can be restarted. All other reactions require discontinuation of the transfusion, and the transfused product and a blood sample from the patient must be sent to the blood bank for further evaluation.

The medical treatment of transfusion reactions is detailed in **Table 17-7**.

**Table 17-7** Treatment for Transfusion Reactions

| Medication | Dosage | Indications |
| --- | --- | --- |
| Diphenhydramine | 0.5-1 mg/kg IV (maximum dose, 50 mg) | Urticaria and hives |
| Acetaminophen/paracetamol | 10-15 mg/kg PO (maximum dose, 1000 mg) | Fever and chills |
| Hydrocortisone | 1-2 mg/kg IV (maximum dose, 100 mg) | Severe urticaria, diaphoresis, rigor, or pallor |
| Epinephrine/adrenaline (1:1000) | 0.01 mL/kg IM (maximum dose, 0.5 mL/dose) | Shock[a], bronchospasm, and hypotension |
| Furosemide | 1-2 mg/kg IV (infants); 0.5-1 mg/kg (older children and adolescents; maximum dose, 40 mg) | Acute hemolytic reaction – maintain urine flow >1 mL/kg/h |
| Oxygen | 100% via non-rebreather face mask | |

IV, intravenous; PO, orally; IM, intramuscular
[a]Patients with shock may require additional therapeutic interventions including fluids, advanced airway management protection, and vasoactive medications.

### 1. Allergic Reactions

Severe allergic reactions can present with urticaria followed by laryngospasm, bronchospasm, and angioedema. These patients require immediate cessation of the transfusion, followed by administration of steroids or possibly epinephrine. Close observation is needed for 4 to 6 hours if the patient's reaction is mild. High-flow oxygen, maintenance of open airway, close cardiac monitoring, and IV access should be considered in asymptomatic patients with a history of serious anaphylactic reaction. Anaphylaxis, an IgE-mediated allergic reaction, is a rare complication but, if not treated immediately, can result in death. Most anaphylactoid reactions (resembling anaphylaxis but caused by a nonimmunologic mechanism) occur in patients with immunoglobulin A deficiency. The transfusion should not be restarted after any severe reaction.

### 2. Febrile Nonhemolytic Reactions

Even after washing or filtering PRBCs, a percentage of leukocytes and cytokines remain. The presence of leukocytes results in the release of cytokines during transfusion in patients with antibodies that react with alloantigens in the blood product. This often results in fever, chills, or diaphoresis. These symptoms can also occur if the blood product is contaminated with bacteria. Individuals receiving transfusions over an extended period should be given leukocyte-depleted blood products to help minimize the development of antibodies that react with foreign WBCs.

The treatment of febrile nonhemolytic reactions is cessation of the transfusion. The patient should be examined, and the vital signs should be monitored. Symptoms should be treated with antipyretics and possibly antibiotics. The transfused product should be evaluated by culture and re-crossmatch.

### 3. Acute Hemolytic Transfusion Reactions

Transfusion of ABO-incompatible blood products results in acute hemolytic transfusion reactions. This is usually a result of mislabeled blood products or the administration of blood products to the wrong patient, resulting in the immunologic destruction of the transfused red cells.

Clinical signs and symptoms of acute hemolytic reactions consist of fever, chills, urticaria, dyspnea, tachycardia, nausea, abdominal or lower back pain, hyper- or hypotension, jaundice, hemoglobinuria (port wine-colored urine), and shock. The hemoglobinuria leads to oliguria and, eventually, renal failure. Laboratory evaluation should include a complete blood count, coagulation studies, urinalysis, and a direct Coombs test. Significant laboratory findings may include anemia, DIC, and hemoglobinuria, and a positive result on the Coombs test.

Therapy for acute hemolytic transfusion reactions involves immediate cessation of the transfusion, fluid support to maintain adequate hemodynamic status, and diuretics (mannitol) if needed to maintain adequate renal blood flow. The urine output should approximate 1 to 2 mL/kg/h. Vasopressors and inotropes may be required for hemodynamic stability. The use of steroids is indicated in the management of acute hemolytic reaction transfusions because of their effectiveness in suppressing the inflammatory reaction.

### 4. Delayed Hemolytic Transfusion Reactions

There are two different types of delayed hemolytic transfusion reactions: primary immunization and anamnestic response. Primary immunization is characterized as a mild reaction tending to occur weeks after the administration of blood products. This type of reaction rarely leads to significant hemolysis. Laboratory evaluation will usually demonstrate a decrease in the hemoglobin level 2 to 4 weeks after transfusion.

The anamnestic response tends to occur in patients with a previous history of sensitization to minor blood group antigens secondary to pregnancy or a previous blood transfusion. This reaction can result in a severe drop in hemoglobin over 3 to 10 days. The clinical signs and symptoms are not as severe as in hemolytic anemia secondary to ABO incompatibility. As with all hemolytic reactions, the diagnosis is confirmed with positive results on a Coombs test and the identification of alloantibodies in the patient's red blood cells. The management of delayed hemolytic transfusion reactions is nonspecific because the symptoms are usually mild. Symptom control is usually sufficient.

### 5. Transfusion-Related Acute Lung Injury

Transfusion-related acute lung injury is a clinical syndrome that presents with dyspnea, hypoxemia, cyanosis, hypotension, fever, chills, and noncardiogenic pulmonary edema. This is a severe and sometimes fatal reaction, the third most frequent cause of transfusion-related mortality. The symptoms ordinarily begin 1 to 4 hours after the administration of blood products. The pathophysiology is secondary to the transfusion of human leukocyte antigen-specific antibodies, the passive transfer of which results in increased capillary permeability and microvascular pulmonary damage. Treatment is respiratory supportive care.

### 6. Transfusion Transmitted Diseases

Significant advances in blood product screening have led to a decrease in the incidence of infections. The common serious culprits of transfusion-related diseases are hepatitis C virus, hepatitis B virus, human immunodeficiency virus, and CMV. Blood donations are routinely screened for both hepatitis viruses and human immunodeficiency virus, but donors who have been recently infected can go undetected. Transfusion recipients may also be at risk for parvovirus B19 and various parasitic infections.

# Oncologic and Hematologic Emergencies and Complications

**Key Points**

- Early admission to the PICU should be considered for children with oncologic complications.

- Preexisting organ dysfunction caused by chemotherapy or its complications is common in pediatric oncology patients.

- Patients with neutropenic fever should be treated aggressively with a single broad-spectrum antimicrobial. Colony-stimulating factors should be considered in the patient with septic shock.

- Resistant bacterial or fungal infections are possible in patients in whom fever persists beyond 3 days despite single broad-spectrum coverage.

- High-resolution CT and bronchoalveolar lavage should be considered early in patients with respiratory insufficiency.

- Early institution of a lung-protective strategy, including the use of high-frequency oscillatory ventilation, may improve the outcome in patients with respiratory failure.

- Early evaluation for cardiac dysfunction or adrenal insufficiency is indicated for patients with shock who do not respond to conventional fluid challenges.

- Tumor lysis syndrome – characterized by hyperuricemia, hyperkalemia, hyperphosphatemia, and hypocalcemia – may result in renal failure, seizures, and potentially fatal cardiac arrhythmias.

- Hyperleukocytosis can cause coagulopathy and hyperviscosity, leading to lung injury and stroke. Prompt initiation of cancer therapy is recommended.

- Emergence of leg weakness, paresthesias in the lower extremities, and/or bowel or bladder dysfunction in children with a history of cancer are symptoms suggestive of spinal cord compression.

- Decreased stamina and the presence of headaches, dyspnea, and pallor are signs of anemia.

- The treatment of DIC focuses on the elimination of the catalyst. Replacement therapy consists of the use of platelets, FFP, and cryoprecipitate. Follow-up laboratory studies are necessary to monitor the correction of deficiencies.

- The standard dose of PRBCs is 10 to 15 mL/kg administered over 2 to 4 hours to avoid congestive heart failure. Rapid replacement of PRBCs is indicated in cases of acute blood loss or shock.

- One unit of random platelets per 10 kg body weight will increase the platelet count by approximately $50,000 \times 10^9$ cells/L, provided there is no active consumptive process (fever, ITP, sepsis, alloimmunization, DIC) or sequestration.

- FFP is administered at 10 to 20 mL/kg and should be infused at a maximum rate of 0.5 mL/kg/min.

- Transfusion-related lung injury presents with dyspnea, hypoxemia, cyanosis, hypotension, fever, chills, and noncardiogenic pulmonary edema. It requires respiratory support.

# Suggested Readings

1. Brierley J, Carcillo JA, Choong K, et al. Clinical practice parameters for hemodynamic support of pediatric and neonatal septic shock: 2007 update from the American College of Critical Care Medicine. *Crit Care Med*. 2009;37:666-688.

2. Coiffier B, Altman A, Pui CH, Younes A, Cairo MS. Guidelines for the management of pediatric and adult tumor lysis syndrome: an evidence-based review. *J Clin Oncol*. 2008;26:2767-2778.

3. Consumptive coagulopathies. In: Hillman RS, Ault KA, Rinder HM. *Hematology in Clinical Practice*. 4th ed. New York, NY: McGraw Hill; 2005:387-392.

4. Fiser RT, West NK, Bush AJ, Sillos EM, Schmidt JE, Tamburro RF. Outcome of severe sepsis in pediatric oncology patients. *Pediatr Crit Care Med*. 2005;6:531-536.

5. Freifeld AG, Bow EJ, Sepkowitz KA, et al. Clinical practice guideline for the use of antimicrobial agents in neutropenic patients with cancer: 2010 update by the Infectious Diseases Society of America. *Clin Infect Dis*. 2011;52:e56-e93.

6. Hagen SA, Craig DM, Martin PL, et al. Mechanically ventilated pediatric stem cell transplant recipients: effect of cord blood transplant and organ dysfunction on outcome. *Pediatr Crit Care Med*. 2003;4:206-213.

7. Hughes WT, Armstrong D, Bodey GP, et al. 2002 guidelines for the use of antimicrobial agents in neutropenic patients with cancer. *Clin Infect Dis*. 2002;34:730-751.

8. Jacobe SJ, Hassan A, Veys P, Mok Q. Outcome of children requiring admission to an intensive care unit after bone marrow transplantation. *Crit Care Med*. 2003;31:1299-1305.

9. Josephson CD. Transfusion formulas. In: Hillyer CD, Strauss RG, Luban NLC. *Handbook of Pediatric Transfusion Medicine*. Philadelphia, PA: Elsevier; 2004:375-377.

10. Klastersky J, Paesmans M, Rubenstein EB, et al. The Multinational Association for Supportive Care in Cancer risk index: A multinational scoring system for identifying low-risk febrile neutropenic cancer patients. *J Clin Oncol*. 2000;18:3038-3051.

11. Kreuz WD. Treatment of consumption coagulopathy with antithrombin concentrate in children with acquired antithrombin deficiency: A feasibility pilot study. *Eur J Pediatr*. 1999;158 (Suppl 3):S187-S191.

12. Lusher JM. Clinical and laboratory approach to the patient with bleeding. In: Nathan DG, Orkin SH, Look AT, Ginsberg D. *Hematology of Infancy and Childhood*. 6th ed. Philadelphia, PA: WB Saunders: 2003:1515-1526.

13. Matthay MA. Severe sepsis – a new treatment with both anticoagulant and anti-inflammatory properties. *N Engl J Med*. 2001;344:759-762.

14. Mejia R, Cortes J, Brown D, et al. Oncologic emergencies and complications. In: Rogers MC, ed. *Rogers Textbook of Pediatric Intensive Care*. Philadelphia, PA: Lippincott Williams & Wilkins; 2008:1710-1724.

15. Porcu P, Cripe LD, Ng EW, et al. Hyperleukocytic leukemias and leukostasis: a review of pathophysiology, clinical presentation and management. *Leuk Lymphoma*. 2000;39:1-18.

16. Rheingold SR, Lange BJ. Oncologic emergencies. In: Fleisher GR, Ludwig S, Henretig FM, Ruddy RM, Silverman BK. *Textbook of Pediatric Emergency Medicine*. 5th ed. Philadelphia, PA: Lippincott Williams & Wilkins; 2005:1202-1230.

17. Sloan SR, Benjamin RJ, Freidman DF, et al. Transfusion medicine. In: Nathan DG, Orkin SH, Look AT, Ginsberg D. *Hematology of Infancy and Childhood*. 6th ed. Philadelphia, PA: WB Saunders; 2003:1709-1756.

18. Transfusion medicine blood component therapy. In: Hillman RS, Ault KA, Rinder HM. *Hematology in Clinical Practice*. 4th ed. New York, NY: McGraw Hill; 2005:431-440.

19. Watson RS, Carcillo JA. Scope and epidemiology of pediatric sepsis. *Pediatr Crit Care Med*. 2005;6(3 Suppl):S3-S5.

20. Wong ECC, Perez-Albuerne E, Moscow JA, et al. Transfusion management strategies: a survey of practicing pediatric hematology-oncology specialists. *Pediatr Blood Cancer*. 2005;44:119-127.

# Chapter 18

# Acute Kidney Injury

## ✓ Objectives

- Recognize patients at risk of acute kidney injury or failure.
- Describe the epidemiology and etiologies of acute kidney injury.
- Review management of acute kidney injury to prevent mortality.
- Identify risks to renal function associated with systemic illnesses.
- Develop a plan to recognize and manage hyperkalemia.
- Discuss current terminology for degrees of kidney impairment.
- Provide an overview for renal replacement therapy modalities.

## 📁 Case Study

A 5-year-old obtunded boy presents with a 5-day history of fever, nausea, and vomiting. His weight at home last week was 20 kg but on arrival is 17 kg. His blood pressure is 80/40 mm Hg and heart rate is 140 beats/min. His capillary refill time is 3 to 4 seconds. Initial laboratory results are as follows: sodium, 147 mEq/L; potassium, 5.2 mEq/L; serum bicarbonate, 15 mEq/L; blood urea nitrogen, 40 mg/dL (14.3 mmol/L); and serum creatinine, 0.9 mg/dL (79.6 µmol/L).

**Detection**
- What is this child's physiologic status?
- What is his likely diagnosis?

**Intervention**
- What are the most immediate treatment strategies?
- What laboratory and imaging studies might be helpful in determining the etiology?

**Reassessment**
- He receives fluid resuscitation with 20 mL/kg of normal saline times 3 doses during his first hour in the emergency department, and then is admitted to the pediatric intensive care unit, where his blood pressure is 90/50 mm Hg and heart rate is 125 beats/min.
- Is the current treatment strategy effective?

- Does he need any other evaluation?
- What next steps are important in preventing further kidney injury?

**Effective Communication**
- When the patient's clinical status changes, who needs the information and how will it be disseminated?
- If renal function declines further, who needs the information?
- Where is the best place to manage the care of this patient?

**Teamwork**
- How are you going to implement the treatment strategy?
- Who is to do what and when?

# I. INTRODUCTION

Although acute kidney injury (AKI) should be a manageable illness, it has significant morbidity and mortality, which may be prevented by healthcare providers who maintain a high index of suspicion and awareness of the variety of clinical AKI. This requires an understanding of the urgency required to stabilize what can be a clinically asymptomatic child who has a potentially life-threatening condition.

AKI is characterized by an abrupt decrease in the renal glomerular filtration (GFR) rate, resulting in decreased ability to eliminate metabolic wastes and regulate electrolyte, acid-base, and fluid homeostasis. The literature has highlighted the importance of the identification of risk, early recognition of the onset, determination of the etiology, and goal-directed therapy as children with AKI are at significant risk from hyperkalemia and/or the underlying disorder. Critically ill children are at particular risk for AKI. This chapter will review current definitions, epidemiology, diagnosis, classification, and management strategies for pediatric AKI.

# II. DEFINING ACUTE KIDNEY INJURY

Current definitions of AKI are based on increases in serum creatinine (SCr) and decreased urine output. In 2004, the Acute Dialysis Quality Initiative established a scoring system that stratifies AKI by progressively worsening levels of renal function. The **R**isk, **I**njury, **F**ailure, **L**oss, **E**nd-Stage Renal Disease (**RIFLE**) criteria classify severity into three distinct categories (risk, injury and failure) based on incremental increases in SCr or progressive decline in urine output during the 48 hours after onset of AKI. It also includes two additional categories (loss, end-stage renal disease) describing two post-AKI clinical outcomes. Subsequently, a modified version of the RIFLE criteria, pRIFLE, was validated for use in the pediatric population (**Table 18-1**). These criteria have provided standardized methods of grading AKI across clinical and research populations, and several studies have now shown a correlation between these scores and clinical outcomes.

### Table 18-1 Pediatric RIFLE Criteria

| Category | Estimated Creatinine Clearance | Urine Output |
| --- | --- | --- |
| Risk | Decreased by 25% | <0.5 mL/kg/h for 8 h |
| Injury | Decreased by 50% | < 0.5 mL/kg/h for 16 h |
| Failure | Decreased by 75% or <35 mL/min/1.73 m$^2$ | <0.3 mL/kg/h for 24 h or anuric for 12 h |
| Loss | persistant failure > 4 weeks | |
| End-stage renal disease | Persistent failure >3 months | |

## A. Risk Factors and Etiology

Prevention and treatment of AKI is aided by the identification of clinical situations which place patients at increased risk for kidney injury. While the underlying cause will be unique to each patient, particular groups at high risk for developing AKI are patients undergoing cardiopulmonary bypass or receiving stem cell transplant, those with severe illness involving multiorgan dysfunction, and patients exposed to toxins. The increased risk in these groups demonstrates the shift in AKI etiology over the last decade from primary renal diseases (e.g., hemolytic uremic syndrome) to systemic illness. It is helpful to differentiate AKI due to primary renal disease from AKI secondary to extrinsic factors affecting perfusion, such as sepsis or toxin exposure. The simultaneous presence of many of these factors in children with critical illness places them at highest risk and highlights the need for a multidisciplinary approach to caring for these patients.

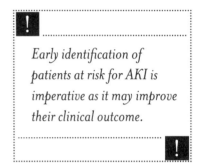

*Early identification of patients at risk for AKI is imperative as it may improve their clinical outcome.*

In the neonate, renal vascular thromboembolism associated with an umbilical artery or vein catheter can cause AKI. It can also arise in an infant with decompensated dehydration. The most frequent causes in neonates, however, are severe perinatal asphyxia, sepsis, and complex surgery affecting hemodynamics. In children, AKI commonly results from comorbid conditions, including hematologic and oncologic diseases, urologic conditions, and hepatic insufficiency, or following cardiovascular surgery or solid organ transplantation. The most frequent causes, however, are ischemia and sepsis. The use of antibiotics, antimycotics, chemotherapy, nonsteroidal anti-inflammatory drugs (NSAIDS), and angiotensin-converting enzyme (ACE) inhibitors also can contribute to AKI. Ischemia is a frequent cause in young children, whereas nephrotoxic causes predominate in school-aged children and adolescents. When AKI occurs in patients with multiorgan failure, multiple contributing factors are possible, including ischemia, sepsis, inflammatory mediators, and nephrotoxic drug effects.

Hypovolemia or a decrease in effective arterial volume restricts renal perfusion and adversely affects renal function. Causes include inadequate intake, hemorrhage, intestinal obstruction, gastrointestinal fluid losses, severe burns, decompensated nephrotic syndrome, and trauma. It can also arise as a result of polyuria, which may be caused by osmotic diuresis in diabetic ketoacidosis, the different forms of diabetes insipidus, a salt-wasting syndrome, or mineralocorticoid deficiency. A fall in effective arterial volume is also found in heart failure and any situation involving a significant decrease in cardiac output. In patients with low effective arterial volume in whom filtration is maintained at the expense of vasoconstriction of the efferent arteriole, vasodilators – like angiotensin-receptor blockers or ACE inhibitors – may cause a sharp drop in filtration.

Hemolytic uremic syndrome (HUS) presents as microangiopathic hemolytic anemia and thrombocytopenia associated with oliguria or anuria, often preceded by bloody diarrhea. The cause is frequently an intestinal infection by a verotoxin-producing strain of *Escherichia coli*. HUS may have a multisystemic course that involves the central nervous system, colonic wall, pancreas, or myocardium. It remains a common cause of intrinsic AKI. Urinary tract obstruction can cause kidney damage and loss of function. Bilateral ureteral obstruction, obstruction of a solitary kidney, or urethral obstruction by valves, a clot, or ureterocele may be responsible.

Evidence strongly suggests an association between sepsis and AKI. Hypotension and shock are often implicated, though usually in the presence of other predisposing factors. Rhabdomyolysis can generate AKI, though it has not been clearly established at what level of creatine kinase and myoglobin this occurs. Myoglobin in the presence of hypovolemia or ischemia is particularly nephrotoxic.

In the postoperative course of cardiovascular surgery, the underlying cardiac pathology, procedure, and duration of cardiopulmonary bypass or aortic cross-clamp are all factors that may increase the risk for AKI. For transplant recipients, risk factors include the duration of the surgery and the amount of blood lost. Organ function and use of calcineurin inhibitors (e.g., tacrolimus and cyclosporine) may also contribute.

The risk of AKI associated with contrast media persists, particularly in patients with preexisting dehydration or renal compromise, and in those who receive a relatively large dose of contrast. Other drugs most commonly associated with nephrotoxicity include NSAIDs, ACE inhibitors, angiotensin-receptor blockers, aminoglycosides, vancomycin, amphotericin B, intravenous (IV) immunoglobulin, acyclovir, and immunosuppressive calcineurin inhibitors.

Tumor lysis syndrome can also precipitate AKI, especially in children with lymphoma (who may develop it before beginning therapy) (**Chapter 17**). Baseline risks, acute clinical conditions, and diagnostic/therapeutic agents associated with the development of in-hospital AKI are shown in **Table 18-2**. New biomarkers – such as neutrophil gelatinase-associated lipocalin, kidney injury molecule-1, or cystatin C, among others – are being evaluated for use in the early diagnosis of AKI.

### Table 18-2  Risk Factors for Acute Kidney Injury

| Baseline Risks | Acute Clinical Conditions | Nephrotoxic Agents |
| --- | --- | --- |
| Chronic kidney disease | Sepsis | Antimicrobial agents |
| Heart failure | Hypotension | Chemotherapeutic drugs |
| Congenital heart disease | Hypovolemia | Immunosuppressive agents |
| Liver failure | Rhabdomyolysis | Nonsteroidal anti-inflammatory drugs |
| Hypoalbuminemia | Nonrenal solid organ transplantation | Contrast media |
|  | Abdominal compartment syndrome |  |
|  | Mechanical ventilation |  |

Adapted with permission. © 2005 Wolters Kluwer Health. Leblanc M, Kellum J, Gibney N, et al. Risk factors for acute renal failure: inherent and modifiable risks. *Curr Opin Crit Care*. 2005;11:533-536.

# B. Classification of Acute Kidney Injury

AKI is typically classified into three broad categories: prerenal azotemia, intrinsic AKI, and post-renal or obstructive AKI. These categories can assist healthcare providers in narrowing the differential diagnosis and allowing for more targeted therapeutic intervention.

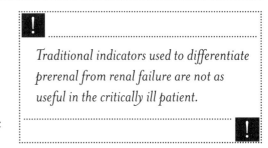

*Traditional indicators used to differentiate prerenal from renal failure are not as useful in the critically ill patient.*

An accurate history provides data on underlying chronic illness, as well as the temporal relationship between acute inciting events and the onset of AKI. The physical exam can give clues regarding underlying systemic diseases involving the kidney. Although urinary output changes can be present in most types of AKI, this readily available information is valuable because the treatment of nonoliguric renal failure is quite different from that of oligoanuric failure. Initial laboratory studies should include the following: serum electrolytes, including phosphorus, magnesium, and ionized calcium; blood urea nitrogen (BUN); SCr; and complete blood cell count. Urine studies should include urinalysis, specific gravity, sediment analysis, electrolytes, creatinine, protein, and osmolality. Many of these laboratory values can be utilized to calculate other indices for the classification of AKI; these indices are straightforward to calculate and are readily available at the bedside.

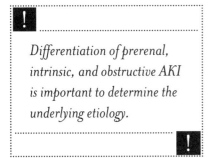

*Differentiation of prerenal, intrinsic, and obstructive AKI is important to determine the underlying etiology.*

The distinction between AKI from decreased renal perfusion (prerenal) and AKI related to intrinsic renal tubular dysfunction is important in determining the underlying etiology of AKI. Under conditions of hypoperfusion, the healthy kidney responds by increasing tubular reabsorption of both sodium and water through multiple mechanisms. One index that points to an appropriate renal response mechanism, and therefore intact tubular function, is an increase in the BUN/creatinine ratio, typically >20:1 in states of reduced renal perfusion. A similar index is the fractional excretion of sodium (FENa). When intrinsic renal function is intact, sodium reabsorption by the renal tubule increases, the urine sodium falls to <20 mEq/L, and the FENa is <1%, indicating the presence of prerenal AKI. In contrast, in acute tubular necrosis or intrinsic forms of AKI, the FENa is typically >3%. The calculation of the FENa requires simultaneous measurements of the serum sodium (SNa) and SCr, urine sodium (UNa), and urine creatinine (UCr) for use in the formula:

$$FENa\ (\%) = (UNa \times SCr) / (SNa \times UCr) \times 100$$

Extrinsic influences, such diuretic therapy, can also disrupt this normal physiologic response, affecting urinary sodium concentrations and decreasing the accuracy of the FENa as a marker for prerenal AKI. In such cases, the fractional excretion of urea (FEurea) can be used. Calculation of FEurea is the same as that for the FENa with the substitution of plasma (PUrea) and urine urea (Uurea) for plasma and urine Na.

$$FEurea\ (\%) = (Uurea \times SCr) / (PUrea \times UCr) \times 100$$

In prerenal AKI, the FEurea is typically <35% (**Table 18-3**).

### Table 18-3. Urinary Indices in Acute Kidney Injury

| AKI Classification | Urine Volume | BUN/Cr Ratio | Urine-specific Gravity | FENa | FEurea |
|---|---|---|---|---|---|
| Pre-renal AKI | ≤0.5 mL/kg/h | >20 | >1.020 | <1% | <35% |
| Intrinsic AKI | Variable | Variable | 1.010-1.020 | >3% | >35% |

AKI, acute kidney injury; BUN, blood urea nitrogen; Cr, creatinine; FENa, fractional excretion of sodium; FEurea, fractional excretion of urea

Urinalysis and microscopic evaluation of the urinary sediment can provide clues to the underlying etiology of AKI. Urinalysis in prerenal azotemia is often normal except for occasional fine granular and hyaline casts. Microscopic evaluation in intrinsic tubular injury, or acute tubular necrosis, shows epithelial cell casts and coarse granular casts. The presence of white blood cells and white blood cell casts is indicative of active inflammatory processes, such as glomerulonephritis, infection, or acute tubulointerstitial nephritis. Urine eosinophils are classically associated with the latter condition but can be seen in many other causes of AKI, such as glomerulonephritis and cystitis. Albuminuria and red blood cell casts indicate underlying glomerular disease. **Table 18-4** lists common causes of AKI according to this classification.

> *Prerenal failure is a high-risk condition that must be identified and corrected promptly to avoid structural damage to the kidney.*

# III. DIAGNOSIS

## A. Clinical Diagnosis

AKI may occur in some patients with clinical conditions leading to hypovolemia, such as dehydration, trauma, sepsis, or exposure to nephrotoxins. The presence of peripheral edema and hypervolemia (heart failure) is suggestive of renal injury. Cutaneous signs, such as petechiae or purpura, may suggest a diagnosis of HUS or vasculitis.

Anuria is indicative of a complete obstructive lesion, vascular lesion, rapidly progressive glomerulonephritis, or bilateral cortical necrosis. When seen with bladder distention, it is suggestive of an obstructive uropathy, although obstruction can cause AKI without causing anuria.

## Table 18-4  Common Acute Kidney Injury Etiologies

**Prerenal**

- Intravascular volume depletion
    - Gastrointestinal losses (diarrhea, emesis)
    - Trauma/hemorrhage/bleeding
    - Severe dehydration
    - Third-space losses (burns, trauma, capillary leak syndrome)
- Urinary losses (central or nephrogenic diabetes insipidus, osmotic diuresis, salt-wasting, diuretics)
- Decreased effective intravascular blood volume
    - Cardiac failure/congestive heart failure
    - Low cardiac output syndrome
    - Tamponade or pericarditis
- Abdominal compartment syndrome
- Drugs
    - Angiotensin-converting enzyme inhibitors, angiotensin II receptor blockers
    - Nonsteroidal anti-inflammatory drugs

**Intrinsic Acute Kidney Injury**

- Acute tubular necrosis
    - Ischemia/progressive prerenal AKI: sepsis or septic shock
    - Exogenous nephrotoxins:
        - Acyclovir
        - Aminoglycosides
        - Amphotericin B
        - Cisplatin
        - Calcineurin inhibitors
        - Foscarnet
        - Ifosfamide
        - Pentamidine
        - Radiocontrast agents
    - Endogenous nephrotoxins: rhabdomyolysis, hemolysis, tumor lysis syndrome
- Pyelonephritis/infection
- Hemolytic uremic syndrome
- Acute interstitial nephritis: drug induced or idiopathic
- Cancer infiltration
- Glomerulonephritis
    - Thrombotic microangiopathy
    - Pauci-immune
    - Systemic lupus erythematosus
    - Goodpasture syndrome
- Vascular injury: cortical bilateral necrosis, renal or arterial thrombosis

**Obstructive Acute Kidney Injury**

- Ureteral obstruction
    - Urinary catheter obstruction
    - Congenital anomalies
    - Posterior urethral valves
    - Ureteropelvic junction obstruction
- Surgical adhesions
- Nephrolithiasis
- Bladder obstruction: neurogenic bladder, tumor
- Bilateral urethral obstruction: tumor or mass

## B. Laboratory Diagnosis

The upper normal creatinine values vary with age. Both creatinine and BUN values can be higher or lower depending on the specific clinical conditions (**Figure 18-1**). Normal values for both are shown in **Appendix 1**. Other metabolic alterations seen in patients with AKI include:

- Metabolic acidosis with wide anion gap due to retention of sulfates, phosphates, and other anions
- Hyperkalemia
- Hyponatremia
- Hyperphosphatemia and hypocalcemia
- Hypermagnesemia

**Figure 18-1.** Clinical Situations That Influence Blood Urea Nitrogen and Creatinine Values

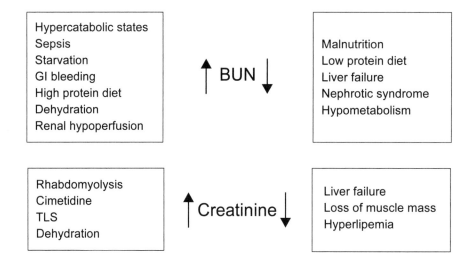

GI, gastrointestinal; TLS, tumor lysis syndrome; BUN, blood urea nitrogen

## C. Diagnostic Imaging

Radiologic imaging of the kidney is also important in the evaluation of a patient with AKI. Renal ultrasound, the most commonly used initial study, provides information on renal length and size, as well as detecting signs of obstruction (hydronephrosis, ureteral and bladder dilatation) and changes in bladder wall contour. Small atretic kidneys can suggest underlying chronic kidney disease. A Doppler ultrasound may be helpful to rule out renal vascular lesions. Scintirenography with technetium diethylenetriamine pentaacetic acid (TcDTPA) is useful for calculating the glomerular filtration rate of each kidney (**Table 18-5**). The initial phase reflects renal perfusion; activity measured after the first few minutes shows functional mass. TcDTPA is eliminated through the urine and may help evaluate the renal excretory system.

| Table 18-5 | Renal Imaging |

- US: size and shape of both kidneys
- Suspicion of urinary tract obstruction (hydronephrosis, renal calculi, bladder distension, and thickness)
- Suspicion of renal vessel occlusion
- Suspicion of chronic renal disease
- Suspicion of unilateral kidney absence
- Radionuclide scanning: TcDTPA (some GFR is required)
- Renal perfusion and renal mass function (glomerular filtration)
- Visualization of the urinary collecting system
- Visualization of small cortical lesions
- TcDMSA: visualization of renal structure (60-70% is retained within the renal cortex)
- Doppler US: assesses renal blood flow velocity patterns and absence or presence of diastolic flow

US, ultrasound; TcDTPA, technetium-labeled diethylenetriamine pentaacetic acid; GFR, glomerular filtration rate; TcDMSA, technetium-labeled dimercaptosuccinic acid

# IV. PREVENTION AND TREATMENT

*The objectives of AKI management in children are to maintain fluid, electrolyte, and metabolic homeostasis; prevent progression of the renal disease; treat the underlying cause of AKI; and provide adequate nutritional support.*

No specific therapy has been shown to effectively treat AKI. Existing interventions are directed at the prevention of AKI and supportive therapies for the related fluid, electrolyte, and hemodynamic abnormalities.

## A. Fluid Volume Management

Strict monitoring of input and output is mandatory for all patients with AKI. Indwelling urinary catheters (i.e., Foley catheters) are not necessary in stable patients and should be avoided to reduce the risk of infection. Urinary catheters are indicated in young children with gastroenteritis and suspected oliguria or anuria. Daily or twice-daily weight measurements should be obtained in all patients.

Maintaining renal perfusion through hemodynamic support is critically important in preventing the onset and progression of AKI. This can be achieved through adequate hydration and the use of vasoactive medications. For euvolemic patients, fluids should be calculated to replace insensible water losses and ongoing losses. Recent data support the concept of early goal-directed fluid resuscitation followed by late conservative fluid management to limit fluid overload. Study results suggest an association between cumulative fluid balance volume and mortality in critically ill patients, highlighting the importance of close monitoring of fluid balance and early intervention in managing critically ill children with AKI.

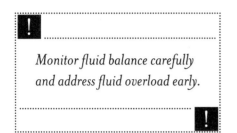

*Monitor fluid balance carefully and address fluid overload early.*

One proposed method for assessing the degree of fluid overload is by examining fluid balance during admission in relation to the child's estimated dry weight through the formula:

$$([\text{Fluid intake in liters}] - [\text{Fluid output in liters}] / \text{Admission weight in kg}) \times 100\%$$

Other potential therapies directed at maintenance of renal perfusion include low-dose dopamine (1-3 µg/kg/min) and fenoldopam, a pure dopamine agonist with effects on the renal vasculature similar to those of dopamine but with less systemic α- and β-adrenergic effects. While some evidence suggests that fenoldopam can reduce AKI risk in specific populations, no data from randomized controlled studies support this. Similarly, no definitive evidence supports a clear benefit for the use of dopamine in patients with AKI. Although low-dose dopamine does not prevent or ameliorate AKI, it may enhance urine volume. Data on the use of diuretics in AKI are either unavailable or have not shown a definite benefit. In addition, none of the drugs are without potential adverse side effects; therefore, any use in specific clinical situations needs close monitoring and discontinuation if the desired response is not achieved and/or adverse effects appear.

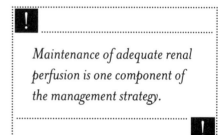

*Maintenance of adequate renal perfusion is one component of the management strategy.*

## B. Avoidance of Nephrotoxicity

The list of pharmacologic agents that are potentially injurious to the kidney is extensive. Some of the most commonly seen nephrotoxins are aminoglycoside antibiotics, antifungal medications, NSAIDS, chemotherapeutics, and radiocontrast dyes (**Table 18-3**). Avoidance of these agents whenever possible is one key to preventing AKI. When use is unavoidable, frequent monitoring is needed, with dosage adjusted based on estimation of kidney function. A quick bedside estimation of GFR can be obtained using the Schwartz formula:

$$\text{GFR} = k \times \text{Height (cm)} / \text{SCr}$$

with *k* values determined by age: infant = 0.45; 1-13 years and adolescent girls = 0.55; adolescent boys = 0.7.

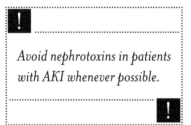

*Avoid nephrotoxins in patients with AKI whenever possible.*

This formula is only an estimate of GFR and tends to overestimate true renal function in many clinical situations. An accurate estimate of GFR can only be obtained when SCr is at a steady state. Therefore, with a rising SCr, a dose should be adjusted to the value for the lowest range of kidney function for that agent.

## C. Electrolyte Management

As noted previously, a hallmark of AKI is the inability to maintain electrolyte homeostasis. Common electrolyte derangements include hyperkalemia, metabolic acidosis, hyperphosphatemia, hypocalcemia, and hypermagnesemia. Treatment measures to address these electrolyte issues are summarized here; please refer to **Chapter 8** for a more in-depth discussion.

**1. Hyperkalemia**

Hyperkalemia, a frequent finding in AKI, is possible with normal intake and metabolism if the kidneys have failed and cannot excrete a normal amount of potassium ($K^+$), or when an excessive load of potassium is present. It can occur essentially without symptoms. The first indication may be a fatal cardiac arrest secondary to cardiac conduction abnormalities.

Inadequate potassium excretion may result from a failure of glomerular filtration or tubular secretion, or both. Some drugs or toxins can produce nonoliguric renal failure. The continuing urine output may mask the progressive uremia and hyperkalemia. In other patients, the lysis of tumor cells, red cells, or muscle cells releases intracellular potassium into the plasma, frequently when kidney function has been compromised by the underlying process. Rapid recognition and aggressive management may be required to prevent hemodynamic collapse or death.

When AKI is suspected or established, prevention and management of hyperkalemia becomes the highest renal priority. A patient with known risk factors for hyperkalemia should be managed presumptively. Potassium intake should be discontinued in both intravenous and enteral forms, in conjunction with continuous electrocardiography (ECG) monitoring. In most situations, undertreatment is more life-threatening than overtreatment.

### a. Mild Hyperkalemia

Potassium levels between 5.1 and 6.0 mEq/L reflect a mild hyperkalemia. A patient without an excessive potassium load and with ongoing urine output may often be managed by stopping potassium intake and administering IV fluids with or without a loop diuretic. Serial monitoring of serum potassium and continuous ECG monitoring are obligatory.

### b. Moderate Hyperkalemia

Potassium levels of 6.1 to 7.0 mEq/L define moderate hyperkalemia. Its management, without ECG changes, includes that of mild hyperkalemia plus consideration of rectal, oral, or nasogastric administration of sodium polystyrene sulfonate and preparation for additional interventions. These might include a glucose and insulin drip and dialysis. Excellent IV access and the bedside availability of IV calcium, albuterol, and bicarbonate are appropriate.

- Calcium gluconate: 100 mg/kg dose IV over 5 minutes
- Sodium bicarbonate: 1 to 2 mEq/kg IV over 5 to 10 minutes
- Insulin: 0.1 U/kg/h concurrently with dextrose 25% 2 mL/kg/h to prevent hypoglycemia
- Sodium polystyrene sulfonate: 1g/kg rectally or orally
- Beta-agonist nebulized solution

### c. Severe Hyperkalemia

As potassium levels increase above 7 mEq/L, the ECG changes and cardiac function are affected. P waves flatten, the PR interval increases, T waves become symmetrically peaked, and the QRS complex widens and approaches a sine wave. When ECG changes are present, cardiac arrest may occur at any moment. This disturbance of cardiac transmembrane potential is corrected most rapidly by administration of calcium, starting with an emergency resuscitation dose administered over 1 to 3 minutes, with continuous ECG observation. Albuterol nebulization may be

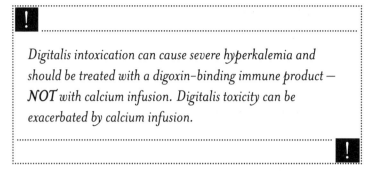

*Digitalis intoxication can cause severe hyperkalemia and should be treated with a digoxin-binding immune product — NOT with calcium infusion. Digitalis toxicity can be exacerbated by calcium infusion.*

started simultaneously as the beta-agonist will also drive potassium into the cell, but this is the least effective intervention. The action of calcium is transient and repeated dosing may be necessary while other measures are employed. A glucose and insulin infusion acts relatively rapidly and may be helpful to stabilize the patient while potassium removal via sodium polystyrene sulfonate or dialysis is arranged. Emergent peritoneal dialysis can be approximated by peritoneal lavage with 10 to 12 mL/kg of warmed, D5W-normal saline infused and drained over 15-minute cycles, when hemodialysis is not available. Ultrasound-guided placement of a pigtail pleural drainage catheter can provide access for peritoneal lavage. If peritoneal dialysate is available, 1.5% or 2.5 % solution would generally be good choices.

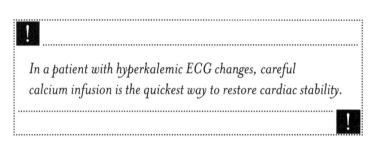

*In a patient with hyperkalemic ECG changes, careful calcium infusion is the quickest way to restore cardiac stability.*

The healthcare provider should be aware that the serum potassium level causing life-threatening cardiac changes will vary among individual patients.

### 2. Metabolic Acidosis

Metabolic acidosis is secondary to an inadequate excretion of hydrogen ions and ammonia. Severe acidosis can increase myocardial irritability and affect peripheral vascular resistance, enzyme activity, and energy production. Treatment of acidosis should be aimed at improving its causes, which include poor cardiac output, exogenous acid administration (e.g., hyperchloremia secondary to sodium chloride administration), and respiratory acidosis. Mild to moderate metabolic acidosis with a pH >7.20 can be treated with oral bicarbonate supplements. Severe metabolic acidosis with pH <7.20 or metabolic acidosis in the presence of hyperkalemia should be corrected intravenously. Correcting a low pH in renal failure risks decreasing ionized calcium, a critical problem, particularly if the calcium is already low due to phosphate retention. If given, IV sodium bicarbonate should be administered slowly (in 1 mEq/kg doses) while monitoring sodium and ionized calcium.

*In the presence of hypocalcemia with hyperphosphatemia, management should be aimed at reducing the phosphorus rather than increasing the calcium levels.*

3. **Hyperphosphatemia**
    - Phosphorus intake should be limited.
    - Phosphorus-binding calcium salts may be utilized.

4. **Hypocalcemia**
    - Correct only in symptomatic patients.
    - Administer calcium gluconate, 100 mg/kg IV, or calcium chloride 10%, 10 mg/kg IV per dose.

5. **Hyponatremia**
    - Calculation of sodium deficit: 0.6 x weight (kg) x (target sodium – measured sodium)
    - Careful sodium correction may be necessary for patients with central nervous system symptoms, although causes other than AKI should be investigated (**Chapter 8**).
    - Fluid restriction

## D. Renal Replacement Therapy

When the fluid and electrolyte abnormalities discussed cannot be corrected with medical management, the patient with AKI will require some form of renal replacement therapy. Additional indications for renal replacement therapies are included in **Table 18-6**. Several modes of dialysis or renal therapies are available.

**Table 18-6** Additional Indications for Renal Replacement Therapies

**Fluid Overload**
- Pulmonary edema
- Congestive heart failure
- Persistent anuria or oliguria with obligatory intake of nutrition or medication
- Refractory hypertension
- Critically ill patient with oliguria and high fluid requirements (e.g., parenteral nutrition, antibiotics, sedation, inotropes)
- Critically ill patient with oliguria needing negative fluid balance

**Electrolyte Or Acid-Base Disorders**
- Severe hyponatremia or hypernatremia
- Hyperkalemia with potassium >7 mEq/L
- Persistent, severe acidosis

**Toxin Removal**
- Urea
- Uric acid
- Exogenous dialyzable toxins

Peritoneal dialysis is a modality in which a catheter is inserted percutaneously or, preferably, surgically into the abdominal cavity, utilizing the peritoneal membrane as a dialysis filter. Solute clearance occurs mainly via diffusion due to concentration differences across the peritoneal membrane between the vascular space and the infused dialysis solution. Similarly, fluid removal is driven by an osmotic gradient created by dextrose contained in the infused dialysate. Peritoneal dialysis does not require central venous access or anticoagulation and can be performed continuously if needed for slower correction of electrolyte derangements and slower fluid removal. Peritoneal dialysis can be limited by prior abdominal surgeries and congenital abdominal wall anomalies and is less well suited for removal of ingested toxins.

The general term *hemodialysis* describes a modality in which an external pump moves a patient's blood through an extracorporeal circuit and across an artificial membrane, allowing for both fluid removal and the correction of metabolic derangements. Hemodialysis can be performed either as intermittent hemodialysis (IHD) or as continuous renal replacement therapy (CRRT).

In IHD, the patient receives therapy during a prescribed period of hours and then is off therapy until the next session. The finite period on IHD requires that solute and fluid removal occur fairly rapidly; therefore, it is more suited to the hemodynamically stable patient who can tolerate rapid changes in volume status. Some benefits of IHD include its efficiency in correcting inborn metabolic abnormalities and toxic ingestions. It also allows patient mobilization for necessary diagnostic testing and conditioning therapies, such as physical therapy.

For those patients with hemodynamic instability or large volumes of fluid overload, fluid removal and solute correction at a slower rate is more appropriate, and CRRT may be a better choice for dialysis. CRRT takes place continuously, 24 hours a day, so that regulation of fluid balance is slower and can be adjusted as needed throughout the treatment based on dynamic changes in the patient's clinical status, such as hypotension or when additional fluids are needed. This feature of CRRT may be ideally suited for critically ill patients in whom hemodynamic instability and frequent changes in fluid input rate are more likely. In addition, anticoagulation is typically required for the CRRT circuit. Although no direct comparison of IHD and CRRT has shown CRRT to be superior in clinical outcomes, the advantages often make it the treatment of choice in the critically ill.

Achieving good vascular access is a key step in the provision of either IHD or CRRT. The preferred site for central venous catheter placement is the internal jugular vein, followed by the femoral vein. The largest lumen catheter that can be safely placed will allow attainment of prescribed blood flows and decrease the risk of clotting. Maintaining vascular access in patients requiring dialysis is a matter of life-saving importance.

The pharmacokinetics of drug clearance on dialysis can be variable, requiring vigilant monitoring of drug levels and adjustment of dosing based on clinical response. Consultation with the intensive care unit pharmacist can be extremely helpful in managing dosing adjustments.

## E. Nutritional Support

Children with AKI have an increased rate of catabolism and are at risk of malnutrition. Adequate nutrition is essential for the treatment of AKI, but providing sufficient nutrition may be difficult because of fluid restrictions.

Concentrated enteral or parenteral nutrition should be used. The enteral route is always preferred when available. Lipids and concentrated glucose solutions improve caloric concentration. Essential amino acids can be used to decrease urea production. Initial protein intake should be limited to 0.5 to 1 g/kg/day. In some situations, dialysis techniques may be used to increase the amount of fluid that can be administered and to decrease nutritional limitations.

## F. Management of Hypertension

Hypertension is often secondary to volume overload in patients with oliguria. Dialysis is indicated in hypervolemic, hypertensive patients failing to respond to antihypertensives, fluid restriction, and diuretics. Those with severe hypertension and encephalopathy or cardiomyopathy should be treated aggressively (**Table 18-7**). Less severe conditions can be treated with nifedipine, 0.25 to 0.5 mg/kg up to 10 mg per dose. Doses of antihypertensive agents may need to be adjusted to the GFR.

### Table 18-7  Medications in Hypertensive Emergencies

| Medication | Loading Dose | Maintenance | Maximum Dose | Route |
| --- | --- | --- | --- | --- |
| Labetalol | 0.2-1 mg/kg (max 20 mg) | 0.4-1 mg/kg/h | 3 mg/kg/h | IV |
| Nicardipine | None | 0.5-5 µg/kg/h | 5 µg/kg/h | IV |
| Nitroprusside sodium (monitor thiocyanate levels) | None | 0.3 µg/kg/min | 10 µg/kg/min | IV |
| Hydralazine | 0.2 mg/kg | 5-20 mg every 4 h | 20 mg | IV |

IV, intravenous

## V. LONG-TERM OUTCOMES

Some children surviving AKI may have increased risk of long-term changes in kidney function, microalbuminuria, and hypertension. In a study following patients 3 to 5 years after AKI, nearly 60% persisted in some degree of underlying renal dysfunction. These data may indicate a significant comorbidity for children surviving AKI, emphasizing the need for methods of early diagnosis, prevention, and treatment. The complexity of managing multiple metabolic disturbances, as well as perhaps uncovering a subtle, underlying diagnosis, requires that consideration is given early to providing nephrology expertise and resources. Medical transport (**Chapter 14**) to a pediatric center may be necessary to give these children the best chance of quality survival.

Finally, **Table 18-8** is offered as a starting point for construction of an AKI algorithm that may be useful in evaluating and stabilizing a patient with signs and symptoms associated with AKI.

### Table 18-8. Acute Kidney Injury Management Strategies Algorithm

1. Evaluate airway, breathing, and circulation and stabilize
2. Determine if patient is hyperkalemic or at risk of hyperkalemia
3. Obtain a 12-lead ECG
4. Obtain laboratory studies:
   a. Creatinine
   b. Hemoglobin
   c. Ionized calcium
   d. Magnesium
   e. Sodium
   f. Potassium
   g. Phosphorus
   h. Serum carbon dioxide
5. Ensure exclusion of further potassium intake enterally or intravenously

**AKF Secondary Checklist**

1. Review CC, HPI, ROS
2. Consider potential etiologies of AKI:
   a. Hypoxic-ischemic event? Trauma, septic shock
   b. Cardiac event of congestive heart failure
   c. Severe dehydration
   d. Gross hematuria
   e. Hypertension
   f. Infection: streptococcal throat or impetigo
   g. Edema
   h. Anemia, thrombocytopenia
   i. GI symptoms
   j. Prolonged use of NSAIDs
   k. Radiographic contrast, other nephrotoxins
   l. Lymphoid malignancy
   m. Acute respiratory failure + hemoptysis
   n. Intra-abdominal hypertension

ECG, electrocardiography; AKF, acute kidney failure; AKI, acute kidney injury; CC, chief complaint; HPI, history of present illness; ROS, review of systems; GI, gastrointestinal; NSAIDs, nonsteroidal anti-inflammatory drugs

## Key Points

## Acute Kidney Injury

- AKI occurs commonly in critically ill children and significantly increases morbidity and mortality.

- Sepsis and nephrotoxic medications are common causes of AKI.

- Traditional indicators used to differentiate prerenal from renal failure may support the diagnosis of AKI during the initial phase, before the patient has received diuretics or vasoactive drugs. They are usually not useful in the critically ill child who needs multiple pharmacologic therapies.

- Metabolic acidosis, hyperkalemia, and hypocalcemia are metabolic conditions frequently found in patients with AKI.

- Preventive strategies to avoid primary or secondary renal injury consist mainly of ensuring adequate renal blood flow and avoiding nephrotoxicity.

- Patients should be monitored for signs of fluid overload. Strict fluid balance and daily weight records are essential.

- Broad indications for renal replacement therapies include fluid overload, electrolyte or acid-base disorders, and toxin removal unresponsive to medical therapies.

- Choice of renal replacement therapy should consider overall clinical status and the goals of the therapy.

- Diligence in drug dosing is required in AKI and dialysis.

- An ideal nutrition plan for AKI patients should offer adequate caloric intake with fluid restriction, limit protein intake, and reduce or eliminate potassium intake.

- AKI can have long-term sequelae.

## Suggested Readings

1. Akcan-Arikan A, Zappitelli M, Loftis LL, Washburn KK, Jefferson LS, Goldstein SL. Modified RIFLE criteria in critically ill children with acute kidney injury. *Kidney Int.* 2007;71:1028-1035.

2. Bagshaw SM, Berthiaume LR, Delaney A, Bellomo R. Continuous versus intermittent renal replacement therapy for critically ill patients with acute kidney injury: a meta-analysis. *Crit Care Med.* 2008;36:610-617.

3. Bailey D, Phan V, Litalien C, et al. Risk factors of acute renal failure in critically ill children: a prospective descriptive epidemiological study. *Pediatr Crit Care Med.* 2007;8:29-35.

4. Barozzi L, Valentino M, Santoro A, Mancini E, Pavlica P. Renal ultrasonography in critically ill patients. *Crit Care Med.* 2007;35(5 Suppl):S198-S205.

5. Bellomo R, Ronco C, Kellum JA, Mehta RL, Palevsky P, Acute Dialysis Quality Initiative Workgroup. Acute renal failure - definition, outcome measures, animal models, fluid therapy and information technology needs: the Second International Consensus Conference of the Acute Dialysis Quality Initiative (ADQI) Group. *Crit Care.* 2004;8:R204-212.

6. Bellomo R, Wan L, May C. Vasoactive drugs and acute kidney injury. *Crit Care Med.* 2008;36 (4 Suppl):S179-S186.

7. Boyd JH, Forbes J, Nakada TA, Walley KR, Russell JA. Fluid resuscitation in septic shock: a positive fluid balance and elevated central venous pressure are associated with increased mortality. *Crit Care Med.* 2011;39:259-265.

8. Chertow GM, Burdick E, Honour M, Bonventre JV, Bates DW. Acute kidney injury, mortality, length of stay, and costs in hospitalized patients. *J Am Soc Nephrol.* 2005;16:3365-3370.

9. Durkan AM, Alexander RT. Acute kidney injury post neonatal asphyxia. *J Pediatr.* 2011;158 (2 Suppl):e29-e33.

10. Flynn JT. Choice of dialysis modality for management of pediatric acute renal failure. *Pediatric Nephrol.* 2002;17:61-69.

11. Foland JA, Fortenberry JD, Warshaw BL, et al. Fluid overload before continuous hemofiltration and survival in critically ill children: a retrospective analysis. *Crit Care Med.* 2004;32:1771-1776.

12. Gotfried J, Wiesen J, Raina R, Nally JV Jr. Finding the cause of acute kidney injury: which index of fractional excretion is better? *Cleve Clin J Med.* 2012;79:121-126.

13. Hoste EA, Clermont G, Kersten A, et al. RIFLE criteria for acute kidney injury are associated with hospital mortality in critically ill patients: a cohort analysis. *Crit Care.* 2006;10:R73.

14. Hui-Stickle S, Brewer ED, Goldstein SL. Pediatric ARF epidemiology at a tertiary care center from 1999 to 2001. *Am J Kidney Dis.* 2005;45:96-101.

15. Kellum JA, Angus DC, Johnson JP, et al. Continuous versus intermittent renal replacement therapy: a meta-analysis. *Intensive Care Med.* 2002;28:29-37.

16. Kellum JA, Levin N, Bouman C, Lameire N. Developing a consensus classification system for acute renal failure. *Curr Opin Crit Care.* 2002;8:509-514.

17. Lassnigg A, Donner E, Grubhofer G, Presterl E, Druml W, Hiesmayr M. Lack of renoprotective effects of dopamine and furosemide during cardiac surgery. *J Am Soc Nephrol.* 2000;11:97-104.

18. Mehta RL, Pascual MT, Soroko S, Chertow GM, PICARD Study Group. Diuretics, mortality, and nonrecovery of renal function in acute renal failure. *JAMA.* 2002;288:2547-2553.

19. Michael M, Kuehnle I, Goldstein SL. Fluid overload and acute renal failure in pediatric stem cell transplant patients. *Pediatr Nephrol.* 2004;19:91-95.

20. Murphy CV, Schramm GE, Doherty JA, et al. The importance of fluid management in acute lung injury secondary to septic shock. *Chest.* 2009;136:102-109.

21. Skippen PW, Krahn GE. Acute renal failure in children undergoing cardiopulmonary bypass. *Criti Care Resusc.* 2005;7:286-291.

22. Tumlin JA, Finkel KW, Murray PT, Samuels J, Cotsonis G, Shaw AD. Fenoldopam mesylate in early acute tubular necrosis: a randomized, double-blind, placebo-controlled clinical trial. *Am J Kidney Dis.* 2005;46:26-34.

23. Uchino S, Kellum JA, Bellomo R, et al. Acute renal failure in critically ill patients: a multinational, multicenter study. *JAMA.* 2005;294:813-818.

24. Varghese SA, Powell TB, Janech MG, et al. Identification of diagnostic urinary biomarkers for acute kidney injury. *J Investig Med.* 2010;58:612-620.

Chapter 19

# Postoperative Management

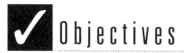

- Discuss anesthetic factors and their relation to the postoperative period.
- Recognize and manage common potential postoperative complications.
- Describe a multimodal approach to postoperative pain management.
- Summarize the management of fluid, electrolyte, and nutritional support.
- Review the management of postoperative nausea and vomiting.
- Discuss thermal regulation and evaluation of postoperative fever.

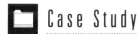

A 4-year-old girl is admitted with fever, tachycardia, and significant physical finding of an acute abdomen. She has a history of well-controlled asthma for which she uses a beclomethasone metered-dose inhaler. She undergoes an exploratory laparotomy with surgical findings consistent with ruptured acute appendicitis and intra-abdominal abscess. Soon after arrival to the ward, she has a heart rate of 160 beats/min, respiratory rate 25 breaths/min, blood pressure 130/80 mm Hg, and a temperature of 103.1°F (39.5°C). She is agitated with inspiratory stridor, and you have been called to the bedside to assist in her management. She is given intravenous (IV) morphine sulfate, 0.1 mg/kg, before your arrival.

**Detection**
- What would you want to know about her preoperative and intraoperative course?
- What is the most likely etiology of her stridor?
- What are the possible reasons the patient appears agitated?

**Intervention**
- What is the treatment strategy for stridor?
- What would be the best approach to her pain management?
- How would you manage her fluid hydration in the first 24 hours postoperatively?

**Reassessment**
- How would you assess the effectiveness of the patient's pain management?

- What are the potential fluid and electrolyte complications you might expect to encounter?
- What are the potential causes of continued postoperative fever?

**Effective Communication**
- What should be communicated in the handoff between the operating room team and the ward assuming care for the patient?

**Teamwork**
- Who else might need to be involved in the care of the patient?
- What are the roles of other healthcare providers in the postoperative management of this patient?

# I. INTRODUCTION

The patient's preoperative clinical condition and management, along with the intraoperative course, determines the postoperative physiologic status and disposition. Key concepts include fluid and electrolyte therapy, pediatric analgesia, and cardiopulmonary evaluation and management. This chapter attempts to integrate these concepts and relate them specifically to the postoperative management of the pediatric patient.

# II. PREOPERATIVE AND ANESTHETIC CONSIDERATIONS

With the advent of modern anesthetic techniques and specialty training in pediatric anesthesiology, anesthetic-related mortality in children is uncommon and estimated at 1 in 185,000 patients. The risk of anesthesia-related cardiac arrest increases in infants who are younger than 1 year and patients with severe underlying disease. Most deaths occur in sick children undergoing emergency surgery. Preoperative severity of illness remains a significant risk factor. The American Society of Anesthesiologists (ASA) developed the physical status classification to estimate severity of illness prior to administration of sedation or anesthesia (**Chapter 20**). The ASA system does not predict risk but allows the anesthesiologist to tailor the anesthetic to the patient's underlying condition. Therefore, the higher the ASA class, the greater the likelihood that the patient will have a complicated postoperative course and require intensive management and monitoring.

The preoperative history is essential for identifying patients with underlying conditions placing them at potential risk for intraoperative, as well as postoperative complications. This history is an essential part of the hand-off communication that should take place between the operating room staff and the intensive care unit or ward team assuming care for the patient. It should include prior medications, allergies, chronic medical conditions (e.g., asthma, epilepsy), and reactions to any anesthetic agents or procedures. Pertinent information about the intraoperative course should be relayed to the medical team providing postoperative care. This would include: (1) procedure performed; (2) anesthetic agents used; (3) type and dose of opioids administered; (4) estimated blood loss and transfusions administered; (5) fluids administered; (6) difficulty in airway and ventilatory management; (7) operative findings; (8) any complications; and (9) presence of tubes, lines, and drains.

# III. RESPIRATORY CONSIDERATIONS

## A. Postoperative Apnea

Postoperative apnea is defined as the cessation of respirations for 15 seconds or more or the cessation of breathing for less than 15 seconds when associated with bradycardia. Premature infants are at increased risk for apnea (central and obstructive) within the first 48 hours after anesthesia. It will usually present in the first 2 to 12 hours postoperatively. This may be due to immaturity of the respiratory center in the brainstem and easy fatigability of the neonatal diaphragm because of low musculature development. In neonates, apnea is a stress response and may be associated with inadequate anesthesia and analgesia.

Premature and full-term infants younger than 44 weeks post-conceptual age are at risk for apnea. The age at which this risk disappears continues to be controversial. Anesthesia should be avoided in the full-term infant younger than 44 weeks postconceptual age, unless emergent surgery is required. Full-term infants younger than 1 month and premature infants younger than 60 weeks postconceptual age should be considered at risk for apnea after general anesthesia and require inpatient monitoring and observation for 24 hours after surgery.

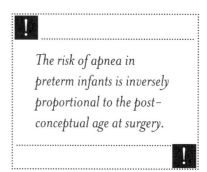

*The risk of apnea in preterm infants is inversely proportional to the post-conceptual age at surgery.*

Anemia is an independent risk factor that increases the chances of postoperative apnea in the neonatal population. It is recommended that infants with a hemoglobin level <10 g/dL should have their elective surgery postponed and be given oral iron supplements until the hemoglobin is >10 g/dL. If surgery cannot be delayed, these patients will require postoperative inpatient observation and monitoring. Children with a known history of obstructive sleep apnea and infants being treated for apnea of prematurity should also be observed for 24 hours postoperatively.

## B. Respiratory Depression

Respiratory depression in the immediate postoperative period is usually caused by opioids, sedatives, residual anesthetic effect, or inadequate neuromuscular blockade reversal. Severe chest or abdominal pain may also cause respiratory splinting with resultant hypoventilation and delay in the elimination of any inhaled anesthetic agents. If an excessive opioid or benzodiazepine effect is suspected, gradual reversal is warranted with naloxone and flumazenil, respectively. The half-life these agents is relatively short compared with most opiates and benzodiazepines, and the patient should be monitored for recurrence of respiratory depression.

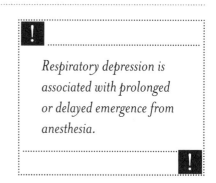

*Respiratory depression is associated with prolonged or delayed emergence from anesthesia.*

## C. Upper Airway Obstruction

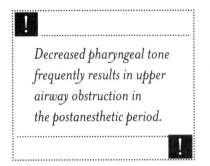

*Decreased pharyngeal tone frequently results in upper airway obstruction in the postanesthetic period.*

Upper airway obstruction is frequently encountered while the child is still somewhat sedated after anesthesia. Protective reflexes are intact, but pharyngeal hypotonia with posterior displacement of the tongue may occur.

This results in airway obstruction with the patient exhibiting paradoxical respiration or seesaw-type breathing (the chest caves in while the abdomen rises). If this respiratory pattern is seen, it should be quickly recognized that the patient has ineffective ventilation. The lack of misting inside an oxygen mask should provide a high level of suspicion that the airway is obstructed. An inability to feel the exhaled breath will confirm the diagnosis. Usually, providing chin lift or jaw thrust and careful suctioning will arouse the patient and open the airway. The use of nasal or oral airway adjuncts may be necessary. In all these situations, the patient must be monitored and the healthcare provider should be prepared to provide a definitive airway and support oxygenation and ventilation (**Chapter 2**).

Postextubation stridor occurs in about 2% of all postoperative pediatric patients. Etiologies include the following: subglottic edema arising from the use of oversized endotracheal tubes, traumatic or repeated attempts at intubation, coughing or bucking with the endotracheal tube in place, or a change in positioning of the endotracheal tube.

*Post-extubation stridor is most often seen in children aged 3 months to 4 years.*

The use of appropriately sized endotracheal tubes with a leak below 30 cm $H_2O$ decreases the risk of airway trauma. If the patient has evidence of significant stridor and increased work of breathing, nebulized racemic epinephrine/adrenaline (0.25-0.5 mL of 2.25% solution in 2-3 mL of normal saline solution) should be administered. The patient will require observation in a monitored environment because of potential rebound edema. Corticosteroids (dexamethasone 0.5 mg/kg intravenously or intramuscularly, maximum dose 12 mg) should be administered for persistent stridor and signs of upper airway obstruction. Patients who do not respond to these interventions and demonstrate marked increased work of breathing, altered sensorium, desaturations, and ineffective gas exchange should be reintubated. When attempting reintubation in this scenario, use an endotracheal tube that is at least a half size smaller in diameter compared to the tube used in anesthesia.

Other reasons for upper airway obstruction may include: laryngomalacia; soft tissue swelling of oropharyngeal structures (e.g., tongue); laryngospasm; uncontrollable bleeding from the nasopharynx, oropharynx, or hypopharynx; or posterior pharyngeal narrowing after cleft palate repair. Usually, these patients will improve with upright positioning, adequate analgesia, suctioning and clearing of secretions, and control of any active bleeding. Intubate when in doubt or if the patient's clinical condition is not improving with these interventions.

## D. Lower Airway Disease

Atelectasis, the most common postoperative respiratory complication, usually occurs in the first 48 hours postoperatively. Alveolar collapse is a result of inhaled anesthetics, high inspired oxygen concentration, and hypoventilation secondary to pain or postoperative narcotics. This leads to retained secretions, which can result in secondary bacterial pneumonia if not expectorated. Deep breathing, coughing, and clearing of secretions can often be accomplished with the aid of incentive spirometry in older children (older than 6 years) or by encouraging younger children to blow bubbles or a pinwheel. This is often effective in the prevention of atelectasis and provision of effective pulmonary toilet.

Hospital-acquired pneumonia is the second most common nosocomial infection and is predominantly seen in ventilated, postoperative, and critically ill patients (**Chapter 7**). The etiology of hospital-acquired pneumonia is microaspiration of bacteria colonizing the oropharynx or gastrointestinal tract. Pneumonia occurs after 48 hours in the postoperative patient who does not have an antecedent infection. The main preventive interventions are elevating the head of the bed 30° to 45° (if no contraindications), early ambulation, and encouraging pulmonary toilet.

## E. Pulmonary Edema

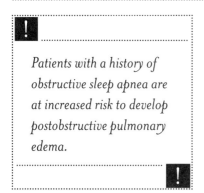

*Patients with a history of obstructive sleep apnea are at increased risk to develop postobstructive pulmonary edema.*

Pulmonary edema is usually rare, unless the patient is known to have congestive heart failure or received an excessive amount of IV fluids intraoperatively. Postobstructive pulmonary edema (previously known as *negative pressure pulmonary edema*) occurs after the acute relief of chronic severe upper airway obstruction or after postextubation obstruction, such as laryngospasm, in which the patient was making forceful inspiratory efforts against a closed glottis. It may be seen in children following an adenotonsillectomy for obstructive sleep apnea.

Management of pulmonary edema is supportive, with mild cases requiring oxygen and possibly 1 dose of IV diuretic (furosemide 1 mg/kg IV). Patients in severe respiratory distress may be managed with noninvasive mechanical ventilation or require intubation and adequate positive end-expiratory pressure. Usually, pulmonary edema in these cases rapidly resolves with appropriate management.

# IV. HEMODYNAMIC CONSIDERATIONS

## A. Dysrhythmias

Children tend to be healthy, and abnormal electrocardiogram results and arrhythmias are uncommon postoperatively in the absence of an underlying cardiac pathology or electrolyte disturbance. Abnormalities of heart rate tend to be the most frequent dysrhythmias seen, and sinus tachycardia is the most common.

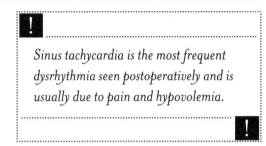

*Sinus tachycardia is the most frequent dysrhythmia seen postoperatively and is usually due to pain and hypovolemia.*

Sinus tachycardia rarely needs specific therapy, but its underlying etiology must be determined. Tachycardia may be an early indicator of compensated shock, with hypovolemia the most common cause in the postoperative patient. Physical examination may detect cool extremities, decreased urine output, and hypotension signaling decompensated shock. Fluid resuscitation should be promptly initiated. Other factors that may result in sinus tachycardia include emergence agitation, pain, anemia, anxiety, hyperthermia, hypercarbia, and the presence of parasympathomimetic agents, such as atropine and glycopyrrolate.

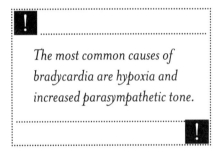

*The most common causes of bradycardia are hypoxia and increased parasympathetic tone.*

Bradycardia in infants requires immediate attention, because this age group depends on heart rate for cardiac output. The most life-threatening cause of bradycardia is hypoxia; thus, administering oxygen and providing assisted ventilation are paramount in the initial management. Tracheal suctioning, nasogastric tube insertion, or the application of ophthalmic pressure can result in increased parasympathetic tone, a common cause of bradycardia in this age group.

## B. Abnormal Blood Pressure

Hypertension in children rarely has a pathologic etiology and, like tachycardia, usually does not require specific therapy, but the underlying cause needs to be determined. Hypertension with associated tachycardia is usually due to increased agitation, anxiety, pain, or parasympathetic effect. When accompanied by normal or decreased heart rate, this may be a sign of hypothermia, increased intracranial pressure, or the effect of α-adrenergic therapy. In all these situations, antihypertensives are not indicated. Antihypertensive therapy is indicated in patients who are known to have chronic renal disease with preexisting hypertension.

Hypotension in the postoperative patient should be considered a medical emergency. This may be seen in the patient who is cold with vasoconstriction and has been rapidly rewarmed. However, the most common cause of hypotension is volume depletion. In all of these situations, volume therapy must be initiated as soon as possible. If the patient does not respond in the expected fashion, the patient may be in shock due to sepsis or cardiac dysfunction. In these situations, vasopressor and/or inotropic support needs to be considered, and the patient should be managed in a monitored setting.

# V. NEUROLOGIC CONSIDERATIONS

## A. Altered Consciousness

Altered consciousness poses a diagnostic dilemma for the anesthesiologist and the medical team managing the patient postoperatively. This is a common reason for unanticipated admission to the pediatric intensive care unit (PICU) from the recovery room. The causes for this can usually be directly traced to prolonged anesthetic effect along with other less common etiologies (**Table 19-1**).

### Table 19-1  Causes of Altered Consciousness in the Postoperative Period

- Prolonged anesthesia or delayed emergence due to residual anesthetic effect
- Prolonged neuromuscular blockade
- Hypothermia
- Metabolic and electrolyte imbalances
    - Hypoglycemia
    - Diabetic ketoacidosis
    - Hypokalemia → severe muscular weakness
    - Hypernatremia and hyponatremia
    - Hypothyroidism
- Hypercarbia secondary to hypoventilation
    - Narcosis with markedly elevated $CO_2$ levels
- Neurologic events
    - Postictal state
    - Embolic event
    - Hypoxic ischemic injury
    - Intracranial mass lesion and raised intracranial pressure or herniation

### 1. Residual Anesthetic Effect

The most common anesthetic agents used in the operating room are inhalational anesthetic agents, the elimination of which is dependent on minute ventilation, cardiac output, drug solubility, and the depth and duration of anesthesia. Therefore, ventilation and cardiac output must be optimized, often requiring a prolonged recovery room stay and possibly observation in an intermediate care unit or PICU admission for mechanical ventilation. As previously noted, excessive opioid administration is a cause of respiratory depression, and this must be evaluated in the patient who fails to awaken. A trial of naloxone can be given; however, it should be used judiciously, because it not only reverses the depressive effects but also the analgesia, resulting in a child who is in pain, agitated, hypertensive, and exhibiting uncontrollable behavior. It is prudent to continue to actively manage the airway and ventilate the

> *It is preferable to actively manage the airway and ventilate the patient until the residual anesthetic effect wears off without acute reversal of analgesia.*

patient until the residual anesthetic or excessive opioid effects abate without the acute removal of analgesia. This can be safely done in a PICU setting. If there is no improvement in the patient's sensorium, then other etiologies must be sought.

**2. Prolonged Neuromuscular Blockade**

Neuromuscular blocking agents are commonly used in general anesthesia during induction and endotracheal intubation. These agents can be divided into two types: depolarizing and nondepolarizing. Succinylcholine is a depolarizing neuromuscular blocking agent that noncompetitively binds to the acetylcholine (ACh) receptors of the motor endplate, resulting in depolarization. It then diffuses from the receptor and is metabolized by hepatic and plasma pseudocholinesterase. Prolonged blockade after administration of succinylcholine is most commonly caused by an abnormal genetic variant of pseudocholinesterase. The patient is managed with supportive ventilation until the effects of neuromuscular blockade (NMB) have dissipated. Other causes of prolonged depolarizing NMB are hepatic dysfunction and hypermagnesemia.

Nondepolarizing neuromuscular blockers, such as pancuronium, rocuronium, vecuronium, and cisatracurium, are commonly used during anesthesia. These drugs competitively inhibit ACh receptors, causing muscular paralysis without depolarization. This type of agent can be reversed or antagonized by administering an inhibitor of acetylcholinesterase (neostigmine, edrophonium, and pyridostigmine); this results in elevated synaptic concentrations of ACh, which then competitively displace the neuromuscular blocking agent from the receptor. Due to the muscarinic effects of these reversal agents, atropine (0.02 mg/kg IV) or glycopyrrolate (0.01 mg/kg IV) should be given concomitantly to prevent bradycardia. The common causes of failure in reversal of nondepolarizing agents are given in **Table 19-2**.

**Table 19-2 Failure of Reversal or Recurring Blockade by Nondepolarizing Agents**

- Respiratory acidosis
- Hypokalemia
- Hypermagnesemia
- Hypothermia
- Drug interactions
    - Antibiotics: aminoglycosides, tetracyclines, polymyxins, lincomycins
    - High-dose corticosteroids
    - Calcium-channel blockers
    - Local anesthetics (quinidine)
    - Alkylating cytotoxic agents
- Myasthenia gravis
- Muscular dystrophies and myotonia

Patients with prolonged NMB will not be able to breathe or move but will retain autonomic and ocular reactivity. They can be evaluated using a peripheral nerve stimulator with the administration of a train-of-four electrical impulses, while observing for corresponding twitches. Usually, the fourth twitch is abolished when >75% of the ACh receptors on the motor endplate are blocked. In adults, when <75% of the receptors are blocked, the patient can still effectively breathe.

Children, on the other hand, have decreased functional residual capacity and a higher incidence of postextubation airway obstruction. Thus, other indications of NMB reversal are the patient's ability to lift the head for more than 5 seconds, exhibit handgrip, and sustain a leg raise.

## B. Emergence Agitation

Emergence agitation (EA) was previously referred to as *emergence delirium.* It is a well-described phenomenon occurring in the immediate postoperative period. These patients exhibit a dissociated state of consciousness in which the child is inconsolable, irritable, uncooperative, typically thrashing, crying, moaning, or incoherent within the first few hours postoperatively. Often these children do not recognize or identify familiar and known objects or people. The incidence of EA in children is greater than in adults (12% vs. 5.3%) and is most commonly seen in children 3 to 9 years of age. These patients pose a risk of harming themselves and often will require restraints, comforting by caregivers, and reduced environmental stimuli in a dark quiet room. Most often EA is self-limiting, but sometimes "rescue" medication (analgesics, benzodiazepines, or hypnotics) is required. However, EA may reoccur after the effects of these sedatives have worn off. Other causes for agitation are pain, hypoxia, hypoglycemia, and anxiety, all of which must be considered.

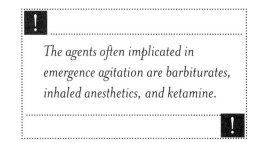

*The agents often implicated in emergence agitation are barbiturates, inhaled anesthetics, and ketamine.*

# VI. PAIN MANAGEMENT

Children of all ages, including premature neonates, experience pain. Approximately 40% to 75% of children will experience moderate to severe pain in the first 24 hours after surgery. In the past, children were denied pain relief as it was felt that they did not have the ability to experience pain or tolerate potent analgesia. This practice resulted in inadequate procedural pain management. No child now needs to experience pain, as we have an armamentarium of medications and techniques available. Their use requires a multidisciplinary and integrated approach throughout the perioperative period, with pain management strategies targeted to the individual patient. The strategies used are determined by the type of surgery, anesthetic technique used, expected duration of the recovery period, and anticipated severity of postoperative pain.

Nociception is the complex process whereby noxious stimuli are sensed, transformed, transmitted, modified, and eventually perceived as pain. The multimodal approach to pain management utilizes pharmacologic and nonpharmacologic therapies to target multiple steps in the process. Use of a combination of analgesics and adjuncts is more effective in pain control than an analgesic that targets a single step in the nociceptive pathway (**Figure 19-1**). This strategy also provides the benefit of reducing opiate use and opiate-related side effects.

**Figure 19-1.** Multimodal Therapy for Postoperative Pain Management

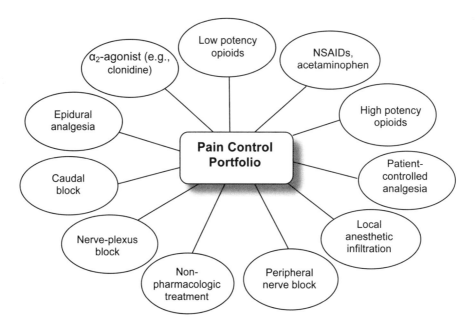

NSAIDs, nonsteroidal anti-inflammatory drugs

## A. Pain Assessment

Determining the appropriate type and dosage of analgesic requires a tool to measure the patient's pain. Pain assessment in children can be difficult; their responses to pain are age-specific and often difficult to distinguish from agitation and anxiety. Many children respond to pain by withdrawing from their surroundings and do not volunteer information out of fear of further painful interventions. This can be misinterpreted by the medical staff as a lack of pain. Validated, developmentally appropriate tools have been developed to objectively assess children (**Table 19-3**). Pain scales that rely on behavioral observations and physiologic changes have been developed for neonates, infants, cognitively impaired children, and ventilated patients. The child between 3 and 7 years can report pain using FACES Pain Rating Scale. Older children can use verbal scales or the adult visual analog scales. Ultimately, what is most important is the consistent application of a pain assessment tool that is specific for the patient population being considered as well as the situation.

## B. Multimodal Strategy of Pain Management

A variety of analgesic drugs can be used in the postoperative pain management of children, including nonopioids, nonsteroidal anti-inflammatory drugs (NSAIDS), opioids, and regional analgesia.

*The combination of analgesic agents should be tailored to the individual child's severity of pain and circumstances.*

| Table 19-3 | Pediatric Pain Assessment Tools | | | |
|---|---|---|---|---|
| Pain Scale | Age Range | Type | Scale Parameters | Uses |
| CRIES | 32-60 weeks | Behavioral and physiologic parameters | Crying, increased $O_2$, increased vital signs, expression, sleepiness | Acute pain; procedural and surgical pain |
| PIPP | Preterm and term infants | Behavioral and physiologic parameters | Gestational age, behavioral state, heart rate, $SpO_2$, facial expression | Procedural pain |
| FLACC | <3 years or nonverbal | Behavioral parameters | Face, legs, activity, cry, consolability | Acute pain; surgical pain |
| Faces scales (e.g., FACES, Wong-Baker) | 3-12 years | Subjects rate pain | Happy to saddest face with 0-10 score | Acute pain; surgical pain |
| Visual Analog Scale (VAS) | >7 years | Subjects rate pain | Horizontal 10-cm line; 0 = no pain, 10 = most pain | Acute pain; surgical pain; chronic pain |
| Numerical scale | >7 years | Subjects rate pain | Integers from 0-10; no pain to most pain | Acute pain; surgical pain; chronic pain |

Single-drug therapy with opioids has been the traditional method by which pediatric postoperative pain was managed. This often resulted in inadequate pain control and the common occurrence of adverse drug effects such as nausea, vomiting, pruritus, constipation, urinary retention, and respiratory and central nervous system depression. The dependence on a single analgesic often results in dosing delays, inadequate dosing, and failure to recognize an individual's pain.

A multimodal analgesia plan (**Figure 19-1**) provides a balanced approach that targets several of the pathways of nociception and encompasses combinations of the following therapies: (1) acetaminophen/paracetamol and NSAIDS acting on the periphery; (2) regional anesthetic blockade of peripheral nerves, nerve roots, or the spinal cord; (3) opioids acting centrally; and (4) nonpharmacological treatments incorporating distraction, and cognitive-behavioral and psychological interventions. This multimodal strategy can minimize the occurrence of adverse drug events by using smaller dosages of each analgesic while still achieving equivalent or superior pain control compared to opioid-only therapy. The weaknesses of opioid-only therapy can be resolved by scheduled dosing of NSAIDS, patient-controlled analgesia (PCA), long-acting regional analgesic techniques, and the use of additional opioids for breakthrough pain. Choices should be tailored to the individual patient's circumstances and pain level.

A stratified method for the use of analgesics in pain management is based on the severity of pain experienced (**Figure 19-2**) and closely follows the Analgesic Ladder model of cancer pain management developed by the World Health Organization. In this approach, nonopioids, including acetaminophen/paracetamol and NSAIDS (e.g., ibuprofen) can be used for mild pain. Lower potency oral opioids (codeine, hydrocodone, and oxycodone) are often used in combination with nonopioids for moderate pain; for severe pain, IV opioids (morphine, fentanyl, hydromorphone, methadone) are utilized in combination with potent IV NSAIDS (ketorolac, 0.5 mg/kg IV every 6 h) and IV acetaminophen/paracetamol (15 mg/kg IV every 6 h or 12.5 mg/kg IV every 4 h).

**Figure 19-2.** Stratified Approach to Analgesic Management of Postoperative Pain

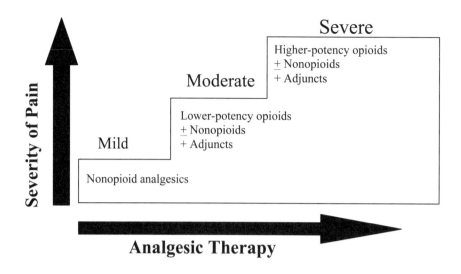

Classified using "The three-step analgesic ladder." In: *Cancer Pain Relief: With a Guide to Opioid Availability.* 2nd ed. Geneva, Switzerland: World Health Organization; 1996:15.

Clonidine is an $\alpha_2$-adrenergic agonist and a useful adjunct in the postoperative pain management plan. When given preoperatively, it can reduce postoperative opioid requirement. It also is a local anesthetic adjunct and can prolong and improve analgesia in peripheral nerve blocks and caudal, epidural, and spinal anesthesia, thereby reducing the need for opiates. Dexmedetomidine, another $\alpha_2$-adrenergic receptor agonist, acts centrally and has 8 times the affinity for the $\alpha_2$ receptor as clonidine. It provides good sedation along with analgesic benefits and can potentially reduce the need for opioids. The other advantage to dexmedetomidine is that it is associated with minimal respiratory depression.

An anesthesia or pain service consultation is highly recommended if a patient is expected to have severe, difficult-to-control, or refractory pain postoperatively.

## C. Patient-Controlled Analgesia

Typically, opioids are administered to patients after they complain or are noted to be in pain. This leads to a vicious cycle of pain followed by delayed administration of an analgesic, with the resultant risk of persistent pain or increased sedation. This places the patient at risk for the side effects of opioids with inadequate pain relief. PCA allows us to break this cycle. It is an excellent delivery system for the control of moderate to severe pain when used with adequate monitoring. It can be used in patients as young as 5 years of age (with proper education) and routinely in children 7 years or older. Any child who can play video games can use a PCA device. The goal is twofold: (1) maintain therapeutic opioid levels to insure adequate analgesia; and (2) utilize a system that is rapidly responsive to the patient's analgesic needs. PCA has a high rate of patient, parent, and

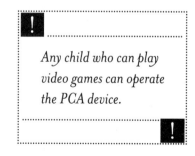

*Any child who can play video games can operate the PCA device.*

staff satisfaction. The PCA regimen usually employs an opioid that can be dosed on demand, continuously (basal infusion), or both (**Table 19-4**).

### Table 19-4  Patient-Controlled Analgesia Dosing Regimen

| Opioid Drug | Demand Dose (µg/kg) | Lock-out Interval (min) | Basal Infusion (µg/kg/h) | 1-Hour Limit (µg/kg) |
|---|---|---|---|---|
| Morphine | 20 (adult dose: 1000 µg) | 8-10 | 0-20 (adult dose: 2000 µg/h) | 100 |
| Fentanyl | 0.5 (adult dose: 50-100 µg) | 6-8 | 0-0.5 (adult dose: 50-100 µg/h) | 2.5 |
| Hydromorphone | 4 (adult dose: 200 µg) | 8-10 | 0-4 (adult dose: 200 µg/h) | 20 |

Adapted with permission. © 2006 Elsevier. Landsman IR, Vustar M, Hays SR. Pediatric anesthesia. In: Grosfeld JL, O'Neill JA, Coran AG, Fonkalsrud EW, eds. *Pediatric Surgery*. 6th ed. St. Louis, MO: Mosby; 2006:242-243.

Continuous basal infusions should only be administered in units where there is close cardiorespiratory monitoring; they should be avoided in the opiate-naive patient except in special circumstances, such as posterior spinal fusion. It has been speculated that basal infusions may facilitate a normal sleeping pattern in the postoperative patient, who is awoken by the experience of pain and then self-administers a dose of opioid. However, no evidence supports this assumption in children, and the risk of adverse respiratory events is increased with continuous opioid infusions. Due to this risk, the routine use of basal infusions is not recommended for nonintubated patients.

Demand dosing is often used as this ensures a margin of safety, while providing adequate analgesia and minimizing opioid side effects. The minimum time interval between demand doses of narcotics is called the *lockout time*, and no drug will be delivered during that time no matter how often the button is pressed. This is intended to prevent narcotic accumulation. A total maximum dose (1- to 4-hour limits) is programmed into the pump to prevent overdosing. To optimize patient safety and prevent adverse events, oxygen saturations, respiratory rate, heart rate, blood pressure, end-tidal $CO_2$, pain, and level of consciousness must be monitored. Rescue orders should be part of the PCA treatment regimen and naloxone (1-2 µg/kg every 5 min to a total of 10 µg/kg) prescribed to reverse the untoward adverse opioid effect of respiratory depression. Severe breakthrough pain is treated with additional IV opioids (same narcotic medication used in the pump) and administered every 3 hours as needed. Pruritus induced by opioids can be treated with nalbuphine (50 µg/kg IV every 4 h) and in the event of severe pruritus, naloxone infusion (0.25 µg/kg/h) can be used.

PCA by proxy allows the parent or nurse to press the PCA button to deliver narcotics to children less than 6 years or with developmental delay. However, different parameters must be set on the PCA pump to prevent accidental overdose by caregivers and should occur in a monitored environment. PCA by proxy has the same incidence of adverse events as PCA by patient but the need for rescue interventions is greater.

## D. Epidural Analgesia

Continuous epidural analgesia (CEA) is an invaluable method of treating severe postoperative pain in neonates, infants, and children. CEA decreases stress response and duration of hospital stay, and may improve outcomes in particular pediatric groups. The epidural catheter is inserted via the caudal approach in infants or can be inserted in the low thoracic or lumbar interspace of L5 and S1. The epidural catheter is threaded to a thoracic or high lumbar level and the catheter tip placed adjacent to the center of the dermatomes to be blocked. This ensures adequate pain control and a continuous infusion of local anesthetic with the added benefit that an opioid can be delivered to provide continuous pain relief. The combined effect of local anesthetics and opioids is synergistic, thus lower doses of each agent can provide adequate analgesia.

A common problem is inadequate pain control due to inaccurate catheter placement, catheter problems (kinking, leaking, dislodgement, breakage), or an insufficient infusion rate or analgesic dose. The possible complications of CEA include: (1) local anesthetic toxicity; (2) motor block as a direct effect of local anesthetics or a late sign of compartment syndrome or epidural hematoma; (3) epidural abscess; and (4) adjuvant opioid side effects. Reducing the concentration or infusion rate of the local anesthetic or using medication to counteract the opioid-induced side effects can usually manage these complications. The patient is routinely monitored for motor block, dermatome block, and fever, along with changes in the patient's hemodynamic and respiratory parameters. Vigilance is needed in monitoring for respiratory depression caused by the level of dermatome block being too high or, more frequently, because IV or intramuscular opioids are used to supplement the epidural opioid.

Patient-controlled epidural analgesia combines the benefits of CEA and PCA and allows the patient to respond in real time to pain exacerbation.

## E. Regional Anesthesia

Regional anesthesia techniques are becoming more popular in pediatric postoperative pain management. With the aid of ultrasound and nerve stimulators, regional anesthesia has improved the success of nerve blocks. These techniques use local anesthetics to block the afferent pathways from nociceptors to the central nervous system and include local infiltration, peripheral nerve blocks, nerve-plexus blocks, and epidural or intrathecal nerve blocks. The anesthetic agent is administered as a single injection or by continuous infusion, and often long-acting local anesthetics are used. Examples of such techniques include penile, femoral, sciatic, axillary, ankle, intercostal, and caudal blocks.

Regional anesthesia can be advantageous in patients who exhibit increased sensitivity to the side effects of opioids, which often occur in neonates and young children. It can also potentially lower the risk of adverse effects frequently encountered with parenterally administered opioids, such as nausea, vomiting, sedation, and respiratory depression. The use of long-acting local anesthetics can reduce the need for high-potency opioids and provide hours of pain relief in the immediate postoperative period when the severity of pain is usually at its greatest.

The most common regional anesthesia block used in children is the caudal block. In this technique, the epidural space is accessed via the sacral hiatus and a single injection of

1 mL/kg of local anesthetic is administered. If available, this block can be performed with the aid of ultrasound guidance. Its success rate is high with a low rate of complication. It usually provides analgesia below the umbilicus and, with the use of only a local anesthetic, the patient is pain-free for several hours. In general, children do not exhibit hemodynamic instability or urinary retention. The addition of opioids will prolong analgesia but increase the risk of side effects. This technique usually works well when severe pain is only anticipated for the first 24 hours postoperatively.

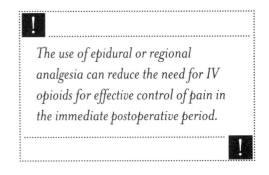

*The use of epidural or regional analgesia can reduce the need for IV opioids for effective control of pain in the immediate postoperative period.*

# VII. FLUID AND ELECTROLYTE CONSIDERATIONS

Fluid and electrolyte deficits are some of the most commonly encountered problems in the care of the pediatric surgical patient. These deficits are usually due to ongoing loss of gastrointestinal fluids (vomiting, nasogastric tubes, and surgical drains), cerebrospinal fluid loss through external ventricular drains, and sequestration of fluids (peritonitis, ileus, burns). Small infants can have extraordinary insensible fluid losses, especially if under radiant warmers or receiving phototherapy. In these conditions, fluid requirements are increased by 10% to 20%. Pulmonary insensible water loss is negligible when patients are mechanically ventilated due to humidity in the circuits.

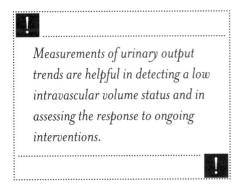

*Measurements of urinary output trends are helpful in detecting a low intravascular volume status and in assessing the response to ongoing interventions.*

The clinical findings in children will depend on the severity of vascular volume depletion and may consist of irritability that progresses to apathy and lethargy, increased heart rate, mottled and cold extremities, and decreased urinary output. Hypotension is a late finding in shock. Laboratory evaluation will usually show increased blood urea nitrogen, with or without elevation in creatinine, and hemoconcentration with an inappropriately elevated hematocrit. In severe volume depletion with significant compromise in oxygen delivery, a metabolic acidosis and increased blood lactate level can be seen.

Children anticipated to have large perioperative fluid shifts or losses and requiring large-volume fluid resuscitation should be monitored invasively with continuous measurement of central venous pressure and arterial pressure. An indwelling urinary catheter should be utilized.

After the acute correction of shock, fluid management should provide for the correction of the remaining deficit, maintenance fluid, and replacement of ongoing losses. In the critically ill postoperative patient, it is safe to assume that any ongoing losses are more likely to be isotonic than hypotonic in composition. It is also safe to assume

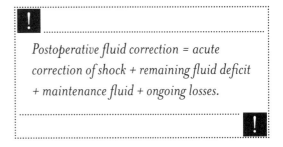

*Postoperative fluid correction = acute correction of shock + remaining fluid deficit + maintenance fluid + ongoing losses.*

that the stressed postoperative patient will experience hemodynamic and nonhemodynamic stimuli for the release of antidiuretic hormone. In this setting, isotonic fluids in the early postoperative period decrease the risk of hyponatremia and potential neurologic complications. The patient should be assessed frequently to check hydration and circulation, to determine serum electrolytes (every 6 to 8 hours), and to adjust electrolyte delivery in the fluids accordingly.

The neurosurgical or head-injured patient who develops the syndrome of inappropriate secretion of antidiuretic hormone poses a special circumstance. These patients are usually euvolemic or have a mild excess of total body water with varying degrees of hyponatremia. They require the provision of maintenance sodium and fluid restriction to 50% of maintenance; the goal is to increase serum sodium at a rate of <0.5 mEq/L/h or 12 mEq/L/day (**Chapter 8**).

## VIII. POSTOPERATIVE NAUSEA AND VOMITING

Nausea and vomiting – distressing aspects of the postoperative period for patients, parents, and healthcare professionals – are responsible for the adverse effects of increased rates of hospital readmission, delay of hospital discharge, postoperative bleeding, aspiration, wound dehiscence, dehydration, and delay of enteral nutrition. Postoperative nausea and vomiting (PONV) are caused by the emetogenic effects of inhaled anesthetics, pain, and opioids. The incidence of postoperative vomiting (POV) in children is estimated to be twice that seen with PONV in adults. Children younger than 3 years have an incidence of POV of 22% to 40%, whereas older children have an incidence of 42% to 51%. The risk factors for pediatric POV are: (1) duration of anesthesia >30 min; (2) age ≥3 years; (3) strabismus surgery; and (4) history of POV, PONV, or motion sickness in the patient, parents, and siblings. The incidence of POV was 9%, 10%, 30%, 55%, and 70% for 0, 1, 2, 3, and 4 risk factors, respectively. Therefore, patients with a higher risk of POV can be identified and treated with a tailored multistep prophylactic and therapeutic antiemetic plan.

PONV is managed using multimodal therapy because of the limited effects of using single-antiemetic drug therapy. An algorithm for the management of POV/PONV (**Table 19-5**) starts with identifying patients with moderate to severe risk, then preemptively employing 2 or more different classes of antiemetics for prophylaxis. With the addition of each antiemetic drug, the risk of PONV decreases by 30%. This is augmented by avoiding or minimizing the use of inhaled anesthetics and postoperative opioids with the use of total IV anesthesia (e.g., propofol), regional anesthesia, and NSAIDS.

Preoperative fasting does not prevent PONV, but hydration and glucose supplementation will ameliorate it. Serotonin antagonists are the mainstay of pharmacologic management of POV/PONV due to their good safety profile and minimal side effects. Ondansetron (0.15 mg/kg IV every 4-6 h) is the most common first-line drug for POV/PONV prophylaxis and treatment, and it is the only serotonin antagonist that is approved for use in children 1 month and older in the United States. The combination of ondansetron and dexamethasone (0.5 mg/kg IV) is very efficacious when used prophylactically in the management of POV/PONV.

| Table 19-5 | Multimodal Approach to Postoperative Nausea and Vomiting |
|---|---|

- Evaluate risk of POV/PONV
- If moderate or severe risk:
    - Reduce baseline risks
        - Avoidance/minimization of inhaled anesthetics, neostigmine, nitrous oxide, and postoperative opioids
        - Total intravenous anesthesia (propofol)
        - Regional anesthesia/analgesia – intraoperative and postoperative
        - Hydration
        - Nonopioid analgesics (NSAIDs)
    - Use ≥2 antiemetics of different classes prophylactically (e.g., dexamethasone + ondansetron[a])
        - Serotonin antagonists (ondansetron[a], granisetron, dolasetron)
        - Ondansetron[a] is usual first-line drug
        - Steroids (dexamethasone)
        - Antihistamine (dimenhydrinate)
        - Antidopaminergic (droperidol[b])
        - Phenothiazine (perphenazine)
    - Treat PONV
        - Serotonin antagonist or antiemetic drug of different class

POV, postoperative vomiting; PONV, postoperative nausea and vomiting; NSAIDs, nonsteroidal anti-inflammatory drugs
[a]Ondansetron is approved in US for POV in children 1 month and older.
[b]In the US, droperidol has a black box warning as it causes a dose-dependent prolongation of the QT interval.

# IX. NUTRITIONAL CONSIDERATIONS

*The unique challenge in the pediatric patient is providing nutrition to meet the increased demands of critical illness and healing as well as the demands of normal growth and development.*

Acute malnutrition is frequently encountered in the postoperative pediatric patient. In this setting, malnutrition is multifactorial and may be caused by prolonged bowel dysfunction or food intolerance after surgery, increased catabolism, lack of aggressive intervention, or missed opportunities to increase nutritional support. To complicate the picture further, many children have long-term malnutrition due to a preexisting chronic condition.

## A. Nutrition Assessment

On admission, all patients should be assessed for evidence of malnutrition. Baseline measures, such as weight, height, and head circumference, should be obtained. Children younger than 2 years should be plotted on normative growth charts, and values can be compared with previous measures from the clinics or prior admissions, if available. Body mass index can de determined in older children. Also, base measures of specific visceral proteins, such as albumin, transferrin, prealbumin, and retinol-binding protein can be obtained. These proteins have a rapid turnover, but during periods of increased catabolism, their synthesis is decreased. Increasing levels are indicative of resolving stress and/or adequate nutrition. Prealbumin and retinol-binding protein, due to their short half-lives (2 days and 12 hours, respectively), are better suited to reflect acute change in the patient's metabolic state. Another readily available biochemical marker is C-reactive protein; in postsurgical patients, a normalizing level is a herald of a returning anabolic state.

## B. Stress Response

During acute physiologic stress, the body's response tends to be similar regardless of the inciting event. The hypothalamic-pituitary axis and the sympathetic nervous system are activated, resulting in an increase in counter-regulatory hormones, including endogenous catecholamines and eventually insulin resistance. Elevated cortisol induces muscle breakdown and promotes gluconeogenesis (conversion of noncarbohydrate energy sources into glucose). The increased levels of catecholamines stimulate glycogen breakdown in the liver and skeletal muscle and mobilization of free fatty acids, all of which fuel the hypercatabolic state.

## C. Nutritional Support

The breakdown of lean body tissue is central during the stress response. Therefore, the goals are to limit protein breakdown during the acute phase of illness by providing amino acids and adequate nonprotein calories (**Table 19-6**).

Carbohydrates in the form of glucose provide 4 kcal/g of energy. Children require a glucose infusion rate of 5 to 8 mg/kg/min to meet metabolic demand. The threshold for ketosis is a glucose infusion rate of <2 mg/kg/min but may be higher in the context of the stress response due to the state of insulin resistance. Overfeeding with glucose delivery rates of more than 10 mg/kg/min should be avoided, because it promotes lipogenesis and increased $CO_2$ production. If hyperglycemia develops despite appropriate glucose delivery, insulin supplementation (starting continuous infusion of regular insulin, 0.05-0.1 U/kg/h) in a monitored environment may be indicated to facilitate cellular uptake. When reintroducing enteral nutrition, a lactose-free formulation may be tolerated best.

**Table 19-6** Nutritional Requirements

| Age (years) | Energy (kcal/kg/day) | Protein (g/kg/day) |
|---|---|---|
| <1 | 50-80 | 2.0-2.5 |
| 1-7 | 45-65 | 1.5-2.0 |
| >7 | 30-60 | 1.5-2.0 |

Fats provide 9 kcal/g of energy. In patients unable to tolerate enteral feedings, fat can be administered parenterally as a 20% emulsion. As little as 0.5 g/kg/day is enough to provide essential fatty acids (linoleic and linolenic acids), but the infusion can be increased by 1 g/kg/day to a limit of 3 g/kg/day, depending upon caloric requirements. Triglyceride levels are best determined at least 4 hours after discontinuing a lipid infusion. Hypertriglyceridemia is frequently caused by an excess caloric load from carbohydrates. When the enteral route is used, the medium-chain triglycerides offered in some formulas are able to enter the portal system directly, facilitating absorption.

The breakdown of protein produces 4 kcal/g of energy. Although unable to prevent the catabolism of proteins during the stress response, amino acids should be provided in an amount sufficient to prevent a deficiency and to facilitate the synthesis of new protein. Maintaining this balance between breakdown and synthesis may require protein intake of 2 to 3 g/kg/day.

# D. Route of Administration

The use of IV delivery devices and central venous catheterization allows the administration of parenteral nutrition to surgical patients who would otherwise suffer the consequences of malnutrition (poor wound healing, infections, even death).

Enteral nutrition is the preferred mode of nutrient intake in critically ill patients with a functional gastrointestinal system, due to its many benefits, lower cost, and lower complication rate compared to parenteral nutrition (**Table 19-7**).

Delayed gastric emptying is common in critical illness. If attempts to feed into the stomach fail or if the risks of aspiration are high, transpyloric tube feeding is usually successful and has the added advantage that feeding can be continued around the period of planned extubation, during surgery or procedures, providing uninterrupted nutrition. Parenteral nutrition continues to play an important role in the support of patients with hemodynamic instability at risk for bowel ischemia and in patients with congenital or acquired abnormalities of the gut, such as necrotizing enterocolitis, bowel atresia, meconium ileus, dysmotility syndromes, bowel obstruction, and short gut syndrome. Complications of prolonged parenteral nutrition are numerous, and every effort should be made to provide some nutrition by the enteral route (**Table 19-8**).

**Table 19-7 Advantages of Enteral Feeding**

- Stimulates release of gut trophic factors
- Maintains enterocyte mass
- Preserves gut motility
- Improves mesenteric blood flow
- Decreases incidence of nosocomial infections
- Lowers costs

**Table 19-8 Complications of Parenteral Nutrition**

- Catheter-related infections
- Electrolyte disturbances
- Hepatic disorders
    - Fatty liver
    - Cholestasis
    - Hepatic fibrosis
    - Biliary cirrhosis (parenteral nutrition-associated liver disease)

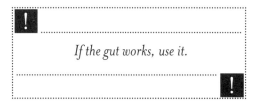

*If the gut works, use it.*

# X. HEMATOLOGIC CONSIDERATIONS

Intraoperative blood loss is carefully monitored by both the surgeon and the anesthesiologist. Most often, the rate of loss is gradual and surgically controlled. Patients usually do not require blood products unless significant blood has been lost or the initial hematocrit was low. Large volumes of blood products given intraoperatively and ongoing bleeding can have a major impact on the patient's status in the postoperative period. When the blood loss has been gradual, the rates at which the hemoglobin and hematocrit fall can be used as an estimation of the extent of the loss. When active bleeding is vigorous, hemodynamic instability is a closer reflection of blood volume depletion. Direct measurement of blood collected from indwelling drains (e.g., thoracostomy tubes) is also used to estimate the extent of ongoing blood loss. Occult bleeding occurring in closed compartments, such as the intra-abdominal compartment and thigh, is an exception to this practice. The etiology of postoperative bleeding must be determined and corrected, especially if it is ongoing and/or brisk. The most common cause for bleeding is poor surgical hemostasis. The other major etiology is coagulopathy due to hemodilution of clotting factors and platelets, increased consumption, massive packed red blood cell (PRBC) transfusion, or other underlying conditions, including sepsis and disseminated intravascular coagulopathy.

The decision to transfuse depends first on the patient's clinical status and the estimated rate of blood loss. The clinical evidence does not support transfusion of PRBCs to hemodynamically stable patients unless the hemoglobin is <7 g/dL. Massive blood loss is defined as the loss of 1 blood volume within a 24-hour period or the loss of 50% of blood volume within 3 hours. Estimated blood volume is 85 mL/kg in infants (0-1 year), 80 mL/kg in children (1-10 years), 70-75 mL/kg in adolescents, and 65 mL/kg in adults. In the event of ongoing massive bleeding, the patient initially should be resuscitated with either crystalloids or colloids via large-bore IV access and PRBCs (10-20 mL/kg) transfused when available. In the meantime, baseline studies should be obtained: complete blood count, coagulation screen, and blood type and screen. Blood product replacement should be guided by the estimated volume loss, rate of ongoing loss, and the patient's response to fluid resuscitation (**Chapter 17**). The combination of crystalloids, colloids, and PRBCs achieves the therapeutic goal of maintaining blood volume or hemodynamic parameters and a hemoglobin >7 g/dL. Fresh frozen plasma and platelets should be used judiciously to prevent or correct any coagulopathy. The trigger for this transfusion (10-15 mL/kg) is an international normalized ratio >1.5, which is typically after 1 to 1.5 times the blood volume replacement. To address coagulopathy early in massive bleeding, a near-equal amount of fresh frozen plasma and PRBCs (1:1 ratio) should be transfused. The need for platelets is variable. A platelet count >20,000/µL may be acceptable in the absence of ongoing bleeding, but a count >50,000/µL is desirable in active bleeding. Patients who have undergone a neurosurgical procedure should maintain platelet counts of ≥100,000/µL. In infants and children, a platelet transfusion of 10 mL/kg will increase the platelet count by approximately 50,000/µL. The priority, however, is to surgically reverse the source of the bleeding.

PRBCs and fresh frozen plasma contain citrate, which chelates calcium and can cause a fall in the serum ionized calcium level. The mobilization of calcium and the hepatic metabolism of citrate are usually rapid enough to prevent a significant fall in the ionized calcium in older children and adults. Neonates have inadequate calcium stores and are susceptible to acute hypocalcemia and its attendant hypotension, and require IV calcium replacement (calcium chloride 10%, 10-20 mg/kg, or calcium gluconate, 100-200 mg/kg). Calcium may also be required if massive amounts of blood products have been transfused. Large transfusions of cold blood products will precipitate hypothermia, so the products should be warmed prior to administration.

# XI. THERMAL REGULATION

As part of the intraoperative management, the anesthesiologist optimizes body temperature control, with the primary goal being normothermia. Some patients are more prone to develop hypothermia or hyperthermia during anesthesia. Hypothermia is a major concern in infants, patients having prolonged procedures, after the administration of large volumes of unwarmed IV fluids or blood products, and in instances that require large areas of surgical site exposure. Hyperthermia is possible when radiant warmers or thermal blankets are used.

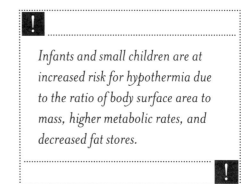

*Infants and small children are at increased risk for hypothermia due to the ratio of body surface area to mass, higher metabolic rates, and decreased fat stores.*

## A. Hypothermia

Shivering is a common occurrence in the immediate postoperative period with the patient often complaining of feeling extremely cold. The use of warm blankets may remedy this and tends to be comforting; subjectively it appears to reduce shivering. Hypothermia, on the other hand, can be a cause of shivering and must be ruled out.

**Table 19-9  Deleterious Effects of Hypothermia**

- Respiratory acidosis
- Apnea
- Hypotension
- Bradycardia
- Prolongation of neuromuscular blockade
- Prolongation of the effects of narcotics

Hypothermia, if not promptly attended to, can lead to life-threatening situations, especially in neonates (**Table 19-9**). During rewarming, cutaneous hyperthermia and burns (especially with improper use of radiant warmers) must be avoided.

## B. Fever

Postoperative fever (temperature >100.4°F or >38°C) is common, managed expectantly with symptomatic treatment, and usually resolves spontaneously. The onset of postoperative fever is important in establishing a differential diagnosis and will determine the workup and management. The causes can be remembered using the five W's of postoperative fever (**Table 19-10**).

Fever in the first 24 hours postoperatively is relatively common and is often due to the inflammatory response from surgery-induced tissue injury, resulting in the release of pyrogens. The patient may have had an occult or known preexisting infection at the time of surgery. Healthcare-associated infections (HAI) are the most common cause of infections that can result in fever. These include hospital-acquired pneumonia, catheter-associated urinary tract infections, catheter-related bloodstream infections, and surgical site infections. Pneumonia usually presents on postoperative day 2 or 3, with urinary tract infections first occurring on days 3 through 5 and surgical infections first becoming apparent on days 5 through 7.

### Table 19-10 The Five W's of Postoperative Fever

POD 2-3: Wind – pneumonia

POD 3-5: Water – catheter-associated urinary tract infection

POD 4-6: Walking – deep venous thrombosis (incidence in children is unknown; should be considered in pubescent adolescents and patients at risk)

POD 5-7: Wound – surgical site infections usually become apparent

POD 7+: Wonder drugs – drugs can cause fever

POD, postoperative day

Interventions that can reduce HAIs in postoperative patients (**Table 19-11**) include extubating mechanically ventilated patients and removing indwelling catheters as soon as possible. Appropriate cultures should be obtained to rule out HAIs and appropriate antibiotics instituted (**Chapter 7**). Persistent postoperative fever may not be due to an infectious agent, and other causes should be sought. Using the process of elimination, the underlying etiology can often be determined and appropriately treated.

Another cause of hyperthermia includes excessive ambient environmental heat with no opportunity for heat loss, seen with the bundling of infants and the use of warming devices. Dehydration secondary to inadequate fluid replacement also predisposes the patient to temperature elevation. In all cases, fever results in increased metabolic demand with resultant tachycardia, tachypnea, and carbon dioxide production, causing increased stress on the patient. Malignant hyperthermia (MH) should be considered in patients who have a rapid increase in temperature in excess of 102.2°F (39°C) during or within hours of having received an inhalational anesthetic.

### Table 19-11  Reducing the Risk of Postsurgical Healthcare-Associated Infections

- Hospital-acquired pneumonia
    - Minimize ventilator days
    - Keep head of bed elevated 30°
    - Ambulate out of bed quickly when age and developmentally appropriate
    - Encourage or improve deep breathing in nonventilated patient
        - Incentive spirometry (4-6 years or older)
        - Blowing bubbles or pinwheel (toddler or older)
- Hospital-acquired infections
    - Minimize use and duration of indwelling catheters and lines
- Proper hand hygiene
- Surgical site infections
    - Administer prophylactic antibiotic 1 h before incision
    - Discontinue prophylactic antibiotics within 24 h after surgery end time (48 h in cardiac patients)
    - Remove hair as appropriate (leave hair intact or remove with clippers)

## C. Malignant Hyperthermia

MH is a familial disorder of muscle hypermetabolism that may complicate the anesthetic course and require further management in the PICU. Its prevalence during general anesthesia varies from 1 in 15,000 children to 1 in 50,000 adults. Children with underlying myopathy are at increased risk. Agents inciting MH include inhalational anesthetic agents and depolarizing muscle relaxants, such as succinylcholine. Exaggerated jaw rigidity (masseter spasms) after succinylcholine use and excessive carbon dioxide production are often the earliest signs; skeletal muscle rigidity, tachycardia, and hyperthermia then ensue. If not controlled, the intense muscle activity leads to rhabdomyolysis, hyperkalemia, and eventual multiple organ system failure. Immediate evaluation for MH would include measurement of arterial blood gases, serum electrolytes, serum creatinine kinase, and urine myoglobin. If MH is suspected, an anesthesia or pediatric intensivist consult should be obtained to assist in its diagnosis and medical management.

Treatment consists of avoidance or removal of triggering agents, muscle relaxation with dantrolene sodium, and supportive care. Dantrolene sodium causes complete and sustained relaxation of skeletal muscles by direct action on calcium release channels. It is given as 1 to 3 mg/kg IV, repeated every 15 minutes as needed, to a maximum dose of 10 mg/kg in the setting of acute MH. Recurrence is prevented by administration of dantrolene sodium 1 mg/kg IV every 6 hours for 24 to 48 hours postoperatively. Supportive care involves airway protection by orotracheal intubation and mechanical ventilation if large doses are needed, active cooling to <100.4°F (<38°C) but avoidance of hypothermia, and correction of acidosis and hyperkalemia. Laboratory testing should include creatine kinase, phosphate, calcium, and myoglobin. In the presence of rhabdomyolysis and myoglobinuria, a brisk urine output should be maintained with IV hydration and osmotic diuretics, such as mannitol. As with other hyperthermia syndromes, coagulopathy, pulmonary edema, and cerebral edema can be potential complications. When MH is suspected based on well-documented clinical events or strong family history, genetic evaluation and muscle testing could secure a diagnosis and indicate appropriate precautions for both the index patient and relatives of all ages.

## Key Points: Postoperative Management

- Postoperative recovery is directly dependent on preexisting conditions, severity of illness, and the duration of anesthesia.

- Adverse respiratory events are the most common complication arising within the first 24 hours after surgery.

- Full-term neonates (younger than 1 month) and premature infants less than 60 weeks postconceptual age should be considered at risk for apnea after general anesthesia, and they require inpatient monitoring and observation for 24 hours after surgery.

- Naloxone should be used if respiratory or central nervous system depression is suspected because of excessive opioid use; however, it should be used judiciously, as it not only reverses the depressive effects but also the analgesia, resulting in a child who is in pain, agitated, hypertensive, and behaviorally uncontrollable.

- Emergence agitation is usually treated with opioids, benzodiazepines, and hypnotics, but other causes – such as hypoxia, hypoglycemia, and severe pain – must be ruled out.

- Children of all ages feel pain and must be aggressively managed in the postoperative period. A developmentally appropriate pain scale is a vital tool in the assessment of the pain intensity.

- A balanced and multimodal approach to pain management, tailored to the patient, delivers effective analgesia and minimizes adverse drug events.

- Volume deficit, the most common fluid problem in the pediatric surgical patient, is usually due to third spacing and ongoing loss of gastrointestinal fluids.

- In the critically ill postoperative patient, it is safe to assume that any ongoing losses are likely to be isotonic in composition.

- Multimodal therapy should be used to prevent and treat PONV in children.

- Early institution of nutrition, preferably by the enteral route, shortens the postoperative period and speeds recovery.

- Fever is common after surgery and is usually self-limiting. Its timing of onset is important in establishing a differential diagnosis and will determine the workup and management.

- If, within hours of receiving an inhalational anesthetic, the patient's temperature rapidly rises in excess of 102.2°F (39°C), and especially if succinylcholine was used, malignant hyperthermia should be considered.

# Suggested Readings

1. Chandrakantan A, Glass PSA. Multimodal therapies for postoperative nausea and vomiting, and pain. *Br J Anaesth*. 2011;107(Suppl 1):i27-i40.

2. Eberhart LHJ, Geldner G, Kranke P, et al. The development and validation of a risk score to predict the probability of postoperative vomiting in pediatric patients. *Anesth Analg*. 2004;99:1630-1637.

3. Gan TJ, Meyer TA, Apfel CC, et al. Society for Ambulatory Anesthesia guidelines for the management of postoperative nausea and vomiting. *Anesth Analg*. 2007;105:1615-1628.

4. Kovac AL. Management of postoperative nausea and vomiting in children. *Paediatr Drugs*. 2007;9:47-69.

5. Kraemer FW, Rose JB. Pharmacologic management of acute pediatric pain. *Anesthesiol Clin*. 2009;27:241-268.

6. Kulaylat MN, Dayton MTPA. Surgical complications. In: Townsend CM, Beauchamp RD, Evers BM, Mattox KL, eds. *Sabiston Textbook of Surgery*. 17th ed. Philadelphia, PA: Elsevier Saunders; 2012:281-327.

7. Landsman IS, Vustar MV, Hays SR. Pediatric anesthesia. In: Grosfeld JL, O'Neill JA, Coran AG, Fonkalsrud EW, eds. *Pediatric Surgery*. 6th ed. Philadelphia, PA: Mosby Elsevier; 2006:221-256.

8. Lehmann KA. Recent developments in patient-controlled analgesia. *J Pain Symptom Manage*. 2005;29(5 Suppl):S72-S89.

9. Letton RW, Chwals WJ, Jamie A, Charles B. Early postoperative alterations in infant energy use increase the risk of overfeeding. *J Pediatr Surg*. 1995;30:988-992.

10. McDonald AJ, Cooper MG. Patient-controlled analgesia: an appropriate method of pain control in children. *Paediatr Drugs*. 2001;3:273-284.

11. Mehta NM, Compher C, A.S.P.E.N. Board of Directors. A.S.P.E.N. clinical guidelines: nutrition support of the critically ill child. *JPEN J Parenter Enteral Nutr*. 2009;33:260-276.

12. Moritz ML, Ayus JC. Prevention of hospital acquired hyponatremia: a case for using isotonic saline. *Pediatrics*. 2003;111:227-230.

13. Vlajkovic GP, Sindjelic RP. Emergence delirium in children: many questions, few answers. *Anesth Analg*. 2007;104:84-91.

14. Voepel-Lewis T, Marinkovic A, Kostrzewa A, Tait AR, Malviya S. The prevalence of and risk factors for adverse events in children receiving patient-controlled analgesia by proxy or patient-controlled analgesia after surgery. *Anesth Analg*. 2008;107:70-75.

15. Wetzel RC. Anesthesia, perioperative care, and sedation. In: Kliegman RM, Stanton BF, St. Geme JW, Schor NF, Behrman RE, eds. *Nelson Textbook of Pediatrics*. 19th ed. Philadelphia, PA: Elsevier Saunders; 2011:359.

# Chapter 20

# Sedation, Analgesia, and Neuromuscular Blockade

## ✓ Objectives

- Identify the indications, risks, and monitoring needs of patients undergoing elective sedation.
- Describe the benefits and appropriate uses of therapeutic analgesia in critically ill patients.
- Explain the benefits and side effects associated with commonly used analgesic medications.
- Outline the benefits and side effects associated with commonly used sedative/hypnotic medications.
- Determine the benefits and side effects associated with commonly used neuromuscular blockade medications.
- Know the reversal medications for benzodiazepine, opioid, and neuromuscular blocking agents.
- Be familiar with the complications of tachyphylaxis and iatrogenic dependence associated with the prolonged usage of benzodiazepine and opioid receptor agonists.

## Case Study

A 4-year-old boy is admitted with a heart rate of 170 beats/min, temperature of 96°F (35.6°C), respiratory rate of 40 breaths/min, and systolic blood pressure of 70 mm Hg. He is mottled, with poor perfusion, and in significant respiratory distress. Several days ago he was diagnosed with influenza A. He is given oxygen by face mask, and fluid resuscitation has begun with isotonic saline.

**Detection**

- What are the most likely diagnoses?
- What are the worst possible diagnoses?

**Intervention**

- What are the most immediate treatment strategies?

**Reassessment**

- If the decision is made to intubate, which medications should be used?
- What medications can be given to provide analgesia and sedation before transfer to the pediatric intensive care unit?
- Which medicines should be avoided?

**Effective Communication**
- When the patient's clinical status changes, who needs to know and how will this information be disseminated?
- Where is the best place to manage the care of this patient?

**Teamwork**
- How are you going to implement the treatment strategy?
- Who is to do what and when?

# I. INTRODUCTION

The treatment of critically ill children would be difficult, if not impossible, without the concurrent use of analgesic, sedative, and neuromuscular blocking agents. When used correctly, these medications not only save lives, they also allow painful and traumatic procedures to be performed on severely ill children. These procedures may include the placement of artificial airways, invasive monitoring devices, central access devices, and even minor surgery. Protection of the child after insertion of these devices may require long-term analgesia and sedation until these treatments are no longer needed. Sedative medications may also be needed for patients undergoing nonpainful procedures like computed tomography scans or magnetic resonance imaging, especially for infants or toddlers who have a difficult time remaining still for prolonged periods.

By definition, a patient who receives a medication to decrease stress or anxiety is receiving sedation or being sedated. Anyone receiving a medication or therapy to relieve pain is receiving analgesia. Some medications provide sedation without analgesia whereas others provide analgesia without sedation; a few provide both. Each practitioner should determine which of these conditions they want to provide and then to choose the appropriate medication, or combination of medications, to accomplish this therapeutic goal.

Sedation in the critical care environment reduces metabolic demands, mortality, morbidity, and hospital costs. More importantly, the treatment of critical illness may not only be painful, but may be frightening as well. In fact, the care of critically ill children can lead to long-term psychological trauma and stress. Therefore, use of appropriate sedation and analgesia can reduce the negative impact of these factors. However, each medication has its own indications and side effects, which must be weighed in terms of benefits and risks for each patient on a case-by-case basis. Used correctly, these medications have incredible benefits. Used incorrectly, or without an appropriate level of caution, they can cause significant harm and even death.

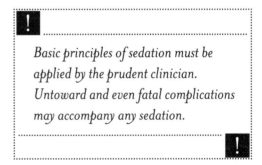

*Basic principles of sedation must be applied by the prudent clinician. Untoward and even fatal complications may accompany any sedation.*

# II. PRE-SEDATION PLANNING

Although different medications may have intrinsic benefits, they can also cause significant harm. Determining the correct medication to use, or avoid, requires careful planning based on the particular patient situation. The overriding goal of any sedation plan should be to use the minimal analgesia or sedation needed to accomplish the therapeutic goal. All patients are different and their responses to any medications can vary. These consequences can be reduced or eliminated by careful assessment and preplanning.

Several questions must be asked before beginning any sedation:

- What is the goal of this sedation?
- What length of sedation is required?
- What complications are possible? Likely?

First, and most importantly: What is the goal of this particular sedation? If only analgesia is needed, the practitioner must determine how long an effect will be required. If the goal is simply to complete a short painful procedure, perhaps the best choice is a short-acting analgesic with minimal or no sedative component. Alternatively, if the procedure requires a prolonged period and is particularly painful or traumatic, perhaps a better choice is a combination of analgesic and sedative medication. What complications are possible? Is the patient at risk of losing the airway during the procedure? If the risk is high, long-acting medications that depress respiration should be avoided, and the practitioner should consider elective intubation before the procedure. If the risk of airway loss is low, a different choice of medications may be made. Is the patient hemodynamically unstable? A radically different choice of medications may be required compared to those used in a patient who is relatively stable. It is recommended that only anesthesiologists or physicians with specialized training perform sedations in hemodynamically unstable patients. Lastly, providers must question themselves and their own skills. What if this child should lose their airway protective reflexes and require an invasive airway? Should a more experienced provider be brought in to help before beginning the sedation? Similarly, how emergent is the procedure? Should an anesthesiologist be performing the sedation? All of these questions must be addressed before any medications are given in order to protect the patient's life and to prevent unnecessary morbidity.

## A. American Society of Anesthesiologists Classification System

The American Society of Anesthesiologists (ASA) Physical Classification System (**Table 20-1**) was developed to classify the severity of illness in patients about to undergo anesthesia. The system has 6 physical status levels, ranging from a healthy individual (ASA PI) to patients who are brain dead (ASA PVI). Although the system is not meant to predict outcomes, it does provide a general assessment of preoperative risk. Most importantly, non-anesthesiologists should be cautious or even avoid electively sedating patients of ASA PIII level and above. Similarly, they should always avoid electively sedating patients of ASA PIV level and above if at all possible.

| Table 20-1 | American Society of Anesthesiologists Classification System |
|---|---|
| **ASA PI:** | Normal healthy patient |
| **ASA PII:** | Mild systemic disease, with no functional limitations |
| **ASA PIII:** | Severe systemic disease which limits activity but is not incapacitating |
| **ASA PIV[a]:** | Incapacitating disease that is a constant threat to life |
| **ASA PV[a]:** | Patients not expected to survive 24 hours with or without an operation |
| **ASA PVI:** | Brain-dead patient being prepared for organ donation |

[a]It is recommended that these patients receive sedation administered by appropriately trained anesthesiologists and intensivists.
Reproduced with permission. © 2008 Macmillan Publishers Ltd. Wilson K. Vital guide to conscious sedation. *Vital.* 2008;5:19-22.

## B. Depth of Sedation

Current classification divides sedation into four levels (**Table 20-2**). The levels are defined by four different parameters corresponding to the presumed "depth" of sedation: responsiveness, airway maintenance, spontaneous respiration, and cardiovascular function. The level of sedation, and the corresponding patient response, is a continuum without clear delineation of transition from 1 level to the next. Likewise, a weight-based drug dosage that provides minimal sedation in 1 patient may cause general anesthesia in another. Similarly, a weight-based dosage that provided minimal sedation to a patient when healthy may cause general anesthesia or cardiovascular collapse in the same patient who develops a critical illness, renal dysfunction, or hepatic failure. For these reasons, providers should attempt to provide the minimum level of sedation required to accomplish the therapeutic goal in each patient. The policy of "start low and go slow" (use low doses and slowly increase as needed) allows the practitioner to titrate to the required, but minimum, level of sedation. While trying to achieve the minimal level, it is also important to use therapeutic dosages. A common mistake is to use sub-therapeutic doses. This results in inadequate sedation but still exposes the patient to potential side effects. A patient can always drift into a deeper than intended level of sedation despite best efforts, and the practitioner must always be prepared to actively manage the airway and ventilation.

## C. Risks of Encountering a Difficult Airway

Anyone performing sedation must be prepared for the patient to lose airway protective reflexes at any time, regardless of the targeted level of sedation. Therefore, the practitioner must always have a plan for advanced airway management in any patient undergoing sedation, as well as the ability and training to execute that plan. For this reason, the provider must attempt to predict how likely any patient is to have a difficult airway prior to administration of any medication. A difficult airway, by definition, is challenging or impossible to maintain by routine or straightforward measures. Any patient, regardless of history, may have a difficult airway. This may result in an increased number of attempts at airway insertion or difficulties with mask ventilation or oxygenation. This cannot be definitively determined until advanced airway management is attempted, but several factors can suggest a high, or at least increased, risk of encountering a difficult airway (**Table 20-3**).

### Table 20-2  Levels of Sedation

| Levels of Sedation | Response | Cardiopulmonary Effects |
|---|---|---|
| Minimal sedation | Normal response to verbal stimulation | Ventilation/airway reflexes intact<br>No cardiovascular effect |
| Moderate sedation/analgesia (formerly conscious sedation) | Responds purposely to verbal commands or to light tactile stimulation | Maintains patient airway, ventilation adequate<br>Minimal cardiovascular effects |
| Deep sedation | Not easily aroused, but responds purposely to repeated or painful stimuli | May require assistance to maintain airway and/or ventilation<br>Cardiovascular function usually maintained |
| General anesthesia | Unconsciousness, unresponsive to physical or verbal commands | Loss of airway reflexes, requires assistance to support ventilation<br>Cardiovascular function may be impaired |

Adapted from Kalinowski M, Wagner HJ. Sedation and pain management in interventional radiology. *C2I2*. 2005;3:14-18.

### Table 20-3  Clinical Conditions and Syndromes Associated with Difficult Airway[a]

- History of difficult intubation
- History of complications with anesthesia
- Family history of difficulty with intubation or anesthesia
- History of obstructive sleep apnea, snoring, tracheomalacia, or laryngomalacia
- Pharyngeal and laryngeal pathology
- Bronchospasm
- Stridor at rest
- Chromosomal abnormalities (trisomy 13, 18, or 21)
- Pierre Robin sequence
- Beckwith-Wiedemann syndrome
- Treacher Collins syndrome
- Micrognathia or retrognathia
- Obesity
- Short neck
- Poor neck extension or fused cervical vertebrae
- High arched palate
- Macroglossia
- Hemifacial microsomia
- Small thyromental or hyomental distance
- Tracheal deviation
- Facial or cervical trauma, mass, or infection
- Trismus
- Mallampati II classification or greater

[a]Bag-valve mask ventilation and/or intubation
Reproduced with permission. © 2002 Wolters Kluwer Health. American Society of Anesthesiologists Task Force on Sedation and Analgesia by Non-Anesthesiologists. Practice guidelines for sedation and analgesia by non-anesthesiologists. *Anesthesiology*. 2002;96:1004-1017.

The Mallampati classification (**Figure 20-1**) is a simple airway assessment technique that involves looking in the patient's open mouth with and without phonation. Higher levels of Mallampati classification are frequently associated with higher grade (level of difficulty) airways found during laryngoscopy. If any features suggestive of a difficult airway are present (**Table 20-3** and **Figure 20-1**), the provider should consider involving an anesthesiologist before sedating a patient, especially if the sedation is elective. In addition, the provider should be familiar with the use of the difficult airway algorithm (**Appendix 8**), regardless of the presence or absence of risk factors. Once a difficult airway is discovered, especially if the patient has received neuromuscular blockade, time is no longer available and a crisis can rapidly ensue. It is far better to plan for a controlled intubation in a patient with a potentially difficult airway than to emergently intubate a child during a procedure.

**Figure 20-1.** Mallampati Classification and Associated Airway Grade

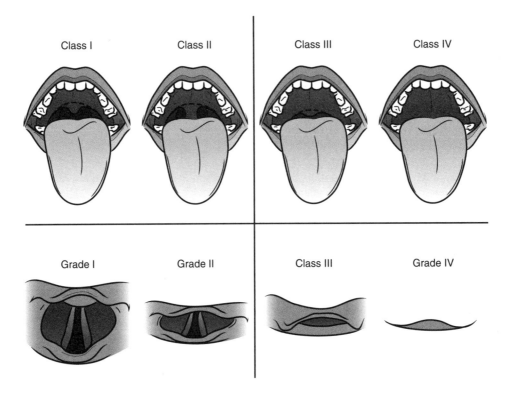

## D. Pre-sedation History

A thorough pre-sedation history should be taken prior to every sedation event to decrease the risk of avoidable complications.

- Does the patient have any history of difficulty with anesthesia? This may include sensitivity to particular drugs, difficulty with obtaining an airway, prolonged effects of anesthesia medications, or any other significant history that may impact safety.

- Is there a history of difficulty with anesthesia or sedation in the parents or other family members? This may uncover common drug allergies or a history suggestive of a difficult airway.

- Is the patient allergic to any drugs that may be given during sedation procedures? Without knowing the history, those medications cannot be avoided.

- Are there other known allergies? This is critical because medications such as propofol cannot be given to people who are allergic to eggs or egg products.

- Have there been any recent illnesses? Especially in elective cases, concurrent upper airway infections can cause prolonged, or difficulties with, ventilation. A positive history may indicate that sedation should not be performed, if possible, until the patient is over the acute illness.

- Does the patient have known renal or hepatic dysfunction? Several medications used in analgesia and sedation utilize liver or kidney metabolism and must be avoided, or have their dosages reduced, in patients with dysfunction.

- Have all available laboratory results been reviewed? Finding a low platelet count or severe coagulopathy after attempted placement of an invasive line can be disastrous.

- Have all imaging studies been reviewed? If the patient is symptomatic because of a large intracranial mass, many drugs should be avoided. Likewise, the presence of a chest mass dictates that even minimal sedation is contraindicated by anyone except a qualified anesthesiologist.

- How long has the patient been fasting? ASA guidelines suggest that patients should have no foods or infant formula 6 hours before sedation. Clear liquids or breast milk can be given up to 4 hours before sedation. The patient should ingest nothing by mouth in the 2 hours before sedation. Vomiting during sedation can turn a routine procedure into a life-threatening event. ASA guidelines apply to elective sedations only. In some situations, emergent sedation may be needed. When the guidelines cannot be followed because of emergent needs, the provider must balance the increased risk of vomiting and aspiration versus the benefit of sedation.

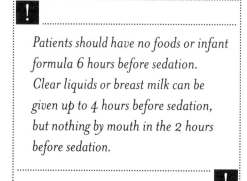

*Patients should have no foods or infant formula 6 hours before sedation. Clear liquids or breast milk can be given up to 4 hours before sedation, but nothing by mouth in the 2 hours before sedation.*

Clearly a small number of targeted questions can avoid a number of life-threatening complications when attempting to provide sedation.

# III. PRE-SEDATION SETUP AND MONITORING

Once a sedation goal has been determined and all risks that can be easily discovered have been found, a successful sedation requires extensive setup before giving any medication. The ASA has carefully defined the minimum equipment and monitoring required prior to any sedation by non-anesthesiologists (**Table 20-4**). Although non-invasive $ETCO_2$ monitoring is only a recommendation, it will signal apnea well before pulse oximetry indicates a fall in $SpO_2$. If all required equipment is not available and set up for use, the sedation induction should not be initiated.

## Table 20-4 Minimal Equipment and Monitoring Necessary for Sedation

Cardiac monitor
- 3- to 5-lead electrocardiography

Pulse oximetry

Respiratory or apnea monitor

$ETCO_2$ monitor

Working access (i.e., peripheral intravenous or central venous line), preferably 2

Resuscitation fluid running (normal saline or lactated Ringer solution)

Oral pharyngeal airway

Nasogastric tube

Bag-mask ventilation
- Appropriate size
- Oxygen flowing

Endotracheal tube
- Correct size
- 1 size larger and 1 size smaller

Drugs appropriate for sedation drawn and labeled

Suction with Yankauer tip, on and running

$ETCO_2$ detector for endotracheal tube placement

Laryngeal mask airway or other backup airway device
- Oral pharyngeal airway
- Nasopharyngeal airway

Laryngoscope blade
- Appropriate size for the child undergoing sedation
- Macintosh or Miller blades

Stylet, size appropriate for endotracheal tube

Reproduced with permission. © 2002 Wolters Kluwer Health. American Society of Anesthesiologists Task Force on Sedation and Analgesia by Non-Anesthesiologists. Practice guidelines for sedation and analgesia by non-anesthesiologists. *Anesthesiology*. 2002;96:1004-1017.

A useful mnemonic for airway equipment setup in all patients is ON BED SCABS:

**O**ral pharyngeal airway

**N**asogastric tube

**B**ag and mask appropriate for this child, with oxygen flowing

**E**ndotracheal tube of appropriate size, 1 size above and 1 size below

**D**rugs appropriate for sedation and reversal, drawn up and labeled

**S**uction on and running with Yankauer tip attached

**C**$O_2$ detector for endotracheal tube placement

**A**lternate airway and alternate plan (i.e., laryngeal mask airway)

**B**lade (laryngoscope) appropriate for this patient, with light working

**S**tylet appropriate for endotracheal tube choice

Or a more familiar mnemonic is SOAPME:

**S**uction

**O**xygen (2 sources)

**A**dvanced airway equipment

**P**harmacy to provide emergency medications and antagonists

**M**onitoring for the level of sedation

**E**quipment for emergency resuscitation

All equipment should be set up for use at bedside and checked before sedation begins. "Nearby" is not close enough and can lead to complications if the equipment and rescue medications are not where they can be immediately used. A conscious effort should be made to administer resuscitation crystalloids (lactated Ringer solution or normal saline) during the procedure so that appropriate boluses can be administered immediately if needed. Likewise, a 3-way stopcock/tap with a 60-mL syringe should be inline so that "pull-push" resuscitation can take place with little loss of time. An adequate amount of fluid should also be prepared so that 20 mL/kg fluid boluses can be immediately administered. No potassium-containing fluids should be in the room as they may be inadvertently used during resuscitation. Lastly, the person monitoring sedation should never be the person performing the procedure. Failure to follow this recommendation can lead to a critical delay in recognizing a change in vital signs requiring immediate intervention. Although this setup may seem excessive to some, planning for every possible contingency can be the difference between life and death in an emergency.

# IV. DRUG ADMINISTRATION DURING SEDATION OR INTUBATION

Medication administration during all sedation and intubation procedures should use a rational and consistent methodology including pre-oxygenation, premedication, sedation, and relaxation.

## A. Pre-oxygenation

Pre-oxygenation is essential for decreasing the risk of hypoxia during intubation or sedation. Not only does this fill all alveoli with oxygen prior to interruption or alteration of ventilation, it also allows for nitrogen washout and maximizes the time available for restoring normal ventilation should that become necessary. Oxygen should be provided, ideally $F_{IO_2}$ 1.0 via face mask, for 3 to 5 minutes before administration of any medications. Oxygen flow should then be maintained throughout the procedure.

## B. Premedication

Premedication of some type is required for most intubations and some sedations. As the term implies, these are medications given before sedatives to optimize sedation, avoid pain, and prevent complications. Selection of premedications is based on the individual patient, clinical situation, and sedation goals determined during pre-sedation planning.

The most common premedication agent is atropine, a vagolytic that can prevent bradycardia induced by sudden increases in vagal tone. These sudden increases may occur during laryngoscopy, airway manipulation, or with increased airway secretions. Most infants maintain cardiac output via an increase in heart rate rather than an increase in stroke volume. Therefore, any drop in heart rate, especially in unstable patients, may result in a catastrophic drop in cardiac output. Because atropine also has drying properties, it prevents secretions from entering the airway during the sedation, possibly decreasing the incidence of micro-aspiration as well as the occurrence of laryngospasm. Atropine, 0.02 mg/kg, should be considered in all infants younger than 1 year. It should never be given below the minimum dose of 0.1 mg as it can cause paradoxical bradycardia. Atropine should also be given prior to the use of succinylcholine as it frequently causes an increase in vagal tone. Glycopyrrolate (4 µg/kg) decreases secretions to a level similar to that of atropine without consequent central nervous system (CNS) effects. It should be considered in all patients undergoing sedation especially when using drugs (such as ketamine) that increase oral or airway secretions.

Analgesia is frequently required as a premedication. This is especially important before painful procedures where sedatives without analgesia (i.e., propofol) are used. Laryngoscopy should be considered a painful procedure; the insertion of a laryngoscope is known to cause transient increased intracranial pressure (ICP). Fentanyl (1 µg/kg) is a good first-line choice because of its rapid onset, short duration, and relatively benign effect on myocardial activity.

Lastly, intravenous (IV) lidocaine (1 mg/kg) is known to blunt the transient increases in ICP that occur with laryngoscopy and should be considered for premedication in all patients with presumed or known intracranial pathology. Although its mechanism is unclear, lidocaine administration before laryngoscopy is considered the standard of care in patients with elevated ICP. IV lidocaine can also suppress the cough reflex and mitigate bronchospasm, and may therefore be beneficial for intubation of the asthmatic patient. Lidocaine is an antiarrhythmic medication, and its benefits must be weighed against potential side effects in each individual patient.

## C. Sedation

After premedication, the sedative chosen during pre-sedation planning can be given. There are numerous medications, each of which has advantages and disadvantages. All medications given for sedation should have a rapid onset, relatively short duration of action, and minimal side effects. As several of the choices can cause vasodilation (i.e., benzodiazepines, propofol, and barbiturates), adequate intravascular volume must be assured before administration. Similarly, isotonic fluids should be immediately available for resuscitation in the event of a rapid drop in blood pressure. Other medications (i.e., benzodiazepines and barbiturates) can cause myocardial depression and should be avoided in patients with marginal cardiac output or shock. Medications that have no intrinsic analgesia (i.e., propofol) must be used in conjunction with adequate analgesia for painful procedures. Lastly, medications with unique side-effect profiles (i.e., ketamine) should only be used after considering the consequences of those side effects in a given patient. There are usually several appropriate choices in every clinical scenario. The agent selected is dependent on the relative balance of positive and negative effects it may, or will, have on a particular patient in a specific situation.

## D. Neuromuscular Blockade

Skeletal muscle relaxation, or neuromuscular blockade (NMB), may or may not be required depending on the clinical situation. These agents may be needed to ensure that the patient remains motionless during a critical procedure, to prevent vocal cord damage during intubation, or to allow ventilation in problematic situations. When needed, these medications have no substitute, but they can also be lethal. If advanced airway management cannot be assured, NMB must be avoided until the airway is secured. In some patients – for example, those with an anterior chest mass – NMB is specifically contraindicated. Each of the paralytic agents has a specific indication and side-effect profile. Careful consideration of the patient, the clinical goal, and the potential side effects of each medication is needed during pre-sedation planning. The dangers associated with these medications cannot be overstated.

# V. SPECIFIC SEDATIVE AND ANALGESIC MEDICATION SIDE EFFECTS AND CONTRAINDICATIONS

Every drug used for sedation and analgesia has a specific indication, side-effect profile, and contraindication. Knowledge of these factors is essential before, during, and after a procedure. The risks and benefits of each medication should be weighed during pre-sedation planning, and the agent chosen should be individualized to each patient and clinical situation. Failure to do so can result in avoidable morbidity and death. This overview is not meant to be all inclusive but rather to highlight aspects of several commonly used medications (**Appendix 7**).

## A. Nonsteroidal Anti-inflammatory Drugs

Nonsteroidal anti-inflammatory drugs (NSAIDs) are highly effective analgesics with numerous applications in clinical practice. All of these medications block inflammation by inhibition of cyclo-oxygenase pathways. In most cases, it is this reduction in inflammation that relieves pain rather than a direct inhibition of pain perception or pain fiber transmission. Because these medications are anti-inflammatory agents, they are also powerful antipyretics. The combination of these effects makes NSAIDs highly desirable in the treatment of postoperative pain. Because they do not cause respiratory depression, constipation, or itching, they are a near-perfect primary or adjunct medication in the treatment of moderate to severe pain. However, several side effects of these drugs limit their usefulness. First, most NSAIDs can inhibit platelet function either directly or indirectly, leading to an increased risk of perioperative and gastric bleeding. In addition, they can cause, or contribute to, renal failure in patients with preexisting renal insufficiency or other predisposing factors, such as concomitant nephrotoxic medications, liver dysfunction, or heart failure. NSAIDs should be used with caution in these patients. For most patients, the use or addition of NSAIDs to nearly every pain regimen will increase pain control and decrease the dosage of other agents needed to treat that pain.

Aspirin (salicylic acid) was the first NSAID developed. Although an effective agent, its use (5 to 10 mg/kg) in most pediatric patients is discouraged secondary to the increased risk of Reye syndrome in those with concurrent viral illness. The "side effect" of platelet inhibition is now the primary reason that aspirin is prescribed. It is the first choice for a daily oral medication for mild anticoagulation in patients at risk for thrombosis, including children.

Acetaminophen/paracetamol (15 mg/kg) is the most commonly used NSAID in pediatric patients. It differs from most NSAIDs in that it is a poor anti-inflammatory agent peripherally, but a powerful anti-inflammatory agent centrally. This makes acetaminophen an ideal antipyretic agent in children because it does not have the associated bleeding and nephrotoxic risks associated with other NSAIDs. In addition, it also appears to have direct central pain-reducing effects independent of its anti-inflammatory properties. Therefore, acetaminophen/paracetamol can be used in conjunction with other NSAIDs to improve pain and fever control via multiple pathways. In hospitalized patients, acetaminophen/paracetamol is now available in oral, rectal, and IV formulations.

Ibuprofen (10 mg/kg) is used frequently to treat fever and pain in children. It is available in several liquid oral preparations, which make it particularly useful in children. It is also available as an IV preparation, primarily used for the closure of a patent ductus arteriosus.

Naproxen is another oral NSAID effective in treating postoperative pain. It has a longer half-life than ibuprofen and is given every 12 hours instead of every 6 hours. It is a useful alternative to ibuprofen but is not available in as many different preparations. In addition, no IV formulation is available, which limits its clinical use.

Ketorolac is a powerful NSAID available in both IV and oral formulations. It has been shown effective in the treatment of postoperative pain even in the absence of adjunctive medications. Concerns of hypersensitivity, renal failure, and increased bleeding in patients younger than 16 years of age have limited its use in pediatrics. However, administration for less than 5 days in patients with no other contraindications to NSAID use is generally accepted as safe, even in the youngest patients.

## B. Opioids

Narcotics are used frequently to prevent pain. All narcotics have similar mechanisms of action. The opioids work as agonists at 3 primary opioid receptors: mu, kappa, and delta. Each medication blocks transmission of pain fiber signals to the brain and thereby prevents the sensation of pain. In choosing the appropriate narcotic agent to use, the practitioner must first determine the clinical goal:

- Is the agent going to be used for short- or long-term pain management?
- Will a continuous infusion be required, or will intermittent dosing be sufficient?
- Are there specific patient factors to consider?

Morphine (0.05 to 0.1 mg/kg) is a good general purpose analgesic. It has a relatively long half-life (2 hours) in most children, but this can increase significantly in small or immature infants. Morphine is metabolized in the liver to generate active metabolites, which are excreted in the urine. For these reasons, morphine must be used cautiously in patients with hepatic or renal dysfunction. Morphine is known to cause vasodilation and hypotension in an immunoglobulin E-independent fashion and should be used with caution in patients with asthma. Additionally, many patients will complain of urticaria due to the associated histamine release. Morphine is also known to cause cardiac depression and should not be used in patients with low cardiac output or shock. Like all narcotics, morphine can cause significant respiratory depression by decreasing minute ventilation and blunting the CNS response to carbon dioxide. Overall, morphine is a good choice for intermittent or patient-controlled analgesia in patients with significant pain. Accumulation of active metabolites and poor clearance in small infants makes it a less desirable agent for continuous infusion in such children.

Fentanyl (1 to 2 µg/kg) is a synthetic opioid with rapid onset (90 seconds) and clearance ($t_{1/2}$ 30 minutes), but it is stored in fat and can have a significantly longer half-life in obese children. It is 100 times more powerful than morphine and must be used at a correspondingly lower dose. Fentanyl is inactivated by the liver and should be used with caution in patients with significant hepatopathy. Like all narcotics, fentanyl causes respiratory depression. Although it does not cause significant myocardial depression, it can cause moderate bradycardia, especially when used with muscle relaxation agents. Unlike morphine, fentanyl does not cause histamine release and is therefore a better choice than morphine for patients with asthma or hypotension. Practitioners should be aware of "rigid chest phenomenon," which can make ventilation difficult or impossible without muscle relaxation. This only occurs with rapid administration and therefore rapid bolus dosing should never be employed. This phenomenon can be reversed by paralysis with NMB, but advanced airway management will be required. Fentanyl does not react with most other medications and is therefore a good choice for continuous infusion analgesia. In addition, its fast onset makes it an excellent choice for rapid sequence intubation or induction.

> *Very significant respiratory depression and hypotension can occur in patients who receive narcotics and benzodiazepines simultaneously.*

Meperidine (pethidine) (0.5 mg/kg) is a synthetic opioid with approximately one-tenth the activity of morphine. It has numerous CNS side effects, including seizures and muscle tremors. For these reasons, it should be avoided when other options are available. In addition, it should not be used as a continuous infusion because of active metabolite accumulation, especially in patients with renal dysfunction.

Methadone (0.1 mg/kg) is frequently used to prevent narcotic withdrawal but can also be used for chronic or intractable pain. It has an extremely long, but frequently variable, half-life (19 hours) and is available in both IV and oral forms. In very small children, the volume per dose in the IV form can be extremely small. Because of its long half-life, the sedative effects of any particular dosage may not be fully appreciated for 1 or 2 days; therefore, its dosage must be adjusted very slowly and the effect of that dosage change must be followed ≥24 hours. For these reasons, methadone should be considered in the prevention of narcotic withdrawal, primarily in its oral form, and caution should be used in very small children. There are better choices for "as needed" pain relief and short-term analgesia.

Codeine (0.5 to 1 mg/kg) is frequently used as an alternative to morphine in patients who can take medications by mouth. It is a synthetic narcotic with approximately one-tenth the potency of morphine. It is rarely given IV as it has led to cardiovascular collapse in some case reports. Its primary usage should remain as an oral, first-line analgesic with intermittent dosing.

Hydrocodone is a synthetic opioid similar to codeine. It appears to be slightly more powerful than codeine, but it is less active than morphine. It is used to alleviate moderate to severe pain in patients who can take oral medications. Like codeine, it can be used as a first-line analgesic with intermittent dosing.

Tramadol, a synthetic opioid available in both oral (1 mg/kg) and IV forms, binds to opioid receptors and blocks pain transmission using the same mechanism of action that all narcotics do. However, it also blocks the effect of the pain-modifying neurotransmitters serotonin and norepinephrine. It is rarely used in pediatrics in the United States as it is not recommended by the Food and Drug Administration in patients younger than 16 years. Tramadol is also known to cause seizures and to lower seizure thresholds in patients who have epilepsy or are taking neuroleptics. For this reason, it must be avoided in these patients. Tramadol is habit forming and will cause respiratory depression if recommended dosing is exceeded.

## C. Benzodiazepines

Benzodiazepines are the most commonly used sedatives in critical care. All benzodiazepines increase CNS gamma-aminobutyric acid (GABA) receptor activity causing global CNS depression and consequently sedation. They are excellent first-choice sedatives in clinical situations ranging from anxiolysis to deep sedation. They are also useful anticonvulsants and potent amnestics. However, like opioids, benzodiazepines cause dose-dependent respiratory depression. Unlike opioids, benzodiazepines blunt both hypoxic and hypercarbic respiratory drive. The concurrent use of benzodiazepines and narcotics can result in a profound depression of respiratory drive secondary to the synergistic effect of these medications. This respiratory depression is much more severe than the predicted effect of cumulative doses for the 2 agents when used independently. In addition, some benzodiazepines can cause substantial myocardial depression and would be contraindicated in patients with borderline cardiac output or shock. As with the narcotics, the appropriate benzodiazepine choice requires a careful assessment of the patient's condition and the clinical goals:

*Appropriate benzodiazepine selection requires a careful assessment of the patient's condition and clinical goals:*
- *Is the agent going to be used for short- or long-term sedation?*
- *Will a continuous infusion be required or will intermittent boluses be sufficient?*
- *Are there specific patient factors to consider?*

- Is the agent going to be used for short- or long-term sedation?

- Will a continuous infusion be required or will intermittent boluses be sufficient?

- Are there specific patient factors to consider?

Midazolam (0.1 mg/kg) is one of the most common benzodiazepines used. It has a rapid onset and relatively short half-life (2 hours). It has extensive metabolism in the liver and is eliminated in the urine. It should be used cautiously in patients with renal or hepatic dysfunction as its half-life can be profoundly increased. Midazolam is a good choice for anxiolysis and long-term sedation by continuous infusion. In addition, it can be titrated rapidly to treat refractory seizures. Midazolam appears to cause the least amount of cardiac depression of the benzodiazepine family and is the best choice of a GABA-nergic agent in patients with unclear cardiac output.

Lorazepam (0.1 mg/kg) has a slower onset than midazolam but has an extremely long half-life (14 hours). For this reason, it is a first-line agent for stopping seizures (**Chapter 15**) and is often used for prolonged sedation. Like midazolam, it undergoes significant liver metabolism and is cleared by the kidneys. With its long half-life, it is a poor choice for use in patients with liver or renal failure. In addition, it is felt to cause more significant cardiac depression than midazolam and should be avoided in patients with persistent shock or low cardiac output. Lorazepam may work well for intermittent dosing in patients requiring long-term sedation. However, it is formulated with propylene glycol and can cause significant lactic acidosis if used for an extended period, especially as a continuous infusion. In addition, its numerous interactions with other medications make it a poor choice for a continuous infusion.

Diazepam (0.2 mg/kg) has an extremely long half-life. It is extensively metabolized in the liver and should not be used in patients with hepatic or renal failure. Like lorazepam, it is also formulated with propylene glycol and may cause pain with peripheral IV administration and contribute to lactic acidosis. For these reasons, diazepam is best used as an oral agent, primarily in the amelioration of benzodiazepine withdrawal.

## D. Barbiturates

Barbiturates are used much less frequently now than in the past because several agents with less significant side-effect profiles are available. However, barbiturates can be ideal agents in some clinical situations, especially with head injury, elevated ICP, and refractory seizures. All barbiturates are powerful GABA agonists, inducing global CNS depression and concomitant decreased cerebral perfusion. These agents can cause profound respiratory depression and the need for advanced airway management should be anticipated whenever they are used. All barbiturates cause cardiac depression as well as vasodilation and should never be used in patients with decreased cardiac output, shock, or volume depletion. Individuals with minimal cardiac reserve may become profoundly hypotensive after only a single dose.

Phenobarbital (loading dose of 20 mg/kg, which may be given in divided doses; maintenance dosing, 5 mg/kg/day divided every 12 h) is frequently used as a third-line agent in the control of refractory seizures. However, it is a second-line agent in patients with refractory seizures who are younger than 6 months due to their immature hepatic metabolism (**Chapter 15**). Phenobarbital has a relatively slow onset but a very long half-life (24 to 96 h). Its clinical use should be restricted to the treatment of refractory seizures, treatment of barbiturate dependence, or as an adjunct in difficult-to-sedate patients who are hemodynamically stable.

Pentobarbital (1 mg/kg) is a fourth-line agent used in the treatment of refractory seizures, usually with the clinical intention of temporary coma induction. It has a half-life of nearly 20 hours, and continuous infusion requires advanced cerebral monitoring such as bispectral index or continuous electroencephalography. It can cause neutrophil inactivation and associated increased infectious risks, as well as profound myocardial depression and should only be used with continuous arterial pressure monitoring. Midazolam infusions have supplanted pentobarbital usage to a large extent, but pentobarbital can still be considered for intubation induction in patients with elevated ICP or for maintenance of medical coma.

## E. Propofol

Propofol (bolus dose, 1-2 mg/kg; continuous infusion, 50-150 µg/kg/min) is an extremely useful short-term medication that avoids many of the problems associated with other drugs described above. Propofol is unrelated to other general use anesthetics but appears to manifest its activity through the potentiation of CNS GABA receptors, similar to benzodiazepines and barbiturates. Propofol has an extremely rapid onset, is cleared quickly by the liver, and exhibits very little respiratory depression, making it ideal for short procedures or anesthesia induction. However, like all medications, propofol has several properties which need to be carefully considered during pre-sedation planning. First, it is compounded in a mixture that contains both egg and soybean products, so it cannot be administered to patients with these allergies. Second, propofol induces vasodilation and significant hypotension in dehydrated patients; therefore, it should never be used in under-resuscitated patients, patients with shock, or those with questionable cardiac output. Third, propofol has been associated with myoclonic movements at low doses but, interestingly, is an effective adjuvant in the treatment of refractory seizures. Fourth, propofol has no intrinsic analgesic properties and must be used in conjunction with narcotics, such as fentanyl, for painful procedures. Lastly, an increased risk of propofol infusion syndrome is associated with long-term use and high doses. This syndrome causes refractory lactic acidosis, cardiac arrhythmia, and hypotension, likely caused by mitochondrial "poisoning." It is possibly not reversible.

Propofol is still an excellent drug in several clinical situations. It is ideal for short procedures in relatively healthy individuals (i.e., setting/reduction of isolated fractures and central line placement) in conjunction with low-dose narcotics. It should also be considered in the initial treatment of refractory status epilepticus. Similarly, it is an excellent intubation induction agent in patients with traumatic brain injury after adequate resuscitation. Practitioners using propofol should have training and experience in its administration, as well as expertise in airway management, as it may cause profound hypotension, transient apnea, and rapid induction of general anesthesia.

## F. Ketamine

Ketamine (1-2 mg/kg IV, 3-4 mg/kg intramuscularly) has several properties that make it an ideal agent in certain clinical scenarios. It is an N-methyl-D-aspartate antagonist providing both analgesia and sedation while preserving both blood pressure and respiratory status. It is metabolized by the liver and is secreted with its metabolites in the urine. It has a rapid onset and is quickly eliminated. Ketamine is a powerful sialagogue and may require concurrent use of an anticholinergic agent (i.e., glycopyrrolate or atropine) to prevent laryngospasm. In addition, its profound dissociative properties and resultant emergence phenomenon may require concurrent usage of low-dose benzodiazepines, such as midazolam.

Ketamine can lower seizure thresholds and should be used with caution in patients with known seizure disorders. Although it has been reported to cause a transient rise in ICP during infusion, recent studies suggest that it may in fact decrease ICP without lowering blood pressure and therefore maintain cerebral perfusion pressure. These studies suggest that ketamine may be safe to use in patients with both traumatic brain injury and intracranial hypertension. Ketamine will also cause a transient rise in catecholamine release, which is useful in the maintenance of blood pressure. In addition, this catecholamine surge results in direct $\beta_2$ stimulation and consequent bronchodilation. Its airway preserving properties, along with its $\beta_2$-stimulation properties, make it an excellent choice for sedation in asthmatic patients. However, its increased α- and β-1 stimulation contraindicate its use in patients with hypertension. Lastly, ketamine is felt to be a negative inotrope and requires its catecholamine surge to maintain blood pressure; failure to recognize this principle can lead to profound hypotension in catecholamine-depleted patients, such as those with catecholamine refractory septic shock.

> *Ketamine is the drug of choice for intubating patients with acute severe asthma or septic shock.*

Ketamine should be considered as a first-line agent for intubation of children with asthma and as both short- and long-term sedation in those children. It is also an ideal agent for short, painful procedures in patients with potentially difficult airways but stable respiratory status.

## G. Dexmedetomidine

Dexmedetomidine is an IV, selective, $\alpha_2$-adrenergic receptor agonist. It is similar in activity to clonidine and works as a sympatholytic at both central and peripheral receptors. It directly inhibits norepinephrine/noradrenaline release and produces both analgesia and sedation. It has a rapid onset and is quickly metabolized by the liver to inactive metabolites. Dexmedetomidine has minimal respiratory depression but does slightly decrease heart rate and blood pressure secondary to its sympatholytic activity. Dexmedetomidine must be given by continuous infusion or slow bolus as it can cause transient hypertension due to antagonism of $\alpha_1$ receptors if given too quickly. It should never be given to patients taking atrioventricular nodal blockers, patients with bradycardia, hypovolemia, or poor cardiac output as it could worsen those conditions by depleting endogenous catecholamines. With these considerations in mind, dexmedetomidine is being used more often in pediatrics as a first-line sedative medication that preserves respiratory function well.

# VI. SIDE EFFECTS AND CONTRAINDICATIONS OF SPECIFIC NEUROMUSCULAR BLOCKING AGENTS

NMB agents are indispensable in several critical care situations. Skeletal muscle paralysis can prevent vocal cord damage during intubation, maintain absolute immobility during critical procedures, and allow ventilation of patients who cannot be ventilated using deep sedation alone. However, relaxation agents are 100% lethal if advanced airway management cannot be assured. For this reason, if the provider is not completely certain of their ability to maintain a patient's airway after paralysis, relaxation agents should never be given. In addition, NMB does not prevent pain transmission and would cause significant terror and stress in an undersedated patient. For these reasons, paralytics should never be used without adequate concomitant sedation and analgesia. Lastly, non-depolarizing NMB agents, especially in conjunction with steroid usage, can cause a prolonged polyneuropathy of critical illness. This can significantly extend hospitalization and increase morbidity.

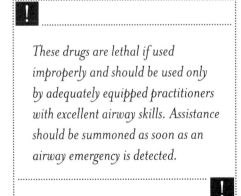

*These drugs are lethal if used improperly and should be used only by adequately equipped practitioners with excellent airway skills. Assistance should be summoned as soon as an airway emergency is detected.*

## A. Depolarizing Agents

NMB medications can be classified into two large groups based on their activity at the neuromuscular junction (NMJ). Depolarizing agents open sodium channels at the post-synaptic membrane and cause rapid membrane depolarization, which prevents further neuromuscular transmission. Once the membrane is depolarized, acetylcholine can no longer propagate action potentials throughout the muscle, inducing paralysis.

Succinylcholine (1 mg/kg IV, 3 mg/kg intramuscularly) is the only depolarizing NMB agent in use today. It is an extremely rapid-acting agent (<1 minute) and is completely metabolized by cholinesterases in minutes, independent of liver and kidney function. Its mechanism of action results in a brief period of fasciculation followed by flaccid paralysis. Fasciculation can be blocked by concurrent administration of a partial dose of a non-depolarizing NMB agent. Although its rapid action and short duration are highly desirable, succinylcholine has several side effects which can be significant:

- Malignant hyperthermia
- Rhabdomyolysis
- Bradycardia
- Hyperkalemia
- Increased intraocular pressure
- Increased ICP

For these reasons, its use is contraindicated in most traumas, neuromuscular disorders, and in cases of elevated ICP, glaucoma, significant acidosis, or metabolic derangement. Outside of these conditions, it is an excellent agent, but it should not be used indiscriminately.

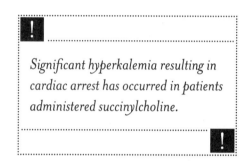

*Significant hyperkalemia resulting in cardiac arrest has occurred in patients administered succinylcholine.*

## B. Non-depolarizing Agents

Unlike the depolarizing agents, the non-depolarizing muscle agents block acetylcholine by binding to its receptor. In this manner, they prevent transmission at the NMJ and induce paralysis until they are metabolized. All non-depolarizing agents have a slower onset than succinylcholine and require a significantly longer period for reversal.

Rocuronium (1 mg/kg) has the fastest onset of all non-depolarizing agents at 1 to 2 minutes. It also has the shortest duration of action at about 30 minutes. Although rocuronium is primarily metabolized by the liver, its effects can be prolonged in patients with renal disease. Due to its short duration of action, rocuronium is a poor choice for long-term paralysis, but the best substitute for succinylcholine when short-term paralysis is needed (i.e., during intubation).

Vecuronium (0.1 mg/kg) provides longer NMB when prolonged paralysis is needed. Vecuronium requires about 60 minutes for reversal, but a single dose may last several hours in infants. Clearance is significantly reduced in patients with liver disease, and renal dysfunction may also compromise its clearance. Vecuronium is probably the best non-depolarizing agent for long-term, continuous sedation.

Pancuronium (0.1-0.15 mg/kg) is the longest acting non-depolarizing agent still in clinical use. A single dose can cause paralysis for more than 2 hours. Like rocuronium and vecuronium, pancuronium clearance is significantly reduced in patients with liver and kidney disease. Unfortunately, the benefits of its long duration of action are outweighed by its vagolytic properties. Pancuronium causes significant tachycardia, which may not be well tolerated in some patients. In light of these considerations, pancuronium is probably only a good choice when vecuronium is not available.

Atracurium (0.5 mg/kg) and cisatracurium (0.1 mg/kg) are clinically useful non-depolarizing agents that are cleared by Hoffman degradation and can be used safely in patients with renal or hepatic failure. Atracurium can cause significant histamine release with resultant hypotension and must be avoided in patients with allergies or asthma. This side effect is greatly attenuated in cisatracurium, which can be considered as a paralytic agent in patients with significant hepatopathy or renal failure.

# VII. REVERSAL AGENTS

Few drugs are available that can reverse the effects of sedative, analgesic, or neuromuscular blocking agents. However, some agents can decrease morbidity or mortality in various clinical situations. They should be immediately available during any sedation, but their usage must be tempered by clinical context.

Naloxone (0.1 mg/kg per dose, up to 2 mg) is a specific antagonist for all opiates. Its action is almost immediate as it displaces opiates from their receptors. All opioid effects are reduced simultaneously at high doses, including respiratory depression and analgesia. At lower doses, naloxone may reverse only respiratory depression and spare analgesia. However, since the medication is usually only given in an emergency, there may not be time available to titrate inadequate dosing. Naloxone's half-life is much shorter than that of most narcotics, and it may need to be re-dosed intermittently until the patient can clear all residual narcotics from the bloodstream. In fact, long-acting narcotics usually require naloxone to be given as a continuous infusion over a prolonged period. Naloxone can be used as an emergency room diagnostic in patients with depressed mental status and poor respiratory effort. When a full reversal dose is given to patients with narcotic overdose, no doubt will remain regarding effect. However, the primary use of naloxone is to reverse narcotic-induced respiratory depression and spare a patient intubation.

Flumazenil (flumazepil), a specific antagonist of benzodiazepines, has a relatively long half-life, approximately 1 hour, but hepatic failure can greatly increase this. Flumazenil completely reverses both the sedative effects and respiratory depression associated with benzodiazepine overdose. Unlike naloxone, flumazenil has several side effects that make it an undesirable medication choice in almost every situation. First, and most importantly, it can trigger seizures in patients with known, or even unknown, seizure disorders. If the patient seizes after flumazenil is given, those seizures cannot be stopped by benzodiazepines, and they may even become refractory to second- and third-line medications as well. Second, flumazenil can cause difficult to control arrhythmias, tachycardia, and hypertension. Lastly, flumazenil can unmask the effects of tricyclic antidepressant overdose associated with polypharmacy overdose. For all of these reasons, flumazenil should never be used diagnostically for benzodiazepine overdose in any situation. In fact, due to its myriad and severe complications, flumazenil should probably be avoided even in known benzodiazepine overdose. The safer alternative would be to support the patient's airway until the benzodiazepines are cleared. The only exception to this would be a patient with respiratory failure and known benzodiazepine overdose who cannot be ventilated or oxygenated by advanced airway maneuvers.

Non-depolarizing NMB agents can also be reversed to some extent, although not directly, as opioids and benzodiazepines. Since non-depolarizing agents work by antagonizing acetylcholine binding to the NMJ, high doses of anticholinesterases, such as neostigmine (0.025-0.1 mg/kg/dose), can be used to reverse their effect. However, neostigmine will increase acetylcholine levels at muscarinic receptors as well as the NMJ. In the high doses of neostigmine given to reverse blockade, the patient would exhibit symptoms of acetylcholinesterase toxicity (increased salivation, hyperpyrexia, miosis, and bradycardia) if given without an anticholinergic agent. Either atropine or glycopyrrolate can be given concurrently with neostigmine reversal doses to prevent these side effects. A variable amount of time is required to reverse paralysis by non-depolarizing agents depending on the percent of acetylcholine receptors occupied by the blocking agent. Therefore, the practitioner must determine that the patient is breathing spontaneously, without assistance, before attempting to remove any advanced airway devices. The method used to reverse non-depolarizing agents will not work with succinylcholine as it has a different mechanism of action. However, it is cleared so rapidly that a reversal agent is usually not needed. This is touted as one of the benefits of succinylcholine, in addition to rapid onset, as compared to non-depolarizing agents.

## VIII. TACHYPHYLAXIS AND IATROGENIC WITHDRAWAL

Tachyphylaxis describes the phenomenon of decreased drug effectiveness as it is used for longer periods of time. This is usually the result of increased drug metabolism or downregulation of the receptor of interest. Most medications exhibit this effect, and each patient will respond differently. Infusion rates or dosages required to obtain adequate levels of sedation and analgesia should be expected to increase the longer the patient is exposed to a drug. In fact, tachyphylaxis can be so significant that the practitioner must add agents to an already complicated drug regimen to achieve the desired clinical goal. This is especially important in the continuously paralyzed patient, as sedation and analgesia levels may become inadequate while the patient is still paralyzed. This would result in an awake, paralyzed patient with significant pain.

## IX. OPIOID AND BENZODIAZEPINE WITHDRAWAL

### A. Pharmacologic Strategies

Opioid and benzodiazepine withdrawal syndromes should be anticipated in all patients requiring ≥5 days of therapy, particularly when synthetic opioids have been administered as a continuous infusion. A long-acting agent, such as lorazepam, can be started 1 to 2 days before anticipated extubation to prevent withdrawal to benzodiazepines; the midazolam infusion can be tapered and stopped gradually once the child is close to extubation. Likewise, methadone can be started at a dosage that approximates the opioid equivalent (while also accounting for pharmacokinetic differences between the 2 agents). It may be initially administered at intervals of 6 hours for approximately 1 day and subsequently decreased to longer intervals. Smaller doses are often effective with careful titration and consultation with a pediatric intensivist or pain specialist. Although methadone is given in 3 to 4 divided doses the first day, the dosing interval is gradually increased and the total daily dose is tapered to avoid drug accumulation.

Lorazepam and methadone are usually tapered on an individualized basis over several days to weeks, depending on the duration of previous treatment with benzodiazepines and opioids, with the goal of preventing physiologically significant complications of withdrawal, such as agitation, seizures, tachycardia, hypertension, diarrhea, and vomiting. Recovery from critical illness and its associated psychological derangements is also expedited by appropriately tapering these agents.

## B. Nonpharmacologic Strategies to Control Agitation

The pediatric intensive care unit environment may be very upsetting to patients and their families. Units that allow privacy, continuous access to a supportive parent, and controlled sound and lighting may decrease anxiety in young patients. Likewise, promotion of a circadian rhythm by encouraging exposure to sunlight during the day and quiet, dark conditions at night may minimize the need to escalate drug therapy. Child life specialists can be very helpful in distracting and entertaining patients in ways that permit reduced doses or brief daytime holidays from opioid and sedative infusions.

## Key Points: Sedation, Analgesia, and Neuromuscular Blockade

- Sedation, analgesia, and neuromuscular blockade are necessary in caring for critically ill patients but, if used improperly, they can cause significant morbidity or mortality.

- Many of the risks associated with sedation, analgesia, and neuromuscular blockade can be eliminated or reduced by careful pre-sedation planning and preparation.

- Drug choices should be made based on the clinical goals and the individual patient. No drug or drug combination is ideal in all situations.

- Each drug has its own side effects and contraindications which must be carefully weighed against the clinical goals the practitioner is trying to achieve.

- A more experienced practitioner should be called for support before initiating sedation if the clinician is uncertain about the ability to maintain an airway, and to ventilate and oxygenate a patient.

- Always "start low and go slow" when choosing the sedation level.

- Clinicians should recognize their own limitations and not initiate sedation when uncomfortable with any patient or scenario. Likewise, they should not use an agent or combination of agents unless confident in doing so.

- Tachyphylaxis should be anticipated with all agents, and dosages should be adjusted for each patient at any time.

# Suggested Readings

1. Bar-Joseph G, Guilburd Y, Tamir A, Guilburd JN. Effectiveness of ketamine in decreasing intracranial pressure in children with intracranial hypertension. *J Neurosurg Pediatr.* 2009; 4:40-46.

2. Cook DR. Neuromuscular blocking agents. In: Fuhrman BP, Zimmerman J, eds. *Pediatric Critical Care.* Philadelphia, PA: Mosby Elsevier; 2006:1729-1747.

3. Heard CMB, Fletcher JE. Sedation and analgesia. In: Fuhrman BP, Zimmerman J, eds. *Pediatric Critical Care.* Philadelphia, PA: Mosby Elsevier; 2006:1748-1779.

4. Kraemer FW, Rose JB. Pharmacologic management of acute pediatric pain. *Anesthesiol Clin.* 2009;27:241-268.

5. Playfor S, Jenkins I, Boyles C, et al; United Kingdom Paediatric Intensive Care Society Sedation; Analgesia and Neuromuscular Blockade Working Group. Consensus guidelines on sedation and analgesia in critically ill children. *Intensive Care Med.* 2006;32:1125-1136.

6. Practice advisory for preanesthesia evaluation: a report by the American Society of Anesthesiologists Task Force on Preanesthesia Evaluation. *Anesthesiology.* 2002;96:485-496.

7. Practice guidelines for management of the difficult airway: an updated report by the American Society of Anesthesiologists Task Force on Management of the Difficult Airway. *Anesthesiology.* 2003;98:1269-1277.

8. Practice guidelines for preoperative fasting and the use of pharmacologic agents to reduce the risk of pulmonary aspiration: application to healthy patients undergoing elective procedures: an updated report by the American Society of Anesthesiologists Committee on Standards and Practice Parameters. *Anesthesiology.* 2011;114:495-511.

9. Practice guidelines for sedation and analgesia by non-anesthesiologists. American Society of Anesthesiologists Task Force on Sedation and Analgesia by Non-Anesthesiologists. *Anesthesiology.* 2002;96:1004-1017.

10. Weingart SD, Levitan RM. Preoxygenation and prevention of desaturation during emergency airway management. *Ann Emerg Med.* 2012;59:165-175.

11. Yaster M, Easley RB, Brady KM. Pain and sedation management in the critically ill child. In: Nichols DG, ed. *Rogers' Textbook of Pediatric Intensive Care.* Philadelphia, PA: Lippincott Williams and Wilkins; 2008:136-165.

Chapter 21

# INVASIVE MEDICAL DEVICES

## ✓ Objectives

- Describe the distinguishing characteristics of various tubes and catheters.
- Compare various age-specific catheter and tube sizes that may be utilized.
- Recognize indications for the implementation of various devices.
- Diagnose potential complications associated with the use of invasive medical devices.

## 📁 Case Study

A 3-month-old male infant with a history of prematurity and placement of a tracheostomy tube, transpyloric feeding tube, and Broviac catheter (C.R. Bard, Inc.) when he was a newborn is brought to the emergency department by his parents after the feeding tube is dislodged and redness and green-colored drainage is seen at the central venous catheter insertion site. The child is irritable, febrile, and tachypneic with increased work of breathing.

**Detection**
- What is this child's physiologic status?
- What are the most likely and the most severe possible diagnoses?

**Intervention**
- Which of the presenting diagnoses need immediate intervention?
- What are the priorities of further assessment and management?
- What additional studies would you like to perform during this patient's evaluation?

**Reassessment**
- Is the current treatment strategy effective?
- Does the patient need cultures to be sent, antibiotic coverage, and/or other therapeutic interventions?

**Effective Communication**
- When the patient's clinical status changes, who needs to know and how will this information be disseminated?
- Where is the best place to manage the care of this patient?

**Teamwork**
- How are you going to implement the treatment strategy?
- Who is to do what and when?

# I. INTRODUCTION

Advances in medical science and technology have helped extend the lives of children with complex medical conditions and healthcare needs. These advances have also made it possible for technology-dependent children to receive complex care outside the hospital setting and to live in the community. Children with chronic health conditions account for a substantial proportion of cases of severe acute illness. Because they have underlying conditions requiring reliance on technology, they are at significant risk for complications associated with invasive medical devices, including malfunction, infection, and displacement, resulting in exacerbation of underlying illnesses. The various tubes and catheters associated with invasive medical devices are not used exclusively in the care of the chronically ill child; they are often employed in the care of a child with acute and critical illness.

# II. TUBES

## A. General Information

Several different types of tubes may be used in the care of critically ill children. These tubes fall into several different categories and provide access to real or potential spaces within the body. They include artificial airways, vascular catheters, gastrointestinal (GI) tubes, peritoneal catheters, internal shunts, bladder catheters. and thoracostomy tubes. Each of the various tube types have a range of sizes, and the selected size is determined by the pediatric patient's age, weight, and anatomical size. Information regarding artificial airways can be found in **Chapter 2**, and neurosurgical shunts are discussed in **Chapter 15**.

## B. Gastrointestinal Tubes

GI tubes are usually made of polyurethane or silicone, have single or double lumens, and may be weighted or vented. The name of the tube generally refers to the anatomical site of insertion and intended use (e.g., nasogastric). Typically, tubes are used to provide direct access, to remove GI contents (air, blood, secretions, or ingested toxins), or to instill products (medications, nutrition, or lavage fluids). Benefits and advantages of utilizing GI tubes include acute decompression; provision of hydration, electrolytes, and nutrition; medication administration; electrolyte removal with exchange resins; and even facilitation of temperature control via lavage fluids. The diameter of a GI tube is measured in French (F) units with each unit equal to 0.33 mm. The pediatric sizes range from 5F to 16F or larger (**Table 21-1**).

### Table 21-1. Nasogastric Tube Size

| Age | Weight (kg) | Nasogastric Tube (F) |
|---|---|---|
| 0 - 6 mo | 3.5 - 7 | 5 - 10 |
| 1 y | 10 | 10 |
| 2 y | 12 | 10 |
| 3 y | 14 | 10 - 12 |
| 5 y | 18 | 12 |
| 6 y | 21 | 12 |
| 8 y | 27 | 14 |
| 12 y | Varies | 14 - 16 |

### 1. Orogastric and Nasogastric Tubes

Orogastric (OG) or nasogastric (NG) tubes are used for both diagnostic and therapeutic purposes. They are frequently indicated for stomach decompression in invasive or noninvasive mechanical ventilatory support and for evacuation of gastric contents after an overdose, hemorrhage, or ileus (**Figure 21-1**).

> *Nasogastric intubation is contraindicated in suspected or confirmed anterior fossa skull fracture or maxillofacial injury.*

**Figure 21-1.** Nasogastric Tube

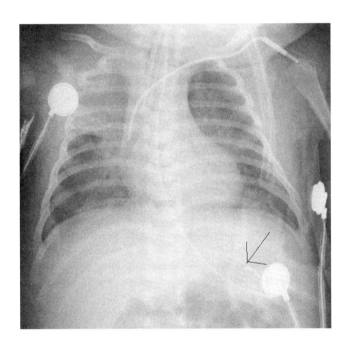

OG intubation is performed by passing a tube through the oral cavity, whereas NG intubation passes the tube inferiorly through the naris, along the top of the hard palate into the nasopharynx; in both instances, the tube is advanced through the pharynx and esophagus into the stomach. OG intubation is specifically recommended for patients with potential head trauma, specifically anterior fossa skull fracture or maxillofacial injury. These patients are at high risk for inadvertent tube placement into the brain via the cribriform plate or ethmoid bone if inserted nasally.

The Salem Sump (Covidien AG) is a vented, non-weighted, double-lumen tube commonly utilized in gastric decompression. The second lumen of the tube allows air to irrigate the distal tip of the tube as suction is applied to the other port. Air irrigation decreases the likelihood of gastric irritation from tube adherence to the gastric mucosa. The Salem Sump tube has an anti-reflux valve that prevents the gastric contents from exiting. The traditional Salem Sump is not optimal for feeding because of the stiffness of tubing material and the presence of venting port; it has more commonly been used for decompression, lavage, or medication administration. However, newer versions of this tube have safe enteral feeding connections.

## 2. Feeding Tubes

A nonsurgical feeding tube is used to provide enteral or tube feeding when patients are unable to obtain sufficient nutrition by swallowing. Placement is usually temporary for the treatment of acute conditions, but these tubes may be used in chronic conditions. Small-bore, weighted or non-weighted, single-lumen tubes are preferred for enteral feeding. Stylets are sometimes included in the packaging to assist in tube placement, after which the stylet is removed and discarded. For long-term use, small-bore feeding tubes are preferable to larger-bore NG tubes because the risk of complications (sinusitis, otitis, and tissue necrosis at the nares) is lower over time. Small-bore feeding tubes are not designed for drainage of gastric contents. They can be used for administration of nutrients, fluid, and medications either for short-term or long-term use, depending upon the child's needs, prognosis, and family preference. The placement of the distal tip of the tube (NG or transpyloric) will dictate the child's feeding regimen. NG placement allows for both bolus and continuous feeding administration. Transpyloric (nasoduodenal or nasojejunal) placement will allow only continuous infusion. Bolus feeding should not be infused transpylorically because the duodenum or jejunum cannot accept large-volume delivery of fluid and nutrients (**Figures 21-2** through **21-4**).

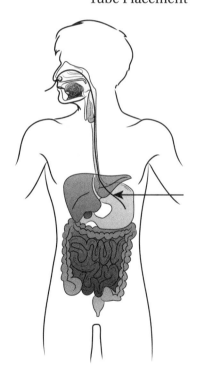

**Figure 21-2.** Nasogastric Tube Placement

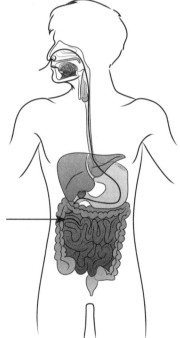

**Figure 21-3.** Nasoduodenal Tube Placement

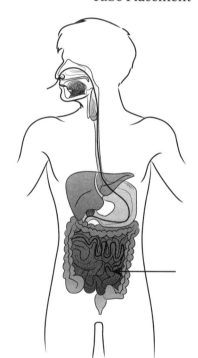

**Figure 21-4.** Nasojejunal Tube Placement

## 3. Complications

The most frequent complications associated with GI intubation are listed in **Table 21-2**. If equipment failure is suspected, remove all connecting materials and flush the feeding tube with 5 to 10 mL of water or air. If the tube flushes easily, the equipment likely has not malfunctioned. The inability to flush the tube probably means it is obstructed and needs to be replaced.

| Table 21-2 | Frequent Complications Associated With Small-Bore Feeding Tube Placement |

- Coughing, hoarseness, or dyspnea, indicating probable bronchial placement
- Epistaxis
- Tube coiled in esophagus or posterior pharynx
- Esophageal tear or intestinal perforation related to trauma of placement
- Dislodgement or removal by patient
- Aspiration of stomach contents despite appropriate placement
- Clogging of enteral tube with formula or medication fragments
- Skin irritation or breakdown at insertion site
- Pneumothorax from inadvertent pleural placement

## C. Surgically Placed Feeding Tubes

An increasingly large population of children now have surgically placed enteral access tubes. These feeding tubes include gastrostomy tubes, gastrojejunal tubes, and jejunostomy tubes. Such tubes also provide the option to decompress or drain stomach contents. Occasionally, incomplete drainage may occur and an additional large-bore NG or OG tube may be needed to facilitate full decompression.

### 1. Gastrostomy Tubes

Gastrostomy or gastric feeding tubes (**Figures 21-5** and **21-6**) are most common and can be placed either surgically (laparoscopic or open laparotomy) or transcutaneously with endoscopic assistance. Percutaneous gastrostomy or percutaneous endoscopic gastrostomy (PEG) tubes avoid the need for laparotomy and initially depend on the traction exerted on the tube as it is anchored to the skin to maintain contact between the gastric opening and the anterior abdominal wall. PEG tubes often have rigid crossbars in the stomach, which preclude traction removal and require a second endoscopy for removal. Unlike in the adult population, these tubes cannot simply be cut and allowed to pass through the GI tract of a young child. Small bowel obstruction and esophageal erosion with perforation secondary to esophageal device "reflux" have been reported. Other potential complications include loss of contact between the stomach and

**Figure 21-5.** Gastrostomy Tube

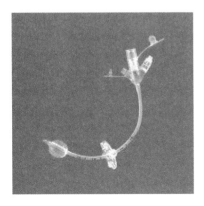

**Figure 21-6.** Gastrostomy Tube Placement

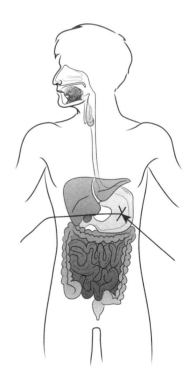

abdominal wall, resulting in intraperitoneal soilage and injury to other viscera in the process of placement.

Tubes used for laparoscopic placement are either primary MIC-KEY tubes (Kimberly-Clark) or other balloon catheters. These are anchored in a manner similar to the PEG. This laparoscopic-assisted procedure, however, avoids laparotomy, while minimizing the risk of injury to adjacent organs, such as the colon, in the process of placing the gastrostomy tube. The types of catheters used in each instance may be different. Operative gastrostomy tubes are generally Malecot or de Pezzer catheters, which are simply removed by traction (**Figure 21-7**).

### a. Complications

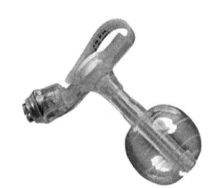

**Figure 21-7.** Mic-Key button

Excessive force should be avoided when replacing gastrostomy tubes, because this may push the stomach away from the anterior abdominal wall and result in a gastric leak into the peritoneal cavity. If any difficulty is encountered in replacing the gastrostomy tube or initial placement was recent (within past 4 to 6 weeks), a contrast study should be obtained to verify correct placement.

If a gastrostomy tube is inadvertently removed, a Foley catheter should be placed to keep the tract open. Simply placing a gauze or dressing over the site may allow it to quickly close spontaneously.

After assessing the thickness of the child's abdomen, a Foley catheter should be selected at a length sufficient to avoid inflating the balloon in the subcutaneous tract (approximately 2-3 cm for most). The catheter should be placed into the stomach wall and the balloon inflated, then gently pulled back snug to adhere to the abdominal wall. The Foley catheter should not be pushed so far that it passes through the pylorus and is inflated in the

> *A Foley catheter needs to be placed promptly into the gastrocutaneous tract to maintain patency for the patient with a dislodged gastrostomy tube.*

duodenum. This will result in gastric outlet obstruction and potentially duodenum rupture. The pylorus is frequently within 5 to 7.5 cm of the site where the tube enters the stomach.

This also is the basis for evaluating feeding difficulties in a child with a Foley catheter used as a feeding tube. If the catheter is not properly secured to the skin, the stomach will propel the balloon forward and through the pylorus as if it were a bolus of food, resulting in a proximal small bowel obstruction (emesis may be bilious) and gastric, but not diffuse, abdominal distension. These children usually present with excessive leakage around the tube site. The diagnosis is determined by examining how much tubing is protruding from the site. The problem is resolved by deflating the balloon, pulling the catheter out, replacing it to the proper depth (inserted 2 to 4 cm), then securing it appropriately with tape. The best solution is a button gastrostomy tube, because this cannot be sucked into the stomach.

### 2. Gastrojejunal Tubes

Gastrojejunal tubes are similar to gastrostomy tubes, but close inspection reveals 3 ports: one to access the stabilizing balloon, one for gastric access, and one for jejunal access. Care and placement are much the same as with gastrostomy tubes. During acute use, the gastric port may be put to drainage, while the jejunal port is used for feeding and medications. Extra care is needed when administering medications via the gastrojejunal port, as blockage of this port may necessitate endoscopic, fluoroscopic, or ultrasound-guided replacement.

### 3. Jejunostomy Tubes

A jejunostomy tube is similar to a gastric tube, though it generally has a finer bore and smaller diameter and is surgically inserted into the jejunum rather than the stomach. Jejunostomy tubes are indicated in medical conditions that require bypassing the upper GI tract. These tubes may be used as soon as 12 hours after surgery (**Figure 21-8**).

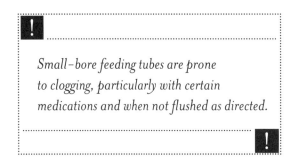

*Small-bore feeding tubes are prone to clogging, particularly with certain medications and when not flushed as directed.*

Commercially prepared formulas are generally used to provide nutrition and to avoid clogging when used with a pump or drip feedings.

## D. Thoracostomy Tubes

A thoracostomy tube (also known as a chest tube, chest drain, or pigtail catheter) is a flexible plastic tube inserted through the chest into the pleural space. These are used to evacuate air (pneumothorax), fluid (pleural effusion, blood, chyle), or pus (empyema) from the intrathoracic space. Depending upon the child's clinical condition and the urgency of the situation, needle thoracostomy may precede the tube thoracostomy because it may be accomplished more quickly.

Chest tubes are sterile, flexible non-thrombogenic catheters made of vinyl or silicone and of varying French sizes and lengths. The size of the tube is dictated by the patient's anatomy and the reason for placement (**Table 21-3**). The insertion site is determined by the indication for the tube. If draining air, the tube is placed anteriorly and toward the apex of the lung; if draining fluid, the tube is directed posteriorly and toward the base of the lung.

**Figure 21-8.** Jejunostomy Tube

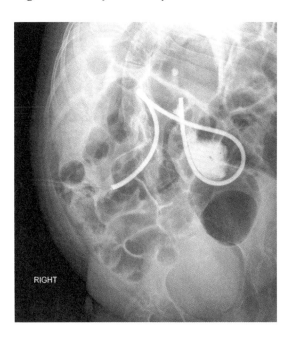

| Table 21-3 Chest Tube Size | | |
|---|---|---|
| Age | 50th Percentile Weight (kg) | Tube size (F) |
| Newborn | 3-5 | 10-12 |
| Infant | 6-9 | 10-12 |
| Toddler | 10-11 | 16-20 |
| Young child | 12-14 | 20-24 |
| Child | 15-22 | 20-32 |
| Older child | 24-30 | 28-32 |

### 1. Complications

The primary complications of tube thoracostomy are similar to those seen with placement of any device through the skin: pain and discomfort, bleeding and infection. Ironically, two additional complications of placement secondary to inadvertent lung injury are also indications for chest tube placement: pneumothorax and hemothorax. Less frequent complications include subcutaneous emphysema, thoracic nerve damage, intercostal vascular injury, and organ damage (lung, heart, diaphragm, liver, stomach, and spleen).

Other complications appear to be directly related to tube location after placement. A tube that is not inserted far enough may cause an air leak and subcutaneous emphysema if any of the side drainage holes are outside the pleural space. A tube inserted too far will press against the parietal pleura or thoracic structures, resulting in pain and further tissue injury.

Complications may also occur after the tube is in place. It may become dislodged or disconnected. Pain at the insertion site may cause the child to splint, leading to atelectasis. The skin at the insertion site may become irritated, erythematous, or excoriated, particularly if the occlusive dressing becomes saturated or requires frequent changing (**Appendix 12**).

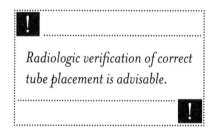

*Radiologic verification of correct tube placement is advisable.*

## III. CATHETERS

A catheter is a tube that can be inserted into a body cavity, duct, or vessel. They allow drainage or injection of fluids and access for surgical instruments. Placement of a catheter (catheterization) may allow for the following:

- Drainage of urine from the urinary bladder
- Drainage of cerebral spinal fluid into a body cavity (**Chapter 15**)
- Administration of intravenous fluids, medications, or parenteral nutrition
- Direct measurement of pressure in an artery or vein

### A. Urinary Catheters

In urinary catheterization, a plastic catheter (e.g., Foley catheter) is either inserted into the patient's urinary tract via the urethra and bladder or via suprapubic catheterization. If the catheter is to remain in place for an indefinite time, a balloon at the end is usually inflated with sterile water to keep the catheter from inadvertently slipping out. In this manner, the patient's urine is collected, measured, and utilized for various medical purposes and tests. Catheters come in a large variety of sizes, materials (latex, silicone, polyvinyl chloride, or Teflon), and types (Foley catheter, straight catheter, or coudé tip catheter). The smallest size is usually recommended for the urethra, although a larger size is sometimes needed to control leakage around the catheter or for continuous bladder irrigation (**Table 21-4**). A large size may also be necessary when the urine is thick, bloody, or contains sediment or clots. Individuals with specific medical conditions (spina bifida or urogenital abnormalities), patients who have undergone repeated or prolonged surgeries or mucous membrane exposure to latex devices, especially early in life, and those with an atopic history or history of food allergy are at a high risk for latex allergies or may have developed allergies or sensitivities to latex after long-term latex catheter use. In such cases, silicone or Teflon types should be used.

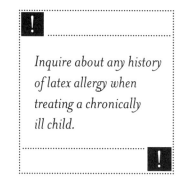

*Inquire about any history of latex allergy when treating a chronically ill child.*

Brief catheterization may be used to collect urine specimens for laboratory testing. Patients with neurologic injuries, especially spinal cord injuries, may require long-term clean intermittent catheterization. A urine collection system is attached to the catheter in circumstances that require the urinary catheter to remain indwelling. The connection of a collecting system maintains a sterile environment.

### Table 21-4 Urinary Catheter Sizes

| Age | 50th Percentile Weight (kg) | Tube size (F) |
|---|---|---|
| Newborn | 3-5 | 5-8 |
| Infant | 6-9 | 5-8 |
| Toddler | 10-11 | 8-10 |
| Young child | 12-14 | 10 |
| Child | 15-22 | 10-12 |
| Older child | 24-30 | 12-14 |

The primary complication of urinary catheterization is infection. Additional problems include bleeding, tissue trauma, false passage, urethral injury, kidney damage (usually in long-term indwelling use), and development of latex allergy.

## B. Indwelling Venous Access Catheters

Indwelling venous access catheters are used to deliver fluid, medication, parenteral nutrition, and blood products directly into a central vein. They may also be used to draw blood samples, and some are designed specifically for chronic intermittent hemodialysis. A variety of catheters are available for long-term use. The type selected is determined by indications for use and the preference of the patient, family, and healthcare team. The catheters are typically classified by manner of placement and device characteristics.

### 1. Tunneled Lines

Catheters that exit the skin after being inserted into a large central vein and tunneled beneath the subcutaneous tissue are typically referred to by brand name, such as Broviac (C.R. Bard, Inc.), Hickman (C.R. Bard, Inc.), and Permacath (**Figure 21-9**). These catheters are most often used for long-term parenteral nutrition, chronic medication administration, and chronic intermittent hemodialysis or apheresis. They are secured by means of a Dacron cuff just under the skin at the exit site, which prevents catheter dislodgement and forms a barrier for infection. These catheters may remain in place for extended periods. Insertion is typically done under sedation or general anesthesia by a radiologist or surgeon. The catheter may have single, double, or triple lumens. External lumens are secured at the exit site with an occlusive dressing. Catheter lumens are typically flushed with an anticoagulant solution on a scheduled basis to prevent blood clots from forming inside the catheter (**Table 21-5**).

**Figure 21-9.** Broviac Catheter

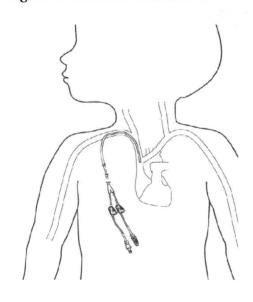

| Table 21-5 | Heparin Flush Table | | |
|---|---|---|---|
| | **Description** | **Site Care**[a] | **Flush** |
| Peripheral IV Catheter | Range in size from 24 gauge to 16 gauge. Always use a T or Y connector. | Every 96 h with site rotation and PRN (as per individual policy) | • Flush amounts for NICU by physician order.<br>• For all other patients, flush capped lines every 8 h and PRN.<br>• Use 2.5 mL NS unless heparin flushes ordered, then use 2.5 mL 10 U/mL heparin. |
| Central Line Catheter | Any venous catheter in which the tip of catheter is lying in or past the SVC. | Once weekly if transparent dressing; every 48 h if gauze used and PRN. Use central line dressing kit. Do not use chlorhexidine on infants <2 mo.<br>• In NICU, use povidone-iodine x3, then rinse with sterile saline solution, apply dressing.<br>• For other infants <2 mo, use alcohol x3, apply dressing.<br>• All >2 mo, use chlorhexidine x1, apply dressing. | • Flush amounts for NICU by physician order.<br>• For all other patients: flush all capped lumens every 12 h and PRN with 2.5 mL 10 U/mL heparin to each lumen.<br>• For blood sampling, discard 2 mL, withdraw specimens, flush with 5-10 mL NS, then heparin per above if capped. |
| Percutaneous Inserted Central Line Catheter | PICC can be either open-ended or Groshong. | Initial gauze dressing removed in 24 h, then once weekly if transparent dressing; every 48 h if gauze used and PRN. Use central line dressing kit. Do not use chlorhexidine on infants <2 mo; use alcohol x3, then povidone-iodine x3, apply dressing. All >2 mo, use chlorhexidine x1, apply dressing. | • Never use anything smaller than a 10-mL syringe.<br>• Flush amounts for NICU by physician order.<br>• For all other patients: PICC, 2.5 mL NS, then 2.5 mL 10 U/mL heparin if <10 kg, 2.5 mL 100 U/mL if >10 kg, every 12 h to each lumen.<br>• Groshong: 3-5 mL NS every 8 h when not in use, and after each use; 5-10 mL NS after blood infusion or withdrawal.<br>• For blood sampling, only if PICC 3F or larger, discard 2 mL, withdraw specimens, then flush with 5-10 mL NS, then heparin per above if capped. |

### Table 21-5  Heparin Flush Table (continued)

| | Description | Site Care[a] | Flush |
|---|---|---|---|
| Tunneled Central Line Cather | Central venous catheters that are tunneled through subcutaneous tissue. | Once weekly if transparent dressing; every 48 h if gauze used and PRN. Use central line dressing kit. Do not use chlorhexidine on infants <2 mo.<br>• In NICU, use povidone-iodine x3, then rinse with sterile saline solution, apply dressing.<br>• For other infants <2 mo, use alcohol x3, apply dressing.<br>• All others >2 mo, use chlorhexidine x1, apply dressing. | • Hickman or Broviac: flush amounts for NICU by physician order.<br>• For all other patients: 2.5 mL NS, followed by 2.5 mL of 10 U/mL heparin every 24 h.<br>• Groshong: 5 mL NS every 7 days when not in use; 5-10 mL NS after each use.<br>• For blood sampling, discard 2 mL, withdraw specimens, then flush with 5-10 mL NS, then heparin per above if capped. |
| Implanted Port | Surgically implanted ports have flat septum; percutaneous Groshong port has domed septum. | Change access every 7 d and PRN. Dressing changes once weekly with access changes; every 48 h if gauze used. Use central line dressing kit, new winged infusion set, 20 or 22 gauge, ¾- or 1-inch needle as per patient. | • Never use anything smaller than a 10-mL syringe on ports.<br>• Flush daily with 2.5 mL NS, then 2.5 mL 10 U/mL heparin if <10 kg, 100 U/mL if >10 kg. At discharge and monthly, use 5 mL of 100 U/mL heparin to all ports.<br>• Groshong port: 5-10 mL NS after each use; 10-20 mL after blood sampling or transfusion. If not in use, flush once monthly with 10 mL NS. May require heparin if valve malfunctions, administer 5 mL heparin 100 U/mL.<br>• For blood sampling, discard 3-5 mL, withdraw specimens, then flush with 5-10 mL NS, then heparin per above if capped. |

IV, intravenous; SVC, superior vena cava; PRN, as needed; NICU, neonatal intensive care unit; NS, normal saline; PICC, peripherally inserted central catheter
[a]All IV tubing and caps are changed every 96 h (or as per individual policy). Total parenteral nutrition/lipid tubing is changed every 24 h with solution changes.

### 2. Ports

Subcutaneous infusion systems require the insertion of a needle through the skin to access a reservoir. The catheter port resides in a subcutaneous pocket in the upper chest, forming a small, palpable bulge under the skin. These catheters, typically Port-a-Cath (Smiths Medical) or PowerPort (C.R. Bard, Inc.), require a flush with anticoagulant only once a month or after completion of access. The risk of infection with this type of catheter is low when not in use. Frequently they are used for intermittent central access, such as for chemotherapy administration, intermittent transfusion needs, or difficult vascular access with predictable recurrent need (**Figure 21-10**).

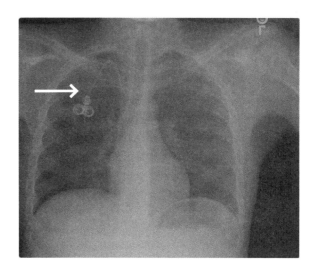

**Figure 21-10.** Port-a-Cath

### 3. Peripherally Inserted Central Catheters

A peripherally inserted central catheter (PICC, or PICC line) is a percutaneously placed small flexible catheter typically inserted in the cephalic, basilic, or brachial vein of the arm, traversing centrally (e.g., via subclavian) to the superior vena cava until the tip of the catheter rests near the cavo-atrial junction. PICCs are usually inserted with the use of local anesthesia or sedation under ultrasound or fluoroscopic guidance and radiographic confirmation of proper placement. A PICC may be used for a prolonged period, typically for chemotherapy, extended antibiotic therapy, or parenteral nutrition (**Figure 21-11**).

### 4. Complications

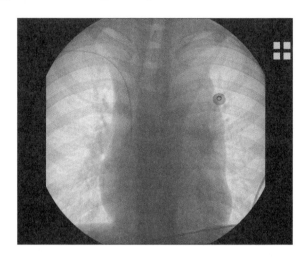

**Figure 21-11.** Peripherally Inserted Central Catheter

Complications associated with indwelling venous access catheters include infection, hemorrhage, occlusion, thrombosis, and phlebitis. These catheters may become displaced, disconnected, dislodged, or obstructed. Bleeding at the exit site may be a presenting sign of developing complication. If the catheter is damaged or separated from an external connection, it may be possible to clamp the catheter near the exit site to prevent further bleeding. If the catheter is dislodged, direct pressure should be applied to the site, and ongoing assessment of the child's airway, breathing, circulation, and hemodynamics should be performed to assess for cardiorespiratory compromise.

The catheter may become obstructed by blood clots or crystals formed by medication or parenteral nutrition. The most serious risk associated with clot formation is the development of pulmonary embolism, which could lead to hypoxemia, respiratory distress, or shock. Signs and symptoms of emboli depend on the organ system affected and may include altered mental status, respiratory distress, cyanosis, dyspnea, chest pain, tachycardia, and shock. Air embolus is another serious risk for the child with an indwelling venous access catheter. Signs and symptoms are the same in blood clot embolism. Treatment involves clamping the catheter, placing the child in a supine position with the left side down and head lower than the body, opening the airway, and administering 100% oxygen. There is a risk for catheter erosion or perforation through the central vein, which may cause pneumothorax, hemothorax, or hydrothorax from infusion of intravenous fluids. Prompt decompression may be necessary. Erosion of the tip of the catheter through the right atrium can result in acute pericardial tamponade.

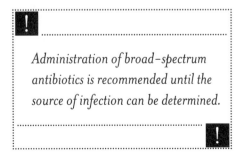

*Administration of broad-spectrum antibiotics is recommended until the source of infection can be determined.*

Infection is one of the most common complications associated with indwelling central access catheters, especially in a child who is immunocompromised. Fever is a symptom of contamination and infection. The presence of swelling, erythema, tenderness, or bleeding at the exit site also may indicate infection. It is recommended that the child's hemodynamic status be assessed, blood be drawn from the catheter for culture, and a complete blood count be performed.

If the source of the infection is determined, the antibiotic spectrum should be narrowed to best treat the specific organism. Prophylactic antibiotics are not useful. Vigilance with insertion, care, and maintenance has proven to be the best defense against infection. Strict adherence to published insertion and maintenance guidelines is strongly recommended.

## C. Hemodynamic Monitoring Catheters

Several types of catheters may need to be inserted to monitor and assess hemodynamic status closely and accurately. These catheters include central venous access catheters and arterial catheters. Because of a lack of benefit, the general trend over the past few decades has been to avoid insertion of pulmonary artery catheters or Swan-Ganz catheters in the pediatric patient.

## D. Central Venous Catheters

Central venous cannulation can be defined as the percutaneous insertion of a vascular catheter within the lumen of a major high-flow vein. The most common insertion sites for access include the internal jugular, subclavian, axillary, and femoral veins (**Table 21-6** and **Appendix 13**). Central venous cannulation provides a more stable and reliable route of venous access than peripheral venous cannulation. It also allows hemodynamic monitoring, sampling of central venous blood for laboratory studies, reliable infusion of vasoactive medications, and the rapid administration of large-volume resuscitation. With a much lower risk of extravasation, central venous access eliminates the complications associated with peripheral administration of potentially caustic medications. Indications for central venous catheter insertion include:

**Table 21-6** Central Venous Catheter Sizes[a]

| Age | Internal Jugular (F) | Subclavian (F) | Femoral (F) |
| --- | --- | --- | --- |
| 0-6 mo | 3 | 3 | 3 |
| 6 mo-2 y | 3 | 3 | 3-4 |
| 3-6 y | 4 | 4 | 4 |
| 7-12 y | 4-5 | 4-5 | 4-5 |
| >12 y | 5-7 | 5-7 | 5-7 |

[a]Selection of catheter length depends upon the operator's use for monitoring purposes or the need to infuse solutions rapidly. Adapted with permission. © 1997 Wolters Kluwer Health. Lavelle J, Costarino A. Central venous access and central venous pressure monitoring. In: Henretig FM, King C, eds. *Textbook of Pediatric Emergency Procedures*. Baltimore, MD: Williams & Wilkins; 1997:251-278.

- Resuscitation of circulatory failure
- Administration of vasoactive medications
- Administration of hypertonic solutions
- Administration of caustic chemotherapy
- Measurement of central venous pressure
- Measurement of estimated mixed venous blood gases
- Access for pacemaker or Swan-Ganz catheter placement

- Hemodialysis access
- Long-term vascular access

**1. Complications**

Complications of central venous catheterization occur more frequently in infants and children than adults (**Table 21-7**). Common complications include pain, infection, thrombosis, vascular perforation, dysrhythmia, air embolus, catheter fragment embolus, and catheter occlusion. Infection can occur with any method or site. In adults, the subclavian location has the lowest incidence of infection. In the pediatric patient, the femoral vein has become the most popular site for central venous cannulation and is associated with a low incidence of infection. The presence of fever, swelling, erythema, tenderness, or bleeding may indicate infection. To prevent infection, maximal barrier precautions must be employed, and stringent cleaning of the catheter insertion site with chlorhexidine should be followed by strict adherence to institutional guidelines for dressing care and maintenance. Prompt evaluation, catheter culture, and narrowing of the antibiotic spectrum to treat the specific organism are essential. Prophylactic antibiotics are not useful. Vigilance with insertion, care, and maintenance has proven to be the best defense against infection.

**Table 21-7 Complications of Central Venous Cannulation**

| Site | Complications |
| --- | --- |
| Internal jugular vein | Carotid artery puncture<br>Carotid artery cannulation<br>Pneumothorax or hemothorax |
| Right subclavian vein | Pneumothorax or hemothorax<br>Tension pneumothorax<br>Thoracic duct puncture<br>Decreased success rate with inexperience |
| Left subclavian vein | Pneumothorax or hemothorax<br>Tension pneumothorax<br>Thoracic duct puncture<br>Decreased success rate with inexperience |
| Femoral vein | Infection<br>Arterial puncture<br>Failure rate during hypotension/shock<br>Inability to thread central catheter |

Adapted with permission. © 2001 Elsevier. Fleck DA. Central venous catheter insertion (perform). In: Lynn-McHale DJ, Carlson K, eds. *AACN Procedure Manual for Critical Care.* 4th ed. Philadelphia, PA: W.B. Saunders; 2001: 503-513.

Accidental entry of the guidewire into the central circulation is a rare complication that can be avoided by ensuring that the proximal end of the wire is secured at all times; if the complication occurs, it may require removal by a surgeon or interventional radiologist. When indications for placement no longer exist, indwelling venous access catheters should be promptly removed. For temporary catheters, need for continued use should be routinely assessed (**Appendix 13**).

## E. Arterial Catheters

Arterial cannulation provides a direct means of continuous measurement of blood pressure, pulse, and sampling for evaluation of arterial oxygenation, carbon dioxide tension, and acid-base balance. In addition to these indications, arterial catheter insertion provides accurate pulse pressure monitoring in surgery, patients with congenital heart disease, or hemodynamically compromised patients. The most common insertion sites are the radial, femoral, posterior tibial, dorsalis pedis, and axillary arteries (**Table 21-8**). The site selection is based on palpable pulses, overall hemodynamic state, and other anatomic and physiologic factors unique to the individual patient. Because of the distance from the heart and the size of the vessel, the posterior tibial and dorsal pedis arteries are less reliable for hemodynamic pressure monitoring.

### Table 21-8 Arterial Catheter Sizes by Site and Patient Weight

| Site | Infants <10 kg | | 10-40 kg | | >40 kg | |
| --- | --- | --- | --- | --- | --- | --- |
| | Catheter Size | French Size (F) | Catheter Size | French Size (F) | Catheter Size | French Size (F) |
| Radial artery, posterior tibial artery, dorsalis pedis artery | Angiocath 22/24 gauge | 2.5 | Angiocath 22 gauge | 2.5/3.0 | Angiocath 20/22 gauge | 3.0 |
| Femoral artery, axillary artery | Angiocath 18/20 gauge | 3.0/4.0 | Angiocath 16/18 gauge | 4.0/5.0 | Angiocath 14/16/18 gauge | 4.0/5.0 |

Single-lumen catheters are manufactured in standard French size and lengths. Only a single lumen should be used for arterial vessel cannulation.
Adapted with permission. © 1997 Wolters Kluwer Health. Torrey SB, Saladino R. Arterial puncture and catheterization. In: Henretig FM, King C, eds. *Textbook of Pediatric Emergency Procedures.* Baltimore, MA: Williams & Wilkins; 1997:783-795.

### 1. Complications

Complications of arterial cannulation include localized or generalized infection, air or particulate matter embolization, hematoma, acute hemorrhage, arterial thrombosis, nerve damage, pain, and arterial pseudoaneurysm. Arterial thrombosis may result in tissue necrosis, tissue ischemia, and growth failure in the affected extremity. In children, the most common complications are minor skin lesions, local necrosis, and radial artery occlusion. The potential for problems increases the longer the catheter remains in place. The need for continued use should be routinely assessed daily.

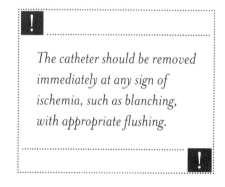

*The catheter should be removed immediately at any sign of ischemia, such as blanching, with appropriate flushing.*

Complications can be minimized by confirming adequate collateral circulation (Allen test) for cannulation of peripheral arteries, selecting an appropriately sized catheter for the artery, performing a careful insertion, exercising vigilant care for the site, and implementing a continuous flush system (**Appendix 16**). The arterial waveform display on the monitor is a safety feature that will help detect catheter occlusion or inadvertent extravasation of blood through an accidentally opened stopcock/three-way tap or break in the system. The extremity with an arterial catheter should be frequently assessed for evidence of ischemia. Placement of an oximeter on the involved extremity/digits can provide a beat-to-beat noninvasive assessment of adequate perfusion via continuous plethysmography. Isotonic (normal saline) flushing, with or without heparin, should be used to maintain arterial line patency. For peripheral arterial catheters, inclusion of papaverine in the flush fluids may prolong catheter life.

## 2. Measurements

The arterial pressure obtained from a properly assembled, positioned, and calibrated monitoring system is the "gold standard" of blood pressure measurement. Noninvasive, indirect measurements or manual determination by auscultation of Korotkoff sounds distal to an occluding cuff may vary somewhat from simultaneous direct arterial measurement and are generally slightly lower.

Waveform analysis and troubleshooting are often required to ensure accuracy of measurement. Several technical and anatomic factors may affect accuracy. Waveforms may display fling or overshoot artifact or a dampened wave. Distortion of the arterial waveform signal may be caused by factors within the blood vessel, hydraulic coupling of the transducer system, and system tubing compliance. Changes in the elasticity of the vessel wall, reflectance of the pulse waveform from the walls or tubing, small air bubbles in the system fluid column, small thrombi around or in the catheter, and stiffness and length of the monitoring tubing are some factors that may result in an incorrect measurement. The arterial blood pressure should also be compared to the noninvasive cuff pressure on a routine basis (**Figure 21-12**).

**Figure 21-12.** Arterial Wave Forms

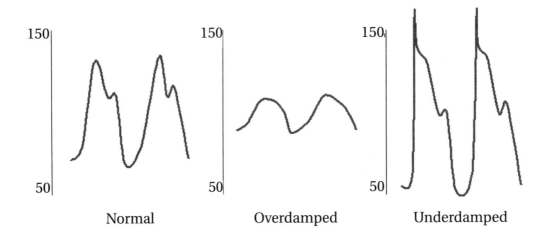

## Key Points

## Invasive Medical Devices

- Children should be checked for the presence of invasive medical devices, which must be evaluated to ensure proper functioning.

- Insertion of invasive devices, especially hemodynamic monitoring catheters, must be performed by individuals who have experience or expertise in the insertion techniques.

- Any monitoring or invasive device requires users to be thoroughly familiar with its operation and potential complications.

- The two primary indications for insertion of an arterial catheter are frequent arterial blood sampling and beat-to-beat blood pressure monitoring. Waveform analysis and troubleshooting are often required to ensure accurate measurements.

- Management of abnormal pleural collections depends upon several factors: the etiology and size of the lesion, the patient's general condition, any associated problems, need for patient transport, and need for mechanical ventilation or general anesthesia. The need for tube thoracostomy should be assessed, as not all pleural collections may require intervention or tube placement.

## Suggested Readings

1. Dev SP, Nascimiento B, Simone C, Chien V. Chest-tube insertion. Videos in clinical medicine. *N Engl J Med*. 2007;357:e15.

2. Franklin C. The technique of radial artery cannulation. Tips for maximizing results while minimizing the risk of complications. *J Crit Illn*. 1995;10:424-432.

3. Graham AS, Ozment C, Tegtmeyer K, Lai S, Braner D. Central venous catheterization. Videos in clinical medicine. *N Engl J Med*. 2007;356:e21.

4. Hazinski MF, ed. *PALS Provider Manual*. Dallas, TX: American Heart Association; 2011.

5. Henretig FM, King C, eds. *Textbook of Pediatric Emergency Procedures*. Baltimore, MD: Williams & Wilkins; 1997.

6. Lacroix LE, Vunda A, Bajwa NM, Galetto-Lacour A, Gervaix A. Catheterization of the urethra in male children. Videos in clinical medicine. *N Engl J Med*. 2010;363:e19.

7. O'Grady NP, Alexander M, Burns LA, et al. Summary of Recommendations: Guidelines for the Prevention of Intravascular Catheter-related Infections. Center for Disease Control and Prevention, Healthcare Infection Control Practices Advisory Committee. Available at: http://www.cdc.gov/hicpac/pdf/guidelines/bsi-guidelines-2011.pdf. Accessed May 11, 2013.

8. Schexnayder SM, Storm EA, Stroud MH, et al. Pediatric vascular access and centeses. In: Fuhrman BP, Zimmerman J, eds. *Pediatric Critical Care*. 4th ed. Philadelphia, PA: Elsevier; 2011:139-163.

9. Schwemmer U, Arzet HA, Trautner H, Rauch S, Roewer N, Greim CA. Ultrasound-guided arterial cannulation in infants improves success rate. *Eur J Anaesthesiol*. 2006;23:476-480.

10. Tegtmeyer K, Brady G, Lai S, Hodo R, Braner D. Placement of an arterial line. Videos in clinical medicine. *N Engl J Med.* 2006;354:e13.

11. Thomsen TW, Shaffer RW, Setnik GS. Nasogastric intubation. Videos in clinical medicine. *N Engl J Med.* 2006;354:e16.

# Appendix 1

# Pediatric Normal Values

### Table A1-1 Vital Signs: Reference Ranges

| Age Group | Respiratory Rate (breaths/min) | Awake Heart Rate (beats/min) | Sleeping Heart Rate (beats/min) | Systolic Blood Pressure[a,b] (mm Hg) |
|---|---|---|---|---|
| Newborn | 30-60 | 100-180 | 80-160 | 60-90 |
| Infant (1-12 months) | 30-60 | 100-160 | 75-160 | 87-105 |
| Toddler (1-2 years) | 24-40 | 80-110 | 60-90 | 85-102 |
| Preschooler (3-5 years) | 22-34 | 70-110 | 60-90 | 89-108 |
| School age (6-12 years) | 18-30 | 65-110 | 60-90 | 94-120 |
| Adolescent (13-17 years) | 12-16 | 60-90 | 50-90 | 107-132 |

[a]50th-90th percentile ranges for boys and girls at 50% height indicated
[b]Lower limit of systolic blood pressure by age calculation for children 1-10 years old: 70 + (age in years x 2)

**Remember:**

- The **patient's** normal range should always be taken into consideration.

- Heart rate, blood pressure, and respiratory rate are expected to increase during times of fever or stress.

- Respiratory rates for infants and children should be counted for a full 60 seconds.

- In clinical decompensation, the child's blood pressure will be the **last** value to change.

- Bradycardia in children is an ominous sign, usually a result of hypoxia. Act quickly.

- Hypotension can be defined as a systolic blood pressure or mean arterial blood pressure below the 5th percentile. In children aged 1 to 10 years at the 50th percentile for height, the predicted 5th percentile systolic blood pressure and mean arterial blood pressure can be quickly determined using the following formulas:

$$\text{Systolic blood pressure (mm Hg)} \; 70 + (\text{age in years} \times 2)$$

$$\text{Mean arterial pressure (mm Hg)} < 40 + (\text{age in years} \times 1.5)$$

Classified using Hazinski MF, ed. Nursing Care of the Critically Ill Child. 3rd ed. Philadelphia, PA: Mosby; 2012. *Pediatric Advanced Life Support (PALS) Provider Manual.* Dallas, TX: American Heart Association; 2011. Haque IU, Zaritsky AL. Analysis of the evidence for the lower limit of systolic and mean arterial pressure in children. *Pediatr Crit Care Med.* 2007;8:138-144.

## Table A1-2  Laboratory Tests: Reference Ranges

| Test | Conventional Unit | SI Unit |
|---|---|---|
| **Acid Phosphatase** | | |
| Newborn | 7.4-19.4 U/L | 7.4-19.4 U/L |
| 2-13 years | 6.4-15.2 U/L | 6.4-15.2 U/L |
| **Alanine Aminotransferase (ALT)** | | |
| Infant | <54 U/L | <54 U/L |
| Child/adult | 1-30 U/L | 1-30 U/L |
| **Albumin** | | |
| Newborn | 3.2-4.8 g/dL | |
| 1 day-1 month | 2.5-5.5 g/dL | |
| 1-3 months | 2.1-4.8 g/dL | |
| 4-6 months | 2.8-5.0 g/dL | |
| 7-12 months | 3.2-5.7 g/dL | |
| 13-24 months | 1.9-5.0 g/dL | |
| 25-36 months | 3.3-5.8 g/dL | |
| 3-5 years | 2.9-5.8 g/dL | |
| 6-8 years | 3.3-5.0 g/dL | |
| 9-11 years | 3.2-5.0 g/dL | |
| 12-16 years | 3.2-5.1 g/dL | |
| **Alkaline Phosphatase** | | |
| Infant | 150-420 U/L | 150-420 U/L |
| 2-10 years | 100-320 U/L | 100-320 U/L |
| 11-18 years, boy | 100-390 U/L | 100-390 U/L |
| 11-18 years, girl | 100-320 U/L | 100-320 U/L |
| **Ammonia** | | |
| Newborn | 90-150 µg/dL | 64-107 µmol/L |
| 0-2 weeks | 79-129 µg/dL | 56-92 µmol/L |
| >1 month | 29-70 µg/dL | 21-50 µmol/L |
| **Amylase** | | |
| Newborn | 0-44 U/L | 5-65 U/L |
| Adult | 0-88 U/L | 0-130 U/L |
| **Aspartate Aminotransferase (AST)** | | |
| Newborn/infant | 20-65 U/L | 20-65 U/L |
| Child/adult | 0-35 U/L | 0-4350 U/L |
| **Bicarbonate** | | |
| Preterm | 18-26 mEq/L | 18-26 mmol/L |
| Full term | 20-25 mEq/L | 20-25 mmol/L |
| >2 years | 22-26 mEq/L | 22-26 mmol/L |

## Table A1-2  Laboratory Tests: Reference Ranges (continued)

| Test | Conventional Unit | SI Unit |
|---|---|---|
| **Bilirubin (Total)** | | |
| 0-1 day | | |
|   Preterm | <8 mg/dL | <137 µmol/L |
|   Term | <6 mg/dL | <103 µmol/L |
| 1-2 days | | |
|   Preterm | <12 mg/dL | <205 µmol/L |
|   Term | <8 mg/dL | <137 µmol/L |
| 3-5 days | | |
|   Preterm | <16 mg/dL | <274 µmol/L |
|   Term | <12 mg/dL | <205 µmol/L |
| >5 days | | |
|   Preterm | <2 mg/dL | <34 µmol/L |
|   Term | <1 mg/dL | <17 µmol/L |
| **Bilirubin (Conjugated)** | | |
| All ages | 0-0.4 mg/dL | 0-8 µmol/L |
| **Calcium (Total)** | | |
| Preterm <1 week | 6-10 mg/dL | 1.5-2.5 mmol/L |
| Full term <1 week | 7-12 mg/dL | 1.75-3 mmol/L |
| Child | 8-10.5 mg/dL | 2-2.6 mmol/L |
| **Calcium (Ionized)** | | |
| Newborn <48 hours | 4-4.7 mg/dL | 1-1.18 mmol/L |
| Adult | 4.52-5.28 mg/dL | 1.13-1.32 mmol/L |
| **Carbon Dioxide ($CO_2$ Content)** | | |
| Infant/child | 20-24 mEq/L | 20-24 mmol/L |
| **Carbon Monoxide (Carboxyhemoglobin)** | | |
| Nonsmoker | 0-2% of total hemoglobin | |
| **Chloride (Serum)** | | |
| Pediatric | 99-111 mEq/L | 99-111 mmol/L |
| **C-Reactive Protein** | | |
| All ages | 0-0.5 mg/dL | |
| **Creatine Kinase (Creatine Phosphokinase)** | | |
| Newborn | 10-200 U/L | 10-200 U/L |
| Adult female | 10-55 U/L | 10-55 U/L |
| Adult male | 12-80 U/L | 12-80 U/L |

## Table A1-2 Laboratory Tests: Reference Ranges (continued)

| Test | Conventional Unit | SI Unit |
|---|---|---|
| **Creatinine (Serum)** | | |
| Newborn | 0.3-1 mg/dL | 27-88 µmol/L |
| Infant | 0.2-0.4 mg/dL | 18-35 µmol/L |
| Child | 0.3-0.7 mg/dL | 27-62 µmol/L |
| Adolescent | 0.5-1 mg/dL | 44-88 µmol/L |
| **Fibrinogen** | | |
| All ages | 200-400 mg/dL | 5.9-11.7 µmol/L |
| **γ-Glutamyltransferase (GGT)** | | |
| Preterm | 56-233 U/L | 56-233 U/L |
| 0-3 weeks | 0-130 U/L | 0-130 U/L |
| 3 weeks-3 months | 4-120 U/L | 4-120 U/L |
| >3 months, boy | 5-65 U/L | 5-65 U/L |
| >3 months, girl | 5-35 U/L | 5-35 U/L |
| 1-15 years | 0-23 U/L | 0-23 U/L |
| **Glucose (Serum)** | | |
| Preterm | 45-100 mg/dL | 1.1-3.6 mmol/L |
| Full term | 45-120 mg/dL | 1.1-6.4 mmol/L |
| 1 week-16 years | 60-105 mg/dL | 3.3-5.8 mmol/L |
| **Iron** | | |
| Newborn | 100-250 µg/dL | 18-45 µmol/L |
| Infant | 40-100 µg/dL | 7-18 µmol/L |
| Child | 50-120 µg/dL | 9-22 µmol/L |
| **Ketones (Serum)** | | |
| Qualitative | Negative | |
| Quantitative | 0.5-3 mg/dL | 5-30 mg/L |
| **Lactate** | | |
| Capillary blood | | |
|   Newborn | <27 mg/dL | 0-3 mmol/L |
|   Child | 5-20 mg/dL | 0.5-2.2 mmol/L |
| Venous | 5-20 mg/dL | 0.5-2.2 mmol/L |
| Arterial | 5-14 mg/dL | 0.5-1.6 mmol/L |
| **Lactate Dehydrogenase (at 98.6°F, 37°C)** | | |
| Neonate | 160-1500 U/L | 160-1500 U/L |
| Infant | 150-360 U/L | 150-360 U/L |
| Child | 150-300 U/L | 150-300 U/L |
| **Lead** | | |
| Child | <10 µg/dL | <48 µmol/L |

## Table A1-2 Laboratory Tests: Reference Ranges (continued)

| Test | Conventional Unit | SI Unit |
|---|---|---|
| **Lipase** | | |
| All ages | 4-24 U/dL | |
| **Magnesium** | | |
| All ages | 1.3-2.0 mEq/L | 0.65-1.0 mmol/L |
| **Methemoglobin** | | |
| All ages | 0-1.3% total hemoglobin | |
| **Osmolality** | | |
| All ages | 285-295 mOsm/kg | 285-295 mmol/kg |
| **Phosphorus** | | |
| Newborn | 4.2-9.0 mg/dL | 1.36-2.91 mmol/L |
| 0-15 years | 3.2-6.3 mg/dL | 1.03-2.1 mmol/L |
| **Potassium** | | |
| <10 days | 4-6 mEq/L | 4-6 mmol/L |
| >10 days | 3.5-5 mEq/L | 3.5-5 mmol/L |
| **Prealbumin** | | |
| Newborn-6 weeks | 4-36 mg/dL | |
| 6 weeks-16 years | 13-27 mg/dL | |
| **Protein (Total)** | | |
| Newborn-1 month | 4.4-7.6 g/dL | |
| 1-3 months | 3.6-7.4 g/dL | |
| 4-6 months | 4.2-7.4 g/dL | |
| 7-12 months | 5.1-7.5 g/dL | |
| 13-24 months | 3.7-7.5 g/dL | |
| 25-36 months | 5.3-8.1 g/dL | |
| 3-5 years | 4.9-8.1 g/dL | |
| 6-16 years | 6.0-7.9 g/dL | |
| **Pyruvate** | | |
| All ages | 0.3-0.9 mg/dL | 0.03-0.1 mmol/L |
| **Sodium** | | |
| Preterm | 130-140 mEq/L | 130-140 mmol/L |
| Older | 135-148 mEq/L | 135-148 mmol/L |

### Table A1-2  Laboratory Tests: Reference Ranges (continued)

| Test | Conventional Unit | SI Unit |
|---|---|---|
| **Triglycerides (Fasting)** | | |
| Male | | |
|     0-5 years | 30-86 mg/dL | 0.3-0.86 g/L |
|     6-11 years | 31-108 mg/dL | 0.31-1.08 g/L |
|     12-15 years | 36-138 mg/dL | 0.36-1.38 g/L |
| Female | | |
|     0-5 years | 32-99 mg/dL | 0.32-0.99 g/L |
|     6-11 years | 35-114 mg/dL | 0.35-1.14 g/L |
|     12-15 years | 41-138 mg/dL | 0.41-1.38 g/L |
| **Troponin** | | |
| All ages | 0.03-0.15 ng/mL | 0.03-0.15 µg/mL |
| **Urea Nitrogen (BUN)** | | |
| All ages | 7-22 mg/dL | 2.5-7.9 mmol/L |
| **Uric Acid** | | |
| 0-2 years | 2.4-6.4 mg/dL | 0.14-0.38 mmol/L |
| 2-12 years | 2.4-5.9 mg/dL | 0.14-0.35 mmol/L |
| 12-14 years | 2.4-6.4 mg/dL | 0.14-0.38 mmol/L |

Adapted with permission. © 2012 Elsevier. Arcara KM. Blood chemistries and body fluids. In: Tschundy MM, Arcara KM, eds. *The Harriet Lane Handbook.* 19th ed. Philadelphia, PA: Mosby; 2012.

Appendix 2

# Intraosseous Needle Insertion

## I. INDICATIONS

1. Emergency vascular access in children if intravenous (IV) access is delayed or after 1 failed attempt at access.
2. Any fluid, blood product or medication that can be given intravenously can be given by the intraosseous (IO) route in the same dosages.

The relative ease of IO line placement allows it to be positioned correctly even under combat conditions.

## II. ANATOMY AND PHYSIOLOGY

Bone is supplied by a major artery. A rich venous network in the bone marrow drains into the central circulation. Blood obtained from an IO aspiration can be used to assess serum pH, $P_{CO_2}$, complete blood count, type and crossmatch, and any electrolyte studies needed. During resuscitation, the onset of action and peak concentrations of medications through the IO route have been shown to be roughly equivalent to the vascular route.

## III. EQUIPMENT

1. Needle selection
   - Jamshidi (CareFusion Corp.)
   - Cook Medical Inc.
   - EZ-IO (Vidacare Corp.): http://www.vidacare.com/EZ-IO/Index.aspx
   - FAST1 (Pyng Medical): http://www.pyng.com/products/fast1/
   - Bone Injection Gun (B.I.G.): http://www.actnt.com/BIG/Bone_Injection_Gun.htm

   See Suggested Readings for comparison of these devices.

2. Sterile syringes and infiltrating needles
3. Sterile 4 × 4 gauze sponges
4. Gloves, sterile drapes
5. Skin disinfectant
6. Supplemental oxygen

7. Pulse oximeter
8. Electrocardiography monitor
9. IV tubing, T connector, and fluid

## IV. SITE SELECTION

1. Proximal tibia 1 to 2 cm distal to the tibial tuberosity on the flat part of the tibia
2. Distal tibial site is entered approximately 1 cm superior to the medial malleolus on the flat part of the tibia
3. Distal femur site is inserted midline 2 to 3 cm above the femoral epicondyles
4. Proximal metaphysis of the humerus
5. Anterior iliac spine
6. Distal radius and distal ulnar

The distal femurs are preferred with infants younger than 2 months old because the proximal tibia is often too thin. If placement is necessary in neonates, insert at proximal tibia, just below the growth plate, distal to the tibial tubercle; in infants 6 to 12 months old, insert 1 cm distal to tibial tuberosity; in children >1 year old, insert 2 cm distal to the tibial tuberosity.

For the older child and adults, in addition to the proximal tibia or distal femur, the area proximal to the medial malleolus, the proximal humerus, or the anterior iliac spine is thin enough for an IO access site. The sternum has been used successfully for adults but is not recommended in children.

## V. JAMSHIDI OR COOK TECHNIQUE (TIBIAL SITE)

1. Apply oxygen, monitor pulse oximeter and electrocardiography.
2. Restrain leg with a small sandbag or IV fluid bag behind the knee for support.
3. Disinfectant skin when time and situation permit. Use povidone-iodine solution or alcohol scrub, 60 seconds of washing and 60 seconds of drying. In children older than 2 months, consider using chlorhexidine, 30 seconds of washing and 30 seconds of drying. To disinfect with a 70 plus percent alcohol solution, 10 seconds of washing and 5 seconds of drying prior to attempting insertion.
4. Infiltrate local anesthetic if the clinical situation permits.
5. Use proximal anterior tibia, midpoint of the medial flat surface, 1 to 2 cm below the tibial tuberosity (**Figure A2-1**).
6. Insert the needle at 60° to 90° to the skin away from the growth plate; advance with a screwing motion.
7. Use the distal tibia only if the proximal tibia is impenetrable (just proximal [1 cm] to the medial malleolus).
8. Confirm entry into the marrow space by noting a lack of resistance after the needle has passed through the cortex.

9. Aspirate marrow into the syringe; this should be accomplished easily. A properly placed IO needle will allow for marrow to be aspirated in only 50% of placements, so failure to do so does not necessarily indicate improper placement.

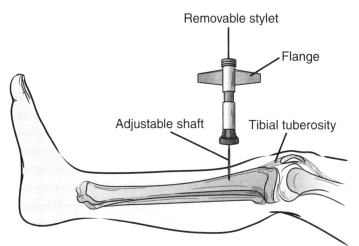

**Figure A2-1.** Intraosseous Needle Insertion

10. Infuse isotonic fluids, which should flow freely with proper placement of IO needle.

11. Secure needle by taping flanges to the skin (may require support of external portion of the needle) or by clamping IO needle near skin insertion site with a hemostat and taping the hemostat to the patient's lower leg.

12. Consider flushing with heparin-saline solution.

13. Infuse IV fluids and critical medications (epinephrine, antibiotics, glucose).

14. Observe for infiltration of fluids continuously to prevent injury.

15. Assign a team member to be solely responsible for preventing inadvertent dislodgement of the IO line until additional secure IV access is obtained.

16. Continue attempts to place IV catheter(s).

17. Discontinue IO infusion and withdraw needle after IV access is established (preferably within 1 to 2 hours) but no longer than 24 hours.

18. Apply pressure to the puncture site for approximately 5 minutes

19. Apply sterile dressing.

20. Do not place the IO needle until medications and fluids are available so as to decrease the risk of dislodgement between placement and infusion.

# VI. PRECAUTIONS/COMPLICATIONS

1. Inability to place needle (approximately 20% of patients)
2. Subcutaneous and/or subperiosteal infiltration of fluid
3. Tibia fracture
4. Compartment syndrome
5. Clotting of marrow within the needle
6. Cellulitis, subcutaneous abscess
7. Osteomyelitis (0.6%)
8. Pain (usually minor)

# VII. CONTRAINDICATIONS

1. Infection at entry site
2. Burn at entry site
3. Ipsilateral fracture of the extremity
4. Osteogenesis imperfecta
5. Osteopenia
6. Previous attempt at the same site
7. Previous attempt in different location on the same bone
8. Unable to locate landmarks

##  Suggested Readings

1. American Heart Association. 2010 Guidelines for Cardiopulmonary Resuscitation and Emergency Cardiovascular Care. *Circulation.* 2010;122(18 Suppl 3):S742, S881.

2. Brenner T, Bernhard M, Helm M, et al. Comparison of two intraosseous infusion systems for adult emergency medical use. *Resuscitation.* 2008;78:314-319.

3. Gazin N, Auger H, Jabre P, et al. Efficacy and safety of the EZ-IO™ intraosseous device: out-of-hospital implementation of a management algorithm for difficult vascular access. *Resuscitation.* 2011;82:126-129.

4. Harcke HT, Crawley G, Mabry R, Mazuchowski E. Placement of tibial intraosseous infusion devices. *Mil Med.* 2011;176:824-827.

5. Hartholt KA, van Lieshout EM, Thies WC, Patka P, Schipper IB. Intraosseous devices: a randomized controlled trial comparing three intraosseous devices. *Prehosp Emerg Care.* 2010;14:6-13.

6. Hoskins SL, Kramer GC, Stephens CT, Zachariah BS. Abstract 79: Efficacy of epinephrine delivery via the intraosseous humeral head route during CPR. *Circulation.* 2006;114:II_1204.

7. Leidel BA, Kirchhoff C, Braunstein V, Bogner V, Biberthaler P, Kanz KG. Comparison of two intraosseous access devices in adult patients under resuscitation in the emergency department: a prospective, randomized study. *Resuscitation.* 2010;81:994-999.

8. Levitan RM, Bortle CD, Snyder TA, Nitsch DA, Pisaturo JT, Butler KH. Use of a battery-operated needle driver for intraosseous access by novice users: skill acquisition with cadavers. *Ann Emerg Med.* 2009;54:692-694.

9. Nagler J, Krauss B. Intraosseous catheter placement in children. Videos in clinical medicine. *N Engl J Med.* 2011;364:e14.

10. Ong ME, Chan YH, Oh JJ, Ngo AS. An observational, prospective study comparing tibial and humeral intraosseous access using the EZ-IO. *Am J Emerg Med.* 2009;27:8-15.

11. Paxton JH, Knuth TE, Klausner HA. Humeral head intraosseous insertion: The preferred emergency venous access (abstract). *Ann Emerg Med.* 2008;52(4 Suppl):S58.

12. Shavit I, Hoffmann Y, Galbraith R, Waisman Y. Comparison of two mechanical intraosseous infusion devices: a pilot, randomized crossover trial. *Resuscitation.* 2009;80:1029-1033.

# Appendix 3

# Acid-Base Balance and Arterial Blood Gas Analysis

Acid-base disorders are common in critically ill children and are due to metabolic and/or respiratory compromise. The arterial blood gas measurement is an important laboratory test in the evaluation of a child's acid-base status.

# I. BLOOD GAS

A blood gas is composed of four basic parts:

1. pH is derived from the logarithmic expression of the hydrogen ion concentration ($H^+$) and is a measure of acidemia (acidosis) or alkalemia (alkalosis). A normal pH is 7.4 ± 0.05. A pH >7.45 is indicative of alkalemia, and a pH <7.35 indicates acidemia. Respiratory and metabolic processes contribute to the pH as described below; acidemia or alkalemia is the summation of one or more of these processes.

2. $Paco_2$ represents the partial pressure of $CO_2$ in arterial blood and is a measure of the adequacy of minute ventilation. It has a significant effect on pH in that for every $Paco_2$ change of 10 mm Hg from the baseline of 40 mm Hg, there is a corresponding pH change of 0.08 in the opposite direction. Hence, looking at an arterial blood gas sample, one can determine whether the pH is attributable solely to the $Paco_2$ level.

   For example, if a patient has a pH of 7.32 and a $Paco_2$ of 50 mm Hg, this is entirely due to the contribution of the respiratory acidosis (elevated $Paco_2$). However, if the pH is 7.28 and the $Paco_2$ is 50 mm Hg, the $Paco_2$ is only partly responsible for the acidosis, so the patient likely has a mixed/combined respiratory and metabolic acidosis.

3. $Pao_2$ represents the partial pressure of oxygen in the arterial blood. This provides an assessment of the patient's oxygenation and should be within the range of 80 to 100 mm Hg for a patient who is breathing room air and has no intracardiac right-to-left shunt. In cases of lung disease, hypoxemia might ensue, and $Pao_2$ levels may decline despite supplemental oxygen.

4. Bicarbonate level ($HCO_3^-$) is a measure of the presence of metabolic acidosis or alkalosis. Assuming a $Paco_2$ of 40 mm Hg, a change in the bicarbonate level for every 10 mEq/L above or below the normal of 24 mEq/L is associated with a pH change of 0.15 in the same direction. This allows an assessment of the metabolic component contributions to the acid-base (pH) status.

Another corollary that can be drawn from this is the calculation of the base excess (metabolic alkalosis) or base deficit (metabolic acidosis). Because the volume of distribution of bicarbonate is 0.3 L/kg body weight, the total body $HCO_3^-$ deficit can be ascertained: $HCO_3^-$ deficit (in mEq) = (calculated base deficit x 0.3 x weight [kg]).

# II. HOW TO EVALUATE AN ARTERIAL BLOOD GAS

When analyzing an arterial blood gas:

A. Determine if the pH is normal (7.35-7.45), low (i.e., acidemia; <7.35), or high (i.e., alkalemia; >7.45).

B. Determine if the $Pa_{CO_2}$ is high (>45 mm Hg) or low (<35 mm Hg). When **high**, think respiratory acidosis if the corresponding pH is low.

C. Look at the bicarbonate level. If it is low (<22 mEq/L) and the pH is low, think metabolic acidosis. If the bicarbonate level is high (>26 mEq/L) and the pH is high, think metabolic alkalosis.

These examples primarily pertain to acute acidosis and acute alkalosis. If the conditions have been present for several hours or longer, the body attempts to compensate for these abnormalities. Hyperventilation occurs to compensate for the profound metabolic acidosis, as seen in diabetic ketoacidosis; alternately renal compensation ensues in cases of chronic respiratory acidosis, seen in chronic lung disease/bronchopulmonary dysplasia. Many times the abnormalities are mixed, having components of each.

Arterial blood gas analysis is the "gold standard" for measuring acid-base status. In patients with indwelling lines with a free flow of blood, venous blood gas analysis has some benefit, but is different; $Pv_{O_2}$ levels might not reflect hypoxemia but can provide information on the circulatory status. If the $Pv_{O_2}$ level is <25 mm Hg, the cardiac output is low. Capillary blood gas analysis is not as helpful due to the potential for hemolysis during sample collection from a heel stick, and the oxygen levels are not predictive of hypoxemia.

### Table A3-1 Arterial Blood Gas Analysis

| Acidosis | Alkalosis | Metabolic | Respiratory | pH (7.35-7.45) | $Pa_{CO_2}$ (35-45 mm Hg) | $HCO_3^-$ (22-26 mEq/L) |
|---|---|---|---|---|---|---|
| X |   |   | X | <7.35 | >45 | normal |
| X |   | X |   | <7.35 | normal | <22 |
|   | X |   | X | >7.45 | <35 | normal |
|   | X | X |   | >7.45 | normal | >26 |

# Appendix 4

# Oxygen Delivery Devices

**Figure A4-1.** Venturi Mask

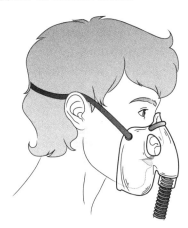

- Delivers humidified oxygen (aerosol adapter can be added)
- $F_{IO_2}$ is set by entrainment dial on mask
- Low concentrations = 24%, 26%, 28%, 31%
- High concentrations = 35%, 40%, 50%

**Figure A4-2.** Oxyhood

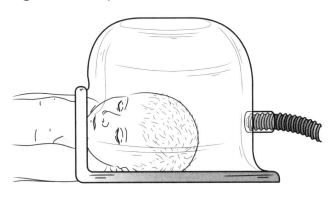

- Delivers heated, humidified oxygen to patients weighing <15 kg
- $F_{IO_2}$ is set by dial on blender
- $F_{IO_2}$ range = 21 - ?100%
- Minimum flow rate = 10 L/min (to clear exhaled $CO_2$ from hood)
- In-line oxygen analyzer will provide oxygen concentration.

**Figure A4-3.** Non-rebreathing Mask

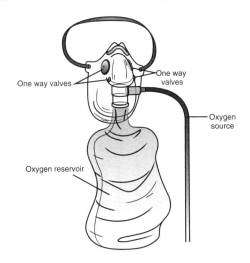

- Delivers non-humidified oxygen
- Used for emergency delivery
- $F_{IO_2}$ range = 60 - ?100%
- Reservoir bag provides 100% $F_{IO_2}$ and minimizes room air dilution
- Flap valves minimize entrainment of room air (which will dilute $F_{IO_2}$)
- Flow rate is adjusted according to the patient's ventilator pattern to keep reservoir bag inflated

**Figure A4-4.** Simple Oxygen Mask

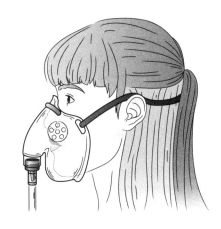

- Delivers humidified oxygen
- Minimum flow rate = 6 L/min (to clear exhaled $CO_2$ from mask)
- Approximate concentrations: 6 L = 40%; 7 L = 50%; 8 L = 60%

**Figure A4-5.** Aerosol Mask

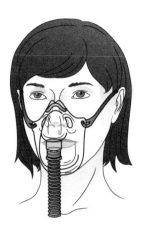

- Delivers cool, aerosolized oxygen or air
- $F_{IO_2}$ is set by dial on oxygen adapter
- Maximum $F_{IO_2}$ = 40%-60%
- Minimum flow rate = 8 L/min

**Figure A4-6.** Tracheostomy Mask

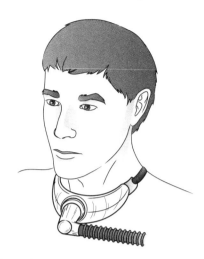

- Delivers heated, aerosolized oxygen or air
- $F_{IO_2}$ is set by dial on blender
- Maximum $F_{IO_2}$ = 40%-60%
- Minimum flow rate = 8 L/min

**Figure A4-7.** Nasal Cannula

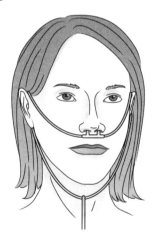

- Delivers humidified oxygen
- Nasal passages must be patent
- Blender setup: $F_{IO_2}$ is set by dial; 1-2 L flow can be used as continuous positive airway pressure for infants
- Wall setup: $F_{IO_2}$ is set by flow rate
- Approximate $F_{IO_2}$ (if respiratory rate and tidal volume are normal):

| Adult | Infant |
|---|---|
| 1 L = 24% | 1/8 L = 28% |
| 2 L = 28% | 1/4 L = 35% |
| 3 L = 32% | 1/2 L = 45% |
| 4 L = 36% | 3/4 L = 50% |
| 5 L = 40% | 1 L = 55% |
| 6 L = 44% | |

**Figure A4-8.** Face Tent

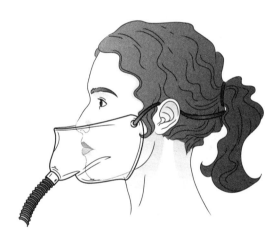

- Delivers cool, aerosolized oxygen or air
- Loose fit under the chin for patient comfort, speaking, etc.
- $F_{IO_2}$ is set by dial on oxygen adapter (concentration is unstable)
- Maximum $F_{IO_2}$ = 40%-50%
- Minimum flow rate = 8 L/min

# Appendix 5

# Airway Adjuncts

## I. OXYGEN DELIVERY DEVICES

A. The *simple oxygen mask* is a low-flow device that delivers oxygen with a flow rate of 6 to 10 L/min. The oxygen concentration delivered to the patient can reach a maximum of 60% because of entrainment of room air. It is important to maintain an oxygen flow rate of at least 6 L/min to sustain an optimal inspired oxygen concentration and prevent rebreathing of exhaled carbon dioxide.

B. A *partial rebreathing mask* consists of simple face mask with reservoir bag. It provides oxygen concentrations of 50% to 60%. During inspiration the patient draws gas predominantly from the fresh oxygen inflow and the reservoir bag, so entrainment of room air is minimized. An oxygen flow rate of 10 to12 L/min is usually required.

C. A *non-rebreathing mask* consists of a face mask and reservoir bag with a valve incorporated into one or both exhalation ports to prevent entrainment of room air during inspiration. Another valve is placed between the reservoir bag and mask to prevent flow of exhaled gas into the reservoir. An inspired concentration of 95% can be achieved with an oxygen flow rate of 10 to 15 L/min and use of a well-sealed mask.

D. A *face tent* is a high-flow soft plastic bucket that is often better tolerated by children than a face mask. Even with a high oxygen flow rate, inspired oxygen concentrations over 40% cannot be reliably provided. A face tent permits access to the face without interrupting oxygen flow.

E. A *nasal cannula* is a low-flow oxygen delivery system that is useful when low levels of supplemental oxygen are required. The net $F_{IO_2}$ depends on the child's respiratory effort, size, and minute ventilation in comparison with the nasal cannula flow.

## II. LARYNGEAL MASK AIRWAY

A. Indications

    1. Provide an airway and ventilation when bag-mask ventilation is difficult

    2. Provide a temporizing airway when endotracheal intubation is unsuccessful

B. Equipment

    1. Bag-mask resuscitation unit with high-flow oxygen source

    2. Pulse oximeter

3. Electrocardiographic monitor
4. Blood pressure monitoring
5. Gloves, mask, eye protection
6. Laryngeal mask airway (LMA) of appropriate size (**Table A5-1**)
7. Syringe for cuff inflation
8. Water-soluble lubricant
9. Qualitative $CO_2$ detector or $CO_2$ monitor
10. Resuscitation cart

**Table A5-1    Laryngeal Mask Airway Size and Cuff Inflation**

| LMA Size | Patient Size | Maximum Cuff Volume | Largest ETT ID (mm)[a] |
|---|---|---|---|
| 1 | Neonate/infant to 5 kg | Up to 4 mL | 3.5 |
| 1.5 | 5-10 kg | Up to 7 mL | 4.0 |
| 2 | 10-20 kg | Up to 10 mL | 4.5 |
| 2.5 | 20-30 kg | Up to 14 mL | 5.0 |
| 3 | >30 kg/small adult | Up to 20 mL | 6.0 cuffed |
| 4 | Average adult | Up to 30 mL | 6.0 cuffed |
| 5 | Large adult | Up to 40 mL | 7.0 cuffed |

[a]Largest endotracheal tube size (ETT ID) that will fit through laryngeal mask airway (LMA) tube lumen.

C. Preparation for insertion
1. Don gloves, mask, and eye protection.
2. Assure patent airway and optimal oxygenation and ventilation.
3. Assure intravenous (IV) access.
4. Apply pulse oximeter, electrocardiographic and blood pressure monitors.
5. Select appropriate size LMA.
6. Check cuff integrity by inflating and fully deflating.
7. Lubricate only the posterior aspect of the deflated mask with a water-based lubricant.
8. Preoxygenate with 100% oxygen for 2 to 3 minutes, if time permits.

D. Technique (**Figure A5-1**)
1. The cuff is deflated completely so that it forms a spoon shape and there are no folds in the mask.
2. The operator stands behind the head of the bed, and the bed is raised to a position of comfort for the operator.
3. The patient is placed in the sniffing position (i.e., head extended, neck flexed), unless potential or definite cervical spine injury prevents neck extension.

**Figure A5-1.** Insertion Technique for Laryngeal Mask Airway

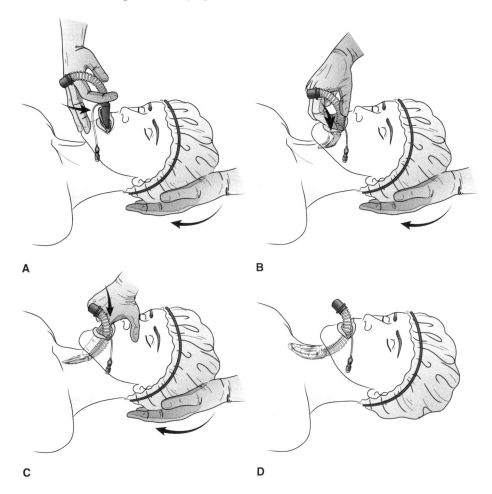

**A)** Insert lubricated and deflated mask into the open mouth with the bowl facing anteriorly. **B)** Hold the device like a pencil, pressing against the palate and pharyngeal wall with the index finger. **C)** Continue inserting the cuff behind the tongue into the hypopharynx until definite resistance is felt. **D)** Without holding the device, inflate cuff with enough air to obtain a seal. Attach manual ventilation device and ensure chest movement.

4. Cricoid pressure is not recommended during placement of the LMA because it may interfere with correct placement.

5. The mask is positioned with the bowl facing anteriorly. Hold the device like a pencil, with the index finger of the dominant hand at the junction of the bowl and tube, pressing against the palate and pharyngeal wall with the index finger.

6. The cuff is inserted into the hypopharynx until definite resistance is felt.

7. Without the operator holding the device, the cuff is inflated with enough air to obtain a seal around the laryngeal inlet. This step results in an outward movement of the tube.

8. The cuff is inflated with enough air to obtain a seal (intracuff pressure of approximately 60 cm $H_2O$). Maximum volumes are listed in **Table A5-1**, but lesser volume may provide an adequate seal.

9. A manual ventilation device is attached, and chest movement and breath sounds are verified in both lung fields. Correct position should be confirmed with a qualitative or quantitative end-tidal $CO_2$ detector.

10. If chest movement is inadequate, or if a large air leak is present, the device should be removed and reinserted.

11. When the LMA is positioned appropriately, the tube is secured with tape.

# III. ESOPHAGEAL-TRACHEAL DOUBLE-LUMEN AIRWAY DEVICE

*Note: The esophageal-tracheal double-lumen airway device is intended for adults and adult-sized children. Pediatric sizes are NOT available.*

A. Indication

    1. Cardiorespiratory arrest and inability to provide an airway by other means

B. Equipment

    1. Bag-mask resuscitation unit with high-flow oxygen source

    2. Pulse oximeter

    3. Electrocardiographic monitor

    4. Blood pressure monitoring

    5. Gloves, mask, eye protection

    6. Esophageal-tracheal double-lumen device (**Figure A5-2**)

    7. Syringe for cuff inflation

    8. Water-soluble lubricant

    9. Qualitative $CO_2$ detector or $CO_2$ monitor

    10. Resuscitation cart

C. Preparation for insertion

    1. Don gloves, mask, and eye protection.

    2. Assure patent airway and optimal oxygenation and ventilation.

    3. Assure IV access.

    4. Apply pulse oximeter, electrocardiographic and blood pressure monitors.

    5. Select appropriate size device. *The esophageal-tracheal double-lumen airway device is intended for adults and adult-sized children. Pediatric sizes are not available.*

    6. Check integrity of both cuffs by inflating and fully deflating.

    7. Preoxygenate with 100% oxygen for 2 to 3 minutes if time permits.

D. Technique

    1. The cuffs should be deflated completely.

    2. The operator stands behind the head of the bed, and the bed is raised to a position of comfort for the operator.

**Figure A5-2.** Esophageal-Tracheal Double-Lumen Airway Device

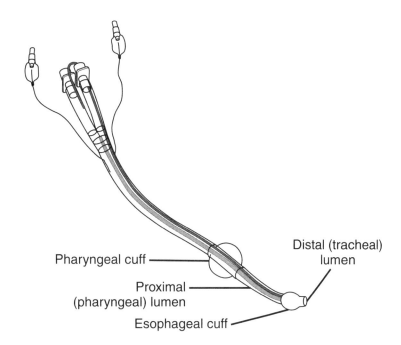

Some tubes have two pilot balloons to allow for independent inflation of the pharyngeal and esophageal cuffs, whereas other tubes have a single pilot port and simultaneously inflate both cuffs. Detection of end-tidal $CO_2$ in the proximal lumen suggests that the tube is in the esophagus. In the rare instance that the tube enters the trachea, ventilation is only possible via the distal lumen and end-tidal $CO_2$ will not be detected from the proximal lumen.

3. The patient is placed in a neutral or sniffing position (i.e., head extended, neck flexed), unless potential or definite cervical spine injury prevents neck extension.

4. The patient's tongue and jaw are grasped between the thumb and index finger, and the device is inserted blindly. It is advanced until the placement ring markers on the tube are positioned as indicated by the manufacturer. Do not force the tube if resistance is met. A laryngoscope can be used to assist with placement.

5. The pharyngeal cuff is inflated first to seal the posterior pharynx.

6. The distal cuff is then inflated.

7. Ventilation should be attempted first through the pharyngeal lumen, and the chest should be auscultated for breath sounds and observed for movement. The tube enters the esophagus approximately 95% of the time.

8. If breath sounds are absent, ventilation should be attempted through the tracheal lumen while auscultating for breath sounds.

9. Use of the correct lumen for ventilation should be confirmed with a qualitative/quantitative end-tidal $CO_2$ or esophageal detector device.

10. When the device is positioned appropriately, the tube is secured with tape.

# IV. VIDEO LARYNGOSCOPE

A. Indications

    1. Endotracheal intubation in known or presumed difficult airway

    2. Known or suspected cervical spine injury

B. Equipment

    1. Bag-mask resuscitation unit with high-flow oxygen source

    2. Pulse oximeter

    3. Electrocardiographic monitor

    4. Blood pressure monitoring

    5. Gloves, mask, and eye protection

    6. Video laryngoscope with appropriate blade

    7. Endotracheal tube (ETT) of appropriate size for patient

    8. Syringe for cuff inflation

    9. Water-soluble lubricant

    10. Qualitative $CO_2$ detector or $CO_2$ monitor

    11. Resuscitation cart

C. Preparation for insertion

    1. Don gloves, mask, and eye protection.

    2. Assure patent airway and optimal oxygenation and ventilation.

    3. Assure IV access.

    4. Apply pulse oximeter, electrocardiographic and blood pressure monitors.

    5. Prepare ETT with stylet and check cuff.

    6. Turn on video laryngoscope power and check light/camera.

    7. Assure proper cable and blade attachment.

    8. Position video screen for optimal viewing during laryngoscopy.

    9. Preoxygenate with 100% oxygen for 2 to 3 minutes if time permits.

D. Technique (**Figure A5-3**)

    1. The operator stands behind the head of the bed, and the bed is raised to a position of comfort for the operator.

    2. The patient is placed in a neutral or sniffing position (i.e., head extended, neck flexed), unless potential or definite cervical spine injury prevents neck extension.

    3. Consider lubricating the tongue side of the laryngoscope blade prior to insertion. Insert the laryngoscope blade into the oropharynx, and advance into the hypopharynx while watching the video screen for anatomical landmarks.

**Figure A5-3.** Video Laryngoscope

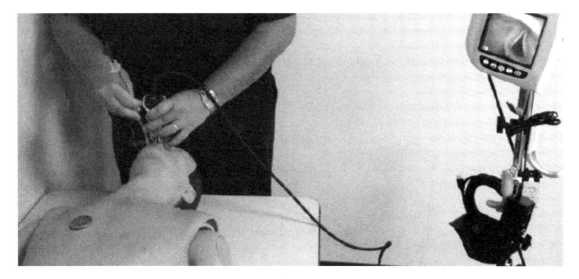

Courtesy of Jason Emerson, Skaneateles Press, Eagle Newspapers, Syracuse, New York, USA.

4. Once positioned in the hypopharynx, lift up and away, then adjust the position until the glottis and vocal cords are seen.

5. Insert and advance the ETT into the hypopharynx until the tip is seen near the end of the laryngoscope blade on the video screen.

6. While watching the video screen, advance the ETT through the glottis opening until the cuff passes the vocal cords. Make small adjustments in the laryngoscope and ETT positioning as necessary to intubate the trachea.

7. Gently remove the laryngoscope blade while holding the ETT in place. Be careful not to kink or pinch the camera cable.

8. Inflate the ETT cuff and remove the stylet. Attach the bag-valve device and provide manual ventilation. Confirm proper placement with bilateral breath sounds and a qualitative/quantitative end-tidal $CO_2$ or esophageal detector device.

9. When the ETT is positioned appropriately, the tube is secured with tape.

# V. OPTICAL LARYNGOSCOPE

A. Indications

1. Endotracheal intubation in known or presumed difficult airway
2. Known or suspected cervical spine injury

B. Equipment

1. Bag-mask resuscitation unit with high-flow oxygen source
2. Pulse oximeter
3. Electrocardiographic monitor

4. Blood pressure monitoring

5. Gloves, mask, and eye protection

6. Appropriately sized optical laryngoscope – color coded

7. ETT of appropriate size for patient

8. Syringe for cuff inflation

9. Water-soluble lubricant

10. Qualitative $CO_2$ detector or $CO_2$ monitor

11. Resuscitation cart

C. Preparation for insertion

1. Don gloves, mask, and eye protection.

2. Assure patent airway and optimal oxygenation and ventilation.

3. Assure IV access.

4. Apply pulse oximeter, electrocardiographic and blood pressure monitors.

5. Prepare ETT, check cuff, and lubricate.

6. Choose appropriately sized optical laryngoscope.

7. Turn on laryngoscope light at least 30 seconds prior to use.

8. Load ETT into optical laryngoscope side channel.

9. Assure ETT tip is seen through eyepiece but is not obstructing view.

10. Preoxygenate with 100% oxygen for 2 to 3 minutes if time permits.

D. Technique (**Figure A5-4**)

1. The operator stands behind the head of the bed, and the bed is raised to a position of comfort for the operator.

2. The patient is placed in a neutral or sniffing position (i.e., head extended, neck flexed), unless potential or definite cervical spine injury prevents neck extension.

3. Consider lubricating the tongue side of the laryngoscope blade prior to insertion. Insert the laryngoscope blade in the midline over the tongue into the oropharynx and advance into the hypopharynx by rotating the laryngoscope along the tongue until it is perpendicular. Use caution not to displace the tongue posteriorly.

4. Once positioned in the hypopharynx, look through the eyepiece and lift up gently. Adjust the position until the glottis and vocal cords are seen. If glottis structures are not seen, gently pull back until seen. Do not tilt back or leverage against upper teeth or gums.

5. Advance the ETT through the glottis opening until the cuff passes the vocal cords. Make small adjustments in laryngoscope positioning as necessary to intubate the trachea.

6. Inflate the ETT cuff and separate from the laryngoscope with a gentle spreading or peeling motion. Be careful not to displace the ETT.

7. Gently remove the laryngoscope blade while holding the ETT in place. Rotate in the opposite direction from insertion.

**Figure A5-4.** Optical Laryngoscope

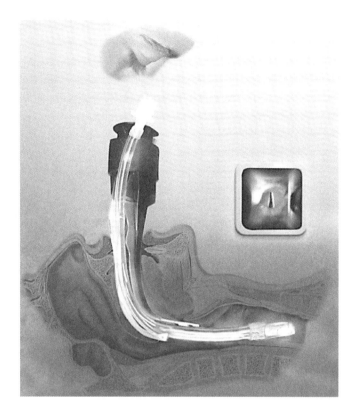

Courtesy of Prodol Meditec SA, Las Arenas Vizcaya, Spain.

8. Attach the bag-valve device and provide manual ventilation. Confirm bilateral breath sounds and use a qualitative/quantitative end-tidal $CO_2$ or esophageal detector device.

9. When the ETT is positioned appropriately, the tube is secured with tape.

 ## Suggested Readings

1. Brain AIJ. The *Intravent Laryngeal Mask Instruction Manual.* Berkshire, UK: Brain Medical; 1992.

2. Danks RR, Danks B. Laryngeal mask airway: review of indications and use. *J Emerg Nurs.* 2004;30:30-35.

3. Krafft P, Schebesta K. Alternative management techniques for the difficult airway: esophageal-tracheal Combitube. *Curr Opin Anaesthesiol.* 2005;17:499-504.

4. Lu Y, Jiang H, Zhu YS. Airtraq laryngoscope versus conventional Macintosh laryngoscope: a systematic review and meta-analysis. *Anaesthesia.* 2011;66:1160-1167.

5. Mace SE. The laryngeal mask airway: guidelines for appropriate usage. *Resid Staff Physician.* 2001;47:30.

6. Niforopoulou P, Pantazopoulos I, Demestiha T, Koudouna E, Xanthos Tl. Video-laryngoscopes in the adult airway management: a topical review of the literature. *Acta Anaesthesiol Scand.* 2010;54:1050-1061.

# Appendix 6

# Endotracheal Intubation

## I. INDICATIONS

A. Loss of protective airway reflexes

B. Alteration or absence of neuronal respiratory drive

C. Increased work of breathing resulting in respiratory distress

D. Airway obstruction to gas flow

E. Alteration in patient's level of consciousness

F. Elective intubation for surgical or nonsurgical procedure

## II. EQUIPMENT

A. Bag-valve-mask resuscitation unit with high-flow oxygen source – appropriate size

B. Airway mask – appropriate size

C. Yankauer and tracheal suction catheters and suction device – appropriate size

D. Monitors: blood pressure device, pulse oximeter, electrocardiography monitor

E. Laryngoscope handle and blade(s)

F. Endotracheal tubes – one size appropriate, one size smaller, and one size larger

G. Stylet – appropriate size: small, pediatric, adult

H. Oral and nasal airways – appropriate size

I. Towel roll or pad for occipital elevation

J. Medication for analgesia/anesthesia, sedation, and neuromuscular blockade

K. 10-mL syringe to inflate cuff, if appropriate

L. Qualitative $CO_2$ detector, $CO_2$ monitor, or esophageal detector device

M. Tape or tracheal tube stabilization device

N. Intravenous tubing and fluid

O. Resuscitation cart

P. Personal protective devices, gown, gloves, mask, and eye protection

# III. OROTRACHEAL INTUBATION VIA DIRECT LARYNGOSCOPY

A. Preparation

    1. Assemble all equipment and ensure proper working order

    2. Don gloves, gown, mask, and eye protection

    3. Confirm optimal oxygenation and ventilation

    4. Establish intravenous access

    5. Apply pulse oximeter, electrocardiographic, and blood pressure devices

    6. Prepare the endotracheal tube

        a. If cuffed tube, check integrity by inflating and fully deflating cuff

        b. Insert stylet into endotracheal tube, bend to configuration predicted to assist glottic entry

    7. Connect laryngoscope blade to handle and assure that light from bulb is bright

        a. Blade selection (operator's choice): larynx of the infant or small child is cephalad, appearing anterior; most clinicians do not use curved blades in infants

            i. Straight blade – used to elevate the epiglottis anteriorly

            ii. Curved blade – inserted into the vallecula

        b. Blade length: must be long enough to reach the epiglottis

    8. Place the patient in the proper head position. A towel placed under the shoulders is usually needed to achieve the sniffing position in infants. Older children and adults may require a towel roll under the head to achieve the sniffing position (if cervical spine injury is not suspected).

    9. Pre-oxygenate with 100% oxygen for 2-3 minutes to build up oxygen reserves, and confirm ability of operator to maintain effective ventilation

    10. Proceed with analgesia and sedation; administer neuromuscular blockade only after confirmed ability to ventilate

B. Technique

    1. The operator stands at the head of the patient and the bed is raised to a position of comfort for the operator. The head of the bed may be flat or raised slightly per operator preference.

    2. When no cervical spine injury is suspected, place the patient in the sniffing position and gently extend the neck (**Figure A6-1**). When cervical spine injury is suspected, the neck is stabilized by an assistant and the anterior portion of the cervical collar is removed.

**Figure A6-1.** Positioning for Orotracheal Intubation

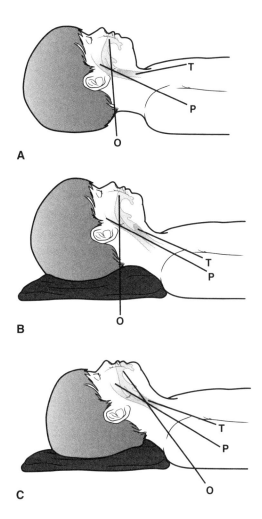

**A**) Maximal opening and visualization of the airway is obtained by aligning the oral (*O*), pharyngeal (*P*), and tracheal (*T*) axes. This is accomplished by placing a patient in the sniffing position. **B**) A folded sheet or towel placed under the occiput aligns the pharyngeal and tracheal axes. **C**) Extension of the neck into the sniffing position then results in approximate alignment of all three axes. Proper positioning places the external ear canal anterior to the shoulder. In children younger than 2 years, a folded towel or sheet is placed under the shoulder rather than under the occiput due to the relatively large forehead-to-occiput distance in this age group.

3. Regardless of the operator's dominant hand, the laryngoscope is always held in the left hand.

4. Cricoid pressure should be gently but firmly applied by an assistant as soon as consciousness is lost, and should be sustained until endotracheal tube placement is confirmed and the cuff is inflated, if indicated.

5. Mouth opening in the sedated/relaxed patient may be assisted by a cross-finger technique, wherein the thumb of the right hand is placed on the front lower teeth or gum of the mandible and the first finger on the upper teeth/gum of the maxilla. The mouth is gently opened by a "reverse scissor" movement of the fingers, and the laryngoscope is introduced into the mouth.

6. The tip of laryngoscope blade is inserted into the right side of the patient's mouth (**Figure A6-2**); the blade is advanced to the base of the tongue.

**Figure A6-2.** Insertion of Laryngoscope Blades

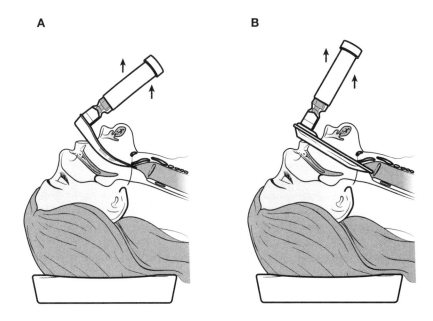

**A)** The curved blade follows the base of the tongue and is inserted into the vallecula. **B)** The straight blade is inserted beneath the epiglottis.

7. The tongue is swept to left; proper tongue control is key to laryngeal visualization.

8. The blade is gently advanced further to its proper position. A straight blade is placed beneath the epiglottis; a curved blade is placed into the vallecula above the epiglottis.

9. Traction should be applied only along the long axis of the laryngoscope handle as the laryngoscope lifts the tongue upward away from the larynx, revealing the glottic opening. A rocking or rotating motion of the blade and handle may damage teeth, gingiva, or lips. The base of the laryngoscope blade should never contact the upper teeth.

10. The vocal cords and glottic opening should be visualized.

11. If the vocal cords and glottis cannot be visualized, it may be helpful to have an assistant grasp the thyroid cartilage between the thumb and index finger and exert pressure until the vocal cords come into view.

12. The endotracheal tube is gently inserted through the vocal cords (**Figure A6-3**), while holding the tube/stylet with the right hand. The proper depth of insertion in centimeters can be estimated by multiplying the internal diameter of the endotracheal tube by 3 (e.g., internal diameter = 4; depth of insertion = 4 x 3 = 12 cm).

13. The stylet and laryngoscope should be removed carefully. The operator must continue to hold the endotracheal tube firmly.

14. The cuff is inflated, if indicated.

15. To ensure proper position of the tube:

    a. Inspect and auscultate the chest to assure equal bilateral gas entry. In addition, auscultate the abdomen to ensure absence of air entry.

**Figure A6-3.** Endotracheal Tube Placement

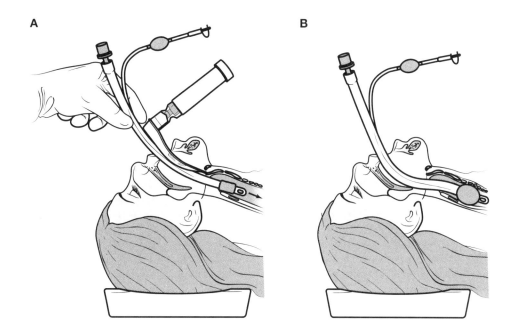

**A**) The endotracheal tube is inserted through the vocal cords until the distal end rests approximately 2 to 3 cm above the carina. **B**) Once the endotracheal tube is in proper position, the laryngoscope and stylet are removed and the cuff is inflated.

        b. Use a qualitative $CO_2$ detector, monitor, or esophageal detector device. Lack of color change with a qualitative $CO_2$ detector or low exhaled $CO_2$ will occur with an incorrectly placed endotracheal tube.

        c. Observe for condensation in the endotracheal tube during exhalation.

        d. Obtain chest radiograph. Tube tip should ideally be seen halfway between the thoracic inlet and carina.

    16. The endotracheal tube should be secured with tape or a tube stabilization device.

# IV. PEDIATRIC CONSIDERATIONS

A. Anatomic differences between adults and children

    1. The larynx is more cephalad in infants than in adults, making it appear more anterior and resulting in a more difficult visualization during laryngoscopy.

    2. Cricoid pressure is valuable during laryngoscopy because of the position of the larynx and assists in preventing aspiration.

    3. In young children, the narrowest part of the airway is at the level of the cricoid cartilage, not at the larynx, making an anatomic "cuff" below the vocal cords.

4. In general, the diameter of the small finger approximates the proper size of the endotracheal tube. A full-term neonate can accept a tube with a 3.5-mm inner diameter.

5. When selecting a cuffed tube for a child <8 years old, the tube size should be one size smaller than the calculated size. Cuffed tubes are usually limited to children >8 years of age (endotracheal tube size >6 mm internal diameter); uncuffed tubes are generally used in younger children. Consideration of a cuffed tube in a younger child may be necessary when a prolonged course of mechanical ventilation or positive pressure ventilation is anticipated.

# V. PRECAUTIONS/COMPLICATIONS

A. Hypoxia, hypercapnia during procedure

B. Cardiovascular compromise during and immediately after procedure

C. Damaged teeth, lips, gingiva

D. Malpositioned tube (right or left mainstem bronchus, esophagus)

E. Pharyngeal, laryngeal, tracheal damage

F. Gastric distension and aspiration of gastric contents

G. Bronchospasm, laryngospasm

H. Upper airway obstruction

I. Inability to visualize vocal cords

J. Inability to ventilate

# Suggested Readings

1. Balk RA. The technique of orotracheal intubation. *J Crit Illness*. 1997;12:316.

2. Gerardi MJ, Sacchetti AD, Cantor RM, et al. Rapid-sequence intubation of the pediatric patient. Pediatric Emergency Medicine Committee of the American College of Emergency Physicians. *Ann Emerg Med*. 1996;28:55-74.

3. McLean B, Zimmerman JL, eds. *Fundamental Critical Care Support*. 4th ed. Mount Prospect, IL: Society of Critical Care Medicine; 2007.

4. Tobias JD. Airway management for pediatric emergencies. *Pediatr Ann*. 1996;25:317-320, 323-328.

# Appendix 7

# Common Medications

### Table A7-1  Analgesics and Sedatitves

| Agent | Dosing | Onset and Duration | Benefits | Cautions |
|---|---|---|---|---|
| **Fentanyl** | *Intermittent Dosing for Sedation/Analgesia:* 1-2 µg/kg/dose IV every 1- 2 h | Onset: Immediate<br><br>Duration: 30-60 min | -Rapid onset of action<br>-Short acting<br>-Reversible with naloxone<br>-Relatively stable hemodynamic profile<br>-Useful for acute and chronic pain | -Chest wall rigidity syndrome<br>-Respiratory depression or apnea<br>-Lacks amnestic properties |
| | *Continuous Sedation/Analgesia:* Bolus: 1-2 µg/kg/dose IV, then infuse at 1-2 µg/kg/h. Titrate upward by 1 µg/kg/h for adequate sedation/analgesia | | | -Narcotic abstinence syndrome and tolerance can occur with prolonged use |
| **Morphine** | *Intermittent Dosing for Sedation/Analgesia:* 0.05-0.1 mg/kg IV every 2-4 h | Onset: 5 min<br><br>Duration: 2 h | -Useful for acute and chronic pain | -Respiratory depression<br>-Histamine release<br>-Hypotension<br>-Pruritus<br>-Angioneurotic edema |
| | *Continuous Sedation/Analgesia:* 0.01-0.03 mg/kg/h IV | | | -Narcotic abstinence syndrome and tolerance can occur with prolonged use |
| **Midazolam** | *Intermittent Dosing for Sedation/Analgesia:* 0.05 to 0.1 mg/kg/dose IV every 5 min, titrate to effect to maximum of 5 mg | Onset: 1-5 min<br><br>Duration: 20-30 min | -Rapid onset<br>-Short acting<br>-Provides amnesia<br>-Reversible with flumazenil | -Lacks analgesic properties<br>-Respiratory depression or apnea<br>-Hypotension and bradycardia |
| | *Continuous Sedation/Analgesia:* 0.05 to 0.15 mg/kg/h IV, titrate upward to achieve adequate sedation | | | -Withdrawal symptoms, tolerance, and myoclonus can occur with prolonged use |
| **Lorazepam** | *Intermittent Dosing for Sedation:* 0.05-0.1 mg/kg IV every 20 min, titrate to effect | Onset: 2-3 min<br><br>Duration: 2-6 hours | -Useful for sedation and status epilepticus<br>-Provides amnesia | -Respiratory depression, apnea<br>-Bradycardia<br>-Hypotension |
| **Ketamine** | *Intermittent Dosing for Sedation:* 0.5 to 1 mg/kg/dose IV every 5 min, titrate to effect | Onset: 1-2 min<br><br>Duration: 15-30 min | -Rapid onset<br>-Airway protective reflexes remain intact<br>-No hypotension or bradycardia<br>-Provides analgesia<br>-Provides bronchodilation | -Increases airway secretions and laryngospasm (blunted with atropine)<br>-Elevates intracranial and ocular pressure<br>-Emergence reactions (blunted with benzodiazepines) |
| | *Continuous Sedation/Analgesia:* 0.5-2 mg/kg/h IV and titrate to effect | | | |

### Table A7-1 Analgesics and Sedatitves (continued)

| Agent | Dosing | Onset and Duration | Benefits | Cautions |
|---|---|---|---|---|
| **Etomidate** | *Intermittent Dosing:* 0.3 mg/kg/dose IV every 5 min, titrate to effect | Onset: 10-20 s<br><br>Duration: 4-10 min | -Rapid onset<br>-Short acting<br>-Stable hemodynamic profile | -Blocks stress-induced increase in cortisol causing prolonged adrenal insufficiency, potentially greater than 24 hours<br>-Myoclonus<br>-No analgesic properties |
| **Thiopental** | 2-3 mg/kg IV, repeat as needed | Onset: 30-60 s<br><br>Duration: 5-30 min | -Ultra-short-acting barbiturate<br>-Decreases intracranial pressure<br>-Anticonvulsant | -Cardiovascular and respiratory depression with apnea<br>-Bronchospasm<br>-Hypotension<br>-No analgesic properties |
| **Pentobarbital** | *Intermittent Dosing:* 1-3 mg/kg IV to a maximum of 100 mg until sedated<br><br>*Continuous Sedation:* 1-2 mg/kg/h IV, titrate upward by 1 mg/kg/h IV to achieve sedation or burst supression on EEG | Onset: 30-60 s<br><br>Duration IV: 15 min | -Rapid onset IV<br>-Useful in status epilepticus and increased intracranial pressure | -Laryngospasm and respiratory depression<br>-Can cause hypotension and bradycardia<br>-No analgesic properties |
| **Dexmedetomidine** | *Intermittent Dosing:* 1 μg/kg over 10 min IV<br><br>*Continuous Sedation:* 0.2-0.75 μg/kg/h IV | Onset: 15 min | -Preserves respiratory status<br>-Stable hemodynamic profile<br>-Prevents delirium and shivering<br>-Lower requirement for benzodiazepines and narcotics | -Hypotension with bolus dosing<br>-Bradycardia<br>-Withdrawal effects if discontinued after prolonged use |
| **Chloral hydrate** | 25-75 mg/kg PO 30 min before procedure, maximum 1 gram for infants, 2 grams for children per dose | Onset: 30-60 minutes<br><br>Duration: 4-8 hours | -Short-term sedative and hypnotic for diagnostic procedures | -May cause "hangover" effect<br>-Paradoxical excitement can occur<br>-Withdrawal effects with prolonged use<br>-No analgesia |

IV, intravenous; EEG, electroencephalography; PO, by mouth
Classified using Taketomo CK, Hodding JH, Krause DM. *Pediatric Dosage Handbook with International Trade Names Index*. 14th ed. Hudson, OH: Lexicomp; 2006-2007.

### Table A7-2  Nonsteroidal Anti-inflammatory Drugs — Recommended[a,b]

| Agent | Dosing | Onset and Duration | Benefits | Cautions |
|---|---|---|---|---|
| **Acetaminophen** | PO: 10-15 mg/kg every 3-4 h<br><br>PR: 15-20 mg/kg every 4 h<br><br>*Newborn dose (< 6 kg or <6 mo):*<br>PO, 10-15 mg/kg every 4-6 h<br>PR, 20-25 mg/kg every 4-6 h | Onset: 10-60 min<br><br>Duration: 1-3 h<br><br>Newborn dosing: 2-5 h | -Analgesic<br>-Antipyretic | -Maximum dose, 75 mg/kg/d<br>-No anti-inflammatory effects |
| **Ketorolac** | IM/IV: 0.5 mg/kg every 6 h<br><br>Maximum dose: 30 mg/dose | Onset: 30 min<br><br>Duration: 4-6 h | -Analgesic<br>-Anti-inflammatory agent<br>-Antipyretic<br>-NSAID | -Maximum 5 d of therapy<br>-Avoid in renal insufficiency<br>-Inhibits platelet aggregation and promotes bleeding<br>-GI bleeding and ulceration can occur with prolonged use |
| **Ibuprofen** | PO: 10 mg/kg every 6-8 h | Onset: 60-120 min<br><br>Duration: 6-8 h | -Analgesic<br>-Anti-inflammatory agent<br>-Antipyretic<br>-NSAID | -Inhibits platelet aggregation and promotes bleeding<br>-Should not be used with with platelet count <50,000/mm$^3$<br>-Avoid in renal insufficiency<br>-GI bleeding and ulceration can occur with prolonged use |
| **Aspirin** | PO: 10-15 mg/kg every 4 h | Onset: 15-20 min<br><br>Duration: dose dependent, ranging 3-10 h with high doses (>1 g) | -Analgesic<br>-Anti-inflammatory agent<br>-Antipyretic<br>-NSAID | -Contraindicated in children with low platelet counts, bleeding disorders<br>-Associated with Reye syndrome in presence of fever or other viral illness<br>-Avoid in renal insufficiency<br>-Avoid if peptic ulcer disease present |

IV, intravenous; IM, intramuscular; PO, by mouth; PR, by rectum; NSAID, nonsteroidal anti-inflammatory drug; GI, gastrointestinal

[a]These doses have a ceiling effect and maximum dose should not be exceeded.
[b]Doses given are for patients weighing <50 kg.
Classified using Taketomo CK, Hodding JH, Krause DM. *Pediatric Dosage Handbook with International Trade Names Index*. 14th ed. Hudson, OH: Lexicomp; 2006-2007.

## Table A7-3  Neuromuscular Blockade Agents

| Agent | Dosing | Onset and Duration | Benefits | Cautions |
|---|---|---|---|---|
| **Succinylcholine** (depolarizing neuromuscular blockade) | 1-2 mg/kg IV to maximum dose of 150 mg | Onset: 30-60 s<br><br>Duration: 4-6 min | -Rapid onset<br>-Short duration | -Bradycardia leading to cardiac arrest in infants <2 months not pretreated with anticholinergic agents (atropine)<br>-Rhabdomyolysis can occur<br>-Causes muscle fasciculations (blunted with low-dose non-depolarizing neuromuscular blocker)<br>-Potentiates hyperkalemia (contraindicated in head trauma, crush injury, burns, hyperkalemia)<br>-May induce neuroleptic malignant syndrome |
| **Vecuronium** (non-depolarizing neuromuscular blockade) | *Intermittent Dosing:* 0.1 to 0.2 mg/kg IV every 30 min to 1 h<br><br>*Continuous Infusion:* 0.1 mg/kg/h IV, titrate upward by 0.05 mg/kg/h to provide adequate muscle relaxation | Onset: 1-3 min<br><br>Duration: 30-40 min | -No fasciculations<br>-Stable hemodynamic profile | -Slower onset<br>-Longer duration of action<br>-No analgesic or sedative properties |
| **Rocuronium** (non-depolarizing neuromuscular blockade) | *Intermittent Dosing:* 0.6-1.0 mg/kg IV every 30 min to 1 h<br><br>*Continuous Infusion:* 10-12 µg/kg/min IV, titrate upward by 1 µg/kg/min to provide adequate muscle relaxation | Onset: 30-60 s<br><br>Duration: 30-40 min | -No fasciculations<br>-Anticholinergic properties | -May cause tachycardia |
| **Cisatracurium** (non-depolarizing neuromuscular blockade) | *Intermittent Dosing:* 0.1-0.2 mg/kg IV every 30-45 min<br><br>*Continuous Infusion:* 1-4 µg/kg/min IV, titrate upward by 0.5 µg/kg/min to provide adequate muscle relaxation | Onset: 2-3 min<br><br>Duration: 35-45 min | -Can be used in renal or hepatic failure<br>-Metabolized through Hofmann elimination | -Potential histamine release<br>-Hypotension<br>-Bronchospasm |
| **Atracurium** (non-depolarizing neuromuscular blockade) | *Intermittent Dosing:* 0.3-0.5 mg/kg IV every 20 to 35 min<br><br>*Continuous Infusion:* 0.4-0.8 mg/kg/h IV, titrate upward by 0.1 mg/kg/h to provide adequate muscle relaxation | Onset: 1-4 min<br><br>Duration: 20-35 min | -Can be used in renal or hepatic failure<br>-Metabolized through Hofmann elimination | -Potential histamine release<br>-Hypotension and bradycardia<br>-Bronchospasm |

IV, intravenous
Classified using Taketomo CK, Hodding JH, Krause DM. *Pediatric Dosage Handbook with International Trade Names Index.* 14th ed. Hudson, OH: Lexicomp; 2006-2007.

# Appendix 8

# Difficult Airway Algorithm

Approach to difficult and failed intubation.

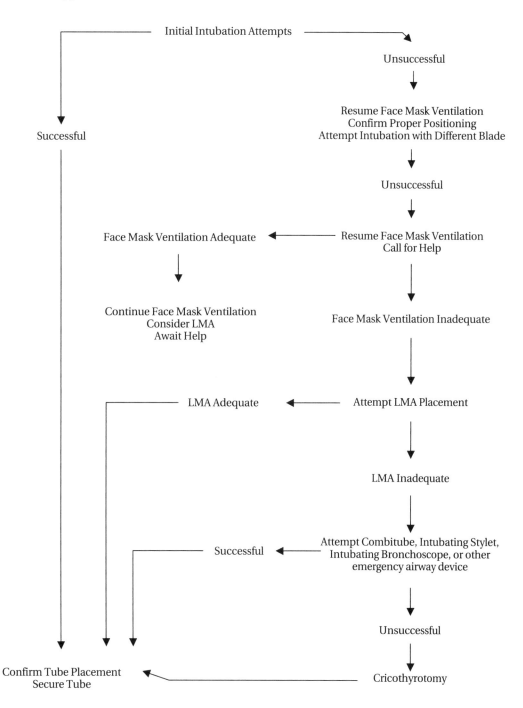

LMA, laryngeal mask airway

# Appendix 9

# Advanced Life Support Algorithms

**Figure A9-1.** Pediatric Cardiac Arrest

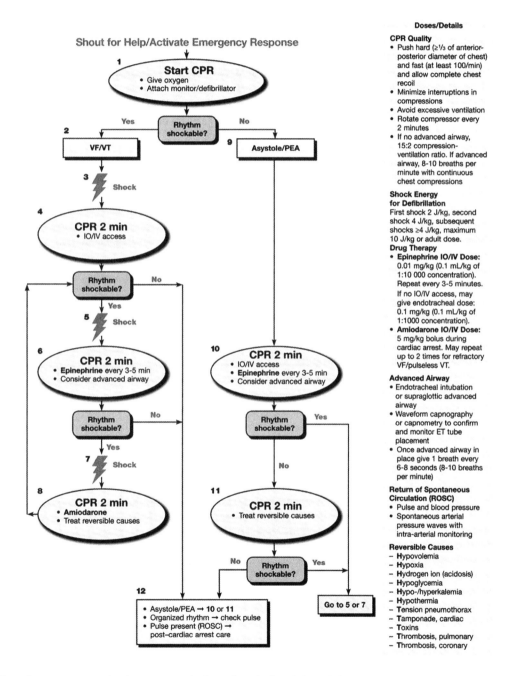

CPR, cardiopulmonary resuscitation; PEA, pulseless electrical activity; IO, intraosseous; IV, intravenous; VF, ventricular fibrillation; VT, ventricular tachycardia; ET, endotracheal tube

Reprinted with permission. © 2010 American Heart Association, Inc. Kleinman ME, Chameides L, Schexnayder SM, et al. Part 14: pediatric advanced life support: 2010 American Heart Association Guidelines for Cardiopulmonary Resuscitation and Emergency Cardiovascular Care. *Circulation*. 2010;122(10 suppl 3) S876-S908.

**Figure A9-2.** Pediatric Bradycardia With a Pulse and Poor Perfusion

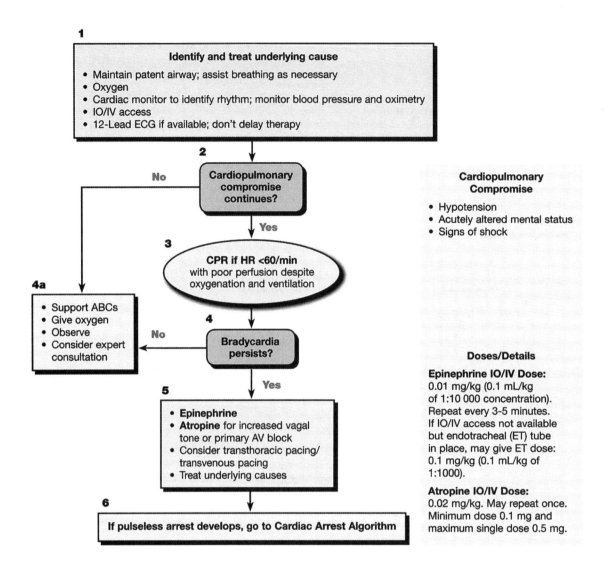

IO, intraosseous; IV, intravenous; ECG, electrocardiogram; CPR, cardiopulmonary resuscitation; HR, heart rate; ABC, airway, breathing, circulation; AV, atrioventricular
Reprinted with permission. © 2010 American Heart Association, Inc. Kleinman ME, Chameides L, Schexnayder SM, et al. Part 14: pediatric advanced life support: 2010 American Heart Association Guidelines for Cardiopulmonary Resuscitation and Emergency Cardiovascular Care. *Circulation.* 2010;122(18 suppl 3):S876-S908.

**Figure A9-3.** Pediatric Tachycardia With a Pulse and Poor Perfusion

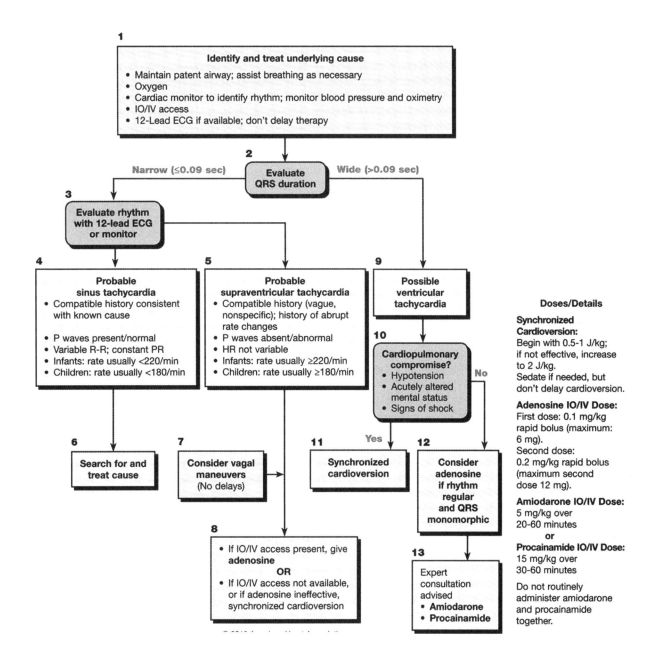

IO, intraosseous; IV, intravenous; ECG, electrocardiogram; HR, heart rate
Reprinted with permission. © 2010 American Heart Association, Inc. Kleinman ME, Chameides L, Schexnayder SM, et al. Part 14: pediatric advanced life support: 2010 American Heart Association Guidelines for Cardiopulmonary Resuscitation and Emergency Cardiovascular Care. *Circulation.* 2010;122(18 suppl 3):S876-S908.

**Figure A9-4.** Pediatric Tachycardia With a Pulse and Adequate Perfusion

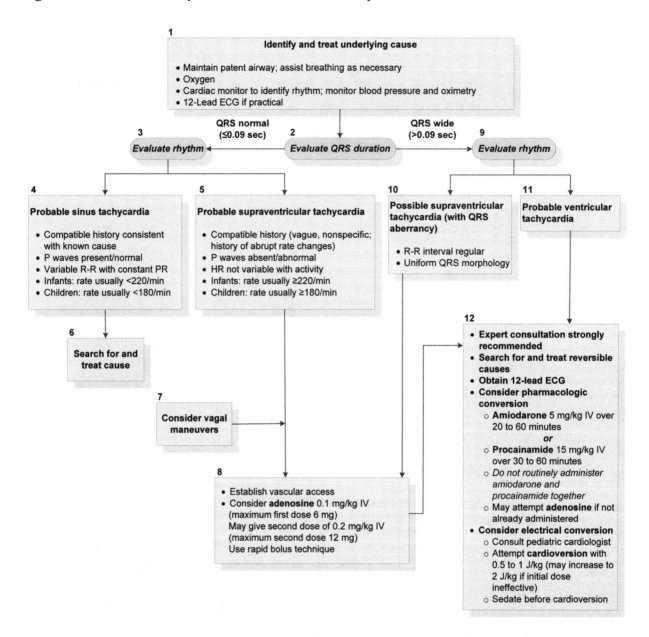

ECG, electrocardiogram; HR, heart rate; IV, intravenous
Reprinted with permission. © 2011 American Heart Association, Inc. Figure 6. Pediatric tachycardia with a pulse and adequate perfusion algorithm. In: *Pediatric Advanced Life Support Manual*. Dallas, TX: American Heart Association; 2011:134.

**Figure A9-5.** Adult Cardiac Arrest

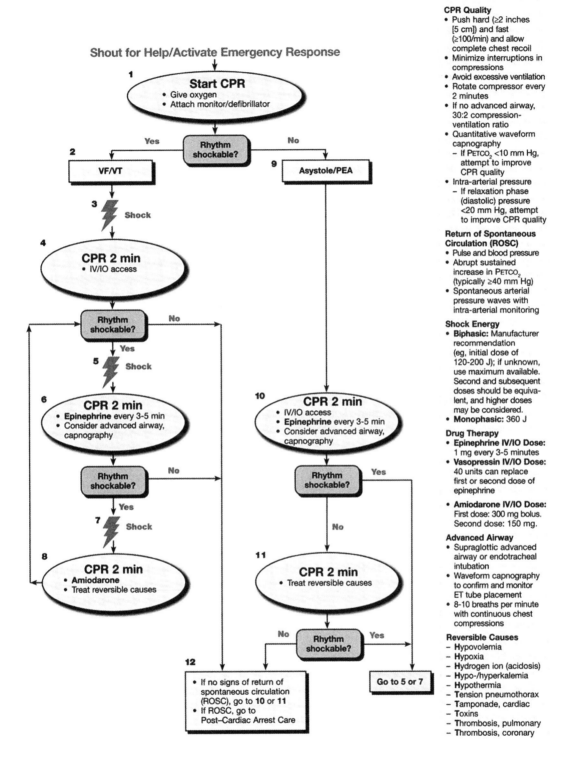

CPR, cardiopulmonary resuscitation; PEA, pulseless electrical activity; IO, intraosseous; IV, intravenous; ET, endotracheal tube
Reprinted with permission. © 2010 American Heart Association, Inc. Neumar RW, Otto CW, Link MS, et al. Part 8: Adult advanced cardiovascular life support: 2010 American Heart Association Guidelines for Cardiopulmonary Resuscitation and Emergency Cardiovascular Care. *Circulation*. 2010;122(18 suppl 3):S729-S767.

**Figure A9-6.** Adult Bradycardia With a Pulse

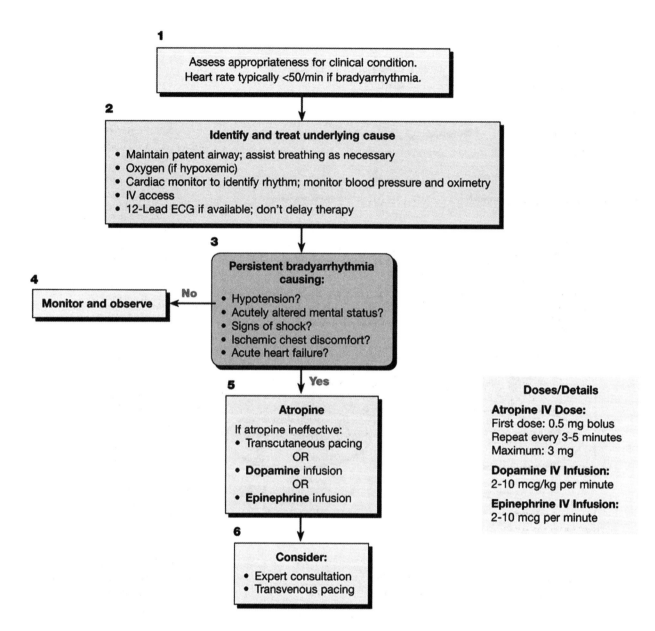

IV, intravenous; ECG, electrocardiogram
Reprinted with permission. © 2010 American Heart Association, Inc. Neumar RW, Otto CW, Link MS, et al. Part 8: Adult advanced cardiovascular life support: 2010 American Heart Association Guidelines for Cardiopulmonary Resuscitation and Emergency Cardiovascular Care. *Circulation.* 2010;122(18 suppl 3):S729-S767.

**Figure A9-7.** Adult Tachycardia With a Pulse

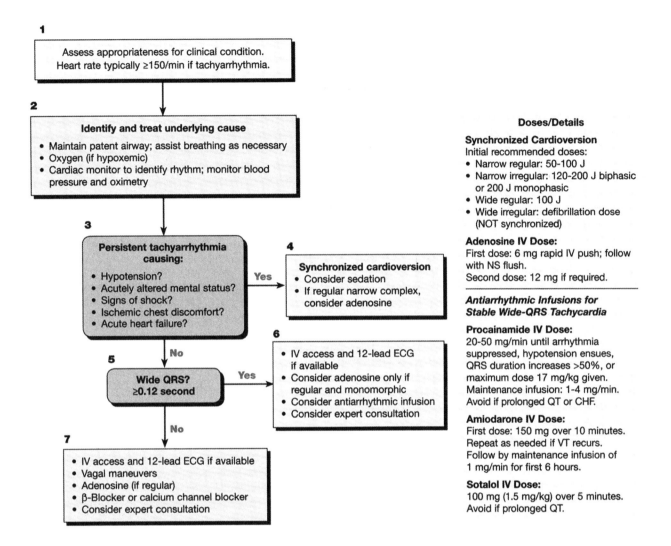

IV, intravenous; NS, normal saline; ECG, electrocardiogram; CHF, congestive heart failure; VT, ventricular tachycardia
Reprinted with permission. © 2010 American Heart Association, Inc. Neumar RW, Otto CW, Link MS, et al. Part 8: Adult advanced cardiovascular life support: 2010 American Heart Association Guidelines for Cardiopulmonary Resuscitation and Emergency Cardiovascular Care. *Circulation.* 2010;122(18 suppl 3):S729-S767.

**Figure A9-8.** Management of Shock After Return of Spontaneous Circulation

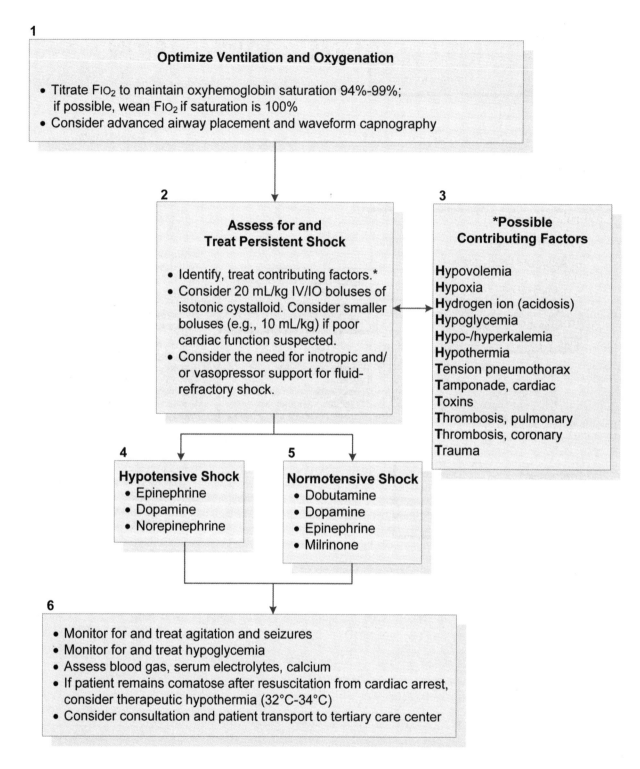

IV, intravenous; IO, intraosseous

Reprinted with permission. © 2011 American Heart Association, Inc. Figure 1. PALS management of shock after ROSC algorithm. In: *Pediatric Advanced Life Support Manual*. Dallas, TX: American Heart Association; 2011:181.

# Appendix 10

# Defibrillation/Cardioversion

## I. INDICATIONS

A. Defibrillation/unsynchronized cardioversion

    1. Ventricular fibrillation

    2. Pulseless ventricular tachycardia

    3. Polymorphic ventricular tachycardia

B. Synchronized cardioversion

    1. Unstable or stable ventricular tachycardia with a pulse

    2. Unstable or stable supraventricular tachycardia, atrial fibrillation, or atrial flutter

## II. EQUIPMENT

A. Conductive gel or self-adhesive defibrillation pads

B. Defibrillator/cardioverter

C. Connecting cable, leads, and electrodes

D. Medication for sedation

E. High-flow oxygen source with bag-mask oxygen delivery device

F. Emergency suction and intubation equipment

G. Pulse oximeter

H. Electrocardiography and blood pressure monitor

I. Intravenous catheter, infusion pump, tubing, fluids

J. Resuscitation cart

# III. TECHNIQUE

A. Recognize cardiac rhythm; determine severity of its physiologic effect.

B. In patients with unstable rhythms or adverse physiologic effects on systemic perfusion, begin immediate defibrillation/cardioversion after initiation of cardiopulmonary resuscitation.

C. Recognize that time delays under the above circumstances decrease the likelihood of conversion to a stable rhythm.

D. Inform and prepare patient as clinical situation dictates; sedate if necessary.

E. Assure intravenous access if time permits.

F. Provide supplemental oxygen or bag-valve-mask ventilation as indicated.

G. Monitor pulse oximeter and electrocardiography.

H. Turn on defibrillator/cardioverter.

I. Attach monitoring electrodes (if needed).

J. Apply conductive gel to paddles or apply conductive pads to chest wall.

    1. Male patients with a hirsute chest may require rapid shaving to ensure adequate contact.

K. Place paddle/electrode: Paddle placement for children is similar to that for adults.

    1. Anterolateral

        a. One paddle/electrode to right of upper sternum below clavicle

        b. One paddle/electrode to lateral of left nipple with center in midaxillary line

    2. Anteroposterior

        a. One paddle/electrode anteriorly over left precordium, below clavicle

        b. One paddle/electrode posteriorly in left infrascapular location, left of thoracic spine

    3. Avoid placement over permanent pacer or implantable cardioverter-defibrillator

L. Apply paddle pressure (if used)

    1. Adult — approximately 25 lb of pressure to each paddle

    2. Pediatric — ensure good contact with chest wall

M. Activate appropriate switch for synchronized cardioversion or unsynchronized defibrillation

N. Set energy level of electrical discharge (in accordance with recommendations of the American Heart Association)

    1. Manual defibrillator

        a. Appropriate paddle size is important; use the largest paddle size possible, assuring good chest contact over its entire area and good separation between the two paddles (about 3 cm)

i. Infants (<10 kg) — 4.5-cm paddles usually used

ii. Children (>10 kg) — 8.0- to 13-cm paddles usually used

b. Be sure that the defibrillator/cardioverter provides a low-dose range for infants. Some defibrillators do not go below 10 J and therefore should not be used for converting infants/children weighing <20 kg (5 to 6 years of age)

c. Pediatric defibrillation

i. 2 J/kg (initial)

ii. Advance to 4 J/kg if rhythm persists.

iii. Subsequent energy levels can be escalated but should not exceed 10 J/kg

iv. Use adult energy levels in children ≥50 kg

d. Pediatric synchronized cardioversion

i. Stable or unstable ventricular tachycardia: 0.5 to 1.0 J/kg

ii. Stable or unstable supraventricular tachycardia: 0.5 to 1.0 J/kg

iii. Advance to 2 J/kg if unsuccessful

e. Adult defibrillation (children >50 kg)

i. Manual biphasic waveform device: energy level is device-specific (typically between 120 and 200 J). If unknown, use 200 J for initial shock. Subsequent shocks should be same or higher energy level as initial shock.

ii. Monophasic waveform device: 360 J, initial and subsequent shocks.

f. Adult cardioversion (synchronized)

i. Ventricular tachycardia (stable): with monophasic or biphasic device, 100 J for initial attempt and advance energy level as needed.

ii. Polymorphic ventricular tachycardia: treat as ventricular fibrillation.

iii. Atrial fibrillation: 200 J with monophasic device, 120 J to 200 J with biphasic device, or consult manufacturer recommendations. Escalate energy levels as needed for subsequent shocks.

iv. Atrial flutter: 50 to 100 J; if rhythm persists advance energy levels as needed.

v. Paroxysmal supraventricular tachycardia: 50 J; if rhythm persists, advance energy levels as needed.

vi. If delays in synchronization occur or conditions are critical, use immediate unsynchronized shocks (defibrillation mode).

2. Automatic external defibrillator

a. >25 kg (age 8 years and older): Use standard adult automatic external defibrillator with adult pad-cable system

b. <25 kg (younger than 8 years): Use attenuated dose if a pediatric system is available. Use adult system if pediatric system is not available

c. Pediatric pads may require anteroposterior placement when used on infants to avoid pad to pad contact

O. Ensure electrical safety (all personnel clear of contact with the patient, bed, and equipment).

P. Charge capacitors through defibrillator/cardioverter.

Q. Depress discharge button(s) on the device or simultaneously on the defibrillator/paddles. (With synchronized cardioversion, the discharge buttons must remain depressed until the energy is released.)

R. If defibrillation performed, immediately resume chest compressions; if cardioversion performed, assess patient (respiration, pulse, and rhythm).

S. If unsuccessful, repeat process, following standard Pediatric Advanced Cardiovascular Life Support protocols.

# IV. PRECAUTIONS/COMPLICATIONS

A. During procedure

1. Skin burn may occur if insufficient gel or improper pads are used, poor contact with the chest wall occurs during discharge, or if the pads/paddles are too close to each other.

2. All metal objects should be removed from the patient to avoid skin burns.

3. Patient's environment and chest must be dry to prevent current from traveling across water, resulting in a decreased amount of delivered energy.

4. Transdermal patches should be removed as they may impede transmission of current.

5. Medical personnel may sustain electrical shock or burn if safety precautions are not followed.

B. After procedure

1. Arterial embolization

2. Pulmonary edema

3. Post-cardioversion arrhythmias; be prepared to institute cardiopulmonary resuscitation

4. Post-shock syndrome (myocardial damage)

## Suggested Readings

1. American Heart Association. *Advanced Cardiovascular Life Support: Provider Manual.* Dallas, TX: American Heart Association; 2010.

2. Part 6. Electrical therapies: Automated external defibrillators, defibrillation, cardioversion, and pacing. 2010 American Heart Association Guidelines for Cardiopulmonary Resuscitation and Emergency Cardiovascular Care. *Circulation.* 2010;122;S706-S719.

3. Wiegand D. *AACN Procedure Manual for Critical Care.* 6th ed. St. Louis, MO: Elsevier Saunders; 2010.

Appendix 11

# Temporary Transcutaneous Cardiac Pacing

## I. INDICATIONS/CONTRAINDICATIONS

A. Indications

    1. Symptomatic bradycardia (hypotension, chest pain, syncope, altered mental status, heart failure, etc.) unresponsive to pharmacologic management

    2. Overdrive pacing of tachycardias, refractory to drug therapy or electrical cardioversion

B. Contraindications

    1. Severe hypothermia

    2. Not recommended for asystole

## II. EQUIPMENT

A. Cardiac pacing electrode pads

B. Pulse generator

C. Connecting leads

D. Medication for sedation and/or analgesia, if necessary

E. Supplemental oxygen (cannula, mask, other as necessary)

F. Pulse oximeter

G. Electrocardiography monitor

H. Intravenous catheter, tubing, fluids

I. Resuscitation cart with pediatric- and adult-sized equipment

# III. TECHNIQUE

A. Recognize cardiac rhythm, determine severity.

B. Prepare patient.

C. Obtain intravenous access if not done previously.

D. Apply oxygen; monitor pulse oximetry and electrocardiography.

E. Attempt pharmacologic management, including atropine, epinephrine, and/or dopamine when appropriate (follow Pediatric Advanced Cardiovascular Life Support guidelines).

F. Assemble equipment.

G. Apply electrode pads.

   1. Anteroposterior

      a. One electrode anteriorly over left precordium as close as possible to maximal cardiac impulse, below clavicle

      b. One electrode posteriorly in left infrascapular location directly behind anterior electrode, left of thoracic spine

   2. Anterolateral

      a. One electrode to right of upper sternum, below clavicle

      b. One electrode to left of nipple with center in midaxillary line

   3. Shave excessive body hair if required to ensure good contact.

H. Administer sedation or analgesia as necessary and tolerated by patient.

I. Connect leads to pulse generator.

J. Turn on pulse generator and monitor.

K. Set rate at 100 beats/min; adjust as needed, based on clinical response

L. Adjust pulse generator output (mA) upward until electrical and mechanical ventricular capture (threshold) occurs (usually 20 to 60 mA). Set output 2 mA above threshold to allow for safety margin. In the setting of severe symptoms or bradycardia, it may be appropriate to start at the maximal output and then decrease if capture is achieved.

M. Be mindful of criteria for proper electrical capture.

   1. Pacer spike followed by a ventricular complex 100% of the time

   2. Wide QRS complex

   3. T wave in an opposite deflection from baseline as the QRS complex

N. Assess efficacy of mechanical capture; obtain blood pressure and palpate pulse distal to carotid site as electrical muscle stimulation from the pacemaker may mimic a carotid pulse.

O. Arrange for temporary or permanent transvenous pacemaker as necessary.

# IV. PEDIATRIC CONSIDERATIONS

A. Bradycardia in children is most often secondary to hypoxemia.

B. Pacing for bradycardic rhythms secondary to hypoxemic insult may be considered after airway management, oxygenation, ventilation, chest compressions, epinephrine bolus (0.01 mg/kg, 1:10,000 concentration) and epinephrine infusion, and possibly atropine bolus (0.02 mg/kg, may repeat; minimum dose 0.1 mg and maximum total dose 1 mg) have been accomplished.

C. The effectiveness of cardiac pacing in this setting is unproven.

D. Even if electrical capture of the heart is accomplished, contractility and myocardial blood flow may not improve without mechanical capture.

E. It is recommended to use the largest available paddles or self-adhering electrode pads that will fit on the chest wall without touching (allow at least 3 cm between paddles or pads).
   1. For children >10 kg (>1 year of age), use large adult paddles.
   2. For children <10 kg (<1 year of age), use small infant paddles (4.5 cm).

# V. PRECAUTIONS/COMPLICATIONS

A. Inability to capture (~20% of patients), usually related to delay in attempting to pace

B. Painful skeletal muscle contraction

C. Skin or tissue damage

D. Temporizing measure only, before transvenous pacing

## Suggested Readings

1. American Heart Association. *Advanced Cardiovascular Life Support: Provider Manual.* Dallas, TX: American Heart Association; 2011.

2. Link MS, Atkins DL, Passman RS, et al. Part 6: electrical therapies: automated external defibrillators, defibrillation, cardioversion, and pacing: 2010 American Heart Association Guidelines for Cardiopulmonary Resuscitation and Emergency Cardiovascular Care. *Circulation.* 2010;122(18 Suppl 3):S706-S719.

3. Wiegand D. *AACN Procedure Manual for Critical Care.* 6th ed. St. Louis, MO: Elsevier Saunders; 2010.

Pediatric Fundamental Critical Care Support

APPENDIX 11-4

# Appendix 12

# Thoracostomy

## I. INDICATIONS/CONTRAINDICATIONS

A. Indications

   1. Tension pneumothorax

   2. Large simple pneumothorax

   3. Penetrating thoracic wound with concurrent need for positive-pressure ventilation

   4. Hemothorax

   5. Symptomatic pleural effusion (recurrent, following thoracentesis)

   6. Empyema

   7. Chylothorax

B. Contraindications

   1. Coagulopathy

      a. Condition must be corrected before nonemergent thoracostomy.

      b. Risk of hemorrhage must be accepted with tension pneumothorax.

   2. Inability to aspirate fluid or air to confirm a patent pleural space

      a. This dictum holds in all circumstances except a penetrating thoracic wound with need for positive-pressure ventilation.

      b. Attempted tube placement in the presence of an obliterated pleural space risks pulmonary injury and potentially fatal hemorrhage.

      c. Aspiration is performed most conveniently through the thoracostomy incision immediately before tube placement.

      d. Aspiration is most important when an apparent effusion presents as a "whiteout" on a chest radiograph, and its free-flowing nature cannot be confirmed radiographically. Such an apparent effusion may be solid tumor, and blunt dissection into such tumor could have devastating hemorrhagic consequences.

# II. EQUIPMENT

A. Needle thoracostomy

      1. 14- to 16-gauge catheter over needle

      2. 23-gauge butterfly needle (infants)

B. Surgical tube thoracostomy

      1. Sterile gloves, gown, eye protection, mask, cap, and drapes

      2. Intravenous catheter, tubing, and fluid

      3. Supplemental oxygen

      4. Monitors (electrocardiographic, pulse oximeter)

      5. Skin disinfectant

      6. Sterile syringes and infiltrating needles

      7. Local anesthetic

      8. Scalpel with #10 or #15 blade

      9. Forceps

      10. Curved clamp

      11. 12F to 40F thoracostomy tube

           a. Approximate sizes for pediatric thoracostomy tubes by age and weight are listed in **Table A12-1**.

           b. 32F to 40F thoracostomy tubes are placed in trauma settings to evacuate an acute hemothorax that potentially contains clots. The largest diameter tube accommodated by the intercostal space is used in this circumstance.

### Table A12-1. Approximate Sizes for Pediatric Thoracostomy Tubes by Age and Weight[a]

| Age | Approximate Weight (kg) | Tube Size (French) |
| --- | --- | --- |
| Newborn to 9 months | 3.5-8 | 12-18 |
| 10 to 17 months | 10 | 14-20 |
| 18 months to 3 years | 12-15 | 14-24 |
| 4 to 7 years | 17-22 | 20-32 |
| 8 years | 28 | 28-32 |
| ≥9 years | ≥35 | 28-38 |

[a]Needle thoracostomy can usually be accomplished on infants with a 23-gauge butterfly needle.

12. If placement the of chest tube is nonemergent and an experienced technician is available, thoracic ultrasound can be a useful adjunct to help localize lung pathology (pleural fluid, pneumothorax) and guide correct positioning of the chest tube.
13. Water-seal drainage system
14. Needle holder
15. 0-silk or 0-polypropylene suture on cutting needle
16. Suture scissors
17. 1/4-inch-wide adhesive tape strips or cable ties with applicator
18. Sterile 4 × 4 gauze sponges
19. Antiseptic ointment
20. 4-inch-wide impervious tape strips
21. 1-inch-wide adhesive tape
22. Resuscitation cart

C. Seldinger technique chest tube

1. Sterile gloves, gown, eye protection, mask, cap, and drapes
2. Intravenous catheter, tubing, and fluid
3. Supplemental oxygen
4. Monitors (electrocardiographic, pulse oximeter)
5. Skin disinfectant
6. Sterile syringes and infiltrating needles
7. Local anesthetic
8. Appropriately sized thoracostomy tube with dilator (**Table A12-1**)
9. Seldinger guidewire
10. Scalpel with #10 or #15 blade
11. Water-seal drainage system
12. Sterile 4 × 4 gauze sponges
13. Antiseptic ointment
14. 4-inch-wide impervious tape strips
15. 1-inch-wide adhesive tape
16. Resuscitation cart
17. If placement of the chest tube is nonemergent and an experienced technician is available, thoracic ultrasound can be a useful adjunct to help localize lung pathology (pleural fluid, pneumothorax) and guide correct positioning of the chest tube.

# III. TECHNIQUE: SURGICAL CHEST TUBE PLACEMENT

A. Analgesia/sedation

    1. Surgical tube thoracostomy is a painful procedure. In nonemergent and semi-urgent circumstances, intravenous narcotic analgesia and a benzodiazepine should be titrated to effect as hemodynamic and respiratory status allow. Local anesthetic should be infiltrated generously throughout the tube thoracostomy tract.

B. Preliminary needle thoracostomy (**Figure A12-1**)

    1. Perform before tube thoracostomy for rapid temporizing treatment of tension pneumothorax.

    2. Select site.

        a. Midclavicular line at the second intercostal space; necessitates that the pectoralis major muscle and possibly breast tissue be penetrated before the intercostal space.

        b. Midaxillary line at the fifth intercostal space; placed in the auscultatory triangle posterior to the pectoralis and anterior to latissimus dorsi muscles where only the thin serratus anterior muscle need be penetrated before the intercostal space.

    3. Don cap, mask, eye protection, and sterile gloves.

    4. Quickly prepare the access site with povidone-iodine solution for children younger than 2 months; if older than 2 months, cleanse site with chlorhexidine solution.

    5. Advance 14-gauge catheter over needle with attached syringe immediately over the superior aspect of the rib while aspirating.

**Figure A12-1.** Sites for Needle Thoracostomy

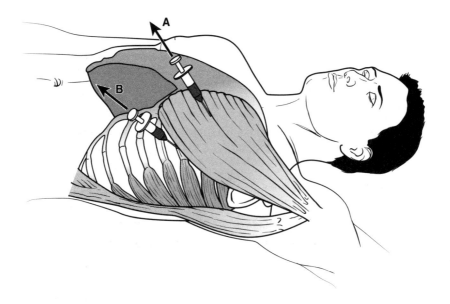

**A**, Second intercostal space, midclavicular line. **B**, Fifth intercostal space, midaxillary line. The latter is also the incision site for placement of a thoracostomy tube and necessitates transgression of much less chest wall musculature and no breast tissue.

6. When air is aspirated, advance catheter completely, and withdraw needle and syringe. Withdraw catheter following completion of tube thoracostomy.

7. Note: 1 mL of saline in the aspirating syringe reveals access of intrapleural air, recognized as bubbles.

C. Preparation for surgical tube thoracostomy

1. Provide supplemental oxygen.

2. In nonemergent circumstances, establish intravenous access, electrocardiographic monitoring, and pulse oximetry.

3. Assemble the following nonsterile materials: water-seal drainage system, 1/4-inch-wide strips of adhesive tape or cable ties to secure thoracostomy tube to drainage system, 4-inch-wide impervious tape strips to secure dressing.

4. Ensure adequate lighting.

5. Place patient in supine position with ipsilateral arm extended.

6. Don cap, mask, eye protection, and sterile gloves.

7. Cleanse patient's anterior and lateral chest wall with antiseptic solution. Remove gloves.

8. Don sterile gown and gloves.

9. On a sterile work space, lay out, from left to right, the following sterile instruments and materials in sequence: syringe with infiltrating needle loaded with local anesthetic, scalpel with blade, forceps, curved clamp, thoracostomy tube, needle holder loaded with suture, suture scissor, dressing composed of gauze 4 × 4 sponges, and antiseptic ointment. These instruments and materials will be used in this sequence.

D. Insertion

| Instrument | Maneuver |
| --- | --- |
| 1. Syringe and needle with local anesthetic | a. Raise the cutaneous wheal at the incision site.<br>b. Deeply infiltrate the underlying subcutaneous tissue. |
| 2. Scalpel | a. Make a 3-cm incision at position B in **Figure A12-1**, through the skin and subcutaneous tissue of the fifth intercostal space.<br>b. Deepen the incision to the level of the chest wall musculature. *Note*: The skin incision parallels the intercostal space. It should be placed one interspace below the intended level of pleural entry so that a tract deep to subcutaneous tissue can be created for the tube. This tract closes spontaneously upon tube removal. |
| 3. Syringe and needle with local anesthetic | a. Through the wound, infiltrate subcutaneous tissue cephalad to the incision. |
| 4. Forceps | a. Using the left hand, retract subcutaneous tissue cephalad away from chest wall to create tension at the junction of subcutaneous tissue and chest wall musculature (**Figure A12-2**). |
| 5. Curved clamp | a. Continue to apply above traction with forceps.<br>b. With curved clamp in the right hand, spread at junction of subcutaneous tissue and chest wall musculature to open this plane (**Figure A12-2**). |

**Figure A12-2.** Blunt Dissection for Thoracostomy

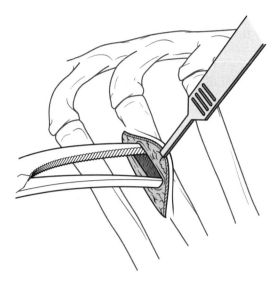

Retraction of skin and subcutaneous tissue with blunt dissection of subcutaneous tissue from chest wall musculature superior to incision.

6. Syringe and needle with local anesthetic
   a. Through the wound, infiltrate musculature and pleura of the fourth intercostal space.
   b. Advance the needle into the pleural space while aspirating syringe.
   c. Confirm the presence of air or fluid in the pleural space.

7. Curved clamp
   a. With curved clamp in the right hand, hold tips against the superior aspect of the fifth rib with concavity of the clamp facing the pleural space.
   b. Perform intercostal dissection immediately superior to a rib to avoid injury to the neurovascular bundle that lies inferior to each rib.
   c. Advance curved clamp through musculature (serratus anterior and intercostal muscles) and pleura into the pleural space (**Figure A12-3**). *Note*: This maneuver may need to be forceful but must always be controlled. A dramatic loss of resistance will signal entry into the pleural space and will be followed by an egress of fluid and/or air.
   d. Ensuring that the tips of the clamp remain on the superior aspect of the fifth rib, widely separate the jaws of the clamp to create a generous opening through the serratus anterior muscle, intercostal muscles, and pleura.
   e. Insert the left index finger into the pleural space as the clamp is withdrawn. Palpation of the smooth pleura confirms the intrapleural location. Sweep the finger through 360° to ensure the absence of adhesions between parietal and visceral pleura. Such adhesions and obliteration of the pleural space would predispose the patient to pulmonary injury during tube insertion.

**Figure A12-3.** Creation of Pleural Opening

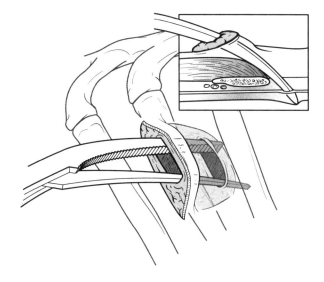

The curved clamp has been advanced into the superior aspect of the incision and advanced through the intercostal musculature and pleura at the superior margin of the fifth rib. The jaws of the clamp are then spread to create a pleural opening. The opening should be generous enough to simultaneously admit a finger and the thoracostomy tube. Insert shows the path of the curved clamp in cross section.

8. Thoracostomy tube
   a. Keep the left index finger in the pleural space.
   b. With the right hand, advance the thoracostomy tube over the tip of the left index finger into the pleural space (**Figure A12-4**). Passage of the tube over the tip of the intrapleural index finger ensures intrapleural placement of the tube.
   c. Advance the tube until resistance is encountered (approximately 15 to 25 cm). The last side hole of the tube should reside 2 cm within the pleural cavity. Ideally, the tip of the tube lies at the pleural apex.

**Figure A12-4.** Placement of Thoracostomy Tube

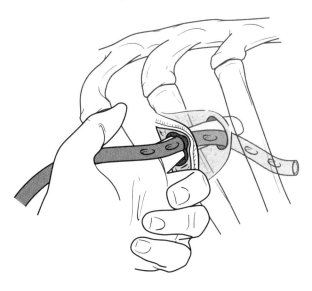

The left index finger replaces the curved clamp and remains within the pleural space as the thoracostomy tube is advanced over the tip of the finger, ensuring intrapleural location.

| | |
|---|---|
| 9. Water-seal drainage system | a. Connect the thoracostomy tube to the drainage system. |
| 10. Needle holder and suture | a. Place a suture of 0-nonabsorbable material through the wound on either side of the thoracostomy tube. |
| | b. Tie each suture to close the wound. |
| | c. Tie each suture about the thoracostomy tube to secure it. |
| | d. Place additional sutures as necessary to close the wound. |
| 11. 1/4-inch adhesive tape or cable tie | a. Secure the connection between chest tube and drainage system tubing (**Figure A12-5**). |
| | b. Do not allow tape to obscure the connection. One must be able to see that the connections are intact at all times. |
| 12. Gauze dressing, 4 x 4 sponges, antiseptic ointment, and impervious tape | a. Place dressing over the thoracostomy site. |
| | b. Secure the dressing with impervious tape. |
| 13. 1-inch adhesive tape | a. Secure chest tube and drainage system tubing to patient's trunk. |

**Figure A12-5.** Connection of Thoracostomy Tube

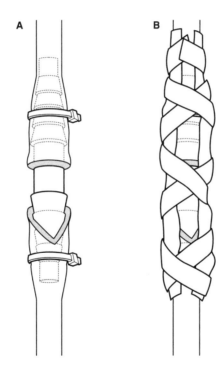

The thoracostomy tube and tubing from the draining system are secured about a conical connecting adaptor with cable ties (**A**) or strips of adhesive tape placed longitudinally and in a spiral fashion (**B**).

# IV. TECHNIQUE: NONSURGICAL CHEST TUBE PLACEMENT (SELDINGER TECHNIQUE)

A. Analgesia/sedation

   1. Nonsurgical chest tubes do not require chest wall dissection to reach the pleural cavity.

   2. Local chest wall anesthetic usually suffices to adequately manage the patient's pain.

B. Preliminary needle thoracostomy (**Figure A12-1**)

   1. Perform as in **Section IIIB**.

C. Preparation for nonsurgical tube thoracostomy

   1. Provide supplemental oxygen.

   2. In nonemergent circumstances, establish intravenous access, electrocardiographic monitoring, and pulse oximetry.

   3. Assemble the following nonsterile materials: water-seal drainage system, 1/4-inch-wide strips of adhesive tape or cable ties to secure thoracostomy tube to drainage system, 4-inch-wide impervious tape strips to secure dressing.

   4. Ensure adequate lighting.

   5. Place patient in supine position with ipsilateral arm abducted.

   6. Don cap, mask, eye protection, and sterile gloves.

   7. Cleanse patient's anterior and lateral chest wall with antiseptic solution. Remove gloves.

   8. Don sterile gown and gloves.

   9. On a sterile work space, lay out, from left to right, the following sterile instruments and materials in sequence: syringe with infiltrating needle loaded with local anesthetic, scalpel, 18-gauge needle, thoracostomy tube with dilators inside, Seldinger wire, needle holder loaded with suture, suture scissors, dressing composed of gauze 4 × 4 sponges, and antiseptic ointment. These instruments and materials will be used in this sequence.

D. Insertion

| **Instrument** | **Maneuver** |
|---|---|
| 1. Syringe and needle with local anesthetic | a. Raise cutaneous wheal at the incision site.<br>b. Deeply infiltrate the underlying subcutaneous tissue and attempt to reach pleural fluid or air. |
| 2. 18-gauge needle and syringe | a. Along the numbed tract, insert an 18-gauge introducer needle over the superior aspect of the rib into the pleural space. Once the pleural cavity is reached, aspirate fluid or air and disconnect needle syringe, making sure not to allow atmospheric air inside needle. |
| 3. Scalpel | a. Make the 1-cm superficial skin incision at entrance to numbed tract to allow the dilator and thoracostomy tube to fit into the pleural space. |

| 4. Seldinger wire | a. Advance wire through a hollow-bore 18-gauge needle until the wire is inside the pleural cavity space, making sure to advance the wire only 2 to 3 cm beyond the length of the needle. Withdraw the needle and place it in a safe location on the tray. |
|---|---|
| 5. Thoracostomy tube and dilators | a. Advance thoracostomy tube and smallest dilator over wire until resistance is felt, then lightly push through the resistance (entering pleural space). Continue to dilate the tract and opening in the pleural space by advancing in sequence (small to large) the supplied dilators over the wire. Advance the chest tube off the dilator until confident that the chest tube holes are in the pleural cavity, then withdraw the dilator. |
| 6. Water-seal drainage system | a. Connect the thoracostomy tube to the drainage system. |
| 7. Needle holder and suture | a. Place a suture of 0-nonabsorbable material through the wound on either side of the thoracostomy tube.<br>b. Tie each suture to close the wound.<br>c. Tie each suture about the thoracostomy tube to secure it.<br>d. Place additional sutures as necessary to close the wound. |
| 8. 1/4-inch adhesive tape or cable ties | a. Secure connection between the chest tube and drainage system tubing (**Figure A12-5**).<br>b. Do not allow tape to obscure the connection from view. One must be able to see that the connections are intact at all times. |
| 9. Gauze dressing, 4 x 4 sponges, antiseptic ointment, and impervious tape | a. Place dressing over the thoracostomy site.<br>b. Secure dressing with impervious tape. |
| 10. 1-inch adhesive tape | a. Secure the chest tube and drainage system tubing to the patient's trunk. |

E. Pleural decompression

    1. Adjust suction to -20 cm $H_2O$.

    2. Consider prophylactic antibiotic coverage.

F. Thoracostomy tube monitoring

    1. Monitor the thoracostomy tube with portable chest radiography to ensure appropriate tube placement and the absence of iatrogenic pneumothorax. The last side hole of the thoracostomy tube lies on a radiopaque line and thus is visible on the radiograph as a gap in this line; the gap should always appear well within the pleural space.

    2. Confirm chest tube patency by the presence of a to-and-fro movement of fluid with respiration (respiratory variation). This may be detected within the thoracostomy tube, the tubing of the collection device, or the water-seal chamber. As the pleural space is definitively decompressed, the thoracostomy tube will become loculated from the general pleural space by visceral and parietal pleural adhesion; respiratory variation will then be lost.

    3. Assess the character and volume of pleural drainage frequently. The significance of diminished drainage volume can only be determined by concurrent chest radiographic

findings. For example, diminishing sanguineous drainage may mean cessation of bleeding or occlusion of the thoracostomy tube by clot; the chest radiograph will reveal increasing effusion/hemothorax in the latter circumstance, but not the former.

    4. Check for air leaks, apparent as air bubbling through the water seal (not the suction regulator). Small air leaks will demonstrate bubbling only during spontaneous expiration or mechanical inspiration. Large air leaks will demonstrate bubbling through both phases of the respiratory cycle. These continuous air leaks may indicate a bronchopleural fistula or tracheobronchial laceration.

G. Thoracostomy tube removal

    1. General criteria for thoracostomy tube removal

        a. Complete radiographic expansion of the lung

        b. Absence of air leak for 24 hours

        c. Drainage volume <100 mL over 24 hours

    2. Prepare a dressing of impervious tape, gauze 4 × 4 sponges, and antiseptic ointment.

    3. With sterile scissors, divide the sutures securing the thoracostomy tube.

    4. Instruct the patient to take a full inspiration, hold the breath, and perform a Valsalva maneuver. Practice this sequence several times.

    5. Repeat the sequence, briskly withdrawing the thoracostomy tube at full inspiration of the Valsalva maneuver, and immediately apply the occlusive dressing to the thoracostomy wound.

    6. Do not close the thoracostomy site with suture or other material.

    7. Obtain an immediate portable chest radiograph to ensure the absence of pneumothorax.

# V. PRECAUTIONS/COMPLICATIONS

A. Possible injury to intercostal artery, vein, or nerve

B. Extrapleural tube position, including subdiaphragmatic placement

C. Subcutaneous emphysema

D. Break in water seal, resulting in pneumothorax

E. Chest wall hematoma/ecchymosis

F. Chest wall or intrapleural hemorrhage

G. Infection

    1. Insertion-site cellulitis

    2. Tract infection

    3. Empyema

H. Laceration of diaphragm or intrathoracic/intra-abdominal viscera

I. Recurrence of pneumothorax (upon removal, secondary to entrained room air or rupture of pulmonary bulla/bleb)

J. Life-threatening tension pneumothorax if chest tube is clamped in the presence of an air leak

# Suggested Readings

1. Etoch SW, Bar-Natan MF, Miller FB, Richardson JD. Tube thoracostomy. Factors related to complications. *Arch Surg.* 1995;130:521-526.

2. Havelock T, Teoh R, Laws D, et al. Pleural procedures and thoracic ultrasound: British Thoracic Society Pleural Disease Guideline 2010. *Thorax.* 2010;65:ii61-ii76.

3. Light RW. Pleural controversy: Optimal chest tube size for drainage. *Respirology.* 2011;16:244-248.

4. Lotano VE. Chest tube thoracostomy. In: Parrillo JE, Dellinger RP, eds. *Critical Care Medicine.* 3rd ed. St. Louis, MO: Mosby, Inc., 2008; 271-279.

5. Martino K, Merrit S, Boyakye K, et al. Prospective randomized trial of thoracostomy removal algorithms. *J Trauma.* 1999;46:369-373.

6. Richardson JD, Spain DA. Injury to the lung and pleura: In: Mattox KL, Feliciano DV, Moore EE, eds. *Trauma.* 4th ed. New York, NY: McGraw-Hill, 2000; 523-543.

# Appendix 13

# Central Venous Access

## I. INDICATIONS

A. Poor peripheral venous access

B. Administration of multiple incompatible medications

C. Administration of vasoactive, irritating, caustic, or hypertonic solutions

D. Hemodynamic monitoring

E. Insertion of a transvenous cardiac pacing catheter

F. Support of rapid infusion of resuscitation fluids

G. Support of frequent blood sampling; minimizing repeated venipuncture

H. Support of hemodialysis

## II. EQUIPMENT

A. Sterile central venous catheter (antibiotic-impregnated catheter is recommended); guidewire; 18-, 22-, or 25-gauge needle, according to catheter size; or central venous catheter kit (single-lumen or multilumen central venous catheter)

B. Consider use of ultrasound for central or peripheral insertion of central catheter: reduces number of attempts, increases rate of success

C. Consider use of peripherally inserted central catheter: may be appropriate for poor or difficult venous access, irritating or hypertonic solutions, or frequent blood sampling

D. Syringe, scalpel, dilator, suture or securement device, infiltrating needles

E. Saline or heparinized saline solution

F. Semitransparent dressing

G. Chlorhexidine-impregnated patch for patients ≥2 months old, per institution-specific protocol

H. Sterile 2x2 and 4x4 gauze sponges

I. Medication for local anesthesia and sedation

J. Sterile gloves, gown, mask, protective eye gear, hat, drapes

K. Chlorhexidine for children ≥2 months old, povidone-iodine for infants <2 months old, or per institution policy

L. Supplemental oxygen

M. Pulse oximeter

N. Electrocardiographic monitor

O. Intravenous tubing and fluid

P. Resuscitation cart available

# III. TECHNIQUE: MODIFIED SELDINGER

A. Obtain consent.

B. Inform the patient using appropriate developmental approach.

C. Notify licensed provider for appropriate timing of sedation.

D. Choose catheter size and site, gather equipment.

E. Ensure appropriate cardiorespiratory monitoring.

F. Conduct final patient verification process.

G. Assure patent peripheral intravenous or intraosseous access, if possible.

H. Assess anatomy of proposed central venous cannulation site with ultrasound, if available.

I. Put on hat, mask, and protective eye gear.

J. Wash hands.

K. Position the patient and identify anatomical landmarks (**Table A13-1**).

L. Wash hands.

### Table A13-1 Insertion Site and Patient Positioning

| Internal Jugular Site | Subclavian Site | Femoral Site |
|---|---|---|
| Patient position: Trendelenburg | Patient position: Trendelenburg | Patient position: Supine with hip abduction and leg in external rotation on side of cannulation |
| 1. Turn patient's head to side opposite of insertion site. | 1. Turn patient's head to side opposite of insertion site. | Place roll under hip side to be cannulated. |
| 2. Extend neck and head by placing a towel under the shoulder on side of insertion site if no cervical spine injury is present. | 2. Place shoulder roll under and parallel along the spine and hyperextend the neck, if no cervical spine injury is present. | |
| **Internal Jugular Site Landmark** | **Subclavian Site Landmark** | **Femoral Site Landmark** |
| 1. Medial and lateral bellies of the sternocleidomastoid muscle form a triangle with the clavicle at the base. | Palpate the clavicle bone. | 1. Palpate the anterior-superior iliac spine and pubic tubercle that delineate the course of inguinal ligament. |
| 2. Internal jugular vein lies within the carotid sheath just beneath the apex of this triangle. | | 2. Palpate the femoral artery that runs beneath inguinal ligament. |
| 3. The carotid artery also lies within the carotid sheath just medial and deep to the internal jugular vein. | | 3. Femoral vein lies ~1 cm medial and parallel to the femoral artery. |

M. Put on a sterile gown and gloves.

N. Create a sterile field; apply a sterile cover to the ultrasound probe if using during the procedure.

O. Open a sterile central venous catheter kit.

P. Prepare the area for cannulation using povidone-iodine for infants <2 months, chlorhexidine for infants and children ≥2 months of age as per institution policy; allow area to dry.

Q. Administer local anesthetic.

R. Flush the needle and catheter with sterile saline or heparinized saline solution, according to manufacturer's recommendations.

   1. With or without ultrasound guidance, insert the needle with an attached syringe at the specified angle and depth, while gently aspirating with a syringe (**Table A13-2** and **Figure A13-1**).

   2. If using a neck approach, the internal jugular is preferred over the subclavian vein for successful cannulation and lower incidence of complications.

S. When backflash of nonpulsatile dark blood is noted, stabilize the needle, disconnect the syringe, and cover the needle hub with a gloved finger.

T. Remove the needle and exert pressure for 5 minutes if pulsatile bright red blood return is obtained on needle insertion.

U. Insert a guidewire through the needle during a positive pressure breath or spontaneous exhalation; minimal to no resistance should be met.

### Table A13-2  Angle of Insertion Based on Anatomical Insertion Site

| Internal Jugular Site | Subclavian Site | Femoral Site |
| --- | --- | --- |
| Anterior Route:<br><br>Aiming toward the ipsilateral nipple, insert needle at midpoint of the anterior margin of the sternocleidomastoid muscle at a 30° angle posteriorly. | Insert the needle under the clavicle bone at the junction of the medial and middle thirds of the clavicle, aiming toward the suprasternal notch at a 45° angle. | Insert the needle 1 finger's width below the inguinal ligament and medial to the femoral artery at a 30° angle, aiming toward the umbilicus. |
| Central Route:<br><br>Aiming toward the ipsilateral nipple, insert needle at apex of the triangle formed by the sternoclavicular heads of the sternocleidomastoid muscle and the clavicle at a 30° angle. | The needle should be parallel to the frontal plane, directed medially and slightly cephalad, beneath the clavicle bone toward the posterior aspect of the sternal end of the clavicle. | |
| Posterior Route:<br><br>Aiming toward the suprasternal notch, insert needle under posterior border of the sternocleidomastoid muscle, approximately halfway between the mastoid process and the clavicle. | | |
| Depth of Insertion: Approximately 1-2 cm | Depth of Insertion: Approximately 2-3 cm | Depth of Insertion: Approximately 1-2 cm |

V. Monitor cardiac rhythm for ectopy when inserting the guidewire, because it may be long enough to reach the heart.

W. Make a small incision with the scalpel adjacent to the needle to slightly enlarge the puncture site and accommodate the dilator and catheter.

X. Remove the needle, while maintaining control of the guidewire.

Y. Pass the dilator over the needle to gently dilate the skin and subcutaneous tissue.

Z. Remove the dilator while maintaining control of the guidewire.

AA. Pass the catheter over the guidewire and advance the catheter to the predetermined landmark, while maintaining control of the guidewire.

BB. Remove the guidewire.

CC. Aspirate blood from all ports of the catheter.

DD. Once blood return is confirmed, flush the ports.

EE. Connect the distal port to the monitor to confirm the central venous position waveform (nonpulsatile).

FF. Suture catheter or use other securement device as appropriate.

GG. Apply chlorhexidine-impregnated patch for infants and children ≥2 months of age.

HH. Apply sterile occlusive dressing.

II. Obtain the chest or abdominal radiograph to confirm proper positioning of the catheter.

JJ. Attach intravenous fluids.

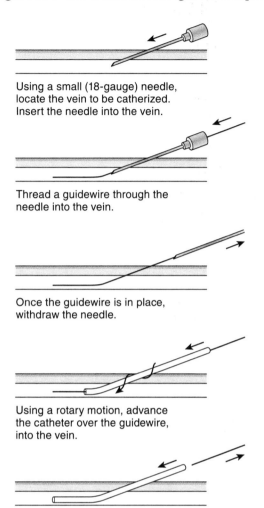

**Figure A13-1.** Modified Seldinger Technique

Using a small (18-gauge) needle, locate the vein to be catherized. Insert the needle into the vein.

Thread a guidewire through the needle into the vein.

Once the guidewire is in place, withdraw the needle.

Using a rotary motion, advance the catheter over the guidewire, into the vein.

Finally, remove the guidewire, leaving the catheter in place.

# IV. PRECAUTIONS/COMPLICATIONS

A. Hemothorax

B. Pneumothorax

C. Chylothorax

D. Bleeding/hemorrhage

E. Venous thrombosis

F. Arterial puncture

G. Heart perforation

H. Air embolism

I. Infection

J. Dysrhythmias

K. Catheter or guidewire embolism

L. Local subcutaneous tissue, nerve, artery, or vein damage

# Appendix 14

# Handoff Mnemonics for Transport and Trauma

## 1. Transport

**SMEAC**

- Situation
  - Location of patient
  - Patient:
    - Past medical history
    - Medications
    - Allergies
    - Fasting/NPO (nothing by mouth) status
  - Pertinent clinical events
  - Treatment(s)
  - Response to treatment/interventions
  - Advice (including preparation of escort)
- Mission
  - Interhospital transfer/Search and Rescue
  - Goals:
    - Retrieve
    - Resuscitate
    - Stabilize
    - Transport
- Expected course/worst case scenario
- Equipment
  - Personnel necessary for transport, including consideration for airway/breathing/circulation
  - Intervention supplies:
    - Standard ABCD equipment
    - Case-specific items (e.g., antibiotics, antivenoms, blood products, orthopedic devices)
  - Monitoring

- Administration (i.e., coordination, team roles, documentation, and timing)
- Communication and Chain of Command (i.e., contact name and number for coordinator, referral site [remember shift changes, ensure handover], transport team)

PRE-RETURN:

Secure and preempt problems with **ABCD**.

– **A**irway/**B**reathing: rapid-sequence intubation equipment readily accessible

– **C** (**AEIOU**): functioning **a**ccess with extension sets, **e**mergency drugs (vasoactive, anesthetics, etc.), (**i**nvasive) monitoring, **o**utput (i.e., indwelling catheters, Foley, naso- or orogastric tube), **u**nexpected problems anticipated (blood pressure derangements, defibrillator/pacing pads in place)

– **D**ocumentation: imaging, results

– **E**scort(s)

## 2. Trauma

**MISTO**

- **M**echanism of injury
- **I**njuries sustained
- **S**igns and symptoms
- **T**reatment(s) and response
- **O**bservation and vital signs
    - Other things:
        – Past medical history
        – Allergies
        – Medications
        – Fasting/NPO status

# Appendix 15

# PEDIATRIC TRANSPORT FORM

Date: _____ Time: _____

NAME: _____ AGE: _____ WEIGHT: _____

DIAGNOSIS: _____

REFERRAL HOSPITAL: _____

REFERRAL MD: _____REFERRAL HOSPITAL PHONE: _____

ACCEPTING MD: _____

MEDICAL CONTROL MD: _____

HISTORY/PE:
VITAL SIGNS: T: _____ HR: _____ RR: _____ BP: _____ $Sp_{O_2}$: _____ $F_{IO_2}$: _____
Hx:


PE:


Labs:


THERAPY/RECOMMENDATIONS:
Discuss possible interventions:



Discussion with transport team:

Medical Control MD:


BED CONTROL: Time contacted _____ Approved by_____ Time_____
                                              (Name)
TIME TEAM DISPATCHED: _____ ☐Helicopter ☐ Fixed Wing ☐ Ground Ambulance

☐ Pediatric/NICU Specialty Team ☐ ACLS Ambulance

TIME ACCEPTED: _____ for admission to ☐ PICU ☐ ER ☐ PEDS FLOOR ☐ NICU

TIME ACCEPTING MD NOTIFIED OF ETA _____

MD, physician; PE, physical examination; T, temperature; HR, heart rate; RR, respiratory rate; BP, blood pressure; Hx, history; NICU, neonatal intensive care unit; ACLS, Advanced Cardiopulmonary Life Support; PICU, pediatric intensive care unit; ER, emergency room; ETA, estimated time of arrival

Pediatric Fundamental Critical Care Support

APPENDIX 15-2

# Appendix 16

# Arterial Catheter Insertion

## I. INDICATIONS

A. Hypertension, hypotension, labile blood pressure

B. Continuous assessment of systolic, diastolic, and mean blood pressure

C. Use of vasoactive agents (vasopressors, vasodilators, or other cardioactive medications)

D. Frequent sampling of laboratory specimens (arterial blood gases or otherwise)

## II. EQUIPMENT

A. Arterial catheter kit with appropriate-sized safety cannula over needle or procedure tray with catheter over guidewire (generally 22- to 24-gauge for radial and 20-gauge for femoral)

B. Ultrasound may be useful to locate artery, increase success rate, and reduce number of attempts

C. 2% chlorhexidine, 10% povidone-iodine, or 70% alcohol

D. Sterile towels, gloves, and gown

E. Mask

F. Protective eyewear

G. Surgical hat

H. Tape

I. Gauze sponges (2 x 2 and 4 x 4)

J. Arm board, if radial artery is being used

K. 3.0 or 4.0 suture and needle driver or other securement device (if not included in arterial catheter kit)

L. Transparent semipermeable dressing

M. Local anesthetic, such as lidocaine

N. Medication for sedation, if necessary

O. Pressure transducer, tubing, and pressure monitor

# III. TECHNIQUE

A. Ensure that child and family understand procedure and all questions are answered.

B. Gather supplies.

C. Assure intravenous access.

D. Wash hands.

E. Perform final patient identification process per institution-specific policy (i.e., time-out).

F. Ensure appropriate cardiorespiratory monitoring.

G. Perform modified Allen test (**Table A16-1**), if using radial artery.

### Table A16-1. The Allen Test

The Allen test is used to test blood supply in the hand. It is performed prior to radial artery blood sampling or cannulation.
1. The hand is elevated and a fist is made for approximately 30 seconds.
2. Pressure is applied over the ulnar and radial arteries so as to occlude both simultaneously.
3. While elevated, the hand is opened. It should appear blanched.
4. Ulnar pressure is released, and the color to the hand should return in approximately 7 seconds.
5. If color does not return or returns after >7 seconds, the ulnar artery supply to the hand is insufficient and the radial artery cannot be safely punctured.

H. Use arm board for immobilization, if using radial artery.

I. Administer analgesia and/or sedation, as appropriate.

J. Position patient appropriately (**Figure A16-1** and **Table A16-2**).

**Figure A16-1.** Catheter-Over-Needle Technique

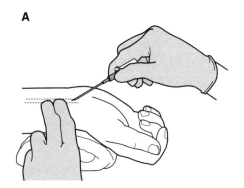 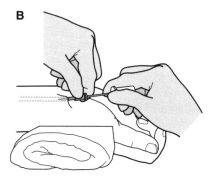

A) After extending and immobilizing the wrist, the radial artery is localized by palpation. The needle is inserted at a 20° to 45° angle. B) After the artery is entered, the catheter is advanced over the needle and the needle is withdrawn.

### Table A16-2  Anatomical Position for Insertion[a]

| Radial Artery | Femoral Artery |
|---|---|
| Position patient appropriately | Position patient appropriately |
| • Dorsiflex wrist 45-60° using small roll under the wrist | • Place towel or blanket under hips and place in frog-leg position |

[a]Axillary, dorsalis pedis, posterior tibial, and umbilical artery catheterizations have been described but will not be discussed here.

K. If available and considered helpful, use ultrasound to identify vessels that may be appropriate for cannulation.

L. Don mask, cap, gown, and sterile gloves.

M. Prepare site using 2% chlorhexidine for infants >2 months of age, 10% povidone-iodine, or 70% alcohol.

N. Scrub site with back-and-forth motion using friction (or as per manufacturer's instructions); allow area to air dry for prescribed period.

O. Prepare sterile field, including use of sterile sheath on ultrasound probe if this equipment will be used during process of cannulation.

P. Identify landmarks; palpate artery.

Q. Infiltrate area with local anesthetic.

R. Puncture anatomical insertion site (**Tables A16-3, A16-4,** and **Figure A16-2**).

### Table A16-3  Anatomical Insertion Site

| Radial Artery | Femoral Artery |
|---|---|
| • Puncture skin at a 30° angle, directing the safety catheter or needle toward the underlying artery. | • Puncture skin at 45° angle, needle bevel up, below the inguinal crease and a few centimeters distal to palpable pulse. |
| • Advance the needle slowly, while watching for flashback. | • Enter through skin, advancing introducer needle into femoral artery. |
| • When blood is obtained, remove syringe and bring needle down against skin. | • When blood is obtained, remove syringe and bring needle down against skin. |

### Table A16-4. Insertion Technique

| Catheter Over Needle | Modified Seldinger Technique |
|---|---|
| Advance the catheter using a rotating motion to the hub and remove needle | • Immobilize needle with free hand.<br>• Advance guidewire through needle slowly; do not force wire in if resistance is met.<br>• Remove needle and wire if unable to remove wire from needle during insertion attempts.<br>• Remove needle while holding guidewire in place.<br>• Pass catheter over guidewire while inserting catheter to the hub; do not force catheter if resistance is met.<br>• Remove guidewire.<br>• Secure catheter to skin after connecting transducer tubing. Ensure that the catheter is not inadvertently dislodged prior to securing with tape or suture material. |

**Figure A16-2.** Modified Seldinger technique

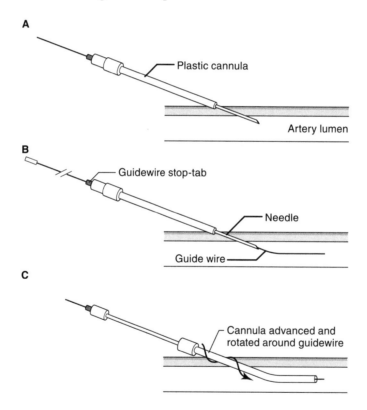

A) The needle is inserted into the artery. B) The guidewire is advanced until the stop-tab reaches the needle hub. C) The catheter is advanced over the guidewire into the artery.

S. Attach catheter to transducer to observe for presence of arterial waveform and for ease of flushing and aspirating blood from catheter.

T. Secure with suture or sutureless securement device.

U. Surround site with chlorhexidine-impregnated sponge, per institution-specific protocol.

V. Cover site with semipermeable transparent dressing, per institution-specific protocol.

W. Dispose of supplies appropriately.

X. Remove personal protective equipment.

Y. Assess circulation to distal extremity.

Z. Wash hands.

AA. Documentation of procedure may include the following:
   1. Type of procedure
   2. Informed consent
   3. Risks/benefits
   4. Skin preparation
   5. Insertion site
   6. Use of local anesthetic or systemic sedation/analgesia
   7. Condition of child at end of procedure
   8. Unexpected outcomes

# IV. VALIDATION OF MEASURES AND SYSTEM CHARACTERISTICS

A. Systolic return-to-flow blood pressure assessment (**Figure A16-3**)
   1. Observe arterial waveform.
   2. Place a manual blood pressure cuff on the same extremity as the arterial catheter and inflate until the arterial waveform flattens.
   3. Release pressure in cuff slowly until the first evidence of pulsatile waveform is again observed, and note pressure on sphygmomanometer.
   4. Sphygmomanometer pressure is the "true" systolic blood pressure and should correlate with pressure measured through the arterial catheter.

**Figure A16-3.** Instructions for Obtaining Systolic Return-to-Flow Blood Pressure

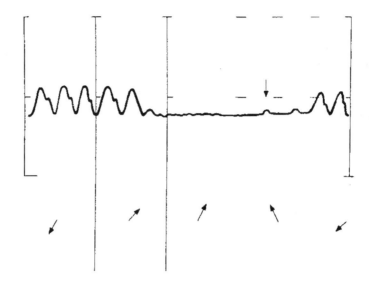

**A)** Observe arterial waveform. **B)** Place a manual blood pressure cuff on the same extremity as the radial or dorsalis pedis arterial catheter and inflate it. Arterial waveform flattens as the cuff is inflated. **C)** Release pressure in cuff slowly until the first evidence of pulsatile waveform is again observed, at which point the pressure on the sphygmomanometer is noted. This sphygmomanometer pressure is the return-to-flow or "true" systolic blood pressure.

B. Square wave test

      1. Use to test system characteristics of tubing (e.g., length, stiffness, presence of bubbles).

      2. Rapidly flush the arterial line tubing (**Figure A16-4**).

      3. Observe waveform for underdamping or overdamping (**Figures A16-5** and **A16-6**).

**Figure A16-4.** Square Wave Test

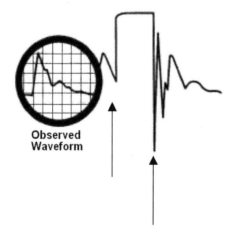

Application of a rapid in-line flush and the correlating evaluation of the monitoring system. First arrow indicates flush applied, and second arrow indicates the rapid frequency response when released. If a neonatal patient is using a pediatric transducer with an infusion pump, a square wave test is not possible using the flush device. Reprinted with permission from Edwards Lifesciences, Irvine, California, USA.

**Figure A16-5.** Overdamping

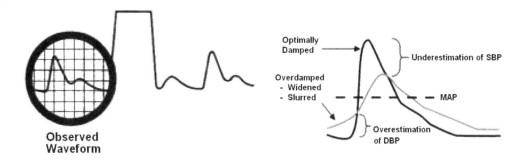

SBP, systolic blood pressure; MAP, mean arterial pressure; DBP, diastolic blood pressure.
An overdamped signal indicates loss of signal related to loose connections, air bubbles in the system, and/or inadequate fluid and pressure applied.
Reproduced with permission from Edwards Lifesciences, Irvine, California, USA.

**Figure A16-6.** Underdamping

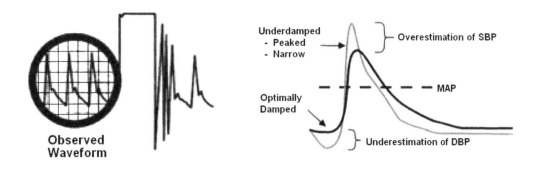

SBP, systolic blood pressure; MAP, mean arterial pressure; DBP, diastolic blood pressure.
An underdamped signal indicates significant increase in frequency response and is generally related to loss of calibration of the transducer, requiring a transducer change.
Reproduced with permission from Edwards Lifesciences, Irvine, California, USA.

C. Factors that may interfere with monitoring accuracy:

1. Connections of stopcocks and interface
2. Constant pressure application (300 mm Hg)
3. Elasticity alterations of the blood vessel wall
4. Reflectance of the pulse wave from the vessel walls or tubing
5. Air bubbles in the fluid column throughout the system
6. Thrombi around or in the catheter
7. Stiffness and length of the plastic tubing

## V. COMPLICATIONS

A. Compromised circulation/ischemia to extremity at insertion site and distal to insertion site

B. Infection

C. Hemorrhage

D. Arterial air embolism

E. Arteriovenous fistula

F. Arterial aneurysm

## VI. Precautions/Contraindications

A. Ischemia of the extremity

B. Infection at the puncture site

C. Raynaud disease

D. Prior vascular surgery or cutdown procedure involving the artery to be punctured

# INDEX

Note: Page numbers followed by *f* and *t* indicate figures and tables, respectively.

## A

A-B-C algorithm, of resuscitation, 3-3–3-4
Abdominal breathing, 2-4
Abdominal compartment syndrome, 9-18
Abdominal injury(ies), blunt, in child abuse, 11-6–11-7
Abdominal pain, acute
    differential diagnosis, 7-24
Abdominal trauma, 9-15–9-18
    evaluation, 9-14*t*, 9-16
    laboratory investigation, 9-16
Abscess. *See also* Retropharyngeal abscess
    brain, altered mental status/coma caused by, 15-16, 15-16*t*
    parapharyngeal, 4-16–4-17. *See also* Retropharyngeal abscess
    peritonsillar, 4-17, 4-21
Accidental injury(ies), patterns, 11-2–11-3, 11-2*t*
Acetaminophen, 20-10
    overdose/poisoning/toxicity, 13-10–13-12, 13-11*t*
    for postoperative pain, 19-11
Acetone poisoning, 13-3*t*
Acetylcholinesterase toxicity, 20-20
Acidosis, 1-12*t*, 1-15. *See also* Diabetic ketoacidosis; Metabolic acidosis; Respiratory acidosis
    management, in shock, 6-18
    in status epilepticus, 15-11*t*
Activated charcoal, 13-5
Acute chest syndrome, in sickle cell disease, 4-43
Acute kidney injury
    causes, 18-6, 18-7*t*
    classification, 18-5–18-6
    definition, 18-2
    diagnosis
        clinical, 18-6
        laboratory, 18-8
    electrolyte management for, 18-10–18-13
    fluid volume management for, 18-9–18-10
    imaging in, 18-8, 18-9*t*
    intrinsic, 18-5
        causes, 18-6, 18-7*t*
        urinary indices in, 18-5, 18-6*t*
    laboratory investigation, 18-5, 18-8
    long-term outcomes with, 18-15
    management, 18-9
        algorithm for, 18-15, 18-16*f*
        metabolic alterations in, 18-8, 18-8*f*
        nutritional support in, 18-14–18-15
        pathophysiology, 18-2
        pediatric RIFLE criteria, 18-2, 18-3*t*
        post-renal (obstructive), 18-5
            causes, 18-6, 18-7*t*
        prerenal, 18-5
            causes, 18-6, 18-7*t*
            urinary indices in, 18-5, 18-6*t*
    RIFLE criteria, 18-2
    risk factors for, 18-3–18-4, 18-4*t*

Acute lung injury
    mechanical ventilation in, 5-16–5-17
    positive end-expiratory pressure in, 5-11*t*–5-12*t*
    transfusion-related, 17-25
Acute respiratory distress syndrome
    adjuvant therapies for, 4-40–4-41
    definition, 4-39
    diagnostic criteria for, 4-39, 4-39*t*
    management, 4-40–4-41
    mechanical ventilation in, 4-40, 5-16–5-17
    pathophysiology, 4-39–4-40
    in pneumonia, 4-36–4-37
    positive end-expiratory pressure in, 4-40, 5-11*t*–5-12*t*, 5-16–5-17
Acyclovir
    for herpes simplex virus (HSV) infections, 7-29
    nephrotoxicity, 18-4
Adenoidectomy, 4-7
Adenosine, 3-15
Adrenaline. *See* Epinephrine
Adrenal insufficiency, 1-22, 6-23–6-24, 8-18–8-19
    primary, 8-18
    signs and symptoms, 8-18–8-19
    tertiary, 8-18–8-19
    treatment, 8-19
α-Adrenergic agents, for neurogenic shock, 1-21
Advanced life support, guidelines for resuscitation, 3-17*f*
Advanced Trauma Life Support, 11-10
Afterload, 1-13, 6-1, 16-20–16-21
    reduction, 1-24
Afterload-reducing agents, 16-20
    for acyanotic congenital heart disease, 16-15*t*
Agitation, 2-6
    emergence, 19-9
    nonpharmacologic management, 20-20
    and postoperative sinus tachycardia, 19-6
Air embolism, with central venous catheter, 21-14
Airflow resistance. *See* Airway resistance
Airway(s), 1-5–1-12, 1-27. *See also* Upper airway disease
    adult vs pediatric, 4-2–4-4, 4-3*t*
    anatomic considerations, 1-10, 2-2–2-4, 4-2–4-4
    compromise, 2-2
    congenital abnormalities, 1-11
    developmental considerations, 2-2–2-4
    diameter, age-related changes in, 4-3
    difficult, 2-23, 2-29, 20-4–20-6, 20-5*t*
    edema, and airflow resistance, 4-4
    equipment setup, mnemonics for, 20-8
    evaluation, 1-8–1-10
        in burn patient, 10-3–10-4
    infant, characteristics, 4-3*t*
    lower, postoperative disorders, 19-5
    Mallampati classification, 20-5, 20-6*f*
    oral, pharyngeal, and tracheal axes, 2-11, 2-11*f*, 2-23

pediatric, characteristics, 4-3*t*
physiologic considerations, 2-2–2-4
pressure and flow tracings, 5-6, 5-7*f*–5-8*f*
radius, and airway resistance, 2-3, 2-3*f*, 4-4
suctioning, 1-9, 1-10
trauma to, 4-17–4-18
Airway adjuncts, 2-10, 2-27–2-28
postoperative, 19-4
Airway disorders. *See also* Lower airway disease, acute; Upper airway disease
anatomic, 4-7–4-10, 4-7*t*
causes, 4-7, 4-7*t*
external or internal compression, 4-7*t*, 4-10–4-11
fever in, 4-21
history-taking in, 4-18–4-19
infectious, 4-7*t*, 4-11–4-17
miscellaneous, 4-7*t*
observation and appearance of patient in, 4-19–4-20
physical examination in, 4-20–4-21
postoperative, 19-5
Airway management, 2-1, 2-2, 2-9–2-30
in anaphylaxis, 3-18
in burn patient, 10-2
in cardiac arrest, 3-5
in interfacility transport, 14-7–14-9, 14-8*f*
in intrahospital transport, 14-6
in neoplastic airway obstruction, 4-11
for neurologic injury, 15-2
and neuromuscular blockade, 2-21
in poisoned patient, 13-2–13-3
postoperative, 19-7–19-8
in respiratory failure, 4-28
in status epilepticus, 15-12*t*, 15-13
in trauma patient, 9-2–9-3
troubleshooting, 2-17
Airway maneuvers, for opening and maintaining airway, 2-11–2-12
Airway obstruction, 1-7, 1-9–1-10, 2-3, 2-5, 2-9, 2-17–2-18
in angioedema, 4-18
and cardiac arrest, 3-2
causes, 1-10, 2-10, 4-7
complete, 2-6
incomplete, 2-5
management, 2-10
neoplastic, 4-10–4-11
observation and appearance of patient in, 4-19–4-20
partial, 4-24
and airway collapse, 4-6
precautions with, 2-17, 2-20
pharyngeal soft-tissue collapse and, 2-11, 2-12, 4-24
posterior movement of tongue and, 2-11, 2-12, 4-3, 4-8, 4-24
post-extubation, 4-18
sedation-induced, 4-24

upper
infectious causes, 4-11–4-17, 4-12*t*
postoperative, 19-4
Airway resistance, 1-6–1-7, 2-2, 4-3–4-4
airway radius and, 2-3, 2-3*f*
Albumin, 19-17–19-18
Albuterol
for hyperkalemia, 18-12
inhaled, for asthma, 4-30–4-31
Alcohol poisoning, 13-3*t*
Alertness, assessment, 1-4*t*, 1-5
Alkalosis, 1-12*t*
Allen test, 21-15
Allopurinol, for uric acid control, 17-11*t*, 17-12
Alprostadil, 1-23
Alveolar hyperventilation, 2-7
Alveolar ventilation, 2-7
American Heart Association, pediatric cardiac arrest algorithm, 3-17*f*
American Society of Anesthesiologists, physical classification system, 19-2, 20-3, 20-4*t*
Aminoglycosides, nephrotoxicity, 18-4
Aminophylline, for asthma, 4-31–4-32
Amiodarone
for cardiac arrest, 3-10*t*, 3-11
overdose/poisoning/toxicity, 13-3*t*
Amodiaquine, for malaria, 7-32
Amphetamine, overdose/poisoning/toxicity, 13-3*t*–13-4*t*, 13-11*t*
Amphotericin B, nephrotoxicity, 18-4
Amrinone, 1-24
Anaerobes
infections in pediatric oncology patient, 17-3, 17-4*t*
necrobacillosis caused by, 7-29–7-31
Analgesia
agents for, 20-2
clinical applications, 20-2
with mechanical ventilation, 5-11*t*, 5-16
planning for, 20-3
for postoperative pain, 19-10–19-11
for premedication, 20-10
in shock, 6-20
Analgesic Ladder, 19-11, 19-12*f*
Anaphylaxis/anaphylactic reaction
signs, 1-21
signs and symptoms, 3-18
triggers, 1-21
Anemia, 17-18–17-20, 17-18*t*
causes, 17-18, 17-19
and postoperative apnea, 19-3
and postoperative sinus tachycardia, 19-6
Anemic shock, 6-7
Anesthesia
for preterm infants, postconceptual age and, 19-3
residual effect in postoperative period, 19-7–19-8
for tracheal intubation, 2-19, 2-20*t*

Anesthetic(s), inhaled
    and emergence agitation, 19-9
    and malignant hyperthermia, 19-23
    and postoperative nausea and vomiting, 19-16, 19-17$t$
Aneurysm(s), and hemorrhagic stroke, 15-23
Angioedema, airway obstruction in, 4-18
Angiotensin-converting enzyme inhibitors, 1-24
    and acute kidney injury, 18-3–18-4
    nephrotoxicity, 18-4
Angiotensin-receptor blockers, 18-4
Anion gap, increased, in poisoned patient, 13-3, 13-3$t$
Anterior mediastinal mass, 4-11
Anthrax, 12-7–12-8, 12-8$t$
Antibiotic(s)
    and acute kidney injury, 18-3, 18-4$t$
    for bacterial meningitis, 7-21–7-22
    for bacterial tracheitis, 4-16
    empiric, 1-26–1-27, 7-9
        for febrile neutropenic patient, 17-3
        for sepsis, 7-11–7-12, 7-12$t$
    for epiglottitis, 4-15
    for malaria, 7-32
    for peritonitis, 7-25
    for pneumonia, 4-36
    for retropharyngeal abscess, 4-17
    for sepsis, 7-11–7-12, 7-12$t$–7-13$t$
    for septic shock, 6-19
    for serious infections in immunosuppressed children, 17-3, 17-4$t$–17-5$t$
    for toxic shock syndrome, 7-15
Anticholinergics
    for asthma, 4-31
    overdose/poisoning/toxicity, 13-3$t$–13-4$t$
Anticholinesterase, 20-20
    poisoning with, 13-11$t$
    antidotes for, 12-6, 12-7$t$
Antidiuretic hormone, 19-16
Antiemetics, 19-16, 19-17$t$
Antifungal therapy, for pediatric oncology patient, 17-4$t$, 17-7
Antihistamines
    for anaphylaxis, 3-19
    overdose/poisoning/toxicity, 13-3$t$–13-4$t$
Antimycotics, and acute kidney injury, 18-3
Antivenoms, 13-13
Antiviral therapy, for pediatric oncology patient, 17-3, 17-4$t$–17-5$t$, 17-6
Anuria, 18-6
Anxiety
    and postoperative agitation, 19-9
    and postoperative sinus tachycardia, 19-6
Aortic cross-clamp, and risk for acute kidney injury, 18-4
Aortic stenosis, 1-23, 16-4
Apnea, 3-3. *See also* Obstructive sleep apnea
    from PGE$_1$, 1-23
    postoperative, 19-3
    in preterm infants, postconceptual age and, 19-3
Apnea of prematurity, 1-11
    and postoperative care, 19-3
Apneustic breathing, 15-8, 15-8$t$
Appearance, patient's, evaluation, 1-4, 2-4
Aromatic hydrocarbon poisoning, 13-3$t$
Arrhythmia(s), 1-14
    after congenital heart disease surgery, 16-17, 16-18$t$
    ECG findings in, 16-17, 16-19$f$
    in hypokalemia, 8-9, 8-10$f$
    postoperative, 19-6
    in status epilepticus, 15-11$t$
    in structural heart disease, 16-17
    in suspected shock, 6-8
    ventricular, 1-14–1-15
Arsenic poisoning, 13-3$t$
Artemether, for malaria, 7-32
Artemisinin, for malaria, 7-32
Arterial blood gas measurement, 1-8–1-11, 1-12$t$, 1-16$t$, 2-6–2-7, 4-21–4-22
    interpretation, 2-7
Arterial catheter(s), 6-10–6-11, 21-14–21-16
    complications, 21-15
    indications for, 21-14–21-15
    insertion sites, 21-15, 21-15$t$
    measurements using, 21-16, 21-16$f$
    sizes, 21-15$t$
Arterial oxygen content, 6-1
Arterial waveforms, 21-16, 21-16$f$
Arteriovenous malformation(s), and hemorrhagic stroke, 15-23
Artesunate, for malaria, 7-32
Arthritis, septic, 7-6$t$
Aspergillus infection, in pediatric oncology patient, 17-3, 17-4$t$, 17-7
Asphyxia
    and cardiac arrest, 3-5, 3-12–3-14
    perinatal, and acute kidney injury, 18-3
Asphyxiation, 11-9
Aspiration, of gastric contents, 2-26
Aspirin, 20-10
    for hypercalcemia, 8-15
Asthma, 1-10–1-11. *See also* Status asthmaticus
    clinical findings in, 4-29–4-30
    diagnosis, 4-29–4-30
    differential diagnosis, 4-30
    laboratory investigation, 4-29–4-30
    mechanical ventilation for, 4-32–4-33
    pathophysiology, 4-28–4-29
    treatment, 4-30–4-33
Asystole, 3-12
Ataxic breathing, 15-8, 15-8$t$
Atelectasis, 4-21–4-22
    in pneumonia, 4-36–4-37
    postoperative, 19-5
Atovaquone-proguanil, for malaria, 7-32
Atracurium, 20-19, 2-21$t$
Atrial flutter, 16-18$t$, 16-19$f$
Atrial septal defect, 16-13
Atrioventricular block, 16-18$t$, 16-19$f$

Atrioventricular septal defect, 16-14
Atropine, 19-8
    for cardiac arrest, 3-10t, 3-11
    dosage and administration, 12-6, 12-7t
    before intubation, 1-14
    with neostigmine, 20-20
    overdose/poisoning/toxicity, 13-4t
    and postoperative sinus tachycardia, 19-6
    for premedication, 20-9
    for vagal-mediated bradycardia, 2-26
Automated external defibrillators, 3-9, 3-12
Azotemia, in adrenal insufficiency, 8-18–8-19

# B

*Bacillus*, infections in pediatric oncology patient, 17-3, 17-4t
Bacteremia
    empiric antibiotics for, 7-11–7-12, 7-12t
    in pediatric oncology patient, 17-5
Bacterial infection(s), 1-26
    in cystic fibrosis, 4-38–4-39
    in pediatric oncology patient, 17-3, 17-4t
Bacterial tracheitis, 1-10
    causative agents, 4-12t, 4-15
    clinical features, 4-12t, 4-15
    treatment, 4-16
*Bacteroides*, necrobacillosis caused by, 7-29–7-31
Bag-mask ventilation, 2-10, 2-12, 2-15–2-16, 2-27
    adequacy, 2-15–2-16
    complications, 2-26
    in CPR, 3-6t
    in intrahospital transport, 14-6
    during intubation, 2-23
    and neuromuscular blockade, 2-21
    technique for, 2-15, 2-15f
    two-person, 2-16, 2-16f
Barbiturate coma, 15-21
Barbiturates, 20-15
    and emergence agitation, 19-9
    for intracranial hypertension, 15-21
Barotrauma, 2-26, 5-13
Basilar skull fracture, 9-6
Benzocaine, overdose/poisoning/toxicity, 13-3t
Benzodiazepines, 20-13, 20-14–20-15
    overdose/poisoning/toxicity, 13-11t
    and respiratory depression, 19-3
    reversal agent, 19-3, 20-19
    selection, 20-14
    for status epilepticus, 15-12t, 15-13, 15-14t
    withdrawal, 20-20–20-21
Beta-agonist(s)
    for anaphylaxis, 3-19
    for asthma, 1-10
    for bronchiolitis, 4-35
    for hyperkalemia, 18-11–18-12
    inhaled, for asthma, 4-30–4-31
    intravenous, for asthma, 4-31
    subcutaneous, for asthma, 4-31

Beta-blocker, overdose/poisoning/toxicity, 13-3t–13-4t, 13-11t
Bicarbonate, 2-7
Bilevel positive airway pressure, 4-7, 4-11, 5-2
    for croup, 4-13, 4-13t
Biologic agents, exposure to, 12-7–12-8, 12-8t
Birth asphyxia, 3-16
Bladder, traumatic injury, 9-17–9-18
Bleeding
    central nervous system, in status epilepticus, 15-11t
    occult, 19-20
    postoperative
        airway obstruction caused by, 19-4
        causes, 19-20
        monitoring, 19-20
Blood culture, 1-26
Blood flow, 3-3–3-4
Blood gas(es), 1-16t. *See also* Arterial blood gas measurement
    analysis, with cardiac arrest, 3-3
Blood loss, intraoperative, 19-20
Blood pressure, 1-15, 1-17, 16-20–16-21
    abnormal. *See also* Hypertension; Hypotension
        postoperative, 19-6
    age-dependent variations in, 7-2, 7-3t
    arterial, direct measurement, 21-16, 21-16f
    measurement, 21-16
    minimal acceptable values, 6-8, 6-9t
    in shock, 6-8–6-9, 6-9t
    systolic, 1-15
Blood products, 17-17–17-25
Bloodstream infection(s), catheter-associated, 19-22
Blood transfusion, 1-13, 17-16, 17-17–17-25, 19-20
    adverse reactions to, 17-23–17-25
        treatment, 17-23, 17-23t
        disease transmission in, 17-17–17-18, 17-25
    in trauma patient, 9-4
Blood urea nitrogen, clinical factors affecting, 18-8, 18-8f
Blood volume, 1-13
    by age group, 19-20
Botulism, 12-8t
Bradycardia, 1-15, 3-2, 6-8
    age-dependent definition, 7-3t
    causes, 19-6
    with hypoperfusion, 3-13–3-14
    with hypoxia, 3-13–3-14
    intubation and, 2-26
    pharmacotherapy for, 3-11
    in poisoned patient, 13-3, 13-4t
    postoperative, 19-6
    in shock, 3-13–3-14
Bradypnea, 1-6, 1-7t
Brain function, assessment, 1-15
Brain tumor(s), altered mental status/coma caused by, 15-16, 15-16t
Breakthrough pain, 19-13

Breathing
- apneustic, 15-8, 15-8t
- assessment, 1-4t, 3-3
- ataxic, 15-8, 15-8t
- in CPR, 3-6, 3-6t
- in trauma patient, 9-3

Breath sounds
- asymmetry, 2-6
    - in intubated patient, 2-26–2-27
- auscultation, 1-7, 2-5
    - in airway disorders, 4-21
    - with intubation, 2-25–2-26

Bronchiolitis, 1-11, 2-6
- acute, differential diagnosis, 4-30
- clinical manifestations, 4-34
- diagnosis, 4-34
- management, 4-34–4-35
- pathophysiology, 4-34

Bronchoscopy, 10-3
Broviac catheter, 21-9–21-10, 21-10f
Brucellosis, 12-8t
Bruise(s), in child abuse, 11-8, 11-8f
Bulla, 7-7t
BUN/creatinine ratio, 18-5, 18-6t
Burn center, referral to, criteria for, 10-8, 10-9t

Burn injury(ies)
- in child abuse, 10-2
- classification, 10-5
- deep partial thickness, 10-5, 10-7f, 10-8
- epidemiology, 10-2
- full thickness, 10-5, 10-7f, 10-8
- and glycemic control, 10-13
- grading, 10-5
- hypermetabolism with, 10-11–10-12
- and hypoalbuminemia, 10-12–10-13
- initial approach to, 10-2
- initial management, 10-3–10-8
- involved body surface area in, estimation, 10-5, 10-6f
- local response to, 10-5, 10-7f
- mechanism of injury in, 10-2
- mortality from, 10-13
- nonaccidental, patterns, 11-2–11-3, 11-3f
- nutritional support with, 10-11–10-12, 10-12t
- outcomes with, 10-13
- pathophysiology, 10-2
- rule of nines for, 10-5, 10-6f
- superficial partial thickness, 10-5, 10-7f, 10-8
- treatment, 10-8–10-13
    - hospital admission for, criteria for, 10-8
    - nonsurgical wound care in, 10-8–10-10, 10-9t
    - topical agents for, 10-8–10-10, 10-9t
    - wound excision and grafting in, 10-10

Butyrophenone poisoning, 13-4t

# C

C-A-B algorithm, of resuscitation, 3-3–3-4
Caffeine, overdose/poisoning, 13-3t–13-4t
Calcineurin inhibitors, nephrotoxicity, 18-4
Calcitonin, for hypercalcemia, 8-15

Calcium
- infusion, precautions with, 18-12
- replacement, in tumor lysis syndrome, 17-11t, 17-12
- serum, 8-13. *See also* Hypercalcemia; Hypocalcemia

Calcium-channel blockers
- intoxication, pharmacotherapy for, 3-11
- overdose/poisoning/toxicity, 13-4t, 13-11t

Calcium chloride, 19-20–19-21
- for cardiac arrest, 3-10t
- for hypocalcemia, 8-14, 18-13

Calcium gluconate, 19-21
- for hyperkalemia, 18-11
- for hypocalcemia, 8-14, 18-13

Calcium salts, in CPR, 3-12
Calciuresis, for hypercalcemia, 8-15
Camphor poisoning, 13-4t
Candida infection, in pediatric oncology patient, 17-3, 17-4t, 17-7
Capillary leak, 6-22
Capillary refill, 1-21, 6-8–6-9
- delayed, 3-2
- in hypovolemia, 1-17

Capnography, 1-8, 1-8t, 1-11, 1-12t, 2-9
Carbamate(s), overdose/poisoning/toxicity, 13-3t–13-4t, 13-11t

Carbon dioxide ($CO_2$). *See also* End-tidal $CO_2$
- arterial, in post-resuscitative care, 3-20
- exhaled, 2-9
    - monitoring, in CPR, 3-7
- minute ventilation, 1-8
- total serum, 1-16t
- transcutaneous monitoring, 1-8

Carbon monoxide poisoning, 2-9, 10-3–10-4, 13-3t–13-4t, 13-11t
Carboxyhemoglobin, 2-9

Cardiac arrest, 3-1–3-23, 4-20, 6-8. *See also* Ventricular fibrillation
- anesthesia-related, 19-2
- asphyxia and, 3-5, 3-12–3-14
- in congenital heart disease, 3-16–3-17
- diagnosis, 3-3
- ethical considerations with, 3-22–3-23
- 6 Hs and 6 Ts, 3-15, 3-16t
- in-hospital, outcomes with, 3-2
- intraosseous access in, 3-8
- medications used in, 3-9–3-11
- out-of-hospital, outcomes with, 3-2
- post-resuscitation care with, 3-2, 3-7, 3-19–3-21
- potentially reversible causes, 3-15, 3-16t
- prevention, 3-2
- recognition, 3-2
- resuscitation for
    - AHA algorithm for, 3-17f
    - family presence during, 3-22
    - prognosis after, 3-22
    - termination, 3-22–3-23
- shock and, 3-12–3-14
- survival, factors affecting, 3-2, 3-22–3-23
- traumatic, 3-19

treatment timeline for, 3-19, 3-19*t*
vascular access in, 3-8
Cardiac contractility, 6-1–6-2, 16-20–16-21
Cardiac contusions, 9-15
Cardiac index, 1-14
Cardiac output, 1-13–1-14, 3-13–3-14, 6-1
    in CPR, 3-6
    decreased, with positive-pressure ventilation, 2-27
    heart rate and, 1-14–1-15
    low. *See also* Low cardiac output syndrome
        evaluation of patient with, 16-21*t*
        in neonate, 16-2–16-6, 16-6*t*
        postoperative, causes, 16-17*t*
    supraventricular tachycardia and, 1-14
Cardiac tamponade, 3-16, 16-20
    postoperative, 16-20
    in trauma patient, 3-19, 9-4, 9-15
Cardiomyopathy(ies), 3-21
    in neonate, 16-5–16-6
Cardiopulmonary arrest, 2-2
Cardiopulmonary bypass, and risk for acute kidney injury, 18-4
Cardiopulmonary monitoring, 2-22
    with cardiac arrest, 3-3
Cardiopulmonary resuscitation, 3-1–3-2, 3-4–3-7, 3-12–3-13. *See also* C-A-B algorithm; Chest compressions
    bag-mask ventilation in, 3-6*t*
    for bradycardic patient, 3-14
    closed-chest, 3-5
    coronary perfusion pressure in, 3-3, 3-6
    goal, 3-7
    high-quality, keys to, 3-5
    medications used in, 3-9–3-11
    monitoring in, 3-7
        quality, 3-7–3-8
    negative intrathoracic pressure in, 3-4
    neonatal, 3-16
    for neonate, 3-6*t*
    open-chest, 3-5
    outcomes with, factors affecting, 3-22–3-23
    quality assessment, 3-7–3-8
    termination, 3-22–3-23
    tracheal intubation in, 3-6*t*
Cardiovascular failure, 1-5, 1-11
Cardiovascular infection, 7-6*t*
Cardiovascular support
    in post-resuscitative care, 3-20
    in status epilepticus, 15-12*t*, 15-13
Cardiovascular system, 1-13–1-24
    anatomy, 1-13–1-15
    evaluation, ancillary studies for, 1-16*t*
    physical examination, 1-15
    physiology, 1-13–1-15
Cardioversion, 3-14–3-15
Carotid artery
    cannulation, with central venous catheter, 21-14*t*
    puncture, with central venous catheter, 21-14*t*
Catecholamines, 1-14

Cathartics, 13-6
Catheter(s), 21-8–21-16. *See also* Indwelling venous access catheter(s); Urinary catheter(s)
    for hemodynamic monitoring, 6-11, 21-13
    heparin flush for, 21-10*t*–21-11*t*
Catheterization, indications for, 21-8, 6-10–6-11
Caudal block, for postoperative pain, 19-14–19-15
Central herniation, 15-8–15-9
Central line catheter, 21-10*t*. *See also* Tunneled lines
Central nervous system disease, respiratory patterns in, 15-8, 15-8*t*
Central nervous system herniation syndromes, 7-21, 15-8–15-9, 15-17–15-18
    prevention, 9-3
Central nervous system infection, 7-6*t*. *See also* Encephalitis; Meningitis
    clinical presentation, 7-20–7-21
    CSF analysis in, 7-21, 7-22*t*
Central venous catheter(s), 6-10–6-11, 21-13–21-14
    complications, 21-14, 21-14*t*
    indications for, 21-13–21-14
    insertion sites, 21-13, 21-13*t*
    sizes, 21-13, 21-13*t*
Central venous pressure, monitoring, 1-14, 1-16*t*
    after cardiac arrest, 3-20
    in shock, 6-11
Cerebral blood flow, 15-5–15-6
    autoregulation, 15-5–15-6, 15-6*f*
    in closed-chest CPR, 3-5
    in open-chest CPR, 3-5
Cerebral blood volume, 15-4
Cerebral edema
    cytotoxic, 15-4
    diabetic ketoacidosis and, 8-17–8-18
    vasogenic, 15-4
Cerebral perfusion, 1-4
Cerebral perfusion pressure, 9-10, 15-20
Cerebral salt wasting, 8-7
Cerebrospinal fluid (CSF)
    analysis, in central nervous system infections, 7-21, 7-22*t*
    culture, 1-26
    flow, 15-4, 15-4*f*–15-5*f*
    increased, 15-5
    physiology, 15-5
    production, 15-4
Cerebrospinal fluid (CSF) shunt(s), 15-25–15-26, 15-26*t*
Cerebrovascular accident, 15-16, 15-22–15-24
Cervical spine
    injury/trauma, 9-6, 9-11–9-12
        and airway management, 2-11–2-12
        evaluation, 9-14*t*
    precautions with, 9-2, 9-6
    stabilization, 1-9, 2-23, 3-19, 15-2
Channelopathy(ies), 3-21
Charcoal hemoperfusion, in poisoned patient, 13-6
CHARGE association, 4-7–4-8
Chemical exposure(s), 12-6, 12-7*t*

Chemotherapy, and acute kidney injury, 18-3, 18-4*t*
Chest
    movement, during respiration, 1-7
        asymmetry, 1-7, 1-7*t*
    shape, during respiration, 1-7
Chest compressions. *See also* C-A-B algorithm; Cardiopulmonary resuscitation
    for bradycardic patient, 3-14
    during cardiac arrest, 3-5
    and coronary perfusion, 3-3, 3-6
    neonatal, 3-16
    rate, in CPR, 3-6, 3-6*t*
    in resuscitation, 3-3
    and ventilation, 3-4
Chest compression-ventilation ratio(s), in CPR, 3-6, 3-6*t*
Chest drain. *See* Thoracostomy tube(s)
Chest radiography, 1-11, 1-12*t*, 1-16*t*
    in airway disorders, 4-22, 4-23*f*
    in intubated patient, 2-27
    with intubation, 2-26
    in pneumonia, 4-37
    in shock, 6-19
    in thoracic trauma, 9-13
Chest tube. *See* Thoracostomy tube(s)
Chest wall
    compliance, 1-5–1-6
    elasticity, 2-4
Cheyne-Stokes respiration, 15-8, 15-8*t*
Child abuse. *See also* Nonaccidental injury(ies)
    injuries suggesting, 11-2–11-3, 11-2*t*, 11-3*f*
Child maltreatment, 1-24–1-25. *See also* Nonaccidental injury(ies)
    acute management, 11-10
    diagnosis, 11-10–11-13
    emergent management, 11-10–11-11
    history-taking in, 11-10
    imaging in, 11-10–11-13
    laboratory investigation, 11-11, 11-11*t*
    medicolegal considerations, 11-13
    patterns, 11-2–11-9
    photographic documentation in, 11-10, 11-13
    reporting requirements, 11-13
    risk factors for, 11-1, 11-2*t*
Chloral hydrate poisoning, 13-3*t*
Chloroquine
    for malaria, 7-32
    overdose/poisoning/toxicity, 13-3*t*
Choanal atresia, 1-9, 4-7–4-8
Choanal stenosis, 4-2, 4-7–4-8
Circulation. *See also* A-B-C algorithm, of resuscitation
    during cardiac arrest, 3-5
    in trauma patient, 9-3–9-4
Circulatory arrest, 1-15
Cisatracurium, 2-21*t*, 19-8, 20-19
Cleft palate, 4-3, 4-8
Clindamycin, for malaria, 7-32
Clonidine
    overdose/poisoning/toxicity, 13-4*t*
    for postoperative pain, 19-12

Closing capacity, 1-6
Coagulopathy(ies), 17-16–17-17
    postoperative, 19-20
Coarctation of aorta, 1-23, 16-4–16-5
Cocaine, overdose/poisoning, 13-3*t*–13-4*t*, 13-11*t*
Codeine, 20-13
    for postoperative pain, 19-11
Cold shock, 1-22, 6-22, 7-10, 7-10*f*
Collagen vascular disease, altered mental status/coma caused by, 15-16, 15-16*t*
Colloids, 1-22
Colony-stimulating factor(s), for febrile neutropenic patient, 17-3–17-4
Color, assessment, 1-4*t*
Coma, 1-24, 15-15–15-18
    differential diagnosis, 15-17
    etiology, 15-15–15-16, 15-16*t*
    evaluation, 15-17
    laboratory investigation, 15-18
    therapy for, 15-18
Compartment syndrome, 9-19
Computed tomography (CT)
    abdominal, in trauma patient, 9-17
    in altered mental status/coma, 15-17–15-18
    in meningitis, 7-21
    in suspected child abuse, 11-11–11-12
Congenital adrenal hyperplasia, 8-18
Congenital heart disease, 1-20
    acyanotic, 16-12–16-14, 16-15*t*
        causes, 16-14, 16-15*t*
        with increased pulmonary blood flow, 16-12–16-14
        initial evaluation and treatment, 16-14, 16-15*t*
    cardiac arrest in, 3-16–3-17
    cyanotic, 16-6–16-11
        with decreased pulmonary blood flow, 16-7–16-9
        with increased pulmonary blood flow, 16-9–16-11
    resuscitation in, 3-16–3-17
Congenital malformation(s), differential diagnosis, 4-30
Congestive heart failure, 1-16, 1-20
    signs and symptoms, 16-5, 16-5*t*
Continuous arterial pressure monitoring, 1-16*t*
Continuous epidural analgesia, 19-14
Continuous positive airway pressure, 4-7, 4-11, 5-4–5-5, 5-7*f*
    for croup, 4-13, 4-13*t*
Continuous renal replacement therapy, 18-14
    in poisoned patient, 13-6
Contrast media, and risk for acute kidney injury, 18-4, 18-4*t*
Co-oximetry, 2-9
Coronary artery(ies), abnormalities, 3-21
Coronary blood flow, 3-3
Corticosteroid(s)
    for acute respiratory distress syndrome, 4-41
    for asthma, 1-10, 4-30
    for croup, 4-13, 4-13*t*
    for distributive shock, 1-22

for intracranial hypertension, 15-21
    postoperative indications for, 19-4
Cortisol, serum levels, in adrenal insufficiency, 8-18–8-19
Cough, 4-21
    in croup, 4-12, 4-12*t*
    in pneumonia, 4-36
Cough reflex, 2-6
Coxsackie virus, 1-26
CPR. *See* Cardiopulmonary resuscitation
Crackles, 1-7, 1-16, 2-6
C-reactive protein, 19-18
Creatinine
    clinical factors affecting, 18-8, 18-8*f*
    serum, 18-5
        and acute kidney injury, 18-2, 18-3*t*
    urine, 18-5
Cricoid pressure, 2-15*f*, 2-22, 2-24, 2-25*f*
Cricothyrotomy, 2-29
CRIES pain scale, 19-11*t*
Croup, 1-4, 1-10, 4-6, 4-12–4-13, 4-13*f*, 4-21
    and bacterial tracheitis, 4-15
    causative agents, 4-12, 4-12*t*
    clinical features, 4-12, 4-12*t*
    clinical scoring tools for, 4-23, 4-23*t*
    differential diagnosis, 4-30
    spasmodic, 4-18
    treatment, 4-12, 4-12*t*, 4-13, 4-13*t*
Cryoprecipitate, 17-23
Crystalloids, 1-22
Cutaneous injury(ies), in child abuse, 11-8, 11-8*f*
Cyanide poisoning, 10-3–10-4, 13-3*t*–13-4*t*, 13-11*t*
Cyanmethemoglobin, 10-4
Cyanosis, 1-7, 4-20
    neonatal, 16-11*t*. *See also* Congenital heart disease, cyanotic
Cystic fibrosis, 4-38–4-39
Cystitis, 7-25
Cytomegalovirus pneumonia, in pediatric oncology patient, 17-3, 17-5*t*, 17-6

# D

Dantrolene sodium, 19-23
Dapsone, overdose/poisoning/toxicity, 13-3*t*
Death(s). *See also* Sudden death
    acute infection and, 7-2
    anesthesia-related, 19-2
    burn injury and, 10-13
    cerebrovascular accident and, 15-22
    gastroenteritis and, 1-17
    from poisoning, 13-2
    respiratory disorders and, 1-6
    shock and, 6-1
    thoracic trauma and, 9-13
Decerebrate posture, 15-7
Decorticate posture, 15-7
Defibrillation, 3-8–3-9, 3-12–3-13
    in cardiac arrest, 3-5

dosing recommendations, 3-8
manual, 3-9
paddle size for, 3-9
Dehydration, 19-22
    in adrenal insufficiency, 8-18–8-19
    signs, 1-4*t*
Dengue fever, 7-32–7-33
Detection, 1-3, 1-3*f*
Dexamethasone
    for adrenal insufficiency, 8-19
    for croup, 4-13*t*
    for intracranial hypertension, 15-21
    postoperative indications for, 19-4
    for postoperative nausea and vomiting, 19-16, 19-17*t*
    for stridulous patient, 1-10
    for subglottic stenosis, 4-7
    for upper airway disease, 4-25, 4-26
Dexmedetomidine, 20-17
    for postoperative pain, 19-12
Dextrotransposition of the great arteries, 16-9–16-10
Diabetes insipidus, 8-8–8-9
Diabetes mellitus, shock in patient with, 6-24
Diabetic ketoacidosis, 8-17–8-18, 13-3*t*
    and cerebral edema, 8-17–8-18
    hyponatremia in, 8-18
    and hypophosphatemia, 8-15
    initial stabilization in, 8-17–8-18
Dialysis, 18-13–18-14
Diaphragm
    anatomy, 1-5
    traumatic injuries to, 9-15
Diaphragmatic excursion, 1-5
Diarrhea, 12-4. *See also* Gastroenteritis
    in burn patients, 10-12
    fluid loss in, 1-17
Diazepam, 20-15
    dosage and administration, 12-7*t*
    for status epilepticus, 15-12*t*, 15-13, 15-14*t*
Difficult airway, 2-23, 2-29, 20-4–20-6, 20-5*t*
DiGeorge syndrome, 16-10
Digitalis, intoxication, 18-12
Digoxin, overdose/poisoning/toxicity, 13-4*t*, 13-11*t*
DIRECT methodology, 1-3, 1-3*f*, 1-26–1-27, 3-2, 8-3
Disability, evaluation, in trauma patient, 9-4
Disaster(s)
    hospital capacity and, 12-2
    pediatric vulnerabilities in, 12-2–12-5, 12-5*f*
Disaster plan(s), adaptation for needs of children, 12-11–12-12
Disaster-related injury/illness, treatment, 12-6–12-10
Disaster response, 12-2–12-3
Disseminated intravascular coagulation, 17-16–17-17
Diuresis, 1-24
    alkaline, in poisoned patient, 13-6
    forced, in poisoned patient, 13-6
    for hypercalcemia, 8-15
    for pulmonary edema, 19-5

Diuretics
    for acyanotic congenital heart disease, 16-15*t*
    hyponatremia caused by, 8-7
Dobutamine, 1-24
    for distributive shock, 1-22
    for shock, 6-14, 6-15*t*–6-16*t*
Dopamine
    for distributive shock, 1-22
    for shock, 6-14, 6-15*t*–6-16*t*, 6-22
Doxycycline, for malaria, 7-32
Drug(s), altered mental status/coma caused by, 15-16, 15-16*t*
Ductus arteriosus, 1-14
Dysrhythmias. *See also* Arrhythmia(s)

# E

E-C clamp technique, 2-15, 2-15*f*
Echocardiography, 1-16*t*
    after cardiac arrest, 3-20
Edrophonium, 19-8
Effective communication, 1-3, 1-3*f*
Electrocardiography
    in arrhythmias, 16-17, 16-19*f*
    with cardiac arrest, 3-3
    in hyperkalemia, 8-10*f*, 8-11, 18-11–18-12
    in hypokalemia, 8-9, 8-10*f*
    in myocarditis, 7-27–7-28
    in pericarditis, 7-27
    in tumor lysis syndrome, 17-11
Electroencephalography, after cardiac arrest, 3-21
Electrolyte(s). *See also specific electrolyte*
    analysis, with cardiac arrest, 3-3
    postoperative deficits, 19-15–19-16
Electrolyte abnormalities, 1-27, 8-4–8-16
    altered mental status/coma caused by, 15-16, 15-16*t*
    in pediatric oncology patient, 17-9
    in tumor lysis syndrome, 17-10
    management, 17-11*t*, 17-12
Embolism. *See also* Pulmonary embolism
    with central venous catheter, 21-14
    with indwelling venous access catheter, 21-12
Emergence agitation, 19-9
Emergency preparedness. *See also* Triage
    and preserving family unit, 12-11, 12-11*t*
    and treatment of disaster-related injury/illness, 12-6–12-10
Empyema, 21-7
    in pneumonia, 4-36–4-37
Encephalitis
    altered mental status/coma caused by, 15-16, 15-16*t*
    clinical presentation, 7-23
    etiologic agents, 7-23
    viral, 7-20
    clinical presentation, 7-23
    CSF analysis in, 7-21, 7-22*t*
    differential diagnosis, 7-24
Endotracheal intubation. *See* Tracheal intubation

Endotracheal tube(s), 2-18–2-19
    airway trauma due to, 19-4
    cuffed, 2-18
        placement, 2-25
    cuff inflation, 2-3, 2-18
    depth of insertion, 2-18–2-19, 9-3
    leak, 2-9
    placement, 2-25, 9-3
    securing, 2-23, 2-26
    size, 2-18–2-19, 2-23, 9-2, 19-4
    stylet for, 2-23
    uncuffed, 2-18
        placement, 2-25
End-tidal $CO_2$
    capnography, 1-8, 1-8*t*, 1-11, 2-9
    for intubation, 2-23, 2-26
    monitoring, 4-22
    in CPR, 3-7
    in post-resuscitative care, 3-20
Energy requirements, 19-18, 19-18*t*
Enteral nutrition, 19-19, 19-19*t*
Enterococcus, 1-26
    infections in pediatric oncology patient, 17-3, 17-4*t*
Enterocolitis, neutropenic, in pediatric oncology patient, 17-7
Epidural analgesia, for postoperative pain, 19-14, 19-15
Epiglottis
    adult vs pediatric, 4-4
    anatomical considerations, 4-4
    anatomy, 2-3
    visualization during laryngoscopy, 2-24
Epiglottitis, 1-4, 1-6–1-7, 1-10, 4-13–4-15, 4-14*f*, 4-15*t*
    causative agents, 4-12*t*, 4-13–4-14
    clinical features, 4-12*t*, 4-14
    incidence, 4-11
    management, 4-14–4-15, 4-15*t*
Epinephrine, 16-21
    for anaphylaxis, 3-18
    for bradycardia, 3-11
    for cardiac arrest, 3-9–3-10, 3-10*t*
    for croup, 4-13, 4-13*t*
    for distributive shock, 1-22
    high-dose, contraindications to, 3-10, 3-11
    postoperative indications for, 19-4
    racemic
        for bronchiolitis, 4-35
        for upper airway disease, 4-25, 4-26
    for shock, 6-15, 6-15*t*–6-16*t*
    for stridulous patient, 1-10
    for subglottic stenosis, 4-7
Equal pressure point, 4-6
*Escherichia coli*, 1-26
    infection, in pediatric oncology patient, 17-3, 17-4*t*
Esophageal injury, 9-15
Esophageal-tracheal double-lumen airway device, 2-28
$ETCO_2$. *See* End-tidal $CO_2$
Ethanol
    poisoning, 13-3*t*–13-4*t*
    withdrawal, 13-8*t*

Ethical issues, with cardiac arrest, 3-22–3-23
Ethylene glycol poisoning, 13-3t–13-4t, 13-11t
Ethyl ether poisoning, 13-3t
Etomidate, 2-20t
Exanthem, 1-26
Exposure, in evaluation of trauma patient, 9-5
Extracellular fluid (ECF) volume, in brain, 15-4
Extremity(ies), trauma to, 9-18–9-19

# F

Face mask, 5-2, 5-3f
FACES Pain Rating Scale, 19-10, 19-11t
Face tent, 2-10
Fasting, pre-sedation, 20-7
Fat emulsion, parenteral administration, 19-18
Feeding tube(s), 21-4
    complications, 21-4, 21-5t
    malfunction, 21-4, 21-5t
    nasoduodenal placement, 21-4, 21-4f
    nasogastric placement, 21-4, 21-4f
    nasojejunal placement, 21-4, 21-4f
    small-bore, 21-4, 21-7
    surgically placed, 21-5–21-7
    transpyloric placement, 19-19, 21-4, 21-4f
Fentanyl, 20-12–20-13
    adverse effects and side effects, 20-12–20-13
    benefits, 2-20t
    dosage and administration, 2-20t
    dosing regimen, for patient-controlled analgesia, 19-13t
    onset and duration of action, 2-20t
    for postoperative pain, 19-11
    precautions with, 2-20t
    for premedication, 20-10
Fever, 1-26, 6-9
    after cardiac arrest, 3-21
    in airway disorders, 4-21
    neutropenic. *See also* Neutropenia, febrile
    definition, 17-2
    in pneumonia, 4-36
    postoperative, 19-22, 19-22t
Fiberoptic intubation, 2-28–2-29
FLACC pain scale, 19-11t
Flail chest, 9-14
Fluid(s), 8-2–8-3
    maintenance, 6-13–6-14, 8-2–8-3
    resuscitation, 8-3
Fluid deficit(s). *See also* Dehydration; Hypovolemia
    in pediatric oncology patient, 17-9
    postoperative, 19-15–19-16
Fluid imbalance, 8-2–8-3. *See also* Dehydration; Hypovolemia
Fluid loss, 1-17
    and hyponatremia, 8-7
    perioperative, 19-15–19-16
Fluid resuscitation, 1-15, 1-22–1-23
    after cardiac arrest, 3-20
    for anaphylaxis, 3-18
    for burn patient, 10-4–10-5
    in hypovolemia, 1-17
    for neurologic injury, 15-2
    planning for, 20-10
    postoperative, 19-6, 19-15
    for postoperative bleeding, 19-20
    setup for, 20-8–20-9
    in shock, 6-11–6-14, 8-3
    in trauma patient, 3-19, 9-4
Flumazenil, 19-3, 20-19
Foley catheter
    as replacement for dislodged gastrostomy tube, 21-6
    for urinary catheterization, 21-8–21-9
    used as feeding tube, 21-6
Fontanelle(s), 1-25
Foreign body
    airway obstruction, 1-4, 1-7, 1-10
    aspiration, 1-9, 1-11
    differential diagnosis, 4-30
Fosphenytoin, for status epilepticus, 15-12t, 15-13, 15-14t
Fractional excretion of sodium (FENa), 18-5, 18-6t
Fractional excretion of urea (FEurea), 18-5–18-6, 18-6t
Fraction of inspired oxygen, in mechanical ventilation, 5-11, 5-11t, 5-12
Frank-Starling curve, 1-13, 1-14f
Free water deficit, 8-8, 8-8t
Fresh-frozen plasma, 17-22, 17-22t, 19-20
Functional residual capacity, 1-6
Funduscopy, in suspected child abuse, 11-13
Fungal infections, 17-3, 17-4t, 17-7
Furosemide, 1-24
    for hypercalcemia, 8-15
    for pulmonary edema, 19-5
*Fusobacterium* spp., necrobacillosis caused by, 7-29–7-31

# G

Gag reflex, 2-6
Gallop, 1-16
Gamma-hydroxybutyrate poisoning, 13-3t
Gasping, 3-2–3-3
Gastric lavage, 13-5
Gastric tube, in trauma patient, 9-5
Gastroenteritis, 1-17
    acute, mortality from, 1-17
    and heart failure, 1-20
    and hyponatremia, 8-6
Gastrointestinal distress, in sepsis, 1-26
Gastrointestinal tube(s), 21-2–21-7
    diameter, 21-2
    indications for, 21-2
Gastrojejunal tube(s), 21-7
Gastrostomy tube(s), 21-5–21-6, 21-5f
    complications, 21-6
    de Pezzer catheter, 21-6
    dislodged, management, 21-6

laparoscopic placement, 21-6
Malecot catheter, 21-6
Mic-Key, 21-6, 21-6f
percutaneous, 21-5
complications, 21-5–21-6
percutaneous endoscopic, 21-5
General examination, 1-4–1-5, 1-4t
Glasgow Coma Scale, 1-25, 6-8, 9-4, 9-9, 15-6, 15-7t
Glidescope, 9-3
Glomerular filtration rate, estimation, 18-10
Glomerulonephritis, 18-6
Glossoptosis, 4-8
Glucocorticoid(s), for hypercalcemia, 8-15
Glucose
 administration, 3-11
 blood
  after cardiac arrest, 3-21
  assessment, 6-9
 infusion, in nutritional support, 19-18
 metabolism, disorders, 8-16–8-17. *See also*
  Hyperglycemia; Hypoglycemia
Glucose testing, point-of-care, 1-25, 6-9
Glycemic control, in burn patients, 10-13
Glycopyrrolate, 19-8
 with neostigmine, 20-20
 and postoperative sinus tachycardia, 19-6
 for premedication, 20-9–20-10
Gram-negative organisms, infections in pediatric oncology patient, 17-3, 17-4t
Gram-positive organisms, infections in pediatric oncology patient, 17-3, 17-4t
Grunting, 1-6, 2-5

# H
*Haemophilus influenzae* (type b), 1-26
 chemoprophylaxis for high-risk contacts, 7-22
 meningitis, 7-22
 vaccine, 4-11
Hagen-Poiseuille equation, 4-3–4-4
Hand hygiene, 19-23t
Head-tilt/chin-lift maneuver, 2-12, 4-24–4-25
 contraindications to, 9-2
Head trauma, 12-4–12-5. *See also* Traumatic brain injury
 abusive, 11-4–11-5, 11-5f
 evaluation, 9-14t
 nonaccidental, 1-24–1-25
 orogastric intubation in, 21-3
Heart block, 16-18t, 16-19f
Heart disease. *See also* Congenital heart disease
 mechanical ventilation in, 5-20
Heart failure, 1-20. *See also* Congestive heart failure
 and acute kidney injury, 18-3, 18-4t
 mechanical ventilation in, 5-20
Heart function, left-right disparity, 1-14
Heart rate, 1-14
 abnormalities, postoperative, 19-6
 age-dependent variations in, 7-2, 7-3t
 and cardiac output, 1-14–1-15

neonatal, 3-16
in poisoned patient, 13-3, 13-4t
at rest, by age group, 1-1–1-2
Heavy metal poisoning, 13-11t
Heliox, 1-10
 for asthma, 4-32
 for croup, 4-13, 4-13t
 indications for, 4-25
 for subglottic stenosis, 4-7
 for upper airway disease, 4-25
Helmet, for noninvasive respiratory support, 5-2, 5-3f
Hematocrit, reference values, by age and gender, 1-13t
Hematology. *See* Oncology/hematology
Hemodialysis, 18-14
 emergency, in hyperkalemia, 8-12
 in poisoned patient, 13-6
Hemodynamic monitoring
 catheters for, 6-10–6-11, 21-13
  measurements using, 21-16, 21-16f
 in shock, 6-11, 6-14
Hemodynamic support, after cardiac arrest, 3-20
Hemoglobin, 1-12t
 oxygen saturation, 1-8, 2-8
 reference values, by age and gender, 1-13t
Hemoglobin concentration, 1-16t
 in shock, 1-22
Hemolytic transfusion reactions, 17-23–17-25
Hemolytic uremic syndrome, 18-4, 18-6
Hemothorax
 with central venous catheter, 21-14t
 chest tube–induced, 21-8
 with indwelling venous access catheter, 21-12
 in trauma patient, 3-19
Heparin, overdose/poisoning/toxicity, 13-11t
Heparin flush, 21-10t–21-11t
Hepatic failure. *See* Liver failure
Hepatomegaly, 1-16
Herniation syndrome(s) (central nervous system), 7-21, 15-7–15-9
 prevention, 9-3
Herpes simplex virus infection, 1-26. *See also*
 Encephalitis; Meningitis, viral
 neonatal, 7-29
Hickman catheter, 21-9
History-taking
 in airway disease, 4-18–4-19
 with cardiac arrest, 3-3
 preoperative, 19-2
 pre-sedation, 20-6–20-7
 in suspected shock, 6-9
Holliday-Segar method, for calculating maintenance fluids, 8-2, 8-2t
Humidification, in mechanical ventilation, 5-12–5-13
Hydralazine, for hypertensive emergency, 18-15, 18-15t
Hydration
 for bronchiolitis, 4-34–4-35
 postoperative management, 19-15–19-16
Hydrocarbons, poisoning, 13-3t

Hydrocodone, 20-13
    for postoperative pain, 19-11
Hydrocortisone
    for adrenal insufficiency, 8-19
    for distributive shock, 1-22
    for hypercalcemia, 8-15
Hydrogen sulfide poisoning, 13-4t
Hydromorphone
    dosing regimen, for patient-controlled analgesia, 19-13t
    for postoperative pain, 19-11
Hydrothorax, with indwelling venous access catheter, 21-12
Hyperbaric oxygen therapy
    for burn patient, 10-11
    for necrotizing fasciitis, 7-19
Hypercalcemia, 8-15
Hypercapnia, and respiratory failure, 4-27–4-28
Hypercarbia, 1-5, 1-12t
    effect on intracranial pressure, 15-20
    and postoperative sinus tachycardia, 19-6
Hypercyanotic spell(s), 16-8
Hyperglycemia, 8-18
    after cardiac arrest, 3-21
    causes, 8-17
    definition, 8-17
    management, 6-13–6-14, 8-17
Hyperkalemia
    in acute kidney injury, 18-8
    in adrenal insufficiency, 8-18–8-19
    with cardiac arrest, pharmacotherapy for, 3-10t, 3-11
    definition, 8-11
    ECG changes with, 8-10f, 8-11, 18-11–18-12
    emergent management, 8-11–8-12
    mild, 18-11
    moderate, 18-11
    overcorrection of hypokalemia and, 8-9
    severe, 18-11–18-12
    signs and symptoms, 8-11
    succinylcholine-induced, 2-21, 2-21t
    treatment, 8-11–8-12, 18-11–18-12
    in tumor lysis syndrome, 17-10, 17-11t, 17-12
Hyperleukocytosis, in pediatric oncology patient, 17-13
Hypermagnesemia
    in acute kidney injury, 18-8
    causes, 8-13
    definition, 8-13
    treatment, 8-13
Hypermetabolism, in burn patient, 10-11–10-12
Hypernatremia, 8-7–8-9
    causes, 8-7
    definition, 8-7
    in diabetes insipidus, 8-8–8-9
    signs and symptoms, 8-7
    treatment, 8-7–8-8
Hyperoxia, 1-10

Hyperphosphatemia, 8-16
    in acute kidney injury, 18-8
    causes, 8-16
    and hypocalcemia, 8-16
    hypocalcemia with, management, 18-12
    management, 18-13
    treatment, 8-16
    in tumor lysis syndrome, 17-10, 17-11t, 17-12
Hyperpnea, 1-5
Hypertension
    postoperative, 19-6
    with volume overload, in oliguria, 18-15
Hypertensive emergency(ies), 18-15, 18-15t
Hyperthermia
    after cardiac arrest, 3-21
    postoperative, 19-22
    and postoperative sinus tachycardia, 19-6
    risk factors for, 19-21
Hypertriglyceridemia, 8-18
Hyperventilation
    after cardiac arrest, 3-20
    central, 15-8, 15-8t
    for intracranial hypertension, 15-20–15-21
    in trauma patient, 9-3
Hypoalbuminemia, in burn patients, 10-12–10-13
Hypocalcemia, 1-25
    in acute kidney injury, 18-8
    blood transfusion and, 19-20–19-21
    with cardiac arrest, pharmacotherapy for, 3-10t, 3-11
    causes, 8-13
    in child, 8-14
    definition, 8-13
    with hyperphosphatemia, management, 18-12
    hyperphosphatemia and, 8-16
    management, 18-13
    in neonate/infant, 8-14
    signs and symptoms, 8-13
    treatment, 8-14, 16-21
    in tumor lysis syndrome, 17-11t, 17-12
Hypoglycemia, 1-5, 1-25, 1-27, 6-9
    in adrenal insufficiency, 8-18–8-19
    after cardiac arrest, 3-21
    causes, 8-16
    definition, 8-16
    laboratory investigation, 8-16
    management, 6-13–6-14, 6-13f
    pharmacotherapy for, 3-11
    and postoperative agitation, 19-9
    prevention, 6-13, 6-13f
    signs and symptoms, 8-16
    treatment, 8-17
Hypoglycemic agent(s), overdose/poisoning/toxicity, 13-3t–13-4t, 13-11t
Hypokalemia, 8-9–8-10, 8-10f
Hypomagnesemia, 3-12, 8-12

Hyponatremia, 1-25, 8-4–8-7
    in acute kidney injury, 18-8
    in adrenal insufficiency, 8-18–8-19
    causes, 8-4, 8-4t
        renal, 8-7
    classification, according to extracellular fluid volume status, 8-4, 8-4t
    definition, 8-4
    in diabetic ketoacidosis, 8-18
    and hypovolemic states, 8-6–8-7
    maintenance fluids and, 8-3
    management, 18-13
    postoperative, 19-16
    signs and symptoms, 8-4
    treatment, 8-5, 8-5f
    in water intoxication, 8-6
Hypoperfusion, and bradycardia, 3-13–3-14
Hypophosphatemia, 8-15–8-16
Hypoplastic left heart syndrome, 1-23, 16-2–16-4
    surgical treatment, 16-3–16-4, 16-3t
Hypopnea, 1-5
Hypotension, 1-15, 1-27
    after cardiac arrest, 3-20
    in anaphylaxis, 3-18
    with initiation of mechanical ventilation, 5-22–5-23
    with positive-pressure ventilation, 2-27
    postoperative, 19-6
    in shock, 6-8–6-9, 6-9t
    in status epilepticus, 15-11t
Hypothermia, 6-9
    after cardiac arrest, 3-21
    deleterious effects, 19-21, 19-21t
    induced, after cardiac arrest, 3-21–3-22
    for intracranial hypertension, 15-21
    risk factors for, 19-21
Hypoventilation, 2-7
    after cardiac arrest, 3-20
Hypovolemia, 1-21, 6-3
    and acute kidney injury, 18-3, 18-4t
    and hyponatremia, 8-6–8-7
    postoperative, 19-6
Hypoxemia, 1-7, 1-12t, 1-15, 2-6, 2-7
    and respiratory failure, 4-27–4-28
    respiratory response to, 1-5
Hypoxia, 1-5, 1-10, 2-7
    in air transport, 14-10–14-11
    and bradycardia, 3-13–3-14
    cerebral, 15-16
    effect on intracranial pressure, 15-20
    in poisoned patient, 13-3, 13-3t
    and postoperative agitation, 19-9
    in status epilepticus, 15-11t

# I

Ibuprofen, 20-10–20-11
    overdose/poisoning/toxicity, 13-3t
Imaging
    in airway disorders, 4-22, 4-23f
    in altered mental status/coma, 15-17–15-18
    in shock, 6-19
Immunosuppressive agents, nephrotoxicity, 18-4
Incentive spirometry, postoperative, 19-5
Indomethacin, for hypercalcemia, 8-15
Indwelling venous access catheter(s), 21-9–21-13
    complications, 21-12–21-13
    heparin flush for, 21-10t–21-11t
Infection(s), 1-27
    abdominal, 7-6t
    acute, 7-2
    airway obstruction caused by, 1-11
    altered mental status/coma caused by, 15-16, 15-16t
    with central venous catheter, 21-14, 21-14t
    criteria for, 7-3t
    cutaneous, 7-6t
    diagnosis, 7-2–7-8
    extrapulmonary, in pneumonia, 4-36–4-37
    general signs, 7-5, 7-6t
    healthcare-associated, 19-22, 19-23t
    in immunosuppressed children, 17-3, 17-4t–17-5t
    with indwelling venous access catheter, 21-12–21-13
    laboratory investigation, 7-5–7-8
    microbiology, 7-8
    risk factors for, 1-26
    severe, empiric antibiotics for, 7-11–7-12, 7-12t
    signs and symptoms, 6-9
    skin manifestations, 7-5, 7-7t
    transfusion-related, 17-17–17-18, 17-25
Infectious mononucleosis, 4-7, 4-17
Influenza
    infection in pediatric oncology patient, 17-3, 17-4t
    pandemic, 12-8
    in pediatric oncology patient, 17-6–17-7
Ingestion(s)
    caustic, in child abuse, 11-9
    in child abuse, 11-9
Inhalant poisoning, 13-3t
Inhalation injury, 10-3
    management, 10-10–10-11
Inotropic support
    for acyanotic congenital heart disease, 16-15t
    indications for, 1-23–1-24
    for shock, 6-14–6-17
Insulin
    for hyperkalemia, 18-11
    in shock patient, 6-13–6-14
Intercostal muscles, 1-5
Intermittent hemodialysis, 18-14
Intervention, 1-3, 1-3f
Intestines, traumatic injury, 9-17–9-18
Intracranial compliance, 15-3, 15-3f
Intracranial hypertension, 15-18
    causes, 15-19, 15-19t
    surgical therapy for, 15-22
    treatment, 15-20–15-22

Intracranial pressure, 15-3–15-5
    in compensated state, 15-3, 15-3f
    elevated, 15-3, 15-3f, 15-5, 15-18. *See also* Intracranial hypertension
        altered mental status/coma caused by, 15-16, 15-16t
        causes, 15-19, 15-19t
        management, 9-9–9-10
        in status epilepticus, 15-11t
    lowering, 15-4
    monitoring, 15-20
    normal, 15-3, 15-3f
    in uncompensated state, 15-3, 15-3f
Intracranial vault, physiology, 15-2–15-6
Intraosseous access
    in cardiac arrest, 3-8
    in trauma patient, 9-4
Intrathoracic pressure, 4-5–4-6
    conversion from negative to positive, and hypotension with initiation of mechanical ventilation, 5-23
Intravenous immunoglobulin(s), nephrotoxicity, 18-4
Intubating stylet(s), 2-28
Intubation, 1-9, 1-11, 1-14, 1-25. *See also* Tracheal intubation
    drug administration during, 20-9–20-10
    effect on intracranial pressure, 15-20
    fiberoptic, 2-28–2-29
    for intracranial hypertension, 15-20
    for neurologic injury, 15-2
    pre-oxygenation for, 20-9
Invasive medical device(s) complications, 21-2
Ipratropium bromide, for asthma, 1-10, 4-31
Iron poisoning, 13-3t, 13-11t
Irritability, 1-5, 2-6
Irritant gas poisoning, 13-3t
Ischemia. *See also* Myocardial ischemia
    and acute kidney injury, 18-3
    cerebral, 15-16, 15-16t
        in status epilepticus, 15-11t
Isocyanate poisoning, 13-3t
Isoniazid, overdose/poisoning/toxicity, 13-3t–13-4t, 13-11t
Isopropyl alcohol poisoning, 13-3t

## J

Jaw-thrust maneuver, 2-11–2-12, 2-12f, 3-19, 4-24–4-25
Jejunostomy tube(s), 21-7, 21-7f
JumpSTART, 12-9–12-10, 12-9f
Junctional ectopic tachycardia, 16-18t

## K

Keratinocytes, 10-5
Ketamine, 20-16–20-17
    benefits, 2-20t
    dosage and administration, 2-20t
    effect on intracranial pressure, 15-20
    and emergence agitation, 19-9
    onset and duration of action, 2-20t
    precautions with, 2-20t
Ketoacidosis, 13-3t
Ketorolac, 20-11
    for postoperative pain, 19-11
Kidney disease, chronic, and acute kidney injury, 18-3, 18-4t
Kidney function. *See also* Acute kidney injury
    assessment, 1-15
Kidney injury, traumatic, 9-17
Klebsiella, infections in pediatric oncology patient, 17-3, 17-4t
Kussmaul respirations, 15-8

## L

Labetalol, for hypertensive emergency, 18-15, 18-15t
Lactate, serum, 1-16t
    monitoring, after cardiac arrest, 3-20
Lactic acidosis, 13-3t
Laryngeal edema, post-extubation, 1-10
Laryngeal mask airway, 2-27–2-28
Laryngomalacia, 4-4, 4-6, 4-20, 19-4
Laryngoscope(s), 2-19, 2-19f, 2-23, 9-3
    insertion, 2-24–2-25, 2-24f, 2-24t
Laryngoscopy, 2-3
    direct, indications for, 4-26
    effect on intracranial pressure, 15-20
    factors affecting, 4-3
    premedication for, 20-10
Laryngospasm, 19-4–19-5
Laryngotracheal reconstruction, for subglottic stenosis, 4-7
Laryngotracheobronchitis, 1-4, 4-20
    viral, 4-12–4-13, 4-13f, 4-13t. *See also* Croup
Larynx
    adult vs pediatric, 4-4–4-5
    anatomical considerations, 4-5
    anatomy, 2-3
    visualization during laryngoscopy, 2-24–2-25, 2-25f
Latex allergy(ies), 21-9
Lead poisoning, 13-11t
Left ventricular dysfunction, after cardiac arrest, 3-20
Lemierre disease, 7-29–7-31
Leukemia(s), hyperleukocytosis in, 17-13
Leukocyte count, age-dependent variations in, 7-2, 7-3t
Level of consciousness, 1-24
    altered
        and airway obstruction, 4-7
        in postoperative period, 19-7–19-9, 19-7t
    emergent evaluation, 15-6
    evaluation, in trauma patient, 9-7
Levetiracetam, for status epilepticus, 15-12t, 15-14t
Lidocaine
    for cardiac arrest, 3-10t, 3-11
    overdose/poisoning/toxicity, 13-3t
    for premedication, 20-10
Lipid infusion, in nutritional support, 19-18
Listeria monocytogenes, 1-26

Lithium poisoning, 13-4*t*, 13-11*t*
Liver failure
    acute, 7-25–7-26
    and acute kidney injury, 18-3, 18-4*t*
Liver injury, traumatic, 9-17
Lockout time, 19-13, 19-13*t*
Loop diuretics, 1-24
Lorazepam, 20-14, 20-20–20-21
    dosage and administration, 12-7*t*
    for status epilepticus, 15-12*t*, 15-13, 15-14*t*
Low cardiac output syndrome, 16-16–16-21
    evaluation, 16-21*t*
    postoperative
        causes, 16-17*t*
            residual lesions and, 16-17*t*
    signs and symptoms, 16-16, 16-17*t*
Lower airway disease, acute, 4-26–4-28
Lower respiratory tract infection, in pediatric oncology patient, 17-5–17-7
Lumbar puncture, 1-26, 7-21, 15-17–15-18
    indications for, 11-5
    precautions with, 11-5
Lumefantrine, for malaria, 7-32
Lund-Browder chart, 10-5, 10-6*f*
Lung(s), 1-6
    hyperinflation, 1-16
Lung disease, asymmetric, mechanical ventilation in, 5-19

# M
Macroglossia, 4-3, 4-7
Macule(s), 7-7*t*
Magnesium
    for cardiac arrest, 3-12
    serum, 8-12. *See also* Hypermagnesemia; Hypomagnesemia
Magnesium sulfate, for asthma, 4-31
Magnetic resonance imaging, in suspected child abuse, 11-12
Malaria, 7-31–7-32
    in pregnancy, 7-32
Malignant hyperthermia, 2-21, 19-22–19-23
Mallampati classification, 20-5, 20-6*f*
Malnutrition, 19-17
Mannitol, overdose/poisoning/toxicity, 13-3*t*
Mean arterial pressure, 1-15
Mechanical ventilation, 1-11. *See also* Pressure-support ventilation; Synchronized intermittent mandatory ventilation
    in acute lung injury, guidelines for, 5-16–5-17
    in acute respiratory distress syndrome, 4-40, 5-16–5-17
    analgesia for, 5-11*t*, 5-16
    assist-control, 5-7*f*, 5-9, 5-9*t*
    for asthma, 4-32–4-33
    in asymmetric lung disease, 5-19
    and auto-positive end-expiratory pressure, 5-11*t*, 5-14–5-15, 5-15*f*
    for burn patient, 10-11
    for cancer patient with respiratory failure, 17-6–17-7
    continuing care during, 5-12–5-16
    controlled, 5-6, 5-9*t*
    flow cycling, 5-6
    fraction of inspired oxygen in, 5-11*t*, 5-12
    in heart disease, 5-20
    humidification in, 5-12–5-13
    indications for, 5-5, 5-5*t*
    initial settings, 5-11, 5-11*t*
        for infants weighing <5 kg, 1-12*t*
    initiation
        guidelines for, 5-11, 5-11*t*
        hypotension with, 5-22–5-23
    inspiratory pressure in, 5-11*t*, 5-13–5-14, 5-13*f*
    inspiratory time/expiratory time relationship in, 5-11*t*, 5-14–5-15
    minute ventilation in, 5-11*t*, 5-15–5-16
    modes, 5-6–5-9
    monitoring, 2-6, 5-21–5-22, 5-22*t*
    neuromuscular blockade with, 5-11*t*, 5-16
    in neuromuscular disease, 5-21
    in obstructive airway disease, 5-18–5-19
    oxygenation in, 5-11–5-16, 5-11*t*
    phase variables, 5-6
    positive end-expiratory pressure for, 1-12*t*
    pressure-controlled (pressure-limited, pressure-preset), 1-11, 1-12*t*, 5-6, 5-7*f*, 5-9, 5-9*t*
    respiratory rate for, 1-12*t*
    sedation for, 5-11*t*, 5-16
    in shock, 6-17–6-18
    in status asthmaticus, 5-18–5-19
    tidal volume for, 1-11, 1-12*t*
    time cycling, 5-6
    time limit for, 1-12*t*
    troubleshooting, 2-27
    ventilator variables, 5-6
    volume-controlled (volume-preset), 1-11, 1-12*t*, 5-6, 5-7*f*, 5-9, 5-9*t*
    weaning from, 5-23–5-24
Meconium aspiration, 1-11
Mediastinal mass(es), 4-11
Medical neglect, 11-9
Mefloquine, for malaria, 7-32
Meningitis
    altered mental status/coma caused by, 15-16, 15-16*t*
    aseptic, 7-22–7-23
    bacterial
        chemoprophylaxis for high-risk contacts, 7-22
        clinical presentation, 7-20–7-21
        CSF analysis in, 7-21, 7-22*t*
        diagnosis, 7-21
        pathogens causing, 7-21, 7-21*t*
        treatment, 7-21–7-22
    fungal, CSF analysis in, 7-21, 7-22*t*
    tuberculous, 7-22–7-23
        CSF analysis in, 7-21, 7-22*t*

viral, 7-20, 7-22–7-23
    CSF analysis in, 7-21, 7-22t
    treatment, 7-23
Meningococcal disease, prevention and control, 7-17, 7-17t
Meningococcemia
    chemoprophylaxis for high-risk contacts, 7-17, 7-17t
    clinical presentation, 7-16
    treatment, 7-16–7-17
Meningoencephalitis, viral, 7-20
Mental status, 1-6
    altered, 1-25, 3-2, 15-15–15-18
        differential diagnosis, 15-17
        etiology, 15-15–15-16, 15-16t
        evaluation, 15-17
        laboratory investigation, 15-18
        therapy for, 15-18
    assessment, 1-15, 2-6
    depressed, 1-5
    in hypovolemia, 1-17
Meperidine, 20-13
    overdose/poisoning/toxicity, 13-4t
Metabolic acidosis, 2-7
    in acute kidney injury, 18-8
    in adrenal insufficiency, 8-18–8-19
    with cardiac arrest, pharmacotherapy for, 3-10t
    in shock, 6-18
    treatment, 18-12
Metabolic alkalosis, 2-7
Metabolic disease, 8-16–8-19
Metal fumes, poisoning, 13-3t
Methadone, 20-13, 20-20–20-21
    for postoperative pain, 19-11
Methanol poisoning, 13-3t–13-4t, 13-11t
Methemoglobinemia, 2-9, 10-3, 13-3t, 13-11t
    in poisoned patient, 13-3, 13-3t
Methylenedioxymethamphetamine poisoning, 13-4t
Methylprednisolone
    for adrenal insufficiency, 8-19
    for asthma, 1-10, 4-30
Methylxanthines, for asthma, 4-31–4-32
Micrognathia, 2-2, 2-23, 4-3, 4-7–4-8
Midazolam, 20-14–20-15, 20-20
    benefits, 2-20t
    contraindications to, 6-17
    dosage and administration, 2-20t, 12-7t
    onset and duration of action, 2-20t
    precautions with, 2-20t
    for status epilepticus, 15-12t, 15-13, 15-14t
Middle mediastinal mass, 4-11
Midface hypoplasia, 2-23
Milrinone, 1-24, 16-20
    for shock, 6-15t, 6-16, 6-16t
Minute ventilation, 1-8, 2-7
    in CPR, 3-6
    in mechanical ventilation, 5-11t, 5-15–5-16
Miosis, 1-25

Mithramycin, for hypercalcemia, 8-15
Monro-Kellie doctrine, 15-3, 15-19
Morphine, 20-12
    adverse effects and side effects, 20-12
    contraindications to, 6-17
    dosing regimen, for patient-controlled analgesia, 19-13t
    for postoperative pain, 19-11
Motor and sensory evaluation
    emergent, 15-7–15-8
    in spinal cord injury, 9-7, 9-7t
Movement, emergent evaluation, 15-7
Musculoskeletal trauma, 9-18–9-19
Mushroom poisoning, 13-4t
Mydriasis, 1-25
Mydriatic drops, 11-6
Myocardial blood flow, in closed-chest CPR, 3-5
Myocardial contractility, drugs and, 16-20
Myocardial dysfunction, 16-20–16-21
    after cardiac arrest, 3-20
    causes, 6-4
Myocardial infarction, and hypotension with initiation of mechanical ventilation, 5-23
Myocardial ischemia
    and hypotension with initiation of mechanical ventilation, 5-23
    mechanical ventilation in, 5-20
Myocardial stunning, after cardiac arrest, 3-20
Myocarditis, 1-20, 7-26–7-28
    clinical presentation, 7-27–7-28
    ECG findings in, 7-27–7-28
    etiology, 7-27, 7-27t
    in neonate, 16-5–16-6
    treatment, 7-28
Myocardium, 1-14

# N

Nalbuphine, for opioid-induced pruritus, 19-13
Naloxone, 13-7, 19-3, 19-7, 20-19
    with patient-controlled analgesia, 19-13
Naphthalene poisoning, 13-3t
Naproxen, 20-11
Narcotics. See Opioids
Nasal breathing, obligate, 4-2–4-3
Nasal cannula, for oxygen delivery, 2-10
Nasal flaring, 1-6, 1-9–1-10, 2-5
Nasal mask, 5-2, 5-3f
Nasal obstruction, causes, 4-2
Nasal passages, suctioning, 1-10, 2-2, 4-2
Nasal pillows, for noninvasive respiratory support, 5-2, 5-3f
Nasogastric tube(s), 21-3, 21-3f
    contraindications to, 21-3
    sizes, 21-2, 21-3t
Nasopharyngeal airway, 2-14, 4-8
    insertion, 2-14f, 2-14t
        with Pierre Robin sequence, 4-8, 4-8f
    in trauma patient, 9-2

Nausea and vomiting, postoperative, 19-16, 19-17*t*
Near drowning, 9-19–9-20
    and cardiac arrest, 3-2
Necrobacillosis, 7-29–7-31
*Necrotizing fasciitis*, 7-19
Neisseria meningitidis, 1-26, 7-16
Neonatal respiratory distress syndrome, 1-11
Neonate(s). *See* Newborn
Neostigmine, 19-8, 20-20
Nephrotoxicity
    and acute kidney injury, 18-3, 18-4*t*
    avoidance, 18-10
Nervous system, 1-24–1-25. *See also* Central nervous system disorders
Neurointensive care, goals, 15-2
Neuroleptic malignant syndrome, 2-21*t*
Neurologic emergency(ies)
    evaluation, 15-6–15-9
    initial management, 15-2
    outcomes with, factors affecting, 15-2
    pathophysiology, 15-2–15-6
    in pediatric oncology patient, 17-13–17-15
    respiratory patterns in, 15-8, 15-8*t*
Neuromuscular blockade, 2-20–2-21, 20-10
    clinical applications, 20-2
    depolarizing, 2-21*t*, 20-17–20-18
    for intracranial hypertension, 15-20
    with mechanical ventilation, 5-11*t*, 5-16
    non-depolarizing, 2-21*t*, 20-18–20-19
        reversal, failure, 19-8, 19-8*t*
    precautions with, 20-17
    prolonged, in postoperative period, 19-8–19-9
    reversal, failure, 19-8, 19-8*t*
Neuromuscular blocking agents, 1-25, 2-21, 2-21*t*
    adverse effects and side effects, 20-17–20-19
    depolarizing, 2-21*t*, 19-8, 20-17–20-18
        and malignant hyperthermia, 19-23
    non-depolarizing, 2-21*t*, 19-8, 20-18–20-19
        reversal, 19-8–19-9, 20-20
    reversal, 19-8–19-9
        failure, 19-8, 19-8*t*
Neuromuscular disease, mechanical ventilation in, 5-21
Neutropenia, febrile
    complications, 17-5–17-7
    definition, 17-2
    laboratory investigation, 17-3
    management, 17-3
    risk factors for, 17-2–17-3
    treatment, 17-3–17-4
Neutropenic enterocolitis, in pediatric oncology patient, 17-7
Newborn
    bradycardia in, 3-14
    CPR for, 3-6*t*
    cyanosis in, 16-11*t*. *See also* Congenital heart disease, cyanotic
    herpes simplex virus infections in, 7-28–7-29
    hypocalcemia in, 8-14

    with low cardiac output, 16-2–16-6
        etiology, 16-6, 16-6*t*
        initial evaluation and treatment, 16-6, 16-6*t*
    resuscitation, 3-16
Nicardipine, for hypertensive emergency, 18-15, 18-15*t*
Nicotine poisoning, 13-4*t*
Nifedipine, for hypertension, 18-15
Nitrates, overdose/poisoning/toxicity, 13-3*t*
Nitric oxide, overdose/poisoning/toxicity, 13-3*t*
Nitrites, overdose/poisoning/toxicity, 13-3*t*, 13-11*t*
Nitrogen dioxide poisoning, 13-3*t*
Nitroglycerine, 16-20
    for shock, 6-16
Nitroprusside sodium, 16-20
    for hypertensive emergency, 18-15, 18-15*t*
    overdose/poisoning/toxicity, 13-3*t*
    for shock, 6-16
Nociception, 19-9
Nodule(s), 7-7*t*
Nonaccidental injury(ies). *See also* Child abuse; Child maltreatment
    patterns, 11-2–11-9, 11-2*t*, 11-3*f*
    risk factors for, 11-1
Nonsteroidal anti-inflammatory drugs, 20-10–20-11
    and acute kidney injury, 18-3, 18-4*t*
    nephrotoxicity, 18-4
    and postoperative nausea and vomiting, 19-16, 19-17*t*
    for postoperative pain, 19-10–19-11
Noradrenaline. *See* Norepinephrine
Norepinephrine, 16-21
    for distributive shock, 1-22
    for shock, 6-15*t*, 6-16, 6-16*t*
Nose, anatomy, 2-2
Numerical pain scale, 19-11*t*
Nutritional requirements, 19-18, 19-18*t*
Nutritional support, 19-18–19-19
    in acute kidney injury, 18-14–18-15
    for burn patient, 10-11–10-12, 10-12*t*
    in shock, 6-20
Nutrition assessment, 19-17–19-18

# O

Obesity, and airway disorders, 4-7
Obstructive airway disease. *See also* Asthma
    mechanical ventilation in, 5-18–5-19
Obstructive sleep apnea, 4-7
    and postobstructive pulmonary edema, 19-5
    and postoperative care, 19-3
Obstructive uropathy, 18-6
Ocular medications, 11-5–11-6
Oliguria, 3-2
Oncology/hematology, complications in. *See also* Hematologic emergency(ies); *specific complication*
    management, 17-2
Ondansetron, for postoperative nausea and vomiting, 19-16, 19-17*t*
Opioids, 20-11–20-12. *See also* Patient-controlled analgesia
    adverse effects and side effects, 19-11

for breakthrough pain, 19-13
overdose/poisoning/toxicity, 13-3t–13-4t, 13-11t
and postoperative nausea and vomiting, 19-16, 19-17t
for postoperative pain, 19-10–19-11
and respiratory depression, 19-3, 19-7
reversal agent, 19-3, 20-19
toxidrome, 13-7, 13-8t
withdrawal, 13-8t, 20-20–20-21
Organophosphate poisoning, 13-3t–13-4t, 13-11t
Organ transplantation, and acute kidney injury, 18-3, 18-4t
Orogastric tube(s), 21-3
Oropharyngeal airway, 2-12–2-13
insertion, 2-12, 2-13f, 2-13t
Orotracheal intubation, 2-24, 2-24f, 2-24t
Orthodromic reciprocating tachycardia, 16-18t
Oseltamivir phosphate, 12-8
Osmolality, serum, 8-4
Osmolar gap, increased, in poisoned patient, 13-3, 13-3t
Osmolar therapy, for intracranial hypertension, 15-21
Osteomyelitis, 7-6t
Ostium primum (atrial septal defect), 16-13
Ostium secundum (atrial septal defect), 16-13
Oxandrolone, for burn patients, 10-12
Oxycodone, for postoperative pain, 19-11
Oxygen. *See also* Arterial oxygen content
administration, 1-9–1-10, 2-9–2-10
for bronchiolitis, 4-34–4-35
for burn patient, 10-11
in cardiac arrest, 3-6–3-7
before sedation/intubation, 20-9
in suspected shock, 6-8
in trauma patient, 9-3
central venous saturation, monitoring, after cardiac arrest, 3-20
delivery systems for, 1-9–1-10, 2-9–2-10
partial pressure, 2-8, 2-8f
Oxygenation, 1-7. *See also* Hypoxemia; Hypoxia
arterial, 1-10
during intubation, 2-23
for intubation, 20-9
in mechanical ventilation, 5-11–5-16, 5-11t
monitoring, 1-11
in resuscitation, 3-7
in post-resuscitative care, 3-20
for sedation, 20-9
Oxygen consumption, 1-10, 1-14, 2-9, 4-22
Oxygen delivery, 6-1
Oxygen desaturation, 4-21–4-22
Oxygen mask, 2-10
Oxyhemoglobin saturation curve, 2-8, 2-8f

# P

Packed red blood cells, 17-18–17-20, 19-20
Pain
assessment, 19-10, 19-11t
breakthrough, 19-13
postoperative, 19-9
and postoperative agitation, 19-9
and postoperative sinus tachycardia, 19-6
Pain management
nonpharmacological approaches for, 19-11
postoperative, 19-9–19-15
multimodal strategy for, 19-9–19-12, 19-10f
stratified approach for, 19-11, 19-12f
Pancuronium, 19-8, 20-18–20-19
Panglottitis, 4-13
Papule(s), 7-7t
Paracetamol. *See* Acetaminophen
Paradoxical respiration, postoperative, 19-4
Parainfluenza
infection in pediatric oncology patient, 17-3, 17-5t
in pediatric oncology patient, 17-6–17-7
Paraldehyde poisoning, 13-3t
Paralysis
pharmacologic. *See* Neuromuscular blockade
vocal cord. *See* Vocal cord paralysis
Parenteral nutrition, 19-19, 19-19t
Patent ductus arteriosus, 1-14, 16-14
Patient-controlled analgesia, 19-12–19-13
dosing regimen for, 19-13t
by proxy, 19-13
Patient-controlled epidural analgesia, 19-14
Peak expiratory flow rate, 1-12t
Peanut allergy, 3-18
Pectus carinatum, 1-7
Pectus excavatum, 1-7
Pediatric Advanced Life Support, 11-10
Pediatric Early Warning Score (PEWS), 1-1, 1-2t, 1-3, 1-9, 1-17, 1-20–1-21, 1-23, 1-27, 3-2
critical, 1-3
Pelvic and extremity trauma
treatment, 9-19
Pentobarbital, 20-15
for status epilepticus, 15-12t, 15-14t
Percutaneous endoscopic gastrostomy tube(s), 21-5
Perfusion status, assessment, 1-27
Pericardial effusion(s), 7-27–7-28
Pericardial tamponade, 9-15
with indwelling venous access catheter, 21-12
Pericarditis, 7-26–7-28
clinical presentation, 7-27
ECG findings in, 7-27
etiology, 7-27, 7-27t
treatment, 7-28
Peripheral intravenous catheter, heparin flush for, 21-10t
Peripherally inserted central catheter, 21-12, 21-12f
Peritoneal dialysis, 18-13–18-14
for hyperkalemia, 18-12
Peritonitis, 7-25
Peritonsillar abscess, 4-17, 4-21
Permacath, 21-9
Petechiae, 1-26, 7-5
Pethidine. *See* Meperidine
Phenazopyridine poisoning, 13-3t
Phencyclidine poisoning, 13-4t

Phenobarbital, 20-15
    for status epilepticus, 15-12*t*, 15-13, 15-14*t*
Phenothiazine(s), overdose/poisoning/toxicity, 13-4*t*, 13-11*t*
Phenylephrine, for neurogenic shock, 1-21
Phenylpropanolamine poisoning, 13-4*t*
Phenytoin, for status epilepticus, 15-12*t*, 15-13, 15-14*t*
Phosphate, serum, 8-15. *See also* Hyperphosphatemia; Hypophosphatemia
Phosphodiesterase inhibitors, 16-20
Physical examination
    in airway disorders, 4-20–4-21
    with cardiac arrest, 3-3
    of cardiovascular system, 1-15
    of respiratory system, 1-6–1-8
    in suspected shock, 6-9
    in trauma, 9-6–9-7
Physostigmine poisoning, 13-4*t*
Pierre Robin sequence, 2-2, 2-14, 4-3, 4-8–4-9, 4-24
    nasopharyngeal intubation with, 4-8, 4-8*f*
Pigtail catheter. *See* Thoracostomy tube(s)
PIPP pain scale, 19-11*t*
Plague, 12-7–12-8, 12-8*t*
Plaque, skin, 7-7*t*
*Plasmodium* spp., 7-32
Platelet transfusion, 17-20–17-21, 17-21*t*, 19-20
Pleura, 4-5
Pleural effusion, 2-6, 21-7
    in pneumonia, 4-36–4-37
Pleural pressure, 4-5–4-6
Pneumocystis jiroveci pneumonia, in pediatric oncology patient, 17-3, 17-5*t*, 17-6
Pneumonia, 1-11, 2-6
    antibiotics for, 4-36
    bacterial, 1-11
    classification, 4-35
    clinical presentation, 4-36
    community-acquired, 4-35
    complications, 4-36–4-37
    diagnosis, 4-36
    hospital-acquired, 4-35, 19-5, 19-22, 19-23*t*
    microbiology, 4-36
    pathophysiology, 4-35
    in pediatric oncology patient, 17-6
    postoperative, 19-5
    recurrent, 4-35
    supportive therapy in, 4-36
    treatment, 4-36
    viral, in pediatric oncology patient, 17-3, 17-5*t*
Pneumoperitoneum, 9-17
Pneumothorax, 2-6, 2-26–2-27, 3-16, 21-7. *See also* Tension pneumothorax
    with central venous catheter, 21-14*t*
    chest tube–induced, 21-8
    in cystic fibrosis, 4-38
    with indwelling venous access catheter, 21-12
    in pneumonia, 4-36–4-37
    in trauma patient, 3-19, 9-3
    traumatic, 9-14–9-15

Poiseuille's law, 1-6, 4-4
Poisoning (child/adolescent)
    acute, 13-2
    antidotes for, 13-11*t*
    causes, 13-3, 13-3*t*-13-4*t*
    in child abuse, 11-9
    chronic, 13-2
    classes of agents causing, 13-2
    enhanced elimination for, 13-6
    external decontamination for, 13-7
    gastrointestinal decontamination for, 13-5
    intentional vs unintentional, 13-2
    laboratory investigation, 13-4, 13-4*t*
    mortality from, 13-2
    recreational drugs causing, 13-9*t*
    resuscitation for, 13-2–13-4
    signs and symptoms, 13-3, 13-3*t*-13-4*t*
    sources, 13-2
    stabilization for, 13-2–13-4
    treatment, 13-11*t*
Port(s), implanted, 21-11, 21-11*f*
    heparin flush for, 21-11*t*
Port-a-Cath, 21-11, 21-11*f*
Position of comfort, 1-8
    patient's, 1-4, 1-6, 1-9–1-10, 1-27, 2-9
    in airway disorders, 4-19–4-20
Positive end-expiratory pressure, 5-4–5-5, 5-11*t*
    in acute lung injury, 5-11*t*–5-12*t*
        guidelines for, 5-16–5-17
    in acute respiratory distress syndrome, 4-40, 5-11*t*–5-12*t*, 5-16–5-17
    and auto-positive end-expiratory pressure, 5-11*t*, 5-14–5-15, 5-15*f*
    and hypotension with initiation of mechanical ventilation, 5-23
    for mechanical ventilation, 1-12*t*
Positive-pressure ventilation
    for cancer patient with respiratory failure, 17-6–17-7
    complications, 2-26–2-27
    noninvasive, 5-2–5-5
        advantages and disadvantages, 5-4
        for asthma, 4-32
        contraindications to, 5-3
        delivery, 5-2–5-3, 5-3*f*
        initial settings for, 5-3, 5-4*t*
        modes, 5-4
        monitoring, 5-4
        for upper airway disease, 4-26
        in pneumonia, 4-36
Postoperative management
    fluid and electrolyte considerations, 19-15–19-16
    hematologic considerations, 19-20–19-21
    hemodynamic considerations, 19-6
    for nausea and vomiting, 19-16, 19-17*t*
    neurologic considerations, 19-7–19-9
    nutritional considerations, 19-17–19-19
    respiratory considerations, 19-3–19-5
    thermal regulation in, 19-21–19-23

Potassium, serum, 8-9. *See also* Hyperkalemia; Hypokalemia
Potassium iodide, 12-7
Pralidoxime, dosage and administration, 12-6, 12-7*t*
Prealbumin, 19-17–19-18
Pregnancy, malaria in, 7-32
Preload, 1-13, 6-1
    positive-pressure ventilation and, 2-27
Premedication, 20-9–20-10
Prerenal azotemia, 18-5
    urinalysis in, 18-6
Pressure-support ventilation, 5-8*f*, 5-9*t*, 5-10
Prilocaine, overdose/poisoning/toxicity, 13-3*t*
Propofol, 6-20, 20-10, 20-15–20-16
    adverse effects and side effects, 20-15–20-16
    benefits, 2-20*t*
    dosage and administration, 2-20*t*, 20-15
    indications for, 20-16
    onset and duration of action, 2-20*t*
    and postoperative nausea and vomiting, 19-16, 19-17*t*
    precautions with, 2-20*t*
Propylene glycol poisoning, 13-3*t*
Prostaglandin(s)
    administration, 1-23
    for cardiogenic shock, 6-5
    $PGE_1$
        for aortic coarctation, 16-5
        for hypoplastic left heart syndrome, 16-3
        indications for, 1-23
        side effects, 1-23
Protein catabolism, in stress response, 19-18–19-19
Protein requirements, 19-18, 19-18*t*, 19-19
Pruritus, opioid-induced, 19-13
Pseudocholinesterase, 19-8
Pseudohyponatremia, 8-18
Pseudomonas, infection, in pediatric oncology patient, 17-3, 17-4*t*
Pulmonary artery catheter, 1-14
Pulmonary edema
    diagnosis, 4-41
    high-pressure, 4-41
    management, 4-42
    negative pressure, 19-5
    neurogenic, 15-8
    non-cardiogenic, 4-41
    pathophysiology, 4-41
    permeability, 4-41
    in poisoned patient, 13-3, 13-3*t*
    postobstructive, 4-41, 19-5
    postoperative, 19-5
Pulmonary embolism, 6-7
    with indwelling venous access catheter, 21-12
Pulmonary hypertension, 1-14
    and cardiac arrest, resuscitation for, 3-17
Pulmonary stenosis, 16-9
Pulse(s), checking, 3-3
Pulseless electrical activity, 3-12
    causes, 3-15, 3-16*t*
    6 Hs and 6 Ts, 3-15, 3-16*t*
    therapy for, 3-15–3-16
Pulselessness, 3-3
Pulse oximetry, 1-8–1-11, 1-12*t*, 2-8–2-9, 4-21
    during intubation, 2-22
    limitations, 2-8–2-9
    in trauma patient, 9-3
Pupillary response, 1-25
    evaluation, in trauma patient, 9-7
Purpura, 1-26
Purpura fulminans, 1-22
Pustule(s), 7-7*t*
pVT. *See* Ventricular tachycardia, pulseless
Pyelonephritis, 7-25
Pyloric stenosis, 2-7
Pyridostigmine, 19-8

# Q

QT prolongation, in poisoned patient, 13-3, 13-3*t*
Quinidine
    for malaria, 7-32
    overdose/poisoning/toxicity, 13-3*t*
Quinine
    for malaria, 7-32
    overdose/poisoning/toxicity, 13-3*t*
Quinsy, 4-17

# R

Raccoon eyes, 9-6
Radiation exposure, treatment, 12-7
Rapid sequence intubation, 2-22
Rasburicase, for uric acid control, 17-11*t*, 17-12
Rash, 1-26
Rash(es), in infection, 7-5
Reassessment, 1-3, 1-3*f*
Recurrent laryngeal nerve injury, 4-7
Red blood cell transfusion, 17-18–17-20, 17-19*t*
    leukocyte-depleted, 17-19
Reflex(es), airway, 2-6
Regional analgesia, for postoperative pain, 19-10–19-11, 19-14–19-15
Rehydration therapy, oral, 1-17
Renal failure, 13-3*t*
    in status epilepticus, 15-11*t*
Renal imaging, 18-8, 18-9*t*
Renal perfusion, maintenance, therapies for, 18-9–18-10
Renal replacement therapy, 18-13–18-14, 18-13*t*
    in tumor lysis syndrome, 17-11*t*, 17-12
Rescue breathing, 3-5–3-6, 3-6*t*
Residual anesthetic effect, postoperative, 19-7–19-8
Respiratory acidosis, 2-7
Respiratory alkalosis, 2-7
Respiratory arrest, 1-5, 4-20
Respiratory compromise, first intervention for, 1-9
Respiratory depression
    benzodiazepines and, 19-3, 20-13, 20-14
    opioids and, 19-3, 19-7, 20-12–20-13
    postoperative, 19-3
Respiratory disorders, mortality in, 1-6

Respiratory distress, 1-5, 2-2. *See also* Acute respiratory distress syndrome; Neonatal respiratory distress syndrome
    longitudinal physical assessment, 2-6
    in sepsis, 1-26
    signs, 1-27
Respiratory failure, 1-5, 1-6, 1-11, 2-2, 2-4–2-5, 2-17, 4-27, 5-2
    acute, causes, 4-28
    acute hypoxemic, 5-17
    causes, 1-11
    clinical indicators, 4-27, 4-28
    in cystic fibrosis, 4-38
    hypercapnic, 4-27–4-28
    hypoxemic, 4-27–4-28
    in infants/toddlers, 1-11
    monitoring in, 4-28
    in older children, 1-11
    in pediatric oncology patient, 17-6–17-7
    in premature neonates, 1-11
    risk factors for, 1-5
    in status epilepticus, 15-11
    in term neonates, 1-11
    treatment, 1-11, 4-28
Respiratory function, monitoring, 2-6–2-9
Respiratory infection, 7-6*t*
Respiratory monitoring, 1-8
Respiratory muscle(s), fatigue, 2-4
Respiratory noise, 4-20–4-21
Respiratory pattern(s), in central nervous system disease, 15-8, 15-8*t*
Respiratory rate
    abnormal, 2-5
    age-dependent variations in, 7-2, 7-3*t*
    assessment, 2-5
    in CPR, 3-6, 3-6*t*
    factors affecting, 1-6, 1-7*t*
    for mechanical ventilation, 1-12*t*
    normal, 1-6
        by age group, 2-5*t*
    at rest, by age group, 1-1–1-2
Respiratory reserve, 1-6
Respiratory status, evaluation, 1-11, 1-12*t*, 2-4–2-6
Respiratory syncytial virus infection, 1-9, 4-2
    bronchiolitis in, 1-10
    in pediatric oncology patient, 17-3, 17-4*t*, 17-6–17-7
    subglottic stenosis in, 4-7
Respiratory system, 1-5–1-12
    anatomic considerations, 1-5–1-6
    physical examination, 1-6–1-8
    physiologic considerations, 1-5–1-6
Resting energy expenditure, 1-10
Resuscitation. *See also* Cardiopulmonary resuscitation
    fluids for, 8-3
    neonatal, 3-16
Retinal hemorrhage(s), 11-5–11-6
Retinol-binding protein, 19-17–19-18
Retractions, 1-6, 2-4–2-5
Retropharyngeal abscess, 4-16–4-17, 4-16*f*
    clinical features, 4-12*t*
    microbiology, 4-16
    treatment, 4-17
Return of spontaneous circulation, 3-19*t*, 3-20
    in cardiac arrest, 3-2–3-3, 3-6
    signs, 3-7
    temperature monitoring after, 3-21
Reversal agents, 20-19–20-20
Rewarming, 19-21
Rhabdomyolysis, and acute kidney injury, 18-4, 18-4*t*
Rib cage, deformity, 1-7
Rib fractures, 9-13–9-14
    in child abuse, 9-13, 11-7, 11-7*f*
*Rickettsia rickettsii*, 7-18
Rocky Mountain spotted fever, 7-18
Rocuronium, 19-8, 20-18, 2-21*t*
Room air resuscitation, 3-16
ROSC. *See* Return of spontaneous circulation
Rubs (breath sound), 1-7
Rule of nines, for burn injuries, 10-5, 10-6*f*

## S

Salbutamol, inhaled, for asthma, 4-30–4-31
Salem Sump, 21-3
Salicylate poisoning, 13-3*t*–13-4*t*, 13-11*t*, 13-12–13-13
*Salmonella*, 1-26
Scoliosis, 1-7
Sedation
    agents for, 20-2
        selection, 20-10
    clinical applications, 20-2
    complications, 20-2
    depth, 20-4, 20-5*t*
    drug administration during, 20-9–20-10
    for emergence agitation, 19-9
    emergent, 20-7
    equipment for, 20-7, 20-8*t*
    fasting before, 20-7
    history-taking for, 20-6–20-7
    for intracranial hypertension, 15-20
    with mechanical ventilation, 5-11*t*, 5-16
    monitoring, 20-7–20-9, 20-8*t*
    planning for, 20-3
    pre-oxygenation for, 20-9
    setup for, 20-7–20-9
    in shock, 6-20
    for tracheal intubation, 2-19, 2-20*t*, 2-21
Sedative/hypnotic
    overdose/poisoning/toxicity, 13-3*t*
    withdrawal, 13-8*t*
Sedative/hypnotic toxidrome, 13-8, 13-8t
Seizures, 1-24–1-25, 1-27. *See also* Status epilepticus
    after cardiac arrest, 3-21
    altered mental status/coma caused by, 15-16, 15-16t
    pathophysiology, 15-10
    pharmacotherapy for, 20-15
    in poisoned patient, 13-3, 13-4*t*
Sellick maneuver, 2-17, 2-24, 2-25*f*

Sepsis, 1-11, 1-26, 7-9–7-13
    and acute kidney injury, 18-3–18-4, 18-4*t*
    antibiotics for, 7-11–7-12, 7-12*t*–7-13*t*
    causative agents, 7-11, 7-11*t*
    criteria for, 7-3*t*
    distributive shock in, 1-21–1-22
    inotropic/vasopressor support in, 17-9
    microbiology, 7-11, 7-11*t*
    organ dysfunction criteria, 7-4*t*
    in pneumonia, 4-36–4-37
    severe, criteria for, 7-3*t*
    signs, 1-26
    treatment, 7-9–7-12
Septic shock, 1-21–1-22
    clinical presentation, 6-22, 7-9
    criteria for, 7-3*t*
    etiologies, 6-23*t*
    fluid resuscitation in, 6-11–6-14, 6-12*f*
    organ dysfunction criteria, 7-4*t*
    in pediatric oncology patient, 17-8–17-9
    treatment, 6-19, 6-22, 7-9–7-12, 17-8–17-9
Sequential Organ Failure Assessment, 12-10, 12-10*t*
Serotonin syndrome, 13-8*t*
Sexual abuse, 11-8–11-9
Shaken baby syndrome, 1-5, 1-24–1-25, 11-4–11-5, 11-5*f*
Shivering, postoperative, 19-21
Shock, 1-15–1-24, 1-27, 12-4. *See also* Septic shock
    ABCs of assessment for, 6-8–6-9
    acidosis in, management, 6-18
    anemic, 6-7
    approach to, 7-10, 7-10*f*
    bradycardia in, 3-13–3-14
    and cardiac arrest, 3-12–3-14
    cardiogenic, 1-19–1-20, 6-4–6-5, 16-5
        clinical presentation, 6-5
        diagnosis, 6-5
        etiologies, 1-20, 6-4, 6-23*t*
        fluid resuscitation in, 8-3
        treatment, 6-5
    clinical presentation, 6-2, 6-8–6-9
    definition, 1-15, 6-1
    in developing countries, 6-24
    in diabetes, 6-24
    distributive, 1-20–1-22
        clinical presentation, 6-6
        definition, 6-6
        etiologies, 6-23*t*
        pathophysiology, 6-6
        in sepsis, 1-21–1-22
        treatment, 6-6
    early (compensated) phase, 1-15
    endotracheal intubation in, 6-17–6-18
    evaluation, 6-8–6-9
    fluid resuscitation in, 6-11–6-14, 8-3
    general care for, 6-19–6-20
    hemorrhagic, in trauma patient, 9-3–9-4
    history-taking in, 6-9
    hypotensive
        after cardiac arrest, 3-20
        in trauma patient, 3-19
    hypovolemic, 1-17–1-18, 1-24–1-25, 6-2–6-3, 8-3
        clinical presentation, 6-3
        etiologies, 6-23*t*
        pathophysiology, 6-3
    in injured patient, 6-21
    inotropic support in, 6-14–6-17
    laboratory investigation, 6-18–6-19
    late (decompensated) phase, 1-15
    mechanical ventilation in, 6-17–6-18
    monitoring in, 6-19
    mortality from, 6-1
    in neonate/young infant, 6-20–6-21
    neurogenic, 1-21
    in trauma patient, 9-4
    obstructive, 1-23–1-24
        causes, 6-7
        clinical presentation, 6-7
        etiologies, 6-23*t*
        pathophysiology, 6-7
        in trauma patient, 9-4
        treatment, 6-7
    in pediatric oncology patient, 17-7–17-9
    physical examination in, 6-9
    in pneumonia, 4-36–4-37
    postoperative management, 19-15
    in postoperative period, 19-6
    radiographic studies in, 6-19
    refractory, 6-24, 7-10*f*, 7-12
    reversal, and survival, 6-1–6-2, 6-2*f*
    signs, 3-2
    survival, factors affecting, 6-1–6-2, 6-2*f*
    treatment, 1-15, 6-10–6-19, 6-22–6-23
        general principles, 6-19–6-20
    types, 6-1
    uncompensated, 1-5
    vasoactive support in, 6-14–6-17
    vasodilatory, after cardiac arrest, 3-20
    vasopressor-resistant, 1-22
Shunt thrombosis, 3-16–3-17
Sickle cell disease, 2-9, 17-19–17-20
    acute chest syndrome in, 4-43
Simple Triage and Rapid Transport (START), 12-9–12-10
Sinus tachycardia, postoperative, 19-6
Sinus venosus (atrial septal defect), 16-13
Skeletal survey, in suspected child abuse, 11-2, 11-12
Skeletal trauma, in child abuse, 11-7, 11-7*f*
Skin
    examination, 1-4*t*
    layers, 10-5
Skin lesion(s), 7-5, 7-7*t*
Sleepiness, in poisoned patient, 13-3, 13-3*t*
Smallpox, 12-8
Smoke inhalation, 13-3*t*
Sniffing position, 1-9, 2-11*f*, 2-12, 2-15, 2-23

Sodium
- increased total body level, with serum hyponatremia, 8-7
- replacement, in hyponatremia, 8-5, 8-5*f*
- serum, 18-5. *See also* Hypernatremia; Hyponatremia
- urine, 18-5

Sodium bicarbonate
- for cardiac arrest, 3-10*t*, 3-11–3-12
- for hyperkalemia, 18-11
- indications for, 6-18
- for metabolic acidosis, 18-12

Sodium deficit, calculation, 18-13
Sodium polystyrene sulfonate, for hyperkalemia, 18-11
Soft-tissue trauma, 9-19
Spinal cord compression, in pediatric oncology patient, 17-14–17-15
Spinal cord injury, 6-6, 9-4
- localization, 9-7, 9-7*t*
- in trauma patient, 3-19

Spinal cord injury without radiographic abnormality, 9-11
Spinal shock, 9-12
Splenic injury, traumatic, 9-17
Staphylococci (*Staphylococcus* spp.), infections in pediatric oncology patient, 17-3, 17-4*t*
*Staphylococcus aureus*, 1-26
- necrobacillosis caused by, 7-29–7-31
- and toxic shock syndrome, 7-14, 7-15*t*

Status asthmaticus
- mechanical ventilation in, 5-18–5-19
- treatment, 4-30–4-33

Status epilepticus, 1-25
- definition, 15-10
- epidemiology, 15-9
- etiology, 15-9, 15-10*t*
- evaluation, 15-11–15-13
- laboratory investigation, 15-12*t*, 15-13
- non-convulsive, 15-13
- organ dysfunction in, 15-10–15-11, 15-11*t*
- pathophysiology, 15-10–15-11, 15-11*t*
- pharmacotherapy for, 15-12*t*, 15-13, 15-14*t*
- refractory, 15-14
- stages, 15-10
- treatment, 15-11–15-13, 15-12*t*
  - common errors in, 15-13, 15-14

Steeple sign, 4-12, 4-13*f*, 4-15
Steroids
- for anaphylaxis, 3-19
- for bacterial meningitis, 7-22
- for bronchiolitis, 4-35
- inhaled, for bronchiolitis, 4-35
- in sepsis, 7-11
- for stridulous patient, 1-10
- systemic, for bronchiolitis, 4-35

Stertor, 4-20–4-21
Streptococci (*Streptococcus* spp.)
- group B, 1-26
- infections in pediatric oncology patient, 17-3, 17-4*t*
- necrobacillosis caused by, 7-29–7-31

*Streptococcus pneumoniae*, 1-26
*Streptococcus pyogenes*, and toxic shock syndrome, 7-14
Stress response, 19-18
Stridor, 1-10, 2-5, 4-7, 4-20–4-21
- in croup, 4-12
- postextubation, 19-4
- with supraglottitis, 4-14

Stroke volume, 1-13–1-14, 6-1
Strychnine poisoning, 13-4*t*
Stylet(s), intubating, 2-28
Subarachnoid hemorrhage, 15-23
Subcutaneous emphysema, chest tube–induced, 21-8
Subglottic edema, 2-3
Subglottic space, 4-4
Subglottic stenosis, 4-4, 4-7
Succinylcholine, 19-8, 20-18, 20-20
- adverse effects and side effects, 2-21, 20-18
- benefits, 2-21*t*
- contraindications to, 20-18
- dosage and administration, 2-21*t*
- effect on intracranial pressure, 15-20
- and malignant hyperthermia, 19-23
- onset and duration of action, 2-21*t*
- precautions with, 2-21*t*
- prolonged blockade with, 19-8

Suctioning
- airway, 1-9, 1-10
- in bronchiolitis, 4-34
- for intubation, 2-22
- nasal, 1-10, 2-2, 4-2
- postoperative, 19-4

Sudden death, evaluation, 3-21
Sudden infant death syndrome, 3-2
Sulfadoxine-pyrimethamine, for malaria, 7-32
Sulfites, food-borne, poisoning, 13-3*t*
Sulfonamide poisoning, 13-3*t*
Superior vena cava obstruction, 4-11
Supraglottitis, 4-13–4-14, 4-14*f*
Supraventricular tachycardia, 16-19*f*
- and cardiac output, 1-14
- hemodynamically unstable, 3-14–3-15
- pharmacotherapy for, 3-10*t*
- therapy for, 3-14–3-15

Surfactant
- for acute respiratory distress syndrome, 4-41
- deficiency, 1-11

Surgery. *See also* Postoperative management
- cardiovascular, and risk for acute kidney injury, 18-4

Surgical site infection(s), 19-22, 19-23*t*
Sweat testing, 4-38
Sympathomimetic poisoning, 13-7, 13-8*t*
Synchronized intermittent mandatory ventilation, 5-8*f*, 5-9*t*, 5-10
Syndrome of inappropriate antidiuretic hormone secretion, 8-6–8-7, 19-16
Syrup of Ipecac, 13-5
Systemic inflammatory response syndrome, 7-9
- criteria for, 7-3*t*

Systemic lupus erythematosus, altered mental status/coma caused by, 15-16, 15-16t
Systemic vascular resistance, 16-20–16-21

## T

Tachyarrhythmia, in poisoned patient, 13-3, 13-3t
Tachycardia, 1-14–1-15, 1-21–1-22, 6-8
    age-dependent definition, 7-3t
    in anemia, 17-18, 17-18t
    in hypovolemia, 1-17
    in poisoned patient, 13-3, 13-4t
    postoperative, 19-6
    in shock, 6-2
Tachyphylaxis, 20-20
Tachypnea, 1-6, 1-7t, 1-8–1-9
    age-dependent definition, 7-3t
    in anemia, 17-18, 17-18t
    in shock, 6-2
Teamwork, 1-3, 1-3f
Temperature. *See also* Fever; Hyperthermia; Hypothermia
    of extremities, in hypovolemia, 1-17
    instability, in sepsis, 1-26
Tension pneumothorax, 2-26–2-27, 9-3–9-4
    with central venous catheter, 21-14t
    and hypotension with initiation of mechanical ventilation, 5-22
    traumatic, 9-14–9-15
Terbutaline, for asthma, 4-31
Terrorist attacks, 12-2–12-3
Tetany, 1-25
Tetracycline, for malaria, 7-32
Tetralogy of Fallot, 16-7–16-8
Tet spell(s), 16-8
Theophylline
    for asthma, 4-31–4-32
    overdose/poisoning/toxicity, 13-3t–13-4t, 13-11t
Thiopental, 2-20t
Third spacing, and hyponatremia, 8-6–8-7
Thoracic duct, puncture, with central venous catheter, 21-14t
Thoracic trauma
    evaluation, 9-14t
    mortality from, 9-13
Thoracostomy
    indications for, 21-7
    needle, 21-7
    for tension pneumothorax, 2-27
    tube, 9-3–9-4
Thoracostomy tube(s), 21-7–21-8, 21-8t
Thorax, in breathing, 1-5
Thrombosis, with central venous catheter, 21-14
Tidal volume, 1-6, 2-4
    for mechanical ventilation, 1-11, 1-12t
Toluene poisoning, 13-3t
Tongue, anatomy, 2-2–2-3, 4-3
Tonsillar-adenoidal hypertrophy, and airway obstruction, 4-7

Tonsillectomy, 4-7
Total anomalous pulmonary venous connection, 16-10–16-11
Total lung capacity, 1-6
Toxic shock syndrome, 7-13–7-15, 7-15t
Toxidrome(s), 13-3, 13-7–13-10, 13-8t
Toxin(s)
    and acute kidney injury, 18-3, 18-4t
    altered mental status/coma caused by, 15-16, 15-16t
    enhanced elimination, 13-6
Trachea, 4-5–4-6
    extrathoracic, 4-5
        closure, forces causing, 4-6
        collapse, 4-20
            with inspiration against subglottic obstruction, 4-5, 4-5f
        internal diameter, 2-3
    intrathoracic, 4-5
        closure, forces causing, 4-6
        collapse, 4-20
    length, 2-4
Tracheal intubation, 2-17–2-27
    anesthesia for, 2-19, 2-20t
    in asthma, 4-32–4-33
    back-up plan with, 2-27, 2-29
    in bacterial tracheitis, 4-15–4-16
    for burn patient, 10-11
    in cardiac arrest, 3-5
    complications, 2-26
    in CPR, 3-6t
    in croup, 4-13, 4-13t
    delayed, with ventricular fibrillation, 3-5
    difficult, 2-23–2-24, 2-29
    DOPE mnemonic, 2-27
    in epiglottitis, 4-15
    failed, 2-27–2-29
    indications for, 2-17–2-18, 2-18t
    monitoring with, 2-26
    positioning for, 2-11, 2-11f, 2-23
    postoperative indications for, 19-4
    rapid sequence, 2-22
    sedation for, 2-19, 2-20t, 2-21
    in shock, 6-17–6-18
    and subglottic injury, 4-4
    supplies and equipment for, 2-22–2-23, 2-22t
    technique for, 2-23–2-26
    in trauma patient, 9-2–9-3
    troubleshooting, 2-27
Tracheobronchial injuries, 9-15
Tracheomalacia, 4-6, 4-20
Tracheostomy, for burn patient, 10-11
Tramadol, 20-13
Transferrin, 19-17–19-18
Transfusion reaction(s), 17-23–17-25
    acute hemolytic, 17-24
    allergic, 17-24
    delayed hemolytic, 17-25

febrile nonhemolytic, 17-24
treatment, 17-23, 17-23*t*
Transport of critically ill child
coordination, 14-3–14-4
interfacility, 14-6–14-12
communication for, 14-12–14-14, 14-13*t*
coordination, 14-12–14-14
delays in, 14-7
equipment for, 14-14, 14-15*t*
indications for, 14-6–14-7
legal considerations in, 14-7
medications for, 14-14, 14-16*t*
mode, 14-9–14-11, 14-12*t*
monitoring during, 14-16
personnel for, 14-14
preparation for, 14-12–14-16
process for, 14-7–14-9, 14-8*f*
referring hospital's responsibilities in, 14-14, 14-14*t*
team for, 14-6, 14-7, 14-11–14-12, 14-11*t*
intrafacility, 14-4–14-6
equipment for, 14-5–14-6, 14-5*t*
monitoring during, 14-5–14-6, 14-5*t*
personnel for, 14-4–14-5
preparation for, 14-4
key elements for, 14-4
mode, 14-3
planning for, 14-2
preparation for, 14-4
risk/benefit analysis, 14-2
system for, 14-3
team for, 14-2–14-3
Transposition of the great arteries, 16-9–16-10
Trauma
airway, 4-17–4-18
altered mental status/coma caused by, 15-15–15-16, 15-16*t*
and cardiac arrest, 3-2
cardiac arrest in, 3-19
in disasters, 12-4–12-5
history-taking in, 9-6
hypovolemic shock caused by, 1-18
nonaccidental, 1-5, 1-24–1-25
ongoing/repeated evaluation in, 9-7
physical examination in, 9-6–9-7
prevalence, 9-1
primary survey in, 1-18, 1-19*t*, 9-1–9-5
ABCDE mnemonic for, 9-1
adjuncts to, 9-5
mnemonic for, 1-19*t*
secondary survey in, 1-19*t*, 6-21, 9-5–9-7
adjuncts to, 9-7
mnemonic for, 1-19*t*
shock in, 6-21
Traumatic brain injury, 1-5
management, 9-8–9-10
mild, 9-9
moderate, 9-9
and secondary brain injury, 9-9
severe, 9-9

Traumatic injury(ies)
evaluation, 9-14*t*
management, 9-8–9-20
Triage, 6-23, 12-9–12-10, 12-9*f*, 12-11–12-12
Tricuspid atresia, 16-8–16-9
Tricyclic antidepressants, overdose/poisoning/toxicity, 13-3*t*–13-4*t*, 13-11*t*
Tripod position, 1-6, 1-9, 4-12*t*, 4-14, 4-20
Tromethamine, indications for, 6-18
Truncus arteriosus, 16-10
Tsunami lung, 12-4
Tube(s), 21-2–21-8. *See also* Endotracheal tube(s)
Tularemia, 12-8*t*
Tumor lysis syndrome, 17-10–17-12
and acute kidney injury, 18-4
clinical manifestations, 17-11
diagnosis, 17-10–17-11
ECG findings in, 17-11
hydration and, 17-12
hyperkalemia and, 17-10, 17-12
hyperphosphatemia and, 17-10, 17-12
laboratory investigation, 17-10
monitoring in, 17-11–17-12
pathophysiology, 17-11
severe electrolyte disturbances in, management, 17-11*t*, 17-12
signs and symptoms, 17-11
treatment, 17-11, 17-11t
uric acid in, 17-10
control, 17-11*t*, 17-12
urine alkalinization and, 17-12
Tunneled lines, 21-9–21-10
heparin flush for, 21-11*t*
Typhlitis, in pediatric oncology patient, 17-7

# U
Ultrasound
FAST, 9-17
in trauma patient, 9-5
renal, 18-8, 18-9*t*
Uncal herniation, 15-9
Unresponsiveness, 3-3
Upper airway disease
diagnosis, 4-22
spectrum, 4-2
treatment, 4-24–4-26
Upper respiratory infection, and heart failure, 1-20
Uremia, 13-3*t*
Urinalysis, 7-24–7-25
in acute kidney injury, 18-6
Urinary catheter(s), 1-16*t*, 21-8–21-9
complications, 21-9
sizes, 21-9, 21-9*t*
in trauma patient, 9-4–9-5
Urinary tract infection(s), 7-6*t*, 7-24–7-25
catheter-associated, 19-22
diagnosis, 7-24–7-25
pathogens causing, 7-24
treatment, 7-25

Urine
        alkalinization, 17-12
                in poisoned patient, 13-6
        culture, 1-26, 7-24–7-25
        specific gravity, 18-5, 18-6t
        volume, 18-5, 18-6t
Urine output, 1-15
        and acute kidney injury, 18-2, 18-3t
        in hypovolemic shock, 1-17
        monitoring
                after cardiac arrest, 3-20
                postoperative, 19-15
                in trauma patient, 9-4

# V

Vagal tone, 1-14
Vagus nerve, 2-26
Valproic acid, for status epilepticus, 15-12t, 15-14t
Vancomycin, nephrotoxicity, 18-4
Vascular access. See also Indwelling venous access
    catheter(s)
        in burn patient, 10-2
        in cardiac arrest, 3-8
        in shock, 6-10–6-11
        in trauma patient, 9-4
Vascular perforation, with central venous catheter, 21-14, 21-14t
Vascular ring, airway obstruction, 1-10
Vasoconstriction, in septic shock, 1-22
Vasodilation, in septic shock, 1-22
Vaso-occlusive crisis, 2-9
Vasopressin, 16-21
        for cardiac arrest, 3-10t, 3-11
        for shock, 6-15t, 6-16–6-17, 6-16t
Vasopressors, 16-21
        for distributive shock, 1-22
        for shock, 6-14–6-17
Vecuronium, 19-8, 20-18, 2-21, 2-21t
Venlafaxine, overdose/poisoning/toxicity, 13-4t
Ventilation
        chest compression and, 3-4
        in CPR, 3-6, 3-6t
        monitoring, 1-11
        physiology, 3-4
        in post-resuscitative care, 3-20
        rate, in CPR, 3-6
Ventilation bag(s), 2-16–2-17
Ventilation-perfusion mismatch, 2-7, 2-9, 4-21–4-22
Ventilator-induced lung injury, 1-11
Ventilatory support. See also Mechanical ventilation;
    Positive end-expiratory pressure; Positive-pressure
    ventilation
        bag-valve-mask/endotracheal tube, 1-11
        for burn patient, 10-11
        in suspected shock, 6-8

Ventricular fibrillation
        cardiac arrest, resuscitation from, 3-8–3-9, 3-12–3-13
        delayed intubation with, 3-5
        pharmacotherapy for, 3-10t, 3-11
        subsequent to resuscitation, 3-12
Ventricular septal defect, 16-9, 16-12–16-13
Ventricular tachycardia, 16-18t
        pulseless
                pharmacotherapy for, 3-10t, 3-11
                resuscitation for, 3-12–3-13
                subsequent to resuscitation, 3-12
Vesicle(s), 7-7t
Vibrio cholerae, diarrhea, 1-17
Viral infection(s), 1-26
        and heart failure, 1-20
        in pediatric oncology patient, 17-3, 17-4t
Viscoelastic coupling, 4-5
Visual Analog Scale, 19-11t
Vital signs, 3-2
        age-dependent variations in, 7-2, 7-3t
Vocal cord paralysis, 4-7
Volume depletion. See also Hypovolemia
        postoperative, 19-15
Volume overload, signs, 1-16
Volutrauma, 1-11, 5-13
Vomiting. See also Nausea and vomiting
        fluid loss in, 1-17

# W

Warfarin derivative poisoning, 13-11t
Warm shock, 1-22, 6-22, 7-10, 7-10f
Water intoxication, hyponatremia due to, 8-6
Westley Croup Score, 4-23, 4-23t
Wheezes/wheezing, 1-7, 1-10, 2-5
        in poisoned patient, 13-3, 13-3t
Whole bowel irrigation, 13-6
Wolff-Parkinson-White syndrome, 16-19f
Work of breathing, 1-5–1-6, 1-11, 2-5–2-6, 4-22
Wound care, in trauma management, 9-19

# Z

Zanamivir, 12-8